Encyclopedia of E–Health and Telemedicine

Maria Manuela Cruz–Cunha
Polytechnic Institute of Cávado and Ave, Portugal & Algoritmi Research Centre, Portugal

Isabel Maria Miranda
Câmara Municipal de Guimarães, Portugal

Ricardo Martinho
Polytechnic Institute of Leiria, Portugal & CINTESIS – Center for Research in Health Technologies and Information Systems, Portugal

Rui Rijo
Polytechnic Institute of Leiria, Portugal & INESCC – Institute for Systems and Computers Engineering at Coimbra, Portugal & CINTESIS – Center for Research in Health Technologies and Information Systems, Portugal

Volume II
Categories: Em – N

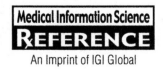

Medical Information Science
REFERENCE
An Imprint of IGI Global

Published in the United States of America by
    Medical Information Science Reference (an imprint of IGI Global)
    701 E. Chocolate Avenue
    Hershey PA, USA 17033
    Tel: 717-533-8845
    Fax: 717-533-8661
    E-mail: cust@igi-global.com
    Web site: http://www.igi-global.com

Library of Congress Cataloging-in-Publication Data

Names: Cruz-Cunha, Maria Manuela, 1964- editor. | Miranda, Isabel Maria,
    1954- editor. | Martinho, Ricardo, 1974- editor. | Rijo, Rui, editor.
Title: Encyclopedia of E-health and telemedicine / Maria Manuela Cruz-Cunha,
    Isabel Maria Miranda, Ricardo Martinho, and Rui Rijo, editors.
Description: Hershey, PA : Medical Information Science Reference, 2016. |
    Includes bibliographical references and index.
Identifiers: LCCN 2015051069| ISBN 9781466699786 (hardcover) | ISBN
    9781466699793 (ebook)
Subjects: LCSH: Medical care--Technological innovations--Encyclopedias. |
    Medical informatics--Encyclopedias.
Classification: LCC R858 .E518 2016 | DDC 610.28503--dc23 LC record available at http://lccn.loc.gov/2015051069

British Cataloguing in Publication Data
A Cataloguing in Publication record for this book is available from the British Library.

All work contributed to this book is new, previously-unpublished material. The views expressed in this book are those of the authors, but not necessarily of the publisher.

For electronic access to this publication, please contact: eresources@igi-global.com.

Editorial Advisory Board

List of Contributors

Table of Contents by Volume

Volume I

Category: Case Studies

Roxana Ologeanu-Taddei, Université Montpellier, France
Isabelle Bourdon, KEDGE Business School, France & Université Montpellier, France
Chris Kimble, KEDGE Business School, France & Université Montpellier, France
Nicolas Giraudeau, Université Montpellier, France

Fernando Almeida, University of Porto Portugal
José Monteiro, Instituto Nacional de Engenharia e Computadores do Porto, Portugal
Mário Lousã, Instituto Superior Politécnico Gaya, Portugal

Marco Nalin, Telbios, Italy
Ilaria Baroni, Telbios, Italy
Maria Romano, Telbios, Italy

Rachid Oumlil, ENCG – Agadir, Morocco

Michelle Monachino, Phoenix JDPUniversidade Nova de Lisboa, Portugal & Linköping
University, Sweden
Paulo Moreira, ISCTE-IUL (IPPS), Portugal & Atlantica School of Business and Industry
(ASIB Europe), Portugal
Filipe Janela, Siemens Portugal, Portugal

Category: Emerging Technologies

Volume II

Alphabetical Table of Contents

Preface

ABOUT THE SUBJECT

According to the World Health Organization (WHO, 2016), e-Health is "the transfer of health resources and health care by electronic means". It encompasses three main areas: 1) the delivery of health information, for health professionals and health consumers, through the Internet and telecommunications; 2) using the power of Information and Communication Technology (ICT) and e-commerce to improve public health services, e.g. through the education and training of health workers; and 3) the use of e-commerce and e-business practices in health systems management. It is broader in definition than Telemedicine, as it includes computer-assisted telecommunications to support management, surveillance, literature and access to medical knowledge. Telemedicine is "the use of telecommunications to diagnose and treat disease and ill-health" (WHO, 2010). These definitions are not consensual. Oh, Rizo, Enkin, and Jadad (2005) found 51 unique definitions with 2 universal themes (health and technology) and 6 less general (commerce, activities, stakeholders, outcomes, place, and perspectives). E-Health itself foresees a range of services, systems and technologies, including Electronic Health Records (EHRs), Computerized Physician Order Entry (CPOE), e-Prescribing, Clinical Decision Support Systems (CDSS), Telemedicine, m-Health, Medical Imaging Processing, and Healthcare Information Systems, among others.

Health informatics began in financial systems in the 60s, helping the billing, payroll and accounting. Clinical departmental solutions arrived in the 70s supporting activities as radiology, laboratory and pharmacy. In the 80s there was a focus on the accounting, material and management systems. The idea of a complete medical EHR arrived in the 90s and the term e-Health appeared with the advent of the Internet.

This evolution and the impact of ICT in health care services and patients suggests the relevance of the study of e-Health and Telemedicine. Therefore, it is important the understanding of its concepts, challenges, technologies, solutions and how to apply them effectively in practice.

One main challenge identified in this Encyclopedia is the need of studying the impact of the use of technology in the patient-doctor relation. Interoperability is also a key concern, due to the heterogeneity of healthcare systems and their supporting devices. In this area, the search for standards for Electronic Health Records is considered an issue requiring combined efforts between the academic and industry communities.

Smart devices, sensors, Patient Area Networks (PAN), augmented reality and serious games are conquering the healthcare area with a huge profusion of intelligent systems for monitoring, diagnosing, supporting the therapy, and education. Also increasing is the apprehensions with the legal framework that regulate these systems, the security, the safety and the privacy of the patients, healthcare professionals and institutions.

New approaches, frameworks and techniques are proposed to deal with the complexity of the circumstances, namely new architectures and software tools. The demographic and epidemiologic transition resulting from ageing and the increase of life expectation means an increment related to chronic conditions. The solution is to restore the consistence between the triple burden of diseases on the health situation and the current system of healthcare practice, with the implantation of healthcare networks. The later is a major concern demanding new policy models and new solutions. In this "network reality", simulation and e-learning take also an important role supporting the spreading of medical procedures and good management practices. The use of Business Process Management (BPM), Enterprise Architectures (EA) and specific Project Management (PM) processes seem to improve the flow of information and the cohesion of these networks.

The intelligent processing and visualization of the huge amount of existing health data are exploited in the works regarding data, text mining and big data, as we can observe regarding pharmacovigilance.

THE MISSION

The mission of the *Encyclopedia of e-Health and Telemedicine* is then to provide a global vision of these areas, offering a comprehensive context and an insight from where the e-Health and Telemedicine come from, the key areas of emerging works and providing useful outlooks of the future. In this way, the book aims to contribute for the theories, practices and policies behind the use of IT and Information Systems for health and social care. Theoretical contributions ground in the solid background work done by the authors, along with the quality of the scientific research expanding the existing knowledge. Practitioners can also take advantage of the innovative developments and solutions presented. These intersect emerging technologies and challenges regarding e-Health and Telemedicine. Finally, numerous case studies and socio-technical experiences will surely help policy makers on an effective adoption of ICT throughout the main health and social challenges in societies.

EXPECTATIONS

Bearing in mind the diversity of the issues and the depth of the content, we believe that this Encyclopedia can be an excellent resource for those who wish to learn more on the challenges and adoption of e-Health and Telemedicine either from the perspective of service providers, academics or researchers. The target audience for this Encyclopedia includes healthcare service providers, policy makers, academics, researchers, Information Systems students and IT managers.

All these works express the desire for a positive contribution to the research area of Information Systems in general and e-Health and Telemedicine in particular. We would like to welcome feedback and comments about this Encyclopedia from readers. Comments and constructive suggestions can be sent to the Editors of IGI Global at the addresses provided at the beginning of this Encyclopedia.

We express our gratitude to IGI-Global for the opportunity to edit this book, and for the excellent support of their team of professionals. We would like to thank all the members of the Scientific Committee, for their commitment and for sharing their knowledge and experience in the support of the decision-making processes. Finally, we would like to show our appreciation and gratitude to all the authors for their excellent contributions: this encyclopedia encloses the result of their relevant work and deep knowledge on the e-Health and Telemedicine domain.

We hope you find it useful. Enjoy your reading!

Maria Manuela Cruz-Cunha
Polytechnic Institute of Cávado and Ave, Portugal & Algoritmi Research Centre, Portugal

Isabel Maria Miranda
Câmara Municipal de Guimarães, Portugal

Ricardo Martinho
Polytechnic Institute of Leiria, Portugal & CINTESIS - Center for Research in Health Technologies and Information Systems, Portugal

Rui Rijo
Polytechnic Institute of Leiria, Portugal & INESCC - Institute for Systems and Computers Engineering at Coimbra, Portugal & CINTESIS - Center for Research in Health Technologies and Information Systems, Portugal

REFERENCES

Oh, H., Rizo, C., Enkin, M., & Jadad, A. (2005). What is eHealth (3): A systematic review of published definitions. *Journal of Medical Internet Research*, 7(1), e1.

WHO. (2010). *Telemedicine*. Retrieved from http://www.who.int/goe/publications/goe_telemedicine_2010.pdf

WHO. (2016). *E-health*. Retrieved from http://www.who.int/trade/glossary/story021/en/

About the Editors

Maria Manuela Cruz-Cunha is a Professor of Information Systems and Project Management at the Polytechnic Institute of Cávado and Ave, Portugal. She holds a Dipl. Eng. (5 years) in Systems and Informatics Engineering, an M.Sci. in Computer Integrated Manufacturing and a Dr.Sci in of Production Systems Engineering. She teaches subjects related with Information Systems, Information Technologies, IT Project Management and Organizational Models to undergraduate and post-graduate studies. She has authored and edited 25 books and her work appears in more than 150 papers published in journals, book chapters and conference proceedings. She is founder and conference chair of the "CENTERIS – Conference on ENTERprise Information Systems", "ViNOrg – Conference on Virtual and Networked Organizations Emergent Technologies and Tools" and "ProjMAN – International Conference on Project Management".

Isabel Maria Miranda is currently the responsible by the Social Services Division of the City Council of Guimarães. She has previously worked as coordinator of continuing education projects at the University of Porto, and simultaneously as lecturer of Management and Social Sciences at higher education institutions. She holds a 5-year degree in Psychology and a Master degree in Psychology of Organizations. Her scientific interests are related with health and social care Information Systems and Technologies.

Ricardo Martinho is an Associate Professor at the School of Technology and Management – Polytechnic Institute of Leiria, Portugal. He teaches several subjects related to enterprise information systems, enterprise application development, software engineering (agile methods) and health information systems. He graduated in Electrical Engineering – Computer Science at University of Coimbra, received his MSc in Computer Science - Information Systems Programming from IST - Technical University of Lisbon, and his PhD from University of Trás-os-Montes and Alto Douro. He is currently the Head of the Healthcare Informatics BSc. degree, and participates as a consultant in several enterprise and health informatics-related research projects. He supervises several MSc and PhD theses in the Computer Science – Health Informatics research areas. He has several publications in conference proceedings, book chapters and journals, related to the Business Process Management, Software Engineering and health informatics research areas. He serves as editor-in-chief, member of editorial board and reviewer for several books and international journals, and has served in several committees of international conferences. He is a co-founder of HCist – International Conference on Health and Social Care Information Systems and Technologies (http://hcist.scika.org).

Rui Rijo is Professor of Computer Science at the Polytechnic Institute of Leiria. He received his Phd in Computer Science from the Trás-os-Montes University and his Engineering degree from Instituto Superior Técnico (Technical University of Lisbon). He has more than ten years of experience as senior information systems consultant in, among others countries, Tokyo (Japan), Macau (China), Hong-Kong (China), São Paulo (Brazil), Kuala Lumpur (Malaysia), Madrid (Spain), Amsterdam (Holland), Madrid (Spain) and Lisbon (Portugal). His publications include book chapters and papers in refereed national and international conferences and journals. He was general chair of HCist - International Conference on Health and Social Care Information Systems and Technologies and associate editor of the International Journal of Web Portals and editor of the International Journal of E-Health and Medical Communications. He was the coordinator of the Healthcare Informatics course and currently is the coordinator of the Master on Healthcare Information Systems Management. His current research interests include health information systems, patient relationship management, serious games, software engineering and project management.

Health Information System to Identify Dermatological Diseases by Software Agent

Eduardo César Contreras Delgado
Autonomous University of Coahuila, Mexico

Isis Ivette Contreras González
Instituto Tecnológico de Saltillo, Mexico

INTRODUCTION

A dermatological diagnosis needs from comparative visual support, which generally becomes by experience and/or it is find in the medical bibliography, due to the great amount of skin affections. Furthermore, great similarity exists between symptoms from a suffering to another. Due to the highly visual nature of specialty, most skin conditions must be diagnosed from an image specially if there is a data bank. (Muir & Lucas, 2008).

One way to reduce the problem is to provide to the general practitioners a didactic tool that allows them to identify skin diseases. This tool is an agent based on goals, that contains the information necessary to identify some of the more common diseases in our region, (Coahuila, México). The conditions differ by geographic region.

This project is a field research, applied to the medical area on the Dermatology specialty related with the Health Information Systems. It is in itself, an automated medical tool to identify skin diseases, based on a Software Agent from Artificial Intelligence specialty, and based on the heuristic compilation of the tacit knowledge of dermatologists.

This study involves education science, medicine and information technologies. In computer science an algorithm is proposed to develop a Software Agent, in education science a research method applied to engineering and in medicine an algorithm to identify skin diseases (Clinical Semiology).

The research objective is to determine the effectiveness of dermatological affections identification aided by a Software Agent, based on tacit knowledge of the Human Agent.

This study also employs an Information Systems Research method, in which concepts are defined; methodological consistency and research variables, linking an architectural design, the model of three layers or levels.

The arrogance of this development, has not as aim to identify all existing skin diseases, instead, just those typical from the Region (Coahuila), because the skin diseases depend on the geographic location, this is to support to our general practitioners in their task of detection of dermatological conditions, in those patients who require medical care in this regard.

DOI: 10.4018/978-1-4666-9978-6.ch045

BACKGROUND

Dermatological Diseases

The study and management of dermatological diseases in a rigorously scientific way has been in charge of the medical specialty of Dermatology.

Definition of the Common Ailments

- **Abscess:** An abscess is an enclosed collection of liquefied tissue, known as pus, somewhere in the body. It is the result of the body's defensive reaction to foreign material (Fauci, 1997).
- **Ulcer:** A local defect, or excavation of the surface, of an organ or tissue, produced by sloughing of necrotic inflammatory tissue (Gale Encyclopedia of Medicine, 2008).
- **Pustule:** A small inflamed skin swelling that is filled with pus; a pimple (The American Heritage, 2007).
- **Comedo:** A plug of keratin and sebum within the dilated orifice of a hair follicle (Miller-Keane, 2003).
- **Candidiasis:** An infection caused by a species of the yeast Candida, usually Candida albicans. This is a common cause of vaginal infections in women (Gale Encyclopedia of Medicine, 2008).
- **Elaioconiosis:** An acneiform eruption that affects metal-industry workers and vehicle mechanics exposed to cutting oils, also known as follicular dermatitis or oil acne (Ministério da Saúde, 2006).

SOFTWARE AGENT DEFINITION

In artificial intelligence, a software agent (SA) is an autonomous entity, which observes and acts upon an environment and directs its activity towards achieving goals (Rich & Knight, 1991). An agent is everything that can be considered that perceives its atmosphere by means of sensors and that response or acts in such atmosphere by means of effectors, (Russell & Norvig, 2003). A sensor is a device that measures a physical quantity and converts it into a signal, which can be read by an observer or by an instrument, for example, voltmeter, thermometer, thermocouple. Effectors are agents or structures that cause an activity, in robotics, an end effector is a device or tool that's connected to the end of a robot arm.

The structure of an end effector and the nature of the programming and hardware that drives it depend on the task the robot will be performing, (Resconi, 2004).

Software agents are often described schematically as an abstract functional system similar to a computer program. On the Internet, an intelligent agent (or simply an *agent*) is a program that gathers information or performs some other service without your immediate presence and on some regular schedule.

MODELS TO CONSTRUCT AGENT'S PROGRAMS

Agents based on goals: besides the states, agents need some kind of information about its goals. Goals will to detail the situations to that it is desired to arrive. The agent program could to combine goals with actions and in this way, to be able to choose those actions that allow reaching the goal. Design of an ideal agent (Russell & Norvig, 2003).

To specify which kind of action should undertake an agent, as an answer to a certain sequence of perceptions constitutes the design of an ideal agent.

- **Agent type:** Medical identification system of dermatological affections.
- General Practitioner's perceptions.
- Symptoms, clinical signs, physical examination, heredity, personal data.
- Actions.
- **Identifies:** Skin state, anatomical region, inflammatory reactions of the skin, wheal.
- How the patient evolves.
- Differentiate diseases.
- Goals.
- Affection identification, time reduction, canalization of patient in case of such another disease.
- Atmosphere.
- Patient, general practitioner.

Of these types we will be based only on: Health Information Systems for Dermatologic Diseases (HISDerD). The actions than this agent undertakes, are based exclusively in an integrated knowledge (provided by the dermatologist), and so, its own perceptions are ignored (it does not count with sensors towards the environment), therefore the agent has not autonomy. Its conduct is defined by the human agent experience. It is reasonable to equip an agent of artificial intelligence with certain initial knowledge and capacity to learn (the dermatology heuristic).

Similar Studies

Within the development of "Healthcare Information Systems (HIS)" several methods as well as different software agents were used, helping the physicians in the process of decision-making and the diagnosis of different diseases and conditions.

The work of Caffery (2012) examines digital imaging and communication in medicine (DICOM) and pictures archiving and communication systems (PACS) and how these concepts relate to teledermatology. They discuss Software requirements for DICOM and presents example workflows showing how they can contribute in teledermatology.

In a report summarizes the key criteria for evaluating Store-and-forward (S&F) Teledermatology applications (Armstrong, 2009).

Al-Tajem & Al-Malaise (2014) in their research objectives integrate different Enterprise Resource Planning (ERP) processes with a centralized ERP database to provide in effective way business intelligence for the dermatologists by applying data mining techniques.

The work of Aggarwal (2002) shows the process of Object-oriented Analysis (OOA) using the Unified Modeling Language (UML) has been used to demonstrate its practical utility in the HIS development for the solution of real problems.

The study of Hazen (2002) demonstrates that Stochastic Trees have also been used as a modeling approach for medical treatment decision analyses.

An application of linear programming discriminant analysis (LPDA) was presented by Kwak, Kim, Lee & Choi (2002), to classify and to predict the symptomatic status of HIV/AIDS patients.

According to Podgorelec (2002, p. 445), "Decision trees are a reliable and effective decision making technique that provide high classification accuracy with a simple representation of gathered knowledge and they have been used in different areas of medical decision making".

The approach presented on the next techniques differs from the previous studies about the way that medical diagnoses are made.

The authors Andonegui et al. (2013) describe the current status of the use of e-Ophthalmology-based models in the screening and follow-up of chronic glaucoma.

In another study, the authors Hernández, Rodríguez & Colomo, (2013) propose a social networks application that allows patients to make contact with their physicians through a Clinical Decision Support Systems (CDSS) list of signs, to obtain clinical diagnosis.

A study is presented in two stages by Ciufudean, Ciufudean & Filote, (2013, p. 892): in the first one, information that links physiology with a patient´s emotional state is gathered; this information allows to make laboratory analysis methods and physicians' diagnoses. "The second stage is focused on the improvement of the automated medical diagnosis based on biological feature selection and classification, as biological features represent patterns of important information".

The authors Angjellari-Dajci, et al., (2013, p. 1045) discuss new developments in telehealth for diagnosis, treatment, and management of Autism Spectrum Disorders (ASDs) in the US, and explain that the cost to society has increased, mostly because autism is hardly detected on early stages, making it difficult to provide an adequate treatment.

Jisha, Simi & Neethu (2014), published an automated melanoma screening system, employee a back propagation neural network where is used with texture distinctiveness lesion segmentation algorithm. The proposed framework achieves higher segmentation accuracy.

Jain & Jain (2012) focused on the development of a skin cancer screening system that can be used in a general practice by non-experts to classify normal from abnormal cases by decomposing images into different frequency sub-bands using wavelet transform.

MAIN FOCUS

Exposition of the Problem

In the community of Saltillo Municipality on Coahuila, there is a population around 850,000 inhabitants. There are 9 clinics hospital, and only 12-specialist in dermatology to take care of typical affections of the region. In 2013, the clinics hospitals have responded around 8100 patients from the total population.

In these diagnoses are not contemplated skin carcinogenic affections, and are only been pointed statistically, those detected for specialist in dermatology, so it's not detected the population taken care by general practitioner, or those from the population that has no access to the health services.

Most of the population in Mexico is served by the main clinics hospitals of Social Security (Social Security Mexican Institute (IMSS). The rightful claimants must request its appointment first instance with the general practitioner, and this as well depending on the disease and also some luck, it will alternate to the specialist doctor: however, the patient waits till three months to obtain an appointment with the specialist doctor.

This without a doubt has consequences, which it can worsen the dermatological disease.

A dermatological diagnosis needs from comparative visual support, which generally becomes by experience and/or it is find in the medical bibliography, due to the great amount of skin affections. Furthermore, great similarity exists between symptoms from a suffering to another; to differentiate them are needed great amount of knowledge in the area, and compare with images. In Mexico the public health hospitals do not have or use Photogrammetry or Dermatoscope, the practitioners have not been used yet DICOM (Digital Imaging and Communications in Medicine) and PACS (Picture Archiving and Communications System) that enables doctors to store all medical data together with relevant images and share.

Definition of variables in dermatological research

- Identification of dermatological affections.
- Information of Human Agent.
- Software Agent.
- Information Technology:
  ◦ Data banks (information and images).
  ◦ User interaction design for the skin affection identification.

Modeling of the Problem

An efficient and right identification of a dermatological affection is in function of the information provided by the dermatologist human agent, as well as, the rules, goals, and algorithms whereupon the intelligent agent is constructed, furthermore of the information on it, and an informatic tool use.

Based on the variables identified previously:

- **Functional Relationship:** Identification of dermatological affections = F (Human Agent's Information, Software Agent + Information Technology).
- **General Objective:** To evaluate the dermatological affections identifications; aided by a Software Agent, based on tacit knowledge of the Human Agent.

Research Method

Method for information systems research employee is Methodological Consistency Table that is developed of the following way: Methodological Consistency Table, where it shows specific objectives, research questions, variables and hypothesis.

Figure 1 relates, for row the first specific objective, with the first group of research questions, with the first independent variable, and the first group of hypothesis. So that there a methodological consistency to each other. The same applies to each variable. See in Table 1.

Development Method for Information Systems Research

Based on the Methodological Consistency Table, have been identified the independent variables, the software agent, the information technology and the human agent knowledge, used to develop the requirements analysis.

Requirements analysis for software agent are:

- Is required, provide a dermatological identification by means of a software agent which contains a knowledge base, and the needed algorithms, to make a search process that allows reaching a defined goal.

Figure 1. User interaction design
Development own, 2014.

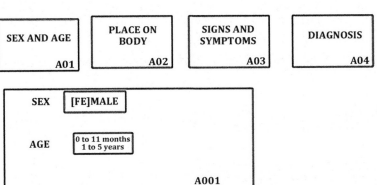

Table 1. Methodological consistency table, where are shown objectives, hypothesis, research questions, and variables

Particular Objective	Research Questions	Variable	Hypothesis
PO1: To value the utility of a Software Agent for dermatological conditions detection by a general physician.	**RQ1:** Rules and goals from the knowledge base related with images will be sufficient to identify the affection?	Software Agent	**H1:** There is a positive relation between the dermatological affection identification by the Human Agent and that provided by the Software Agent.
PO2: To determine the Software Agent effectiveness of dermatological affections identification provides by the Human Agent experience.	**RQ2:** Information provides by the human agent based on symptoms and observation would obtain a correct identification?	Human Agent Information	**H2:** If the information provided by the human agent is precise, the correct dermatological affection identification could be obtained.
PO3: To determine the Information Technology utility on dermatological affections search, to ensure that the general practitioner makes an approximate identification of the disease.	**RQ3:** General practitioners will adopt Information Technology, if this manages to identify the common affections?	Information Technology	**H3:** If the physician experienced through educational information technology, it will facilitate the identification of skin diseases.

Development own, 2014.

- Is required, create a data bank which contains the information of general data of the patient, visual data (rash, grain, color, anatomic location, and so on), signs, symptoms, and descriptive images of several sufferings.
- The human agent (dermatologist) requirements are: provide the information to elaborate the structured questions, the initial evidences, rules and goals to that it is desired to arrive.
- The requirements for the independent variable Information Technology are: a user interaction design that allows it to capture the needed information on a structured form, and that shows the same way an answer by means of a text file and images.

Design Specifications

The Methodological Consistency Matrix achieves establishing the design specifications. This matrix take in count factors, indicators, and dimensions, see in Table 2. They are qualitative and quantitative characteristics that set criteria to be satisfied the software agent design.

Human Agent

This agent, provide information for the table of initial evidences, that table is a flat file, which contains references to text files, where different sufferings are described, and the references to the descriptions than links to the corresponding suffering images.

Interaction template, this template, is the guide to develop the questionnaire to evaluate the interaction between the human agent, and the software agent performance, related with the quality of the dermatological affection identification, so that the general practitioner could emit the diagnosis.

Software Design

Architectural design. The model of three layers or levels is used.

- **D0 User Interaction Design:** In this layer a template was design to allow the physician to interact with the software agent, see Figure 1, this template simultaneously is related with a flat file, which

Table 2. Methodological consistency matrix, where are shown variables, factors, indicators, and dimensions

Variable	Factor	Characteristic	Measurable
Information Human Agent	Symtoms	Burning	True/False
		Itching	
		Pain	
		Sweeling	
	Observation	Color	Red
			White
			Violet
		Size	Big
			Medium
			Small
Software Agent	Knowledge base	Goals	True/False
		Rules	True/False
	Images	Real	yes/no
		correct	s/n
Information Tecnology	Images Text	Quality Information	User interaction
			Image quality
			Usability Facility
			Easy visualization of answer
			Easy data capture

Development own, 2014.

contains all information of several skin affections and images which are flat files with properties and attributes to describe the defined image by review the skin affections types, which allow to identify the image related with the affection. This file function is that the algorithm realizes a search in the text, according to the selected goal, when a coincidence is encountered, then compare factors that address an image or a group of them, which are shown with the referring texts to the affection, so that the physician settles down a comparison between the image emitted by the tool, software agent and the presented/displayed dermatological affection in the patient, and with that the physician can identify a disease and emit his diagnosis.

- **D1 Domain Logic:** In this layer are developed the search algorithms that link to the tables of the data bank, which contains the rules, actions, and goals, to allow identify the affection. See algorithm HISDerD.
- **D2 Data Bank:** This layer contains all tables and flat files, see the group of tables in data design which describes them.

Data Design

Development of tables to set database:

1. **Table of Questions:** Table-containing information about the anatomic region, signs and symptoms.
2. **Table of State Update:** Table containing the identifier of the question related with the initial evidences identifier.
3. **Table of Conditions:** Table that relates the option identifier with the topic identifier, to connect to the table of rules later.
4. **Table of Rules:** The topic identifier based on the evidence, and the positive state determines the property rule, according to the condition, to refer the goal.
5. **Table of Actions:** Table that contains the property rule identifier, and the goal identifier.
6. Table of goals contains the goal identifier; the goal description; the goal level; the goal status and the evidence percent.
7. Table shows the pre-diagnosis and information; this is a flat file, which addresses a text file, and an images file.

SOFTWARE AGENT ALGORITHM

Health Information Systems for Dermatologic Diseases (HISDerD)

The algorithm consists of a narrative related with a diagram and a tables group, named knowledge base, in order to obtain its understanding of didactic way.

Algorithm HISDerD

```
1. Start
```

First the user is asked to identify if the disease is specific of the region. When the human agent (general practitioner) initiate its interaction with the

Health Information Systems to Dermatology, shows the dermatological affections group that could be identify by this tool, in order not to generate expectation of a false diseases identification not specific of the region.

2. Input percepts.

Call for the data

{

        Age and sex

        Onset Type

        Signs

        Symptoms

        Region affected (body)

           If it is grain, abscess, comedones, …

           Size of affection

           Color of affection

}

This data are contained in Table of questions.

3. State Update

The knowledge base is initialized; all the states are turned to 0 or false on tables 2 to 6.

The patient data are requested to capture them into the table state update, which contains: gender, age, part of the body affected, grain, rash, color, size, etc., (symptoms and signs data are entering).

To have entered the age and sex, is looked for in the Data Base diseases that match the age and sex that the user entered and stored. Result1 = Percepts1 $\cap$ **A**, where are the diseases recorded in the table knowledge base, percepts1 data entered above.

To have entered the onset type is looked for in the database diseases to coincide with the start type that the user entered and stored. Result2 = percept2 $\cap$ **A**.

To have entered the part of the body affected, a disease that matches the region affected that the user entered is sought in the database and is stored. Result3 = percept3 $\cap$ **A**.

To have entered change of the skin (rash), a disease that matches skin eruption that the user entered is sought in the database and is stored. Result4 = percept4 $\cap$ **A**.

To have entered the color and size of affected region seeks a disease that matches the affected region that the user entered in the database and saved. Result5 = percept5 $\cap$ **A**.

To have admitted the sign or signs is sought in the database diseases matching the sign or signs that the user entered and stored. Result6 = percept6 $\cap$ **A**.

To have admitted the symptom or symptoms database is search diseases that match the symptom or the symptoms that the user entered and stored. Result7 = percept7 $\cap$ **A**.

Thus the sum of partial results is: Partial Result (PR)

PR = Result1 ∩ Result2 ∩ Result3Result4 ∩ Result5 ∩ Result7 Result6

4. Formulate Goal

With the partial result, it obtained a first goal, performs a preliminary identification, at the moment the software agents known to the goal to be achieved, in other words, so far has identified a group of diseases that share common characteristics.

There is a conditions search, (a relation between answers to the questions are search, where are selected all those coincidences of the table of questions (1), with the table of state update (2)).

There is a conditions selection (selecting in agreement with the coincidences of the table of questions (1) + all the coincidences in the table of state update (2)).

The possible coincidences of the table of questions + the coincidences of the table of state update, pass a validation at the table of conditions (3), from which is obtained a preliminary answer on first purification of: selected questions + initial evidences.

The purified result is taken from the done purification by the table of conditions; to go to the table of rules (4), see Table 3. The table of conditions has a topic identifier, and a description of the initial evidence related with the table of rules (4), on this table the topic id coincidences with the rules id are selected, and with this data goes to the table of actions (5), this is in charge to relate rules with a previous goal, establishing probabilistic weights and selecting the goal with major value on the evidence. If there is no coincidence or the value is too low, is going back to the table of rules, selecting another rules group, which are registered on the table of actions to find a new goal, through this algorithm acts like a sieve filter between conditions and rules, establishing probabilistic weights (select 1 of x number that can be selected), to be considered by the algorithm just those of great weight, being selected only those who are in possibility to be an answer.

From the table of goals (6), see Table 4. The goal with an approximation of probability close to 100% is selected. A search is made on the flat text file (which has two information groups, file texts describing the dermatological affection and an attributes bank describing the image) according to the attributes obtained from the algorithm, and then compare the flat file attributes that describe the images and the attributes of the flat text file, that match the goal.

5. Formulate Problem

If the algorithm find coincidences, the image and descriptive text are deploy, in answer to the data provide by the human agent.

6. Plan

He or She will establish a plan to select one of the diseases of the identified group (general practitioner). What happens if I take action A? Or if I take action B?

If taken to action leads to a goal to which we do not know if it is correct. This forces us to create a search-space (Nilson, 2004).

If there is ambiguity with the situation of the dermatological affection the patient presents, and the answer provided by the software agent. The human agent, request a new affection proposal inside the possibilities set by the software agent in agreement to the weight set by the algorithm.

The difference for these software agents is the use of a Bank of images for general practitioner so they can compare the injury of the patient with the disease that is shown in the image and software agent compares these features to perform the search.

7. Search

while (plan **not** empty) **do {**

If (agree state == true) then {

If there are similarities with the provided data (state) establishes an action leading to a recommendation, by selecting an option in the space of search (search-space), considering the rules that are specific to each disease (these are those that allow us to do a proper identification). Emits a response through the effectors (user interaction) to the environment (general practitioner, patient).

If one accepts the answer ends.

}

Else {

If does not return to do a new search

It establishes a new plan calling for new data (creates a new state) to have options to generate new actions that would lead us to a new target from the selected groups of diseases (remainder), in every new search, it will decrease the (remainder) until exhausted. }

8. Output action

Displays the name of disease found. If there is a coincidence, the physician accepts the proposal, and then issues the diagnosis by himself. If it is accepted, ends.

Else if there are no more actions to take and there is not a coincidence, displays a message that does not have sufficient information to identify a disease of this kind.

Message: "There's not enough information to identify the required affection".

9. End

Programming Stage: The codification of the algorithms is realized aided by SQL searches. User interaction design related with logic and data in a tables group.

Table 3. Table of rules, the topic identifier based on the evidence, and the positive state determines the property rule, according to the condition, to refer the goal

idRules	idTopic	Status	Evidence	numConditions	Rule Description
1	1	T	100	12	Acne Vulgaris
2	1	F	100	4	Acne Conglobata
3	1	F	100	2	Acne Queloidea
4	1	F	100	6	Acne Fulminans
5	1	F	100	10	Elaioconiosis
6	1	F	100	5	Nodular Elastoidosis (Favre-Racouchot)
7	1	F	100	4	Demodecidosis
8	2	T	100	4	Cutaneous vascular complex of the leg
11	2	F	100	3	Arterial Ulcer
12	3	T	100	9	Perioral dermatitis
13	3	T	100	4	Periorial dermatitis pink
15	3	F	100	6	Atopic dermatitis
16	3	F	100	6	Jock itch (Tinea cruris)
17	4	T	100	12	Acute Dermatitis
18	4	F	100	10	Chronic Dermatitis
19	4	F	100	2	Subacute Dermatitis

Development own, 2014.

Table 4. Table of goals, contains the goal identifier; the goal description; the goal level; the goal status, and the evidence percent

IdGoal	Description	Level	Status	Evidence
1	Acne Vulgaris	1	S	100
2	Acne Conglobata	1	S	10
3	Acne Queloidea	1	S	10
4	Acne Fulminans	1	S	20
5	Elaiconiosis	1	S	0
6	Nodular Elastoidosis (Favre-Racouchot)	1	S	0
7	Demodecidosis	1	S	0
8	Cutaneous vascular complex of the leg	1	S	0
11	Arterial Ulcer	1	S	100
12	Perioral dermatitis	1	S	100
15	Atopic dermatitis	1	S	100
16	Jock itch (Tinea cruris)	1	S	100
17	Acute Dermatitis	1	S	100

Development own, 2014.

SOLUTIONS AND RECOMMENDATIONS

Information to the Population and Physicians

Modifying the culture of the population in terms of popular beliefs of the dermatologic disorders are cured with home remedies or self-medicate, to alleviate ailments people fall into apathy and let the time pass to receive adequate professional attention.

General practitioners who have years on practicing commonly received little information on dermatologic diseases, there is an especial need to offer them courses through the medical institution to which they belong. In this way it can improve its approach to identify a dermatologic condition to ensure that the patient receives timely specialized medical attention. As mentioned above the general medical depends on the detection and prompt attention, which has become a vital part to address the problem in time.

In Educational Institutions

Medical schools promote specialists in dermatology to meet the demand of the population and to comply with the ratio of inhabitant/physician (50/1) that in our country is not enough.

Encourage the use of Health Information Systems as alternative didactics; in our country this is an educational problem for the lack of resources and training to the medical teaching tools.

Create multidisciplinary Workgroups. Physician, Dermatologist, CIT's engineering, students that still are in the formative stages of engineering.

Recommend promote the development of applications that focus to Health Information Systems to address some of the demanding problems in our country in students and teachers in conjunction with specialists from the sector health.

Physician Dermatologist

Our country (México) usually the physician dermatologist provides medical care in his Office and very few are involved in research projects. It is recommended that they be supported by government agencies or of private initiative for research activities. On the other hand medical specialists are encouraged to increase the participation in events that allow the publication of information in books of texts, journals, magazines, proceedings, etc.

FUTURE RESEARCH DIRECTIONS

Perspective

In the future the new trends are to deploy applications using HIS in the medical sector to enable decision-making based on the knowledge of specialists.

In Mexico the social aspect has lagged behind in the development of the technology because it has focused on productivity, development of quality and economic improvements with cost-cutting in enterprises and the labor and productive sector.

From the technological aspect, using HISDerD propose new solutions based on technologies that will improve social and health services to treat a patient in time and take effective control of their disease.

Model

On the way in which it is proposed the use of the model goal-based agents related to the medical area, can be very useful for students of computer science with application in artificial intelligence that helps to understand the algorithm and the structure of software agents and allows them later to develop such applications. Use of HIS in their professional development, as well as software developers are to be considered an alternative resource for medical researchers.

Paradigm

Some public institutions of health and in the majority of private institutions electronic formats are used to take control of the record of the patient, consultation to pharmaceutical dictionaries, existence of medicines at the pharmacy of the institution itself, but not on computer auxiliary diagnosis processes. This tells us that in the future the general practitioner can accept computer programs to improve their job performance and to enable them to make a reliable diagnosis with high expectations of accepting a new paradigm.

Future Research

A proposal for future research opportunities using software agent in medicine is the application:

- **Physical Medicine:** The goal of software agents is to suggest to the general practitioner when he should send the patient for attention by the specialist in physical medicine and to receive physical rehabilitation therapy. Physical rehabilitation is considered as alternative medicine, for this reason not all physicians resort to it. The areas of medicine that frequently require management by physical medicine as support are Traumatology and orthopedics, Neurology and Rheumatology, however other areas can benefit from its use. An algorithm with the characteristics of the disease that afflicts the patient can achieve a timely delivery to a rehabilitative treatment to enable the recovery of a patient.

Similar to the previous proposal, apply the same algorithm with appropriate amendments, in this case the treatment received by the patient (cold, ultrasound, heat, infrared, hydrotherapy, physical exercise) that the patient needs is going according to the conditions of the joints or the affected part of the body.

The development of a medical diagnosis requires the mental processing of data provided by the patient, the exploration the physician, clinical semiology, would take and support studies. For this reason any area of medicine could benefit from the creation of tools similar to which is intending in this chapter.

CONCLUSION

The use of HISDerD as a tool to solve social and health problems, leads to the following:

1. The tests were made with classic examples where taken seven from the common diseases of the region. Software agent finds the right answer, it was verify, than the flat files contain the correct information, and also that the relation with the goals exists.

2. The software agent finds the right answer if the affection is common, this means, diseases that presents very little, won't find results, because they have not been included the rules to arrive the goals, neither the complete information. For this will be necessary to enlarge the knowledge base.

3. The project development and its completion through HISDerD, did not require many financial resources, most valuable resource was the human resource.

4. This tool is an effort between researchers, physicians and students to improve the patients in health care, which are invited to participate in a future in collective projects to solve society's problems.

5. Considers that the software agent tool is a guide, the physician determines the diagnosis.

6. There is a large backlog in the use of HIS in the institutions of public health in our country; there is the possibility that HISDerD will support telemedicine to apply it in places where there are no Dermatologists.

7. The algorithm may be useful for general practitioners, professors, and computer science students, as an assistance that would help them to solve similar problems

8. This is neither the only solution nor the only tool, but new applications must be developed where the HIS sector is highly present in this context.

9. The dermatologist's knowledge is lost; the knowledge contained in the software agent is not lost.

REFERENCES

Aggarwal, V. (2002). The Application of the Unified Modeling Language in Object-Oriented Analysis of Healthcare Information Systems. *Journal of Medical Systems, 26*(5), 383 - 397.

Al-Tajem & Al-Malaise. (2014). Integrated Business Intelligent System for E-Health: A Case for Dermatology Diseases. *Journal of Cosmetics, Dermatological Sciences and Applications*, 53-59. Retrieved from http://www.scirp.org/journal/jcdsa

Andonegui, J., Eguzkiza, A., Auzmendi, M., Serrano, L., Zurutuza, A., & Pérez de Arcelus, M. (2013). E-Ophthalmology in the Diagnosis and Follow-Up of Chronic Glaucoma. In M. Cruz-Cunha, I. Miranda, & P. Gonçalves (Eds.), *Handbook of Research on ICTs and Management Systems for Improving Efficiency in Healthcare and Social Care* (pp. 88–108). Hershey, PA. doi:10.4018/978-1-4666-3990-4.ch005

Angjellari-Dajci, F., Lawless, W. F., Agarwal, N., Oberleitner, R., Coleman, B., & Kavoossi, M. (2013). Telehealth-Based Systems for Diagnosis, Management, and Treatment of Autism Spectrum Disorders: Challenges, Opportunities, and Applications. In M. Cruz-Cunha, I. Miranda, & P. Gonçalves (Eds.), *Handbook of Research on ICTs and Management Systems for Improving Efficiency in Healthcare and Social Care* (pp. 1044–1065). Hershey, PA. doi:10.4018/978-1-4666-3990-4.ch055

Armstrong, A. W. (2009). *Store-and-Forward Teledermatology Applications, California HealtHCare Foundation*. Retrieved September 11, 2014, from http://www.chcf.org/~/media/MEDIA%20LIBRARY%20Files/PDF/S/PDF%20StoreForwardTeledermatologyApplications.pdf

Caffery, L. J., Soyer, H. P., Binder, M., Smith, A. C., & Wurm, E. (2012). *Teledermatology PACS. Telemedicine in Dermatology*. Springer Science & Business Media.

Ciufudean, C., Ciufudean, O., & Filote, C. (2013). New Models for ICT-Based Medical Diagnosis. In M. Cruz-Cunha, I. Miranda, & P. Gonçalves (Eds.), *Handbook of Research on ICTs and Management Systems for Improving Efficiency in Healthcare and Social Care* (pp. 892–911). Hershey, PA: IGI Global. doi:10.4018/978-1-4666-3990-4.ch046

Fauci, A. S. (1997). *Harrison's Principles of Internal Medicine*. New York: McGraw-Hill.

Gale Encyclopedia of Medicine. (2008). The Gale Group, Inc.

Hazen, G.B. (2002). Stochastic Trees and the StoTree Modeling Environment: Models and Software for Medical Decision Analysis. *Journal of Medical Systems, 26*(5), 399 – 413.

Hernández-Chan, G. S., Rodríguez-González, A., & Colomo-Palacios, R. (2013). Using Social Networks to Obtain Medical Diagnosis. In M. Cruz-Cunha, I. Miranda, & P. Gonçalves (Eds.), *Handbook of Research on ICTs and Management Systems for Improving Efficiency in Healthcare and Social Care* (pp. 306–320). Hershey, PA: IGI Global. doi:10.4018/978-1-4666-3990-4.ch015

Jain, Y. K. & Jain, M. (2012). Comparison between Different Classification Methods with Application to Skin Cancer. *International Journal of Computer Applications, 53*(11).

Jisha, M. J., Simi, S. S. & Neethu, M. J. (2014). Segmentation of Skin Lesions from Digital Images using Texture Distinctiveness with Neural Network. *International Journal of Advanced Research in Computer and Communication Engineering, 3*(8).

Kwak, N.K. (2002). An Application of Linear Programming Discriminant Analysis to Classifying and Predicting the Symptomatic Status of HIV/AIDS Patients. *Journal of Medical Systems, 26*(5), 427-438.

Miller-Keane. (2003). Encyclopedia and Dictionary of Medicine, Nursing, and Allied Health (7th ed.). Elsevier, Inc.

Ministério da Saúde. (2006). *Secretaria de Atenção à Saúde. Departamento de Ações programáticas Estratégicas*. Retrieved September 13, 2014, from http://bvsms.saude.gov.br/bvs/publicacoes/protocolo_dermatoses.pdf

Muir, J., & Lucas, L. (2008). *Tele-Dermatology in Australia. In Current Principles and Practices of Telemedicine and e-Health*. R. Latifi.

Podgorelec, V., Kokol, P., Stiglic, B., & Rozman, I. (2002). Decision trees: An overview and their use in medicine. *Journal of Medical Systems, 26*(5), 445-463.

Pressman, R. S. (2002). *Ingeniería del Software. Un enfoque práctico*. Madrid: McGraw-Hill.

Resconi, G., & Jain, L. (2004). *Intelligent agents theory and applications*. Germany: Springer-Verlag.

Rich, E., & Knight, K. (1991). *Artificial Intelligence*. Mc Graw-Hill.

Russell, S., Norving, P. (1996). *Inteligencia artificial un enfoque moderno*. Prentice Hall Hispanoamericana, S.A.

The American Heritage Medical Dictionary. (2007). Houghton Mifflin Company.

KEY TERMS AND DEFINITIONS

Clinical Semiology: Semiology is the mainstay of clinical medicine. It is an art and a science. It is the group of knowledge that deals with the identification of the various pathological manifestations (signs and symptoms).

Functional Relationship: The function that relates the dependent variable to the independent research variables.

IMSS: Government medical institution that serves the majority of the Mexican population.

Measurement Instrument: Instrument for determining various quantities such as temperature, mass, length. In a research method that can be a questionnaire.

Methodological Consistency: Research method of linking the basic elements, so that there is a methodological congruence between them. There is a logical relationship between the independent variable, hypothesis, objective and research question.

Methodological Consistency Matrix: Table that contains the necessary elements to develop the measurement instrument to be used in research methods.

Research Variables: Logical grouping of attributes. The operational measures of the indicators.

A Holistic Infrastructure to Support Elderlies' Independent Living

Marco Nalin
Telbios, Italy

Ilaria Baroni
Telbios, Italy

Manuel Mazzara
Service Science and Engineering Lab, Innopolis University, Russia

INTRODUCTION

This chapter starts from a literature analysis of definitions, indices and scales related to fragility and pre-fragility, to identify all those aspects which can be monitored unobtrusively and remotely from a person. In this respect, an holistic profile has been defined, which includes vital signs, information related to behaviors (e.g., daily habits, elderly person's mobility level, etc.), and information related to the environment (with ambient assisted living solutions). The SITAD project, co-funded by Lombardia Region, proposed a scalable and extendable architecture, which allows the integration of heterogeneous set of devices, sensors and actuators, through a variety of wireless and wired connections and protocols.

Such platform, which will be described in this chapter, will allow the monitoring and the early identification of meaningful variations in the daily habits, and the possible decline of the functional and cognitive abilities of the elderly person. This will hopefully create alternative diagnostic tools which will be cheaper than those currently used (PET, MRI, etc.), less invasive (being invisibly installed in the house or in the worst case worn by the person), remote (the person doesn't need to go to the hospital) and continuous (it's not a one-shot analysis, but it's continuously generating data).

BACKGROUND

In a common medical sense, the frail elderly have an advanced age, chronic pathologies, clinical instability, social isolation and a certain degree of disability. The condition of "pre-frailty" is present when only a few frailty factors are observed.

In Italy, there are one million of frail patients, and this number will double in next 20 years, with a consequent proportional increase in healthcare spending related to their management. Therefore, it is a fundamental goal for scientific research to define objective and standardized criteria of classification for these patients and for prediction of the temporal evolution of their frailty in order to implement appropriate forms of early diagnosis, monitoring of disease status and of intervention at the local and national level.

Within the framework of the EU initiative "Innovation Partnership on Active and Healthy aging" (EIP-AHA), the document "Prevention of functional decline and frailty", action plan number 3 "Prevention and early diagnosis of frailty and functional decline, both physical and cognitive, in older people" issued at the 1st Conference of Partners on November 6th, 2012 in Brussels, clearly shifts the objective from

DOI: 10.4018/978-1-4666-9978-6.ch046

"frailty" to "pre-frailty", revealing the necessity not only to define diagnostic criteria but also prediction models with the "active elderly" population as their target. Moreover, the document reveals the need to add cognitive performance indicators, currently not always included in clinical status scales and in the frailty evaluation models, defining the "multidimensional and functional decline" due to physical and cognitive causes or their combination.

The need to implement indices and clinical practices for the collections of information related to cognitive functions comes from the dramatic increase in the probability of developing Alzheimer's disease (AD), a neurodegenerative process which extends for several years without any manifestations of cognitive decline (pre-clinical phase). Then, for some years, there is a slight objective cognitive decline, called mild cognitive impairment (MCI). In a remarkable percentage of cases (approximately 50%) amnesic MCI subjects can be considered as prodromal AD that, after a few years, progresses into a serious cognitive impairment and loss of functional autonomy. To diagnose AD in the pre-clinical or prodromal phase, distinguishing it from benign cognitive deficits related to reversible psycho-physical condition, instrumental tests have been developed, such as the examination of beta and tau amyloid proteins in the cerebrospinal fluid, the volume of the hippocampus and of the cerebral cortex through magnetic resonance imaging (MRI), the assessment of cerebral metabolism and of the accumulation of beta amyloid through positron emission tomography (PET).

The goal of creating an effective screening for cognitive frailty, which in some cases could contribute to an early AD diagnosis and to the identification of reversible conditions (based on nutrition, relate to mood disorders, co-morbidity, etc.) requires a revision of the currently validated instruments and a reconsideration of the areas of frailty data collection, which cannot be connected only to the hospital/clinical setting. EIP-AHA also recommends the implementation of validated tools, tests and protocols with low cost ICT equipment to be used on populations defined on a EU basis and for co-morbidity groups, and on data gathered not only in a healthcare environment, but also in a "holistic" ecological environment.

The SITAD project, co-funded by Lombardia Region, represents a scalable and extendable architecture allowing the integration of a heterogeneous set of devices, sensors and actuators, through a variety of wireless and wired connections and protocols. The SITAD system is an advanced home care platform for elderly people and operates through the synergic actions of domotic and biomedical tools. Data are continuously collected and analyzed in order to identify potentially critical (life threatening) situations. SITAD architecture is based on the integration of both hardware and software components of heterogeneous nature and provenance. Such heterogeneity is partly due to technical choices and partly to the presence on the market of project participants or manufacturers related with them in business terms.

In the SITAD system multiple devices work together to monitor specific event related to users' needs and profile.

REFERENCE MODELS

Frailty and Pre-Frailty Definitions

The prediction and identification of possible frailty or pre-frailty condition is an important issue in the elderly social and health care. As visible in Figure 1, frailty represents a period in which the patient suffers from a functional decline (a sort of "accelerated" aging) which leads quickly to disability, with increasing patient's management costs (Akner 2013).

Figure 1. Aging patterns and their flow

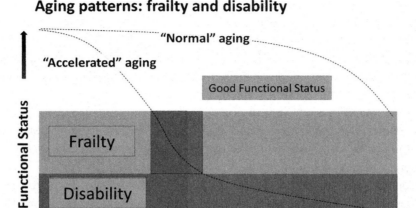

A list of frailty definitions, index and parameters is reported below, to try to describe how this concept is classified and recognized by different authors in literature. The purpose is to determine which factors should be included in the patients' profile and which ones should be monitored by the SITAD platform.

There isn't a universal definition of frailty because this status is represented by multiple conditions on autonomy, ability, physical and mental health, and co-morbidities, that all together creates the critical status.

Wingrad enunciates one of the first definition in 1991 (Winograd, 1991), affirming that from some pathologies it is possible to identify frailty conditions, like with cerebral stroke or chronic disabling disease. Moreover, Wingrad said that there are multiple autonomy boundaries that can increase the risk of frailty, which are: confusion episodes, repeated falls, reduced mobility, incontinence, malnutrition, bedsores, prolonged bed rest, use of restraints, sensory issues, and socio-economic problems or familiar problems.

In 1992 Buchner (Buchner, 1992) described the frailty as the reduction of physiological reserve in neurological control systems, in physical performances and in energy metabolism, which gives a point of view more focused on physical constitution than on diseases (other researchers followed the same approach, as Chin, 1999 and Roubenoff, 1999).

Schultz claimed in 1993 (Schultz, 1993) that the frailty level is established by the discrepancies between what is offered by the environment and the abilities of the subject (according with Brown, 1995), both at physical and cognitive level, while for Ory (Ory, 1993), the definition is focused on strength, resistance and mobility of the subject.

A couple of years later Gloth (Gloth, 1995) started to put in evidence the age of the elderly, as a threshold of frailty and institutionalization, and this concept moved on with Sager and Siu which added also questionnaires with evaluations and symptoms detection purposes (Sager, 1996). Another strong point of frailty is the depression factor, which is added by Maly (Maly, 1997), nearby urinary incontinence, falls and functional problems, in the same time Wieland add to his definition the cognitive impairment, and the disabilities in daily activities (Wieland, 2003).

A work made in 2001 (Fried, 2001) tried to give another universal definition of frailty, based on a study with 4,735 subjects of age 65 and older, for which the clinical syndrome is defined by at least three of the following situations at the same time: unintentional weight loss, self-reported exhaustion, weakness, slow walking speed, low physical activity. A different approach was used by Rockwood in 2005 (Rockwood, 2005), where he defined a frailty scale composed by seven levels, depending on the abilities, the activities and the autonomy of the patient.

Even if there is not a global definition of frailty, nowadays the early diagnosis is done for elderly with more than 80 years, or with physical dependencies, that have at least three of the following comorbidities: urinary incontinence, postural instability, bandages or immobilization, depressive syndrome or cognitive decline. Some points of these definitions are easy to assess, as the age of the subject, or a possible bandage, but some others need specific diagnosis (e.g. postural instability, depressive syndrome). In this case, the evaluation can be completed with the use of other instruments, like questionnaires, indexes, scales, tests, etc., now discuss more in depth.

To be able to design predictive strategies for frailty, it's useful to analyze the most spread indexes in this field. As suggested by previously reported definitions, there are some recurring parameters: autonomy, depression, comorbidity, cognitive perception, movement capability and nutritional information. The idea behind SITAD is to investigate which indexes can be monitored in a domestic environment, with the purpose to understand how far one can go in the prediction of these risk factors.

Starting from autonomy, the most used indexes are the ADL (Active of Daily Living) (Katz, 1963), IADL (Instrumental Activity of Daily Living) (Lawton, 1969), AADL (Advanced Activity of Daily Living) (Reuben, 1990) and Barthel (Mahoney, 1965). The purpose is to evaluate the autonomy during the daily activities at home or in a normal day, and the common actions measured are: bathing, dressing, use of health services, moving between bed and armchair, taking the stairs, continence, housework, taking drugs, hobbies, meet people and physical activity. Moreover in 2011 Vermeulen (Vermeulen, 2011) found other physical indicators as frailty predictors, based on ADL: weight loss, lower extremity function, balance, muscle strength. To monitor these activities there are multiple solutions that can be introduced in a domotic system: movements' sensors to assess home paths (stairs included), drug pills counter, humidity sensors to evaluate the activities in the bathroom, permanence on sofas, armchairs and bed, and activities in the kitchen. With an adequate support by inferential algorithms, it is possible to distinguish between occupants and analyze the support of other people or caregivers.

As far as concern the specific analysis of movement abilities, the Tinetti index (Speechley, 1991) might be approached, which analyzes specific values, like the size and the length of a step, the symmetry, the gait study, etc. To collect these information it's necessary to have complex equipment, which is not so easy to be replicated for a collection of information at home.

Depression is mentioned by several frailty definitions and it is quite common. It affects patients of all ages, and it can be analyzed in different ways, always with the diagnosis of a psychologist or pshychiatrist. Other two scales related to frailty are the Cornell index (Alexopoulos, 1988) and the GDS (Geriatric Depression Scale) (Yesavage, 1982). In the first the assessment is focused on the mood, behavioral disorders, cyclic functions and attempted suicide, and it's filled in third person, which means that a specialist will complete the questionnaire based on patient's conditions. As opposite, the GDS scale is a simple self-assessment questionnaire with Y/N answers for the patient, which fills the questionnaire in first-person and reports his perception. As far as concern an automation of the depression measurement, it's clear that the system is not able to (and should not) substitute a specialist, but it could be helpful to provide some self-assessment questionnaires, leaving the final judge to the specialist.

Another questionnaire used not only in generic frail people, but also in patients affected by dementia, is the MMSE (Mini Mental State Examination) (Folstein, 1975). The purpose is to evaluate the lucidity and the mental capacity of the subject with frailty risk by his cognitive perception. The patient is evaluated through some questions on simple topics like dates, counting, mnemonic questions, tongue twisters, simple actions and orientation exercises in the environment. This index seems to be easily implementable at home through touch screens with all the questions and tasks which can be replicated every day. Moreover, the same screen can be used to offer small daily questionnaires to examine the mental condition or to provide small exercises.

Another important element to monitor deterioration of elderly is nutrition. It often happens that aged people stop to eat, or reduce the amount of food ingested, repeating the same foods and meals. The MNA (Mini Nutritional Assessment) index takes care of the loss of appetite (Vellas, 2006), weight and water and food taken per day, and also the perceptions of the patients about his health status, BMI, and how he manages the preparation of meals. Domotic sensors could be inserted in the kitchen to monitor the food habits and when and where the elderly is moving in this room.

Finally, another aspect which is frequent in frailty indexes is the presence of co-morbidities: there are indexes like CIRS (Cumulative Illness Rating Scale) that take care of the chronic diseases of the patient, and give a result based on the their severity (Linn, 1968). In this case, questionnaires are filled by specialists, and it's not so easy to assess this risk through home monitoring solutions. The only way to collect some information is to pick some data from medical devices, to provide feedbacks that can be used by doctors to consider the severity and the evolution of each known disease.

After all these considerations, below there's a collection of all the parameters that can be used to monitor the frailty risk at home. The first column represents the topic, the second collects some examples, the third refers to some measurable parameters, and the last one indicates some indexes correlated.

A control panel available to the Service Centre with alerts system can monitor all the parameters listed above: if one of the condition is over a predefined threshold for that patient, it can contribute to the assess the frailty risk, which is constantly monitored by the system and periodically reported to the doctor. In this way it's possible to monitor the elderlies' conditions and if they're degrading. Appropriate actions can be timely taken either by the Service Centre or by the doctor to prevent possible deteriorations, before of the patient falls into frailty or disability condition.

The Personal Profile and Service Levels

Users are clustered based on an initial assessment (which can be updated and refined over time), to be stratified based on their fragility level (thus on their social or health needs), which can be high, medium or low.

Evidences from medical literature demonstrated that some risk factors are important to be considered to predict the possibility of falls, which is one of the main cause of deaths among fragile patients. Thus the following information were considered by the system in the personal profile of the person:

- **Previous Falls Record:** One of the most frequent fall risk factors in an elderly patient reported in prospective studies is a previous fall event. For this reason it is important to consider in the patient profile previous episodes, frequencies, characteristics and contexts in which fall happened (e.g., during night).
- **Multiple Pharmacological Therapies or Usage of Particular Drugs:** It is important for the system to track the pharmacological prescriptions, with particular attention with what concerns benzodiazepines, psychotropic drugs, diuretics, antidepressants, antihypertensive, narcotics, pain

Table 1. Parameters which can be used by SITAD system to assess frailty

Fields	Examples	Measurable Parameters	Indexes Involved
Personal hygiene	Brush your teeth, shower, toilet	• Dwell time in bathroom • Number of people • Number of times • Water consumption	ADL Barthel
Autonomy in moving	Transfers at home, long distances, stairs, transfers bed/chair, balance	• Dwell time in the different spaces • Distance travelled in a single ride • Number of people that are doing together the same route	ADL AADL Barthel
Domestic autonomy	Dressing, housework, laundry, hobbies, reading, listening to music	• Dwell time in dressing places • Number of people • Microphones	ADL IADL AADL Barthel
Continence Capacity	Continence	• Dwell time in bathroom • Number of people • Number of times	ADL Barthel
Nutrition	Eating, cooking, drinking, food shopping, food quality, number of meals	• Dwell time in kitchen (refrigerator/stove zones) • Number of times • Number of peoples	ADL IADL Barthel MNA
Diseases management	Drugs assumption	Pills counter	IADL MNA
Social life	Phone, see friends and family, go out of house (cinema, church, bar, etc)	• Number of people • Activities (phone, intercom) • Time spent out of home	IADL AADL
Physical activity	Walks, bike rides, gymnastic	• Time out of home • Use equipment • Steps counter	AADL
Psychological factor	Anxiety, sadness, irritability, behavioral disorders, sleep problems, ideological disorders	• Questionnaires on depression • Switching lights during the night • Movements in the house during the night	Cornell MNA
Weakening	Weight loss, appetite, energy, IMC	• Weight of the person • Amount of daily physical activities	Cornell MNA
Cognitive abilities	Memory of information, computing capacity, contextualization, command execution, dementia	Mnemonic tests	MMSE MNA
Abilities of movement	Trigger gait, step length and height for left and right side, symmetry and continuity of the walk, deviations, ripple trunk	Tests on movements	Tinetti
Sedentary lifestyle	Bedsores, bed rest	Time spent in bed	MNA
Self-assessment of health status	It is considered well nourished, judgment, general health	Questionnaires	MNA

killers and antiepileptic. Furthermore several studies reports that patients treated with three or more drugs simultaneously have higher risk of recurrent falls with respect to patients treated with less drugs.

• **Mobility Problems:** Test carried out in several studies reveal that alterations in speed, distances and vacillations are important indicators to predict fall risk.

- **Lack of Physical Exercise:** This is a risk factor both for frail and non-frail patients. Studies conducted in the past (O'Loughlin 1993) demonstrated the effect of physical activity in elderlies, with improvements in physical abilities (functional abilities and stamina), cognitive performances (memory, processing speed, etc.) and quality of life (global quality of life, psychophysical wellbeing, social relationships, etc.).
- **Sight Alteration:** Several studies conducted both at patients' homes and in hospitals revealed that elderlies with sight impairment have higher fall risk.
- **Social Isolation:** Elderlies which live alone as well those with poor income have higher risk associated to falls.

To complete the picture, there are a number of risks which are associated to domestic accidents as well, but they were out of the scope of the SITAD platform, because of the lack of appropriate sensors and devices or reliable data sources (e.g., use of open flippers, etc.).

As already mentioned, depending on the risk profile, patients are clustered into different service levels. The services offered by the SITAD platform are basically of three types:

- **Initial Assessment:** As already mentioned this is called initial, but it can be seldom repeated in case of significant changes in the patient's health or social condition. It includes a physical assessment (blood pressure Holter monitor, physical abilities assessment, questionnaires, etc.), and an environmental assessment (risk areas identification in the house, questionnaires on domestic risks, etc.).
- **Continuous Monitoring:** A lifelong monitoring of patients' physical activity, drug therapies, vital signs and behaviors (e.g., habits patterns, mobility level, social relationships, etc.)
- **Emergency Management:** Upon identification of an emergency (which can be automatic or manually triggered by the patient through a "panic button" device) the system will react activating appropriate emergency response protocols.

The services are composed depending on the risk level of the patient, which can be low, medium or high:

- **Low Risk Level:** The initial assessment is done through questionnaires, educational services are proposed, there is a "manual" management of emergencies (patients are provided with "panic button" device, but no automatic means for fall detection are provided), and patients are prescribed with a personalized training plan.
- **Medium Risk Level:** The initial assessment is done through devices for what concerns the physical dimension (e.g., blood pressure Holter monitor for one week), and a continuous monitoring is provided for physical activity, drug compliance and vital signs monitoring.
- **High Risk Level:** The initial assessment includes an environmental assessment at the house of the patient, domotic technologies are installed and there is an automatic fall detection, plus all the services provided to the other risk levels.

The assessment of the risk level is done by a clinician, based also on the data collected in the period previous to the visit.

HOLISTIC INFRASTRUCTURE TO SUPPORT ELDERLIES' INDEPENDENT LIVING

Home-Care Systems

Remote home care systems are used to constantly monitor elderly patients - typically the only occupiers of the house - who suffer from degenerative pathologies. The house is equipped with sensors for environmental monitoring that are placed at strategic points, according to the type of data that have to be collected and the type of pathologies that are intended to be kept under control. Doors, windows, appliances are some of the critical points of the house that may need monitoring.

Domotic sensors are typically associated with biomedical devices in order to determine, store and transmit in real time the major vital signs of the patient under observation. By means of a synergy between domotic and biomedical data, daily habits of individuals with chronic diseases can be observed and analyzed by a remote operator, who may submit part of this information to nursing and medical staff. Each telemedicine system must therefore be associated with a service center capable of providing the technology platform.

These modern systems allow following patients at home and offering greater security along with the possibility of following a particular treatment while remaining at home and with minimal changes in daily habits. The objective of these systems is improving the quality of life of the elderly and, at the same time, reduce the rate of hospitalization and health care costs.

Remote home care systems work on an interaction model between patients and the facilities offering healthcare. The telecommunications infrastructure should provide:

- Monitoring of physical and cognitive condition of the patient;
- Monitoring of vital parameters;
- Moral and psychological support to the patient and his family;
- Specialist support for medical treatment applied locally;
- Support for chronic patients;
- Communication with the family;
- A reminder of commitments and activities of the day (medicines to take, analysis to do etc.).

The SITAD System

The system includes the following domotic and biomedical devices:

User Devices

- **Body Guardian (ECG, Respiration Rate):** Observation of cardiac and respiratory systems rates;
- **Tracker (Accelerometer, GPS):** It follows the physical activity of patients and allows the pressure of a button for requesting assistance;
- **Oximeter:** Portable instrument for measuring the amount of hemoglobin in the blood;
- **Scale:** The patient's weight is a matter of particular importance for the traceability of certain pathologies;
- **Blood Pressure Monitor:** A portable instrument for blood pressure traceability;

- **Drugs Dispenser:** It adjusts the delivery of one or more drugs (timed and able to detect dispenser inclination through accelerometer). Medication has to be monitored to ensure that the patient is following the prescribed therapy.

Home Devices

- **Communication Device:** It is a connection standing between patient and service center. It is equipped with an emergency button;
- **Camera:** Allows the transmission of images of the patient in cases of emergencies;
- **Infrared Presence Detector:** It can determine the presence of an individual in a specific room;
- **Doors/Windows Opening Devices:** They allow an analysis of patient behavior.

During their daily activities, patients wear a small portable device (tracker) equipped with an emergency button. This mobile device is connected to the gateway and includes an accelerometer and a blood pressure monitor in order to collect major data on the individual. The goal of this section is presenting in more detail the overall architecture of the system as described by Figure 2.

Figure 2. SITAD architecture

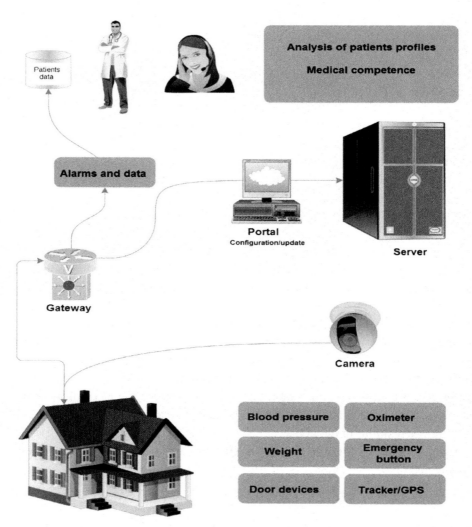

The SITAD System Architecture

The analysis of the requirements phase of the SITAD project led to the system architecture as shown in Figure 3 by UML component and deployment diagrams. The component diagram by itself provides the specification of all the modules, their interfaces and dependencies. The modules of the systems are represented as rectangles and the functionalities they offer as circles. When other modules join these circles by an arrow whose head is a semicircle that means they are exploiting such a functionality. The component diagram contains all the high-level information on the system, with the exception of the deployment of components onto their physical locations or devices, which is instead represented by the deployment diagram. The functions, as shown in Figure 3, provide the following interfaces:

- **Detection Devices Management:**
  - **Ping ():** Verifies device functioning.
- **Monitoring:**
  - **Diagnostic ():** Requires a diagnostic device.
  - **CollectData (d):** Collects data from devices.
  - **Set (Pi):** Sets a configuration parameter.
  - **Get (Pi):** Gets a parameter configuration.
- **Camera Management:**
  - **Ping ():** Verifies device functioning.
  - **GetImg ():** Get images from the camera.
- **Service Center:**
  - **Signal (code):** Signals an event to the Service Center.
- **Portal Service:**
  - **Configure ():** Allows configuration of the system.
  - **Report (uc):** Generates reports for a specific user.
- **Database:**
  - **Read (d):** Queries to the data base.
  - **Write (d):** Updates the database.

Deployment

SITAD is a distributed system, so the functionality offered has to be deployed onto geographically different places and the modules actually implemented in different hardware locations. Deployment of functionalities has been performed according to the following considerations for each of the devices.

- **Devices and Camera:** The house is equipped with several devices, including a portable oximeter and an emergency button, which are connected via radio to a gateway physically present in the house too. The communication between the gateway and the devices takes place via radio on a frequency regulated by Italian laws on social emergencies.
- **Monitoring:** The monitor is responsible for collecting data coming from the house in order to manage the peculiar medical condition of the patient. The monitoring module has to be deployed onto the gateway residing in the house.
- **Service Center (Management of the Patient):** Service center activities can be distinguished in two dimensions:

Figure 3. UML and deployment component diagrams of SITAD

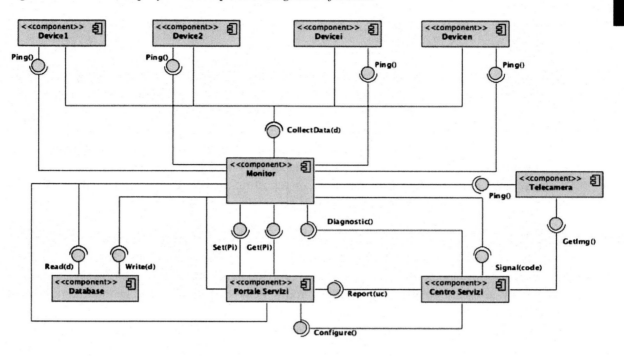

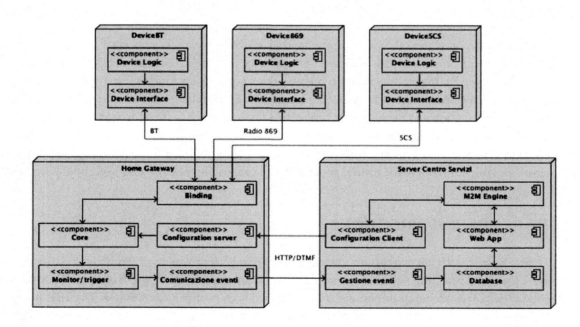

- ○ **Biomedical Tracking:** Biomedical devices allows the reconstruction of patient's story and analyze critical issues;
- ○ **Behavioral Tracking:** Home automation devices allow to identify variations from the standard pattern of user's behavior and identify, based on rules of "common sense," dangerous behavior such as falls or inactivity.

Filtering and data aggregation occur at the level of the monitoring function. The service center focuses on managing emergencies only. The module Service Center has to be therefore deployed onto the physical location where the operators are.

- **Portal Services (Management of the House):** The data collected by the monitoring module require filtering, aggregation and analysis. This part of the algorithmic functionality is implemented in the reporting of the Portal Services. Not all events and data collected from the monitor are in fact forwarded to the Service Center that is only alerted in case of potential life threatening situations. Instead, the data are stored in the database in order to be analyzed. The module Portal Services is deployed onto the gateway located inside the house.
- **Database:** The database stores information for reporting purposes. It is only used by modules residing in the gateway and it is located outside the home, at the service center.

The deployment diagram shown in Figure 3 describes the physical allocation of functionality on the hardware nodes, and the way in which they are related. This diagram together with the component diagram represent how software modules are distributed onto the hardware resources of the system. Nodes are represented by cubes and relationships between nodes are described as lines. The modules allocated on a node are described as rectangles into cubes.

The devices supported by the system use the following protocols as shown in Figure 3:

- Bluetooth ®, for biomedical devices;
- Radio 869MHz, for signaling (European Social Alarm Frequency);
- Bus SCS (Simplified Wiring System by Bticino) for domotic devices.

The devices collect raw data that are communicated by the gateway to the server in the form <data, device, timestamp>. For each triplet of this type a priority may be associated that will be adequately managed by the server. In this architecture the gateway does not host any kind of intelligent logic and data analysis is only performed server side. The communication is client/server with the gateway acting as initiator of the conversation and periodically connecting to the central system through its identifying ID. The server maintains a database of associations between gateway ID and user profiles and is therefore able to determine to which patient raw data has to be associated. These data are communicated in push mode to the server on which the database resides together with the graphical front end used by the operator.

FUTURE RESEARCH DIRECTIONS

Research has made significant progresses toward usability and effectiveness of Ambient Assisted Living solutions, yet without reaching solid results which are convincing and allow the widespread adoption of such technologies. Two research directions should be pursued, probably in parallel. The first being on usability studies, which ensures acceptance of the proposed solution from elderly people and the assurance that the technology simplifies their life (improving the quality), instead of adding superfluous burden. The second being on the development of intelligent algorithms which can process multi-dimensional data and can correlate them to find reliable and important outcome indicators.

CONCLUSION

The chapter presented an infrastructure which is able to capture data from an heterogeneous set of devices, sensors and data sources, and provide services supporting elderly and frail people to live longer, healthier and more independently. The key take away is not on the single forms of monitoring, but on the integration of all of them, which provides an added value to the end users. In other words, the final value of the set of the different types of monitoring is higher than the sum of the values of the single ones. The underlying reason is that complex patients requires an holistic approach, which takes into account the whole person with a systemic approach, rather than just one of his characteristic (e.g., a chronic disease).

Fragmented approach will fail, because will result in technology push of overwhelming solutions for a class of patient that is becoming slowly open to technology, but it's not yet.

Ambient Assisted Living solutions will facilitate the process, but only if they are seamlessly integrated in the environment and transparent for the end users.

Furthermore, service design should be carried out in parallel to technology development, otherwise technology alone will fail if it is not properly supported by effective clinical and social assistive protocols.

ACKNOWLEDGMENT

The work has been supported by the Russian Ministry of education and science (agreement 14.612.21.0001), and by Italian Ministry of University and Research and Lombardia Region through the project SITAD (project ID: 30221379).

REFERENCES

Akner, G. (2013). Frailty and multimorbidity in elderly people: a shift in management approach. *Clinical Geriatrics, 21*(9).

Alexopoulos, G. S., Abrams, R. C., Young, R. C., & Shamoian, C. A. (1988). Cornell Scale for Depression in Dementia. *Biological Psychiatry, 23*(3), 271–284. doi:10.1016/0006-3223(88)90038-8 PMID:3337862

Brown, I., Renwick, R., Raphael, D. (1995). Frailty: constructing a common meaning, definition, and conceptual framework. *Int J Rehabil Res., 18*(2), 93–102.

Buchner, D. M., & Wagner, E. H. (1992). Preventing frail health. *Clinics in Geriatric Medicine, 8*, 1–17. PMID:1576567

Chin, A., Paw, M. J., Dekker, J. M., Feskens, E. J., Schouten, E. G., & Kromhout, D. (1999). How to select a frail elderly population? A comparison of three working definitions. *Journal of Clinical Epidemiology, 52*(11), 1015–1021. doi:10.1016/S0895-4356(99)00077-3 PMID:10526994

Folstein, M. F., Folstein, S. E., & McHugh, P. R. (1975). "Mini-mental state". A practical method for grading the cognitive state of patients for the clinician. *Journal of Psychiatric Research, 12*(3), 189–198. doi:10.1016/0022-3956(75)90026-6 PMID:1202204

Fried, L. P., Tangen, C. M., Walston, J., Newman, A. B., Hirsch, C., Gottdiener, J., & McBurnie, M. A. et al. (2001). Cardiovascular Health Study Collaborative Research Group: Frailty in older adults: evidence for a phenotype. *The Journals of Gerontology. Series A, Biological Sciences and Medical Sciences, 56*(3), M146–M156. doi:10.1093/gerona/56.3.M146 PMID:11253156

Gloth, F. M. III, Walston, J., Meyer, J., & Pearson, J. (1995). Reliability and validity of the Frail Elderly Functional Assessment Questionnaire. *American Journal of Physical Medicine & Rehabilitation, 74*(1), 45–53. doi:10.1097/00002060-199501000-00008 PMID:7873113

Katz, S., Ford, A. B., Moskowitz, R. W., Jackson, B. A., & Jaffe, M. W. (1963). Studies of Illness in the Aged. the Index of Adl: a Standardized Measure of Biological and Psychosocial Function. JAMA, 185, 914–919.

Lawton, M.P., & Brody, E.M. (1969). Assessment of older people: self-maintaining and instrumental activities of daily living. *Gerontologist, 9*(3), 179–186.

Linn, B. S., Linn, M. W., & Gurel, L. (1968). Cumulative illness rating scale. J Am Geriatr Soc, 16(5), 622-6.

Mahoney, F. I., & Barthel, D. W. (1965). Functional Evaluation: The Barthel Index. *Maryland State Medical Journal, 14*, 61–65. PMID:14258950

Maly, R. C., Hirsch, S. H., & Reuben, D. H. (1997). The performance of simple instruments in detecting geriatric conditions and selecting community-dwelling older people for geriatric assessment. *Age and Ageing, 26*(3), 223–231. doi:10.1093/ageing/26.3.223 PMID:9223719

O'Loughlin, J. L., Robitaille, Y., Boivin, J. F., & Suissa, S. (1993). Incidence of and Risk Factors for Falls and Injurious Falls among the Community-dwelling Elderly. *American Journal of Epidemiology, 137*(3), 342–354. PMID:8452142

Ory, M. G., Schechtman, K. B., Miller, J. P., Hadley, E. C., Fiatarone, M. A., Province, M. A., & Kaplan, M. (1993). Frailty and injuries in later life: The FICSIT trials. *Journal of the American Geriatrics Society, 41*(3), 283–296. doi:10.1111/j.1532-5415.1993.tb06707.x PMID:8440853

Reuben, D. B., Laliberte, L., Hiris, J., & Mor, V. (1990). A hierarchical exercise scale to measure function at the Advanced Activities of Daily Living (AADL) level. *Journal of the American Geriatrics Society, 38*(8), 855–861. doi:10.1111/j.1532-5415.1990.tb05699.x PMID:2387949

Rockwood, K., Song, X., MacKnight, C., Bergman, H., Hogan, D. B., McDowell, I., & Mitnitski, A. (2005). A global clinical measure of fitness and frailty in elderly people. *Canadian Medical Association Journal, 173*(5), 489–495. doi:10.1503/cmaj.050051 PMID:16129869

Roubenoff, R. (1999). The pathophysiology of wasting in the elderly. *The Journal of Nutrition, Health & Aging, 4*, 140–142. PMID:10936900

Sage, M. A., Franke, T., & Inouye, S. K. (1996). Functional outcomes of acute medical illness and hospitalization in older persons. *Archives of Internal Medicine, 156*(6), 645–652. doi:10.1001/archinte.1996.00440060067008 PMID:8629876

Schultz, R., & Willanson, G. M. (1993). Psychosocial and behavioural dimensions of physical frailty. *Journal of Gerontology, 48*(Special), 39–43. doi:10.1093/geronj/48.Special_Issue.39 PMID:8409239

Speechley, M., & Tinetti, M. (1991). Falls and injuries in frail and vigorous community elderly persons. *Journal of the American Geriatrics Society*, *39*(1), 46–52. doi:10.1111/j.1532-5415.1991.tb05905.x PMID:1987256

Vellas, B., Villars, H., Abellan, G., Soto, M. E., Rolland, Y., Guigoz, Y., & Garry, P. et al. (2006). Overview of the MNA--Its history and challenges. *The Journal of Nutrition, Health & Aging*, *10*(6), 456–463. PMID:17183418

Vermeulen, J., Neyens, J. C., Van Rossum, E., Spreeuwenberg, M. D., & De Witte, L. P. (2011, July 1). Predicting ADL disability in community-dwelling elderly people using physical frailty indicators: A systematic review. *BMC Geriatrics*, *11*(1), 33. doi:10.1186/1471-2318-11-33 PMID:21722355

Wieland, D. (2003). The effectiveness and costs of comprehensive geriatric evaluation and management. *Critical Reviews in Oncology/Hematology*, *48*(2), 227–237. doi:10.1016/j.critrevonc.2003.06.005 PMID:14607385

Winograd, C. H., Gerety, M. B., Chung, M., Goldstein, M. K., Dominguez, F. Jr, & Vallone, R. (1991). Screening for frailty: Criteria and predictors of outcomes. *Journal of the American Geriatrics Society*, *39*(8), 778–784. doi:10.1111/j.1532-5415.1991.tb02700.x PMID:1906492

Yesavage, J. A., Brink, T. L., Rose, T. L., Lum, O., Huang, V., Adeym, M., & Leirerm, V. O. (1982). Development and validation of a geriatric depression screening scale: A preliminary report. *Journal of Psychiatric Research*, *17*(1), 37–49. doi:10.1016/0022-3956(82)90033-4 PMID:7183759

KEY TERMS AND DEFINITIONS

AD: Alzheimer's disease, also known in medical literature as Alzheimer disease, is the most common form of dementia. There is no cure for the disease, which worsens as it progresses, and eventually leads to death.

Ambient Assisted Living: It's a relatively new ICT trend to embed intelligent objects in the environment to support people (mostly elderly) in living independently and monitored.

Fragility: Condition common to many elderly, which are frail from the point of view of health and/ or social conditions.

Independent Living: Ability for elderly people to live longer without the need of assistance from other persons.

Internet of Things: Machine to machine communication among smart objects spread into the environment.

MCI: Mild cognitive impairment (MCI) is an intermediate stage between the expected cognitive decline of normal aging and the more serious decline of dementia.

Telehealth: Set of telecommunication technologies which support the delivery of health-related services and information.

Telemonitoring: Remote data collection from a patient. Data are usually sent to someone which supervise the patient, being it a Service Centre or directly a doctor.

Information and Communication Technology for Mental Health:
A Systematic Literature Review

Shrutika Namle
Griffith University, Australia

Amir Hossein Ghapanchi
Griffith University, Australia

Alireza Amrollahi
Griffith University, Australia

INTRODUCTION

Information and Communication technology (ICT) is the tool of choice for a range of problems that exist around us. On the other hand, "health care is described as a complex, often cumbersome mix of community and hospital – based services, provided by a bewildering array of health professionals located in public and private facilities and organizations across the country"(Whetton, 2005). The need to manage the surge of expectations gives rise to the use of ICT in health care (Whetton, 2005). Gradually, the adoption of ICT in the various clinical departments of health has taken strength. There has been a reasonable amount of improvement since then.

There is an abundance of research available about the use of ICT in mental health. Literature demonstrates that ICT has been used for a variety of purposes in mental health. Mental health is an umbrella term covering a vast number of disorders and diseases. Also, technology has a wide range covering the simplest telephone to the most advanced smartphone and the simplest computer to the super computers that we have today. Due to the above variability, abundance of information and data is available on the use of ICT in mental health. However, there is no uniformity of the studies and of the data that is available. Thus, this systematic review on the various information and communication technologies associated with mental health is necessary in order to summarize the vast amount of literature available. The study aims to establish the effectiveness of the information and communication technologies used in the field of mental health. It will clarify what particular technologies are more commonly utilized to achieve various outcomes in mental health. Also, it will highlight what types of mental health problems could be better targeted, with the help of information and communication technology. The study will point out the areas which lack adequate research and would prove to be a good starting point for further studies. The following questions have been addressed in the study:

RQ1: What different types of information and communication technologies have been used for different types of mental health problems?
RQ2: Which mental disorders have been targeted for treatment with ICT?
RQ3: For which purposes ICT have been used in mental health area?

DOI: 10.4018/978-1-4666-9978-6.ch047

The remainder of this paper is organized as follows. Section 2 gives an overview of the literature. Section 3 describes the methodology used for conducting the literature review. Section 4 illustrates the results of the systematic literature review. We discuss the results of the study in Section 5 and provide some recommendations for future research.

BACKGROUND

Mental Health

Mental health disorder consists of a range of diseases including psychotic illnesses and other disorders, eating disorders and personality disorders. The scope of mental health is not well defined and there is a thin line between mental disorders and brain disorders. Mental health does not depend on clinical biomarkers but on a cluster of symptoms for the diagnosis of a condition unlike the other physical conditions. The mental disorders are currently classified by the Diagnostic and Statistical Manual of Mental Disorders, (DSM) (APA, 1980), currently in its fourth edition, and the International Classification of Disease (ICD) (WHO, 1992)

The nature of mental health disorders is such that these disorders co-exist and are inter-related with other mental disorders or physical disorders.(AIHW, 2010) This involves multiple health interactions at the different levels in the health care system. This requires for an accelerated system of information and communication management to ensure a proper and coordinated system for delivering health care services. Thus, technology plays a crucial role by enhancing communication paths in this respect (Cleary et al., 2008).

Mental health in Australia is one of the seven National health Priority areas, which concentrate on diseases causing the highest morbidity and mortality in the country. The proportion of mental health patients has been increasing steadily from 2001 to 2011- 2012 ("Australia's Health 2012," 2012).

The Global burden of disease study, 2010 states that depression, anxiety and substance use accounts for one quarter of years lived adjusted to disability (GBD, 2010). Mental health problems are a leading cause of disability in Australia. Over 27.3% of the people receiving disability- support pensions have a psychiatric or psychological disorder (AIHW, 2010). According to the ABS 2003 report, the prevalence of psychiatric disability was 5.2% of the Australian population (AIHW, 2010).

A broad range of medical and rehabilitative services are available for the mental disorders. These include hospitals, residential care units, hospital out–patient units, general practitioners and community health care services (Ghanbarzadeh et al., 2014). The amount of psychiatrists working in Australia during 2011, were 2813 and mental health nurses amounted to 17,916. The total amount of subsidized mental health medications accounted for 11.2% of the total subsidized medications (AIHW, 2013b).

Literature suggests that there has been a higher prevalence of mental health illness in the rural areas due to socio-economic conditions, harsher climatic conditions, social environment and isolation (Morrissey and Reser, 2007).

There are certain underserved communities that are unable to reap the benefits of the mental health services provided. These communities include veterans and prison inmates. The prison health census suggests that almost one third of the prison entrants were reported to be suffering from a mental health problem (AIHW, 2010).

In Australia, at least $28.6 billion dollars per year, excluding the capital expenditure, is spent on supporting people with mental health. This $28.6 billion occupies 2.2% of the Gross Domestic Product

(Medibank, 2013). Almost $6.9 billion dollars were spent on mental health services during the year 2010-2011. The expenditure on mental health has increased by 5.7% as compared to 2005 ("Australia's Health 2012," 2012).

The 'National Survey of Mental Health and well' being have collected data on the extent of use of the available mental health services. Almost 35% people with a 12 month period of mental disorder had made use of the mental health services (AIHW, 2013a). There were around 2.1 million people with a 12 month period of mental health disorder who did not make use of the mental health services available but who perceived that they had an unmet need (ABS, 2008).

In a study conducted in South Australia in 2012, it was highlighted that almost 60% of the population, residing in rural areas of Australia, perceived access to mental health services difficult. The most likely reason for the above fact could be the smaller choice of health service providers and community clinics (Mills et al., 2012). Another reason for the poor utilization could be the inability of retaining the staff in rural areas for longer period of time (Wilks et al., 2008). It is apparent from the above scenario that overcoming the challenges would benefit the health care system significantly.

Information and Communication Technology for Mental Health

There have been various studies discussing the different aspects of ICT in mental health with respect to their benefits. These benefits are highlighted in terms of accessibility (Griffiths & Christensen, 2007), utilization and workforce (Wendel et al., 2011), expenditure, (Farhadi et al., 2012) and improving the quality of life (Cleary et al., 2008; Najaftorkaman et al., 2014). In order to gain a better understanding about the various types of technologies available in the market, a short review is provided.

The ICT tools that are used in the health care industry are more or less similar to the recently developed technology. However, these tools have been seen to be modified to suit the specific requirements of health care. These tools include text messaging, patient web portals, patient education websites, Smart phones, Tablet PC's, Electronic prescribing and Telemedicine (Robert E Hoyt, 2012).

The existing studies on ICT in mental health are inconsistent and disorganized with respect to the benefits. Due to the small scale and short term studies, it was difficult to generalize the studies (Whitten et al., 2002). A need for further research is highlighted as the data available is inconsistent and weak (Reger & Gahm, 2009). The existing studies have failed to prove the clinical benefits of ICT though it was suggested as a feasible and satisfactory method (Garcia-Lizana & Munoz-Mayorga, 2010).

Another study conducted on depression stated that there is poor evidence to show the effectiveness of the ICT in mental health. The study clearly shows that there are benefits of using ICT in depression in terms of patient accessibility and satisfaction, though the effectiveness, efficiency and cost–effectiveness of ICT is yet unclear (García-Lizana & Muñoz-Mayorga, 2010).

On the other hand, there are many studies that exist which provide evidence that the use of ICT in mental health is effective in terms of treatment engagement and improved care management (Meglic et al., 2010), workforce shortages, (Benavides-Vaello et al., 2013), improved access, expenditure and workforce (Toperczer, 2011).

As a result, ICT may act as a solution and try to minimize the problems. Evidence suggests that there have been studies investigating the various technologies in the different type of mental health problems. These studies highlight different areas of research like the effectiveness, feasibility and acceptability of such techniques. There have also been studies exploring the cost-effectiveness, time-effectiveness and labor-effectiveness of the ICT in mental health. Studies detailing the challenges and barriers to ICT use in mental health also exist. On the other hand, there are studies that suggest that greater research is required to provide the evidence that such techniques are effective. This emphasizes that the available knowledge and research of ICT in mental health is not uniform and needs revision. This points to the fact that a well-defined and systematic analysis of the available literature is essential to understand the benefits and advantages of Information and Communication Technology in mental health.

RESEARCH METHODOLOGY

A Systematic literature review was undertaken to find published articles about information and communication technology used in "mental health" problems. Figure 1 illustrates the stages of study selection for the systematic review in this paper using Kitchenham's (2004) guidelines. The first stage involved searching the keywords on 5 scientific databases. As a result, 4552 primary studies were identified. Subsequently, stages 2-4 were undertaken. A detailed search of five electronic bibliographic databases was undertaken (Scopus, ProQuest, ISI web of science, Association for information systems electronic library, and Science Direct) (Amrollahi et al., 2013; Najaftorkaman et al., 2013).

Keywords

Titles and abstracts of papers were searched with the following keywords.

(Technology OR "information and communication technology" OR ICT OR Telemedicine OR ehealth OR Telehealth) AND ("mental health" OR "mental disorder" OR psychiatry OR "mental illness" OR "mental deficiency" OR "mental deficiencies" OR "mental problem" OR "mental problems" OR "mental imbalance" OR "mental sickness" OR "mental instabilities" OR "mental instability" OR "behavioural problems" OR "behavioral problem" OR "behavioural disorder" OR "behavioural illness" OR "behavioural deficiency" OR "behavioural disabilities" OR "behavioural disability" OR "behavioural

Figure 1. Stages of study selection

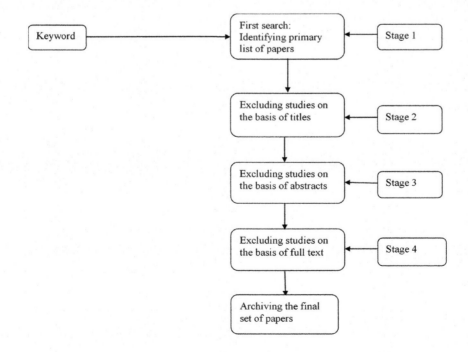

instabilities" OR "behavioural instability" OR "behavioral disorder" OR "behavioral illness" OR "Behavioral deficiency" OR "behavioral disability" OR "behavioral disabilities" OR "behavioral instability" OR "behavioral instabilities" OR "neurotic disorders" OR "neurotic disease" OR "neurotic instability" OR "neurotic instabilities" OR "neurotic health" OR "neurotic illness" OR "neurotic disabilities" OR "neurotic disability" OR "neurotic deficiency" OR "neurotic deficiencies" OR "neurotic problems" OR "psychiatric disorders" OR "psychiatric diseases" OR "psychiatric illness" OR "psychiatric disabilities" OR "psychiatric disability" OR "psychiatric imbalance" OR "psychiatric deficiency" OR "psychiatric deficiencies" OR "psychiatric problems" OR "psychiatric instabilities" OR "psychiatric instability")

Inclusion/Exclusion Criteria

We used the method which have been used in the literature (Amrollahi, Ghapanchi, & Najaftorkaman, 2014; Amrollahi, Ghapanchi, & Talaei-Khoei, 2014; Amir Hossein Ghapanchi & Aybuke Aurum, 2011; Ghapanchi et al., 2013) and limited our search to articles which have been published after 2000. The first set of papers (4552) was obtained after searching with this criterion the keywords in the databases. A 'Title Search' Strategy was used to exclude the irrelevant articles from this set of papers which gave the second set of papers. In this stage we attempted to exclude papers which were not related to the mental health and use of ICT. The total number of papers in the second set was 1102. Then the abstracts of the remaining papers were studied to shortlist the relevant papers from the second set of papers, pertaining to the topic which gave the third set of papers. The total number of papers in the third set was 551. This set of 551 papers was skimmed through to get the fourth set of papers which was 70 papers. The papers were read in detail and were further reduced. At this stage, duplicate articles were excluded as well. Thus, the final list of papers obtained was 44. In the last two stages we checked the papers to see if they had made use of any kind of technology for treatments or any other therapeutic purposes and if they were addressed to any kind of mental health problem. Table 1 provides the details of the search findings.

DATA ANALYSIS

Following the identification of the relevant papers, we attempted to label them with appropriate terms regarding the above mentioned research question. After finishing the first round of labelling, we con-

Table 1. Research findings

Database	Initial Number of Papers	After Exclusion Base on Title	After Exclusion Base on Abstract	After Exclusion Base on Abstract	Final Set of Papers
Science direct	57	9	5	0	0
Scopus	3747	678	348	43	36
ProQuest	484	237	117	11	1
Association for information systems electronic library	83	17	3	0	
ISI web of science	181	161	78	16	7
Total	4552	1102	551	70	44

tinued to second and third rounds in order to gain a better classification. We revised some labels with better vocabulary or merged some of the categories in the second and third rounds to achieve our final classification, which is depicted in the results section of the paper.

RESULTS

The above search strategy gave back a final set of 44 papers. All the 44 studies were read in detail and the data with respect to the research questions was extracted and classified for analysis.

Technology Used

In order to answer the first research question, different types of technologies are employed in mental health problems. The findings from the study reported that video technology, phone, mobile phone technology and internet were the predominant technologies used. Table 2 provides details of the various technologies used, their type and the number of papers reporting them.

Video Technology

Video technology consisted of 37.5%, used in almost 18 studies. Video technology was further divided into one way communication technology and 2 way communication technologies. One way video technology was reported in two studies whereas two way video technologies were reported in 16 studies.

Telephone

The findings from the study reported that the use of telephone was 14.58% of all the technologies. This was also further divided into one way communication and two way communications. There was only one study with a one way communication, whereas the studies with two way communication were 6.

Table 2. Technologies used

Technology Used	Type of Technology		Number of Papers
Video technology (18)	2 way communication		16
	1 way communication		2
Telephone (7)	2 way communication		6
	1 way communication		1
Mobile technology (9)	2 way communication	Calls	1
		SMS	3
		Apps	4
	1 way communication	Calls	0
		GPS	1
Internet (14)	2 way communication	Patient web portals	5
		Networked communication systems	7(emails, chats)
	1 way communication	Web portals	2

Mobile Technology

The use of mobile technology in the studies was 18.75%. Mobile technology was also further divided into one way communication and two way communications. One way communication included calls and GPS technology, whereas two way communications included calls, SMS and apps. Eight studies made use of two way communication. On the other hand, only one study made use of one way technology. Of the two way communication technology, 4 studies were reported on apps, with 3 and 1 studies on SMS and calls respectively.

Internet

The use of Internet as tool of choice was made in 29.16%of all the technologies used. These were again divided into one way communication and two way communication technologies. One way technology consisted of web portals and had 2 studies making use of it. Two way technologies, on the other hand, had patient web portals, interactive games, chat rooms and emails. Five studies made use of patient web portals, 3 of them made use of interactive games or video games while emails and chats were used in two studies each.

From the above findings, it can be deduced that Video technology and Internet are the two broad areas of technology that are used in mental health. Overall, the use of two way technologies was significantly more compared to that of one way technology. In terms of video technology and telephones, there was no further classification. In the use of mobile phone technology, the use of apps predominated as compared to phone calls and SMS technology whereas in the case of internet, patient web portals occupied the majority as compared to emails, chats and interactive games.

Figure 2 shows a pictorial presentation of the facts and figures of the technologies used in mental health representing the more employed two way communication technology as compared to one way technology.

Figure 2. Technologies used

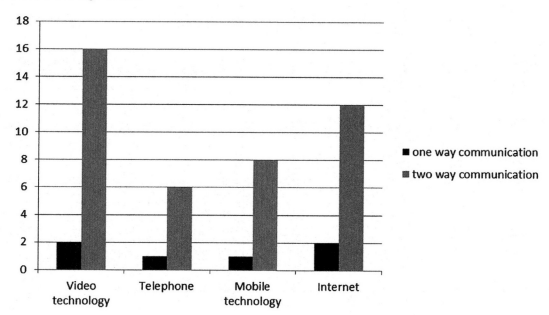

Mental Disorders Targeted

Various mental health disorders in which technology has been employed are reported here. The mental health disorders identified were divided into two groups:

1. A case mix group consisted of a mixture of the different types of mental health cases. This group covered 22.64% of the total number of mental health disorders found in the studies.
2. Individual cases.

This group case group consisted of cases with a single diagnosis of any disorder. This group accounted for 77.35% of all the papers studied. Studies on Schizophrenia were 14.63% with 6 studies. Depression accounted for 21.95% of all the individual cases with 9 cases. Substance use disorders were reported to be 9.75% of the individual cases. Obsessive compulsive disorders and anxiety disorders, both accounted for 12.19% of the cases with 5 cases of each. Post-traumatic stress disorders were studied in 3 cases where 2 cases of eating disorders were studied representing 7.31% and 4.87% respectively. Other disorders like mania, panic disorders, sleep disorders, dementia, attention deficit hyperkinetic disorder, mood disorders and disruptive disorders were clustered up together as each disorder had one study undertaken. These together resulted in 7 studies which occupied 17.07% of all the cases. See Table 3 and Figure 3 for details.

It is apparent from the above findings that technology related studies in mental health have been conducted in almost all types of mental health disorders. The findings show that the amount of studies conducted on depression, are greater as compared to the other types of mental health disorders. The number of studies on depression is followed by Schizophrenia studies. Overall, the studies reported on substance use disorders, anxiety, Obsessive compulsive disorders, eating disorders, post-traumatic stress disorders reported to be more or less the same in number. The disorders listed in 'others' were reported to have less number of studies on them.

Purpose of Study

The findings from this group suggest the use of technology in mental health has been done for a variety of purposes. This study reports the use of ICT for assessments of various symptoms or diseases, treat-

Table 3. Mental disorders targeted

Mental Problems Targeted	Number of Papers
Schizophrenia	6
Depression	9
Substance use disorders	4
Obsessive compulsive disorders	5
Anxiety disorders	5
Post-traumatic stress disorders	3
Eating disorders	2
Others (Mania, Panic, sleep disorders, Dementia, Attention hyperkinetic disorder, other disruptive disorders, mood disorders)	7
Case mix	12

Figure 3. Mental health disorders targeted

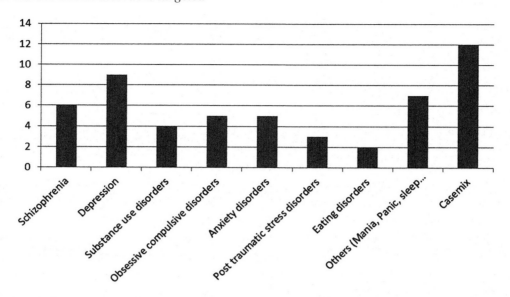

ments in its various forms, preventive activities, educational programs, communicating data and reports, monitoring of symptoms and prognosis of diseases and improving functional independence. Table 4 and Figure 4 indicate detail information on various purposes.

The findings show that a total of 55 different purposes were reported in the 44 papers for the use of ICT in mental health disorders. The "assessments" consisted of 12.72% of all the purposes. "Treatment" consisted of almost half the studies i.e. 47.27%. "Educational activities" were reported in 10.9% of the studies. "Monitoring of disease prognosis and severity" constituted of 7.27% of cases whereas "treatment adherence" constituted 9.09% of all the studies. The use of ICT in data collection and preventive activities has been expressed in 3.63% each. Communication, functional independence assessment and prescription contributed to 1.81% each with reporting only one case for each.

Table 4. Purpose of the study

Purpose of the Study	Number of Papers
Assessment	7
Treatment	26
Education	6
Functional independence	1
Communication	1
Monitoring	4
Data Collection	2
Prescription	1
Prevention	2
Treatment adherence	5

Figure 4. Purpose of the study

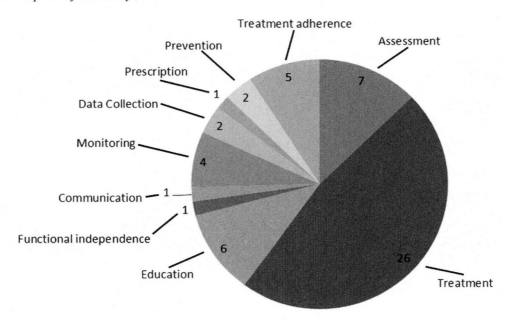

CONCLUSION

Information systems and technologies have been used in several various contexts up to now (Ghapanchi & Amrollahi, 2014; Amir Hossein Ghapanchi & Aybüke Aurum, 2011; Ghapanchi & Aurum, 2012a, 2012b; Ghapanchi et al., 2008; Najaftorkaman et al., 2014; Vichitvanichphong et al., 2013; Zarei et al., 2010). The aim of the study was to investigate the various information and communication technologies associated with mental health. It also aimed to determine the various purposes for which ICT has been used and the disorders which have been targeted.

According to the findings, ICT has been adopted in mental health on a large scale. This fact is evident from the different types of mental health conditions, it caters. A lot of studies have been done on depression, being one of the mood disorders. The technologies used are mostly networked connections and stand-alone computers were rarely used in the studies. This indicates to the replacement of standalone computers by the more advanced networked computers. Mental health researchers have made attempts to explore the recent technologies like smart phones and tablets.

The use of ICT promises to resolve a portion of the workforce issues in the underserved population where accessibility is jeopardized. The cost-effectiveness of ICT is a concern, though, that still needs attention. There have not been enough studies reporting on the cost- benefit analysis of the ICT use

The study has paved way for some further studies in different aspects of mental health. This includes studies to investigate the effect of ICT use in individual mental health disorders. Also studies investigating the utility of specific recent technologies like smart phones and tablets in mental health could be conducted. The effect of ICT on the cost-effectiveness of the system is another area that needs attention. An in depth study of the barriers associated with ICT use will help reduce them and eventually result in better outcomes.

A great amount of heterogeneity was demonstrated in the papers studied with respect to the technology used and mental health population targeted. This deemed as a limitation to the analysis of the data. Some of the papers did not comment about the effectiveness and the acceptability of ICT whereas there were only a few papers commenting on the cost, time and labor effectiveness of ICT.

REFERENCES

ABS. (2008). *National Survey of Mental Health and Well-being.* Canberra: Australian Bureau of statistics.

AIHW. (2010). Canberra: Australia's Health.

AIHW. (2013). *Mental health services in Brief 2013.* Canberra: Australian Institute of Health and Welfare.

Amrollahi, A., Ghapanchi, A. H., & Najaftorkaman, M. (2014). *A Generic Framework for Developing Strategic Information System Plans: Insights From Past Three Decades.* Paper presented at the 18th Pacific Asia Conference on Information Systems, Chengdu, China.

Amrollahi, A., Ghapanchi, A. H., & Talaei-Khoei, A. (2013). A Systematic Literature Review on Strategic Information Systems Planning: Insights from the Past Decade. *Pacific Asia Journal of the Association for Information Systems, 5*(2), 39–66.

Amrollahi, A., Ghapanchi, A. H., & Talaei-Khoei, A. (2014). Three Decades of Research on Strategic Information System Plan Development. *Communications of the Association for Information Systems, 34*(1), 84.

Australia's Health 2012. (2012). *Australia's health series no. 13 Cat. no. AUS 156.* Canberra: Australian Institute of Health and Welfare.

Benavides-Vaello, S., Strode, A., & Sheeran, B. (2013). Using Technology in the Delivery of Mental Health and Substance Abuse Treatment in Rural Communities: A Review. *The Journal of Behavioral Health Services & Research, 40*(1), 111–120. doi:10.1007/s11414-012-9299-6 PMID:23093443

Cleary, M. R. N. B. M., Walter, G. M. B. B. S. B. P. F., & Matheson, S. B. (2008). What Is the Role of e-Technology in Mental Health Services and Psychiatric Research? *Journal of Psychosocial Nursing and Mental Health Services, 46*(4), 42–48. PMID:18478808

Farhadi, M., Ismail, R., & Fooladi, M. (2012). Information and communication technology use and economic growth. *PLoS ONE, 7*(11), 12. doi:10.1371/journal.pone.0048903 PMID:23152817

Garcia-Lizana, F., & Munoz-Mayorga, I. (2010). What about telepsychiatry? A systematic review. *Primary Care Companion to the Journal of Clinical Psychiatry, 12*(2). PMID:20694116

García-Lizana, F., & Muñoz-Mayorga, I. (2010). Telemedicine for Depression: A Systematic Review. *Perspectives in Psychiatric Care, 46*(2), 119–126. doi:10.1111/j.1744-6163.2010.00247.x PMID:20377799

GBD. (2010). Global Burden of Disease: Country profiles. Institute of Health Metrics and Evaluation (IHME).

Ghanbarzadeh, R., Ghapanchi, A. H., Blumenstein, M., & Talaei-Khoei, A. (2014). A Decade of Research on the Use of Three-Dimensional Virtual Worlds in Health Care: A Systematic Literature Review. *Journal of Medical Internet Research, 16*(2), e47. doi:10.2196/jmir.3097 PMID:24550130

Ghapanchi, A. H., & Amrollahi, A. (2014). Serious Games in an Information Technology Course: Opportunities, Challenges, and Outcomes. *The International Technology Management Review*, 4(2), 78–86. doi:10.2991/itmr.2014.4.2.2

Ghapanchi, A. H., & Aurum, A. (2011). Antecedents to IT personnel's intentions to leave: A systematic literature review. *Journal of Systems and Software*, 84(2), 238–249. doi:10.1016/j.jss.2010.09.022

Ghapanchi, A. H., & Aurum, A. (2011). *Measuring the effectiveness of the defect-fixing process in open source software projects.* Paper presented at the System Sciences (HICSS), 2011 44th Hawaii International Conference on. doi:10.1109/HICSS.2011.305

Ghapanchi, A. H., & Aurum, A. (2012a). Competency rallying in electronic markets: Implications for open source project success. *Electronic Markets*, 22(2), 117–127. doi:10.1007/s12525-012-0088-0

Ghapanchi, A. H., & Aurum, A. (2012b). The impact of project capabilities on project performance: Case of open source software projects. *International Journal of Project Management*, 30(4), 407–417. doi:10.1016/j.ijproman.2011.10.002

Ghapanchi, A. H., Ghapanchi, A. R., Talaei-Khoei, A., & Abedin, B. (2013). A Systematic Review on Information Technology Personnel's Turnover. *Lecture Notes on Software Engineering*, 1(1), 98–101. doi:10.7763/LNSE.2013.V1.22

Ghapanchi, A. H., Jafarzadeh, M. H., & Khakbaz, M. H. (2008). An Application of Data Envelopment Analysis (DEA) for ERP system selection: Case of a petrochemical company. *ICIS 2008 Proceedings*, 77.

Griffiths, K. M., & Christensen, H. (2007). Internet-based mental health programs: A powerful tool in the rural medical kit. *The Australian Journal of Rural Health*, 15(2), 81–87. doi:10.1111/j.1440-1584.2007.00859.x PMID:17441815

Hoyt, & Bailey. (2012). *Health Informatics: Practical guide for healthcare and information technology professionals.* Academic Press.

Medibank. (2013). *The case for mental health reform in Australia: A review of expenditure and system design.* Medibank Private Limited.

Meglic, M., Furlan, M., Kuzmanic, M., Kozel, D., Baraga, D., Kuhar, I.,... Brodnik, A. (2010). *Feasibility of an eHealth service to support collaborative depression care: results of a pilot study.* Academic Press.

Mills, V., Van Hooff, M., Baur, J., & McFarlane, A. C. (2012). Predictors of Mental Health Service Utilisation in a Non-Treatment Seeking Epidemiological Sample of Australian Adults. *Community Mental Health Journal*, 48(4), 511–521. doi:10.1007/s10597-011-9439-0 PMID:21994023

Najaftorkaman, M., Ghapanchi, A. H., Talaei-Khoei, A., & Ray, P. (2013). Recent Research Areas and Grand Challenges in Electronic Medical Record: A Literature Survey Approach. *The International Technology Management Review*, 3(1), 12–21. doi:10.2991/itmr.2013.3.1.2

Najaftorkaman, M., Ghapanchi, A. H., Talaei-Khoei, A., & Ray, P. (2014). A taxonomy of antecedents to user adoption of health information systems: A synthesis of thirty years of research. *Journal of the Association for Information Science and Technology*.

Reger, M. A., & Gahm, G. A. (2009). A meta-analysis of the effects of internet- and computer-based cognitive-behavioral treatments for anxiety. *Journal of Clinical Psychology, 65*(1), 53–75. doi:10.1002/jclp.20536 PMID:19051274

Toperczer, T. (2011). Telepsychiatry in the cloud. *Health Management Technology, 32*(8), 28–29. PMID:21905491

Vichitvanichphong, S., Kerr, D., Talaei-Khoei, A., & Ghapanchi, A. H. (2013). *Analysis of Research in Adoption of Assistive Technologies for Aged Care.* Paper presented at the 24th Australasian Conference on Information Systems 2013.

Wendel, M. L., Brossart, D. F., Elliott, T. R., McCord, C., & Diaz, M. A. (2011). Use of technology to increase access to mental health services in a rural Texas community. *Family & Community Health, 34*(2), 134–140. doi:10.1097/FCH.0b013e31820e0d99 PMID:21378510

Whetton, S. (2005). Health Informatics: A socio - technical perspective. Academic Press.

Whitten, P. S., Mair, F. S., Haycox, A., May, C. R., Williams, T. L., & Hellmich, S. (2002). Systematic review of cost effectiveness studies of telemedicine interventions. *BMJ (Clinical Research Ed.), 324*(7351), 1434–1437. doi:10.1136/bmj.324.7351.1434 PMID:12065269

Wilks, C. M., Oakley Browne, M., & Jenner, B. L. (2008). Attracting psychiatrists to a rural area - 10 years on. *Rural and Remote Health, 8*(1), 14. PMID:18284309

Zarei, B., Merati, E., & Ghapanchi, A. (2010). Project process reengineering (PPR): A BPR method for projects. *International Journal of Information Systems and Change Management, 4*(4), 299–313. doi:10.1504/IJISCM.2010.036914

Integrated Care in Europe:
New Models of Management of Chronic Patients

Francisco Ródenas
Polibienestar Research Institute – University of Valencia, Spain

Jorge Garcés
Polibienestar Research Institute – University of Valencia, Spain

Elisa Valía
Polibienestar Research Institute – University of Valencia, Spain

Ascensión Doñate
Polibienestar Research Institute – University of Valencia, Spain

INTRODUCTION

The demographic change entails an increase in the number of people with chronic conditions who have higher requirements on health and social services (Garcés et al., 2005). In this context, and to promote stratification, integrated care services and active and healthy ageing programmes have become a priority for the European Commission, who has launched strategies as EIP-AHA (European Innovation Partnership on Active and Healthy Ageing). In this process, the information and communications technologies (ICTs) and e-Health approaches can improve organizational and management aspects in the healthcare system on chronic patients that require long-term care (LTC). In this regard the European Innovation Partnership on Healthy and Active Ageing (EIP-AHA) through the Digital Agenda for Europe highlights the need to empower and socially include informal and formal caregivers through ICTs.

The objective of the current chapter is to present an approach to a transferable and easily implementable model for the future primary health care centres in urban contexts, which should move towards proactive, anticipatory and integrated care services. The chapter will focus on the proposal of integrative health and social services for elderly people in order to promote active and healthy ageing in the framework of the European project UHCE. Important benefits for end-users, service providers and other stakeholders can be achieved by implementing these innovative solutions, mainly consisting of early detection of frailty, management of polypharmacy, prevention of falls using ICT and integrated health and social care pathways. The target group for this model is independent elderly people living at home in urban environments. The expected benefits of the implementation of this model are the improvement of quality of life, the reduction in the use of health services and the decrease in costs.

BACKGROUND

Europe is currently facing a scene characterized by the necessity to cope several kinds of social challenges (Garcés & Monsonis-Payá, 2013); firstly, the well-known socio-demographic change, which prognosticates a notable increase of elders as a share of the global population. Thus, according to *The*

DOI: 10.4018/978-1-4666-9978-6.ch048

2012 Ageing Report (European Commission, 2012) the population aged 65 and above from the European Union will almost double, rising from 87.5 million in 2010 to around 160 million in 2060. Also, the number of older people aged 80 years and above is projected to increase by even more, almost tripling from 23.7 million in 2010 to over 65 million in 2060.

Elderly people often suffer chronic diseases or comorbidity – as diabetes, cardiovascular diseases, chronic respiratory diseases or stroke –, which entail the need of provision of LTC, with high health needs and costs (Geneau et al., 2010). According to the World Health Organization chronic conditions are by far the main cause of mortality in the world, representing 60% of all deaths (WHO, 2005); and, for example in Spain their care accounts for 70% of the healthcare expenditure (García-Goñi et al., 2012). This complex situation is worsening – in some countries more notably than in others around Europe – by the current context of austerity and fiscal policies triggered by the economic crisis (Ifanti et al., 2013). Governments and entities are searching measures aimed to assure the efficiency and sustainability of public systems, without having a negative impact on the quality of the care provision to patients.

In this sense, nowadays the care of elderly people is a major challenge for public administrations in almost all countries around Europe. The management of patients, especially of those with chronic diseases and morbidity, is usually carried out from primary settings for treatment, monitoring and prevention (Smith et al., 2012). So, the coordination of both health and social community-based services within primary care settings represents a good opportunity to explore the threefold benefits of integrated care in the quality of life of patients, in the quality of care provided by multidisciplinary professionals and, at the end, in the cost-benefit impact to the sustainability of the system (Garcés et al., 2013). The authors have already worked in this research line in the framework of European networks as CORAL – Community of Regions for Assisted Living (over 20 regions working together to promote independent living along Europe), ENSA – European Network of Social Authorities (network of cities and European regions that has the aim of promoting international cooperation in social welfare), ISCH COST Action IS1102 Social Services, Welfare State and Places (the restructuring of social services in Europe and its impacts on social and territorial cohesion and governance) and the European Innovation Partnership on Active and Healthy Ageing promoted by the European Commission. Furthermore, the authors were actively involved in European projects regarding this topic as INTERLINKS or HOST. The aim of INTERLINKS project, funded by 7th Framework Programme, was to help people in Europe who work with elderly in need of LTC by means of a framework for Long Term Care containing a set of tools and practice examples to guide the future development of long-term care systems in Europe. The approach of INTERLINKS is very interesting since it places users needing integrated long-term care at the interfaces between social and health care, and formal and informal care (Liechsenring et al., 2013). The project HOST 'Smart technologies for self-service to seniors in social housing' (http://www.host-aal.eu/) was funded by the Ambient Assisted Living (AAL) Joint Programme. This project aims to develop a digital infrastructure of the social housing with access to a package of services to improve the elders' quality of life and in-dependence. Social housing has been trying to provide a comfortable and friendly context to enable the integration of elders - especially for frail people- into the self-serve society, founded on the awareness of ICT (easy-to-use technologies). The HOST project highlights the need to integrate care and services with the support of ICT by experimenting a European model of "flats connected" for older people.

The integration of new technologies in the provision of LTC is an urgent challenge and necessity to support the care of older people and/or people with disabilities since sustainable and cost-effective approach. In this field we find the CARICT project – co-financed by DG CNECT and JRC-IPTS of the European Commission – which is aimed to study the impact of ICTs on LTC provided by informal and formal caregivers to older people living in the community. Its results suggest (Carretero et al., 2012) that ICT-based services make existing services more effective, varied, accessible and with more quality being part of an integrated group of services from different agencies. Many of these ICTs do not require high investments, so they are financially viable, accessible and sustainable; especially as they facilitate the reduction of the need for formal home care. Another example of the benefits of the introduction of ICTs on LTC is they support for informal caregivers remain active in the labor market.

Research groups as Polibienestar Research Institute from the University of Valencia - which has developed the Social Sustainability Theory (Garcés et al., 2003; 2006; 2011) - are currently working on integrated care programmes (Ródenas et al., 2008), simulation tools for LTC (Grimaldo et al., 2014; Grimaldo et al., 2013) and strategies pursuing improvements in efficiency of the management of chronic patients (Ródenas et al., 2014; Doñate-Martínez et al., 2014). The interest of these topics for funding entities both at national and international level is manifest by projects and initiatives as *Valcronic* (improvement on care of chronic patients in the Valencian Region using ICTs in 2012) or *Continuity-Care* (improvement on continuity of care between different health and social resources addressed to patients with LTC needs and their management) in Spain. At European level it is worth to highlight projects as *UHCE (Urban Health Centres Europe)* aimed to contributing to innovative urban health centres integrating health and social care pathways or *ASSEHS (Activation of Stratification Strategies and Results of the interventions on frail patients of Healthcare Services)* aimed to improve the management of chronic patients and interventions for frail patients (both funded by the II Health Programme of the European Commission during 2014-2016).

THE LACK OF INTEGRATION BETWEEN HEALTH AND SOCIAL CARE

Integrated care can be defined as <<*a coherent and coordinated services delivery to individual service users across a board range of health and social care organizations, different professionals and informal caregivers*>> (Leichsenring, 2004; Mur-Veeman et al., 2008). In many European countries there is a lack of integration of LTC systems; with health resources on one hand, and social services on the other without any link between them. According to the review of Mur-Veeman et al. (2008), in the opposite side there are the experiences from Finland, Sweden, The Netherlands and England, where legislation, financial incentives and other measures have encouraged providers to establish integrated care methods and adjustments and supported their efforts.

In Spain, the situation regarding the current regulatory framework is a fragmentation between health and social services. There is not a law that regulates joint benefits for people who require LTC. Laws do not define joint mechanisms or tools for the assessment of the health and social needs, and they do not consider a unique portfolio of resources. As a consequence the coordination between different social and health care resources is not as effective as expected in covering the wide variety of needs of dependent older adults, and this has evidenced the lack of adaptation of supply and of service planning to meet these needs (Garcés et al. 2003). The adjustments proposed to reduce or control public spending have led to an absence of growth in the supply of public resources and to a shift to private supply and/ or family or informal care. This lack of integrated care policies and practices has as a consequence the inefficiency in the provision of different kinds of care and interventions, higher costs for the administrations, lower users' satisfaction rate and poor quality of the different services and resources involved within the health and social systems (Gröne & García-Barbero, 2004; Lloyd & Wait, 2006). The gaps can be specified as follows:

1. Deficiencies in the traditional organizational model of care to address chronic diseases. The traditional model is focused mainly on acute care; a chronic patient is only treated when his health worsens. The traditional approach is face to face, reactive, focused on healing, in which the patient is passive, and is not suitable for treating chronic patients. It is required a proactive model of medicine, more focused on prevention and care (including long term care). This new approach is based on the segmentation of patients, necessary to determine the risk of disease and identification of care needs, by assigning individualized care plans (Garcés et al., 2013).

2. Increased health care costs associated with the care of chronic patients. The costs of care for patients with more than one chronic disease, is up to 6 times higher than for those who have no chronic disease or have only one. In this line, in Spain two thirds of health expenditure of some organizations are due to treatments of patients with five or more chronic conditions, multiplying by twenty-five hospital expenditure (Regional Ministry of Health from Valencia, 2012). If this problem is not suitably dealt with, it can lead to the consumption of the majority of health system resources and contribute to bankruptcy of its sustainability.

3. The lack of information in real time and of the possibility to share this information among professionals of different levels of care (hospitals and primary). For professionals, the introduction of eHealth in the field of chronic care is associated with an improvement in the access to relevant information, electronic prescribing or bio-measurements control, all through the electronic health record. For healthcare managers eHealth can help to control the efficiency and sustainability of the system, redirecting it towards preventive models (Grimaldo et al, 2014). And for citizens eHealth provides information that helps them promote their health and self-care and even getting alternative diagnoses.

The answer to this problem is the restructuring of both health and social care systems with the aim of making them more efficient and effective. A theoretical solution for this gap is the *Sustainable Social and Healthcare Model (SSHM)* that consists of a joint reorganization of both protection systems providing an answer to the needs of people requiring LTC; increasing, so, their welfare and quality of life (Garcés, 2000). This model was developed and validated using case management methodology to link the network of health and social resources with the support of multidisciplinary teams (Ródenas et al., 2008; Garcés et al., 2011). The application of SSHM implemented new care pathways in primary care systems contributed to decrease the use and cost of health services and to improve the integration and efficiency of social and health care for elderly people with LTC needs in a Mediterranean Welfare State scenario.

In the Spanish context – among other European systems – general practitioners (GPs) are the first and most frequent contact with patients with chronic conditions, so their role in screening specific needs and problems associated with these diseases is very relevant. In this way, according to the SSHM, as well as to other approaches (e.g. Brand et al., 2004), one of the first strategies to improve the management of patients with comorbidity is the segmentation of the population in risk groups by means of standardized tools (Doñate-Martínez et al., 2014).

The Valencian Region has implemented a pilot initiative, called *Valcronic programme*, aimed to efficiently manage chronic patients from the primary care system. This programme offered different levels of telemonitoring and telecare according to the users' risk of a future hospital admission previously identified through a joint strategy based on clinical criteria and standardized screening tools (Ródenas et al., 2014; Doñate-Martínez et al., 2016). For patients at moderate and high risk of suffering hospitalizations the programme offered telemonitoring of biologic variables through biomedical devices according to their diseases (as blood pressure or heart and respiratory rates). These data were sent to the health centres through different ICT devices (Tablet, computer or smartphone).

Going one step beyond in this field, it is very important to promote primary care centres able to provide comprehensive answers to general needs of citizens, as:

1. Encouragement of autonomy and capacity to decide on their own health;
2. Development of initiatives to promote patients' empowerment and self-care; or
3. Promotion of health and prevention.

A Solution Based on Integration of Services within Primary Care Centres: The UHCE Project

Polibienestar Research Institute develops research aimed at enhancing primary health care by the integration of health and social care services by means of different projects at European level as the UHCE (*Urban Health Centres Europe*), which will contribute to the redefinition of the current role and services offered by primary health centers. The project UHCE promotes innovative integrated health and social care pathways, early detection of frailty, management of polypharmacy and prevention of falls for active and healthy ageing in European cities. It is focused on innovations with regard to the primary care setting at the local level.

The aspects on which the project is focused represent a concern affecting all countries across Europe. Table 1 presents some data that outlines the significance of these factors in the participating countries. Pharmaceutical expenditure accounted for almost a fifth (19%) of all health expenditure on average in Europe in 2010; meaning the third biggest spending component after inpatient and outpatient care (OECD, 2012). Likewise, according to data from the European project ADHOC, 22% of people aged 65 years and over reported polypharmacy in Europe – defined as nine and more medications (Fialová & Onder, 2009). Other data suggests that prevention of hip fracture through programmes based on physical activity is very relevant as patients aged between 55 and 64 and sustaining a primary fracture of the hip have a much greater risk of further fracture than the rest of the population (Lawrence et al., 2010).

The project is funded by the European Commission, within the II Health Programme. It is currently running and it is expected to end in December 2016. The UHCE consortium is made up of universities, municipalities, small and medium-sized enterprises (SMEs) and networks of professionals from 5 different European countries:

Table 1. Relevant factors

	Spain	Netherlands	United Kingdom	Italy	Croatia	Greece
Expenditure on pharmaceuticals per capita and as a share of GDP [1]	1.8%	1.1%	1%	1.6%	n.a	n.a
Prevalence of polypharmacy in older adults (65+) [2]	n.a	13.1%	20.1%	7%	n.a	n.a
Feelings of loneliness in people aged 65 and over [3]	14%	9%	n.a	18%	n.a	21%

Source: Own elaboration.

[1]Data retrieved fromOECD (2012). The expenditure on pharmaceuticals is expressed as expenditure per capita and as a share of GDP in 2010 (or nearest year).

[2]Data retrieved fromFialová et al. (2005). Polypharmacy is defined as nine and more medications.

[3]Data retrieved fromSundström et al. (2009). Percentage of people aged 65 and over reporting substantial loneliness (feelings of loneliness almost all of the time or most of the time over the last week) from SHARE project (Survey of Health, Ageing and Retirement in Europe)

n.a. Data not available.

- Erasmus MC (Netherlands).
- City of Rotterdam (Netherlands).
- University of Applied Science Rotterdam (Netherlands).
- Polibienestar Research Institute – Universitat de València (Spain).
- AGE Platform Europe.
- European Local Inclusion and Social Action Network – ELISAN.
- VIDAVO A.E. (Greece).
- Municipality of Pallini (Greece).
- University of Manchester (The United Kingdom).
- Croatian Society for Pharmacoeconomics and Health Economics (Croatia).
- Zorg Op Noord (Netherlads).
- University of Rijeka, Faculty of Medicine (Croatia).

Main Goals

UHCE is conceived to produce and disseminate a transferable and easily implementable model for innovative community integrated care in European cities, which contributes to the pillar on prevention, screening and early diagnosis of the Strategic Implementation Plan adopted by the Steering Group of the EIP-AHA. Thus, UHCE contributes to the following actions: 'Prescription and adherence action at regional level', 'Personal health management, starting with a falls prevention initiative', and 'Action for prevention of functional decline and frailty'.

The project aims to develop, implement and evaluate the UHCE in 5 varied cities from Europe (Rotterdam, Netherlands; Rijeka, Croatia; Pallini, Greece; Valencia, Spain; and Manchester, The United Kingdom) that will act as pilot sites.

The specific objectives to be achieved are:

1. To develop a platform characterized by:
    a. Integrated health and social care in the community.
    b. Population oriented approach focused on anticipatory care.
    c. Deployment of nurse practitioners/physician assistants to provide standardized care.
2. To implement existing evidence-based protocols supported by ICTs aimed to promote active and healthy ageing and based on empowerment as the following:
    a. Early detection of frailty.
    b. Patient-carer-shared decisions on and execution of integrated care pathways.
    c. Management of polypharmacy.
    d. Prevention of falls.
3. To integrate general interventions to be adapted to the local context and preferences from the different European sites involved.
4. To evaluate the implementation of the UHCE with regard to process and effects from different perspectives: older citizens/patients; relatives or carers; neighborhood or organizations; health and social sector; professionals and volunteers; and financing and policy. The specific issues to be taken into consideration are reach, implementation integrity, independence, empowerment and health-related quality of life, use-of-care, costs and appreciation by patients, professionals and stakeholders involved.

E

5.   To produce a transferable and easily implementable model for UHCE in Europe through a tool box with instruments and protocols and concise policy documents.

Target Group

The primary end-users of the project are citizens of 65 years and older living independently (non-institutionalized) at risk of multimorbidity and/or frailty. Moreover, other relevant secondary end-users who will benefit from the outcomes are informal caregivers and care providers.

For the development of UHCE demands and preferences of the different stakeholders have been assessed through focus group interviews from June to July of 2014. Each pilot city has carried out 2 focus groups with older citizens/patients; 2 groups with health care professionals; and 2 groups with informal caregivers (as relatives or volunteers).

By way of illustration, the intervention programmed for the pilot in Valencia (Spain) will be carried out in around 600 elderly people from two primary health care centres (see Figure 1).

Methods

In an early stage of the project, in order to gather existing knowledge on the universal context and specific characteristics of UHCE the researchers of the project have carried out systematic reviews of the literature, with special emphasis in integrated health/social care, population-oriented approach and deployment of nurses/assistants. Different focus groups have been set up to know which are the demands and preferences of older people and other stakeholders. All this information will lead to the development of a generic UHCE template.

Taking into consideration the results of the systematic reviews, focus groups and additional desk research/interviews, existing evidence-based protocols supported by ICT tools on detection of frailty, integrated care pathways, management of polypharmacy and prevention of falls have been identified and optimised.

The generic template of UHCE will be adapted in a later stage by each pilot site to enable the implementation of the programme according to the local preferences that might have emerged during the previous stages.

Before starting the implementation of the UHCE, each pilot site - Rijeka, Pallini, Valencia, Manchester and Rotterdam - will invite 417 75+ citizens in the community to provide informed consent. Assuming a participation rate of 60%, 250 per site will be involved in the deployment of the programme in each

Figure 1. Intervention in Valencia

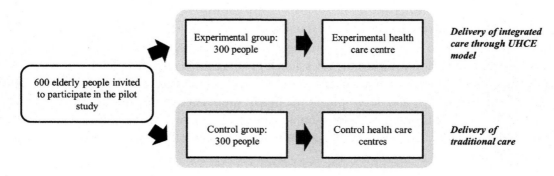

pilot site, so a total of 1250 citizens. Nurses or assistants will be asked to do screening according to the protocols established in earlier stages. Nurses, assistants and physicians will make a shared decision with the patient regarding the most appropriated integrated care pathways he/she should follow. These integrated care pathways which include management of polypharmacy, fall prevention and management of frailty will be monitored and will end after a 12 months follow-up.

The CDC-Framework for Programme Evaluation (MMWR, 1999) will be used, applying 2 perspectives: end-users (older citizens); and care providers/services/volunteers. The design: a specific pre-post controlled design (Miller et al, 1989). A control group, i.e. 75+ citizens from a comparable neighbourhood (without specific innovations) will be established at each pilot. Measurements will be collected at baseline, and during/after 12 months follow-up.

The Programme

The programme is composed by four main phases:

1. Assessment;
2. Shared decision making process;
3. Referral to specific pathways; and
4. Intervention with follow-up.

First of all trained research assistants or nurses will carry out a screening assessment of patients (individually or in groups depending on the decision of each pilot site). Besides an evaluation of clinical and social needs a home safety assessment will be done in order to provide advice for improving the accessibility at home and thus reducing the risk of falls. With the subsequent results, a nurse and/or physician, the elderly patient and a family member (if necessary) will jointly make a shared decision to decide the most appropriate health and social pathways the patient should be involved in. The available pathways are focused in the following aspects:

1. Clinical, to adapt the usual care according to patient's needs (frequency of visits, schedule blood tests, etc.);
2. Falls, based on a multifactorial intervention, including exercise programme, home safety adjustments and aids;
3. Polypharmacy, a self-management programme including devices, like simplified dosing regimens and the application of a protocol by the health professionals to review the drugs prescribed to the patients in order to evaluate if these could be reduced;
4. Loneliness, through the establishment of social activities within a group and social support advice.

The duration of the intervention will be 12 months. At the end of this period a comprehensive assessment will be carried out to assess the impact of the different pathways in the health, physical and social status of the participants. Moreover, health professionals involved in the implementation of this programme will do frequent monitoring, especially of those patients with a high risk of falls in the basal analysis.

In the programme design and development the needs, preferences and requirements of every local setting where the project is going to be pilot-implemented have been taken into consideration. So, the instruments and pathways have been adapted to the different cultural contexts and translated into the different languages.

Expected Impact

UHC2.0 will contribute to the innovation in primary care systems specifically addressed to elderly patients as this share of the population is the one requiring most health and social services. UHC2.0 will generate a population oriented approach with a special focus on proactive, anticipatory and preventive care pursuing the ultimate objective of contributing to the sustainability of Health Systems.

In this sense, it is planned to deploy home visits by nurses or assistants to provide standardized preventive integrated care; especially for older people with multimorbidity. Nurses or assistants will apply protocols for early detection of frailty. UHCE model aims at empowering patients and their relatives to be able to make shared decisions with the healthcare professionals regarding which integrated care pathways are needed, and so assuming an active role in their own care pathway. Moreover the healthcare professionals will support and monitor these pathways, including management of polypharmacy, management of frailty and prevention of falls.

The project will generate a transferable and easily implementable model for UHCE for integrated health and social care pathways in European cities. The model will be incorporated into a practically useful tool box with instruments and protocols and a concise policy document, which will help policymakers and stakeholders to plan interventions and introduce structural changes in Health Care Systems regarding frail older citizens. At the same time, this toolbox will contribute to the priorities of the EIP-Active and Healthy Ageing.

UHCE is aligned with Action Plans A2, A3 and B3 from the European Innovation Partnership on Active and Healthy Ageing. Action Plan A2 works on "Personalized health management and prevention of falls", and this project aims to prevent falls of elderly people at their own homes through the provision of health and social support, as well as recommendations to be introduced at their houses as architectural improvements. UHCE contributes to the Action Plan A3 "Prevention of functional decline and frailty" as frail patients or those at risk of frailty will be early detected to be included in intervention or monitoring to improve their wellbeing (e.g. through physical exercise programs, diets, information and awareness activities). Action Plan B3 focuses on "Integrated Care for chronic diseases" and UHCE will take into consideration the complexity and heterogeneity of situations of these patients with multimorbidity face in their daily life by integrating both health and social resources.

The outcomes of UHCE by achieving the pursued objectives will have a great impact on the Health Care Systems by offering better care to European citizens at lower costs. By providing tailored care to groups of population or individual patients, UHCE will optimize the services provided and thus contribute to a better quality of life for patients and more efficient and sustainable Health care Systems. Both patients and Health Care Systems will benefit from the reduction of avoidable emergency admissions and relapses and the improvement of the health status of the population, and their associated costs, respectively.

Furthermore, the implementation of the UHCE model will also lead to raised awareness among health and social professionals and policy makers on the benefits of the integration of health and care services for managing polypharmacy, prevention of falls and frailty for elderly patients.

FUTURE RESEARCH DIRECTIONS

One of the key elements Europe and its health care systems should work on is developing new models based on prevention. Prevention entails a double benefit, increasing the quality of life of the population and reducing the needs for health care services and thus the costs of the services provided. In this sense, the authors´ next projects will try to develop preventive approaches at different levels.

Moreover, to promote even more a health care model centred in the patient it is necessary to develop and implement initiatives and strategies taking into consideration specific LTC needs of patients with chronic conditions. Thus, it is very relevant the establishment of models of prevention and early detection of patients at risk through stratification of the population (Doñate-Martínez, et al., 2014; Ródenas et al., 2014). In this line, Polibienestar Research Institute is currently developing algorithms to screen and detect elderly patients with chronic conditions at risk of suffering future hospital admissions combining different kinds of variables (socio-demographic, clinical and related to the use of health and social resources). These tools will support the clinical decision of health professionals as they will be able to identify which patients have high risk of suffering relapses or frailty; and they will be able to design and put into practice individualized care pathways including prevention, monitoring and management programmes (Nuño et al., 2012).

Another key point to take into consideration for future efforts is focused on the management and integration of services. For this purpose, building on the above stratification of the population into risk groups it will be possible to design care pathways according to the specific needs and requirements of patients in general. Moreover, it is also important to design individualized interventions for patients with specific diseases as respiratory or cardiovascular conditions (e.g. Shepherd & While, 2012), as they present a symptom picture, a progress and complications associated with the own nature of every disease.

Finally, through advances in R&D it is important to support the work of policy makers and public administrations as well providing numbers and predictions about the future LTC needs. In this sense, Polibienestar has developed the Simulator of Integrated Long-Term Care Systems for Elderly People (LTCMAS) aimed to simulate LTC systems for large populations using a single standard computer platform (Grimaldo et al., 2014; Orduña et al., 2013). This tool will increase the prediction capacity of decision-makers for the LTC policies, improving the decision making process in short, medium and large term in different European regions. Thus, the simulator will be able to provide results of the modelled health systems and the cost savings achieved with respect to the standard health system. At this stage, the simulator does not consider cost-benefit variables but along this project those variables will be analysed and included. The proposed simulator goes towards the personalisation of LTC for elderly people, in such a way that patients perceive a better quality of the health and social system, and at the same time the costs of public health and social systems are reduced by means of avoiding unnecessary tests and identifying inefficient services.

CONCLUSION

During the last decades, in many European countries, administrations and governments have done a great effort to improve the net of health services, especially those addressed to elderly and dependent people. However, the integration of health services jointly with social resources did not take the same relevance (Garcés & Ródenas, in press). In this sense, in the last years, the integration of both health and social services through programmes with multidisciplinary teams and interventions has become a priority for public administrations and other kind of care providers especially regarding the care of people with chronic conditions (EIP-AHA, 2012). So, having these two levels operating in parallel and following a coordinated procedure entails changes in professional activities, in care settings and in communication between the different stakeholders involved as well (for example, GPs, nurses, social workers and patients). So, this integration of services may lead to LTC systems characterized by effectiveness and efficiency, having a positive impact in the quality of life of their users and meaning an opportunity to reduce the burden of clinical professionals and expenditures on care.

Besides this integration of services from health and social welfare systems it is necessary to implement strategies that take into consideration the long-term and progressive nature of chronic conditions. In this regard, preventive and proactive approaches are key factors to guarantee an efficient and sustainable care model of quality. Thus, the work of GPs would benefit from the introduction of tools that help them to identify patients at risk of frailty, which would entail a support in their clinical decision.

The restructuring health care model should begin in the primary care level, where users find a more closed relationship and interaction with health professionals. In this regard, within the aforementioned UHC2.0 project, from the groups interviewed in Spain it is possible to draw some preliminary results about the preferences of different stakeholders to improve the services within primary care centres.

Older citizens and patients indicate a need of a closed management and monitoring of their diseases (e.g. control blood sugar level for diabetics), as for example through an established schedule of visits at home for those patients with reduced mobility. In this sense, one of their main requirements is the necessity of specific care pathways for elder people, taking into consideration their needs and barriers. Moreover, although elder patients consider that the work of health care professionals is excellent, they also manifest complaints related to the consequences of the latest cutbacks, such as the retirement of some subsidies to buy medicaments or the lack of enough resources in some hospitals.

Relatives and informal caregivers express that within the current system there is a lack of a comprehensive answer to the social needs of families with elders with LTC needs and requiring home care, as well as a lack of adequate resources in primary health centres related to social assistance resources.

Health care professionals consider that their daily work is stressful as they do not have enough time to attend to patients. Moreover, they express the necessity of more initiatives related to the care of elderly and chronic patients (e.g. training on care or promotion of physical activity, etc.), as well as the necessity for relative and informal caregivers of patients to get training too in order to be able to adequately carry out the instructions provided by professionals. In this regard, they are interested in new technologies which facilitate the contact and monitoring of patients; for example the monitoring of clinical tests carried out by patients at home and whose results can be sent to the centre by means of a tablet or similar devices. They also express that the current care system has several gaps and consider the Nordic healthcare Model as a good reference point to improve our current Spanish system.

The authors of this article are very committed to propose innovative solutions that help to face the different challenges of the European population, in particular the great challenge of achieving more efficient and sustainable health and social care systems in order to reduce or even avoid the consequences of the cuts triggered by the economic crisis. The main pillar of the future research of the authors is to contribute to a mature relationship between citizens and health care providers conceived as a mutual commitment on prevention and integrated provision of services, taking into consideration preferences and demands of citizens, care services providers and policy makers. Likewise, policy makers will also need to promote citizens´ behavioural change by raising awareness on the importance of adopting healthier lifestyles and preventive attitudes.

REFERENCES

Brand, C. A., Jones, C. T., Lowe, A. J., Nielsen, D. A., Roberts, C. A., King, B. L., & Campbell, D. A. (2004). A transitional care service for elderly chronic disease patients at risk of readmission. *Australian Health Review*, 28(3), 275–284. doi:10.1071/AH040275 PMID:15595909

Carretero, S., Stewart, J., Centeno, C., Barbabella, F., Schmidt, A., Lamontagne-Godwin, F., & Lamura, G. (2012). *Can Technology-based Services support Long-term Care Challenges in Home Care? Analysis of Evidence from Social Innovation Good Practices across the EU: CARICT Project Summary Report.* European Commission Joint Research Centre Institute for Prospective Technological Studies. Retrieved March 27, 2015 from http://ftp.jrc.es/EURdoc/JRC77709.pdf

Doñate-Martínez, A., Garcés, J., & Ródenas, F. (2014). Application of screening tools to detect risk of hospital readmission in elderly patients in Valencian Healthcare System (VHS) (Spain). *Archives of Gerontology and Geriatrics*, 59(2), 408–414. doi:10.1016/j.archger.2014.06.004 PMID:25022713

Doñate-Martínez, A., Ródenas, F., & Garcés, J. (2016). Impact of a primary-based telemonitoring programme in HRQOL, satisfaction and usefulness in a sample of older adults with chronic diseases in Valencia (Spain). *Archives of Gerontology and Geriatrics*, 62, 169–175. doi:10.1016/j.archger.2015.09.008

EIP-AHA. (2012). *Action Plan on 'Replicating and tutoring integrated care for chronic diseases, including remote monitoring at regional level'*. Retrieved September 20, 2014, from http://ec.europa.eu/research/innovation-union/pdf/active-healthy-ageing/b3_action_plan.pdf#view=fit&pagemode=none

European Union. (2012). *The 2012 Ageing Report. The Economic and budgetary projections for the 27 EU Member States (2010-2060)*. Luxembourg: Publications Office of the European Union.

Fialová, D., & Onder, G. (2009). Medication errors in elderly people: Contributing factors and future perspectives. *British Journal of Clinical Pharmacology*, 67(6), 641–645. doi:10.1111/j.1365-2125.2009.03419.x PMID:19594531

Fialová, D., Topinková, E., Gambassi, G., Finne-Soveri, H., Jónsson, P. V., Carpenter, I., & Bernabei, R. et al. (2005). Potentially inappropriate medication use among elderly home care patients in Europe. *Journal of the American Medical Association*, 293(11), 1348–1358. doi:10.1001/jama.293.11.1348 PMID:15769968

Garcés, J. (2000). *La nueva sostenibilidad social*. Valencia, Spain: Ariel.

Garcés, J., Carretero, S., & Ródenas, F. (2011). *Readings of the social sustainability theory*. Valencia: Tirant lo Blanch.

Garcés, J., & Monsonís-Payá, I. (2013). *Sustainability and Transformation in European Social Policy*. Bern: Peter Lang International Academic Publishers. doi:10.3726/978-3-0353-0475-6

Garcés, J., & Ródenas, F. (in press). Towards a Sustainable Welfare and Healthcare System in Spain: Experiences with the Case Management Program. In J. Broerse & J. Grin (Eds.), *Towards system innovations in health systems: Understanding historical evolution, innovative practices and opportunities for a transition in healthcare*. New York: Routledge.

Garcés, J., Ródenas, F., & Hammar, T. (2013). Converging methods to link social and health care systems and informal care - confronting Nordic and Mediterranean approaches. In K. Liechsenring, J. Billing, & H. Nies (Eds.), *Long Term Care in Europe - Improving policy and practice*. London: Palgrave MacMillan. doi:10.1057/9781137032348.0012

Garcés, J., Ródenas, F., & Sanjosé, V. (2003). Towards a new welfare state: The social sustainability principle and health care strategies. *Health Policy (Amsterdam)*, *65*(3), 201–215. doi:10.1016/S0168-8510(02)00200-2 PMID:12941489

Garcés, J., Ródenas, F., & Sanjosé, V. (2006). Suitability of the health and social care resources for persons requiring long-term care in Spain: An empirical approach. *Health Policy (Amsterdam)*, *75*(2), 121–130. doi:10.1016/j.healthpol.2005.01.012 PMID:16226336

Garcés, J., Ródenas, F., Sanjosé, V., & Carretero, S. (2005). An efficient alternative care scenario for long term care bases on the principles of social sustainability and quality of life in Spain. In J. Yfantopoulos (Ed.), *The economics of health reforms*. Athens: The Athens Institute for Research Education and Research.

García-Goñi, M., Hernández-Quevedo, C., Nuño-Solinís, R., & Paolucci, F. (2012). Pathways towards chronic care-focused healthcare systems: Evidence from Spain. *Health Policy (Amsterdam)*, *108*(2-3), 236–245. doi:10.1016/j.healthpol.2012.09.014 PMID:23116631

Geneau, R., Stuckler, D., Stachenko, S., McKee, M., Ebrahim, S., Basu, S., & Beaglehole, R. et al. (2010). Raising the priority of preventing chronic diseases: A political process. *Lancet*, *376*(9753), 1689–1698. doi:10.1016/S0140-6736(10)61414-6 PMID:21074260

Grimaldo, F., Orduña, J. M., Ródenas, F., Garcés, J., & Lozano, M. (2014). Towards a simulator of integrated long-term care systems for elderly people. *International Journal of Artificial Intelligence Tools*, *23*(1), 1–24. doi:10.1142/S0218213014400053

Grimaldo, F., Ródenas, F., Lozano, M., Carretero, S., Orduña, J. M., Garcés, J., & Fatas, E. et al. (2013). Design of an ICT tool for decision making in social and health policies. In M. M. Cruz-Cunha, I. M. Miranda, & P. Gonçalves (Eds.), *Handbook of Research on ICTs for Human-Centered Healthcare and Social Care Services*. IGI Global Publication. doi:10.4018/978-1-4666-3986-7.ch042

Gröne, O., & Garcia-Barbero, M. (2004). *Approaches towards measuring integration and continuity of care*. Copenhagen: World Health Organization.

Ifanti, A., Argyriou, A., Kalofonou, F., & Kalofonos, H. (2014). Financial crisis and austerity measures in Greece: Their impact on health promotion policies and public health care. *Health Policy (Amsterdam)*, *113*(1-2), 8–12. doi:10.1016/j.healthpol.2013.05.017 PMID:23790265

Lawrence, T. M., Wenn, R., Boulton, C. T., & Moran, C. G. (2010). Age-specific incidence of first and second fractures of the hip. *The Bone & Joint Journal*, *92-B*(2), 258–261. PMID:20130319

Leichsenring, K. (2004). Developing integrated health and social care services for older persons in Europe. *International Journal of Integrated Care*, *4*(3), e10. PMID:16773149

Liechsenring, K., Billing, J., & Nies, H. (2013). *Long Term Care in Europe - Improving policy and practice*. London: Palgrave MacMillan. doi:10.1057/9781137032348

Lloyd, J., & Wait, S. (2006). *Integrated care. A guide for policymakers*. London: Alliance for Health and the Future.

Miller, J. N., Colditz, G. A., & Monsteller, F. (1989). How study design affects outcomes in comparison of therapy. II: Surgical. *Statistics in Medicine, 8*(4), 455–466. doi:10.1002/sim.4780080409 PMID:2727469

MMWR. (1999). Framework for Program Evaluation in Public Health. Centers for Disease Control and Prevention. 48(No. RR-11).

Mur-Veeman, I., van Raak, A., & Paulus, A. (2008). Comparing integrated care policy in Europe: Does policy matter? *Health Policy (Amsterdam), 85*(2), 172–183. doi:10.1016/j.healthpol.2007.07.008 PMID:17767975

Nuño, R., Coleman, K., Bengo, R., & Sauto, R. (2012). Integrated care for chronic conditions: The contribution of the ICCC Framework. *Health Policy (Amsterdam), 105*(1), 55–64. doi:10.1016/j.healthpol.2011.10.006 PMID:22071454

OECD. (2012). *Health at a Glance: Europe 2012*. OECD Publishing. Retrieved March 27, 2015, from http://ec.europa.eu/health/reports/docs/health_glance_2012_en.pdf

Orduña, J. M., Grimaldo, F., Lozano, M., Ródenas, F., Carretero, S., & Garcés, J. (2013). Design of and ICT tool for decision making in social and health policies. In Handbook of Research on ICTs for Healthcare and Social Services: Developments and Applications. IGI Global.

Regional Ministry of Health from Valencia. (2012). *Plan de atención a pacientes con enfermedades crónicas de la Comunidad Valenciana 2012. Líneas de actuación*. Generalitat Valenciana, Valencia. Retrieved October 01, 2014, from http://iv.congresocronicos.org/documentos/plan-de-atencion-pacientes-cronicos-valencia.pdf

Ródenas, F., Garcés, J., Carretero, S., & Megia, M. (2008). Case management method applied to older adults in the primary care centres in Burjassot (Valencian Region, Spain). *European Journal of Ageing, 5*(1), 57–66. doi:10.1007/s10433-008-0073-9

Ródenas, F., Garcés, J., Doñate-Martínez, A., & Zafra, E. (2014). Aplicación de The Community Assessment Risk Screen (CARS) en centros de Atención Primaria del Sistema Sanitario Valenciano. *Atencion Primaria, 46*(1), 25–31. doi:10.1016/j.aprim.2013.07.010 PMID:24332509

Shepherd, C., & While, A. (2012). Cardiac rehabilitation and quality of life: A systematic review. *International Journal of Nursing Studies, 49*(6), 755–771. doi:10.1016/j.ijnurstu.2011.11.019 PMID:22197653

Smith, S. M., Soubhi, H., Fortin, M., Hudon, C., & O'Dowd, T. (2012). Managing patients with multimorbidity: Systematic review of interventions in primary care and community settings. *BMJ (Clinical Research Ed.), 345*, e5205. PMID:22945950

Sundström, G., Fransson, E., Malmberg, B., & Davey, A. (2009). Loneliness among older Europeans. *European Journal of Ageing, 6*(4), 267–275. doi:10.1007/s10433-009-0134-8

WHO. (2005). *Preventing chronic diseases: a vital investment*. WHO Library Cataloguing-in-Publication Data.

KEY TERMS AND DEFINITIONS

E

Integrated Care: The integration of care entails a coherent and coordinated services delivery to individual service users across a board range of health and social care organizations, different professionals and informal caregivers.

LTCMAS (Long-Term Care Multi-Agent Systems): LTCMAS is a simulator that, as a starting point, used a holistic model of care systems for people that need long-term care, the Sustainable Socio-Health Model (SSHM). The implementation of the simulator on the Jason multi-agent platform allows the tool to include human interactions, preferences and social abilities that take place between older people and the staff of healthcare systems (health and social workers). The closed-loop design of the proposed simulator permits repeated simulation of successive interactions of the target population with the healthcare system.

Social Sustainability: The first principle of the Social Sustainable Healthcare Model, which takes on the value of solidarity between generations, and is legitimized ethically through a wider and deeper re-analysis of the fundamental social values of freedom and equality: a) freedom and responsibility, insofar as our present freedom implies the responsibility of taking into account our successors in our actions or the conditions of life we nurture; b) equality of rights and obligations, as a consequence of our actions, no present or future citizen should have their freedom, their options or their decision taking capacity impaired.

Internet and Social Network as Health/ Physical Activity Information Sources

Dulce Esteves
Beira Interior University, Portugal & CIDESD - Research Center in Sports Sciences, Health and Human Development, Portugal

Paulo Pinheiro
Beira Interior University, Portugal & NECE - Research Center in Business Sciences, Portugal

Kelly O'Hara
Beira Interior University, Portugal & CIDESD - Research Center in Sports Sciences, Health and Human Development, Portugal

Rui Brás
Beira Interior University, Portugal & CIDESD - Research Center in Sports Sciences, Health and Human Development, Portugal

INTRODUCTION

The Internet increasingly serves as a platform for the delivery of health information and its potential use as health information source has been demonstrated across a wide range of conditions (Bennett & Glasgow, 2009).

The Internet has been acknowledged as a valuable channel of health promotion, with information in web spread throw static health educational sites, peer support groups, online health consultations and delivery of Internet interventions (Vandelanotte, Spathonis, Eakin, & Owen, 2007).

Health information seeking is defined as the purposive acquisition of information from selected information sources to guide health-related decision making (Johnson & Case, 2012).

Health information seeking behavior comprehends intentional or active efforts to obtain specific information not found by the normal patterns of media exposure or by interpersonal sources (Atkin, 1973; Griffin, Dunwoody, & Neuwirth, 1999).

Lambert and Loiselle (2007) consider two main dimensions when defining the concept of Health information seeking behavior: (1) the information dimension, that emphasizes the characteristics of the information sought, namely the type (content and diversity of the search) and the amount (how much information about a given topic one seeks) and (2) the method dimension, focused on the discretionary actions individual use to obtain health related information and sources of information used (include direct and indirect questioning, asking for clarifications, discussing and exchanging information with others, reading and using information technologies).

Considering the information dimension of health information seeking behavior, Weaver et al. (2009) consider the existence of two main groups: one more related to medicine (with high loadings on the medications, illness or disease, treatments and insurance measures) and other related with wellbeing (with high loadings on the exercise and diet measures). Physical Activity (PA) information seeking on the Internet is considered as a sub-level of health information seeking by Pew Surveys (Jones & Fox, 2009). This article intends to present the potentialities, problems and future trends of the use of the

DOI: 10.4018/978-1-4666-9978-6.ch049

Internet and online Social Networks (SN) as PA information sources and promoting channels and the actual perspective of associated technology to become active.

BACKGROUND

Regular moderate-intensity PA influences health status and wellbeing, with important role in the prevention of various chronic diseases (Klavestrand & Vingård, 2009). In fact, the benefits of PA on health have been extensively reported by World Health Organization, Centers for Disease Control and Prevention (USA), American College of Sport Medicine, American Heart Association, European Community (EU Working Group "Sport & Health"). Embracing an active lifestyle is broadly seen as an important step to achieve good health status and wellbeing, among all ages.

The exponential growth and penetration of new information technologies may affect the PA patterns, since those technologies

1. May be an adequate channel to delivery PA promotion policies, and
2. They are an important information repository that individuals can use to seek for exercise and fitness information.

Considering the importance of exercise on health status, Fox and Jones (2009) report a huge interest in information about exercise and fitness by Internet users. The percentage of American adults getting PA information online increased from 21% in 2002 to 38% in 2009, the major evolution of the health topic covered in the survey. Pew Project report showed that 72% of online 18-29 year olds use SN websites, and 31% of online teens (aged 12-17) get their information on health, dieting or PA from the Internet (Gabarron, Fernandez-Luque, Armayones, & Lau, 2013).

McCully, Don, and Updegraff (2013), consider that when analyzing the Internet use for seeking PA information, people generally search for PA associate with healthy dietary, and weight control. Internet users seeking information about weight, dietary and PA, show a higher level of PA and more fruits and vegetables intake than those who do not use the Internet to seek this kind of information (Mcully et al., 2013).

Indeed, the Internet is an interesting medium for seeking and promoting Health and PA, since

1. It provides the option of delivering versions of individualized computer-tailored interventions at any time and place (Brouwer et al., 2009);
2. Have the potential to service large numbers of the population (Vandelanotte et al., 2007);
3. Have convenience, novelty, appeal and flexibility of use (Leslie, Marshall, Owen, & Bauman, 2005);
4. Permit automated data collection (Brouwer et al., 2009);
5. Allows proactive recruitment (contacting potential participants and offering them services) (Leslie et al., 2005);
6. Can be delivered through various non-face-to-face channels, thus reducing the influence of barriers associated with face-to-face interventions (e.g., time constraints, childcare) (Marcus et al., 2007);
7. Allows participants to access large amounts of information and choose the time to interact and receive information (Brouwer et al., 2009); and
8. Offer the advantages of cost savings (Steele, Mummerey, & Dwyer, 2007).

Web applications that facilitate collective knowledge creation and exchange (referred to as "web 2.0") have become increasingly popular, including weblogs, wikis, online social networks (SN) social bookmarking, tags and tag clouds (which give rise to folksonomies), pod- and vod-casts, mash-ups and RSS feeds (Adams, 2010). These tools emphasize the value of user-generated content, collective knowledge production and the exchange of personal experiences. The use of web 2.0 channels to retrieve exercise information and to promote an active lifestyle offers immense potential for the delivery of both information and behavior change campaigns, but it is unclear how those technologies may be used to achieve effective health behavior change (Maher et al., 2014).

INTERNET, ONLINE SOCIAL NETWORKS, AND PHYSICAL ACTIVITY PATTERNS

Issues, Controversies, Problems

Maibach (2007) points out that recently the number of media delivery platforms and channels available has increased dramatically, including personal computers and Internet access, mobile and stationary video game platforms and mobile phones. The author considers that to understand the potential impact of these trends on PA, two opposite effects should be considered: a positive effect is the potential use of those channels to promote PA (creation and dissemination of content that may somehow influence thoughts or feelings about PA, which, in turn, may have influence on PA level) ; a negative effect is the sedentary behavior potentially promoted by using those media, (spending time surfing the Web or on online social networks may displace time previously spent being physically active).

The positive effect referred by Maibach (2007) may be enhanced considering three approaches: specific Internet based interventions, online social networks and specific technologic devices to promote PA. In spite of technologic potentialities to contribute to the adoption of an active lifestyle, problems related to online PA information seeking are also analyzed, in the next sections.

1. Specific Internet Based Interventions to Promote an Active Living

Internet-based PA interventions aim to change individual behavior towards a more active lifestyle (Joseph, Durant, Benitez, & Pekmezi, 2013) and may vary from static informative webpages to specific designed, interactive and integrative (with other delivery channels) interventions (Vandelanotte et al., 2007).

Unlike the promotion of some other health behaviors, providing information has been found to be an advantageous method to increase individual PA level (Pinheiro, Esteves, & Brás, 2011). In fact, if people lack knowledge about the health risks of physical inactivity and benefits of an active lifestyle, they may not have enough motivation to change their sedentary habits (Hirvonen, Huotari, Niemelä, & Korpelainen, 2012). Increasing knowledge of the risks and benefits can be considered a precondition for behavioral change, although, this does not necessarily lead to improvements in behavior (Hirvonen et al., 2012).

Webb, Joseph, Yardley, and Michie (2010) reported that over 30% of Internet webpages regarding increasing PA use only one mode of delivery, with the main goal to provide an enriched information environment. Since providing information of the behavior consequences is a commonly used behavior change technique (Webb et al., 2010), disseminate information regarding PA benefits and unhealthy consequences of inactivity may contribute to behavioral change.

E

More interactive website-delivered interventions for health behavioral change may be effective and may overcome many barriers associated with traditional face-to-face PA programs, since user can seek advice at any time, any place, and often at a lower cost compared with other delivery modalities. Among these interventions, considerably differences were found, regarding mode of delivery, such as

- Interactivity;
- Integration with other delivery modes (e.g., telephone, interactive voice response, short message service, email or videoconferencing);
- Use of automated functions (automated tailored feedback; automated follow-up messages);
- Communicative functions, access to an advisor/expert or peer-to-peer access (Webb et al., 2010).

The successful web-based PA interventions must include personalized interventions, numerous participant contacts and social support elements. Web-based interventions that provide personalized advices result in improved engagement and behavioral outcomes compared to interventions providing generic advices (Alley, Jennings, Plotnikoff, & Vandelanotte, 2014). Vandelanotte et al. (2007) and Soetens, Vandelanotte, de Vries, and Mummery (2014) corroborate this idea, considering that personally tailored information is better remembered, read, and perceived as more relevant, compared with generic information.

These personalized interventions may be achieved through coaching or computer-tailoring advice: coaching is based on interaction between an expert (coach) and each individual and computer-tailored advice is automatically produced using a computer-based expert system that delivers feedback based on participant's responses to a questionnaire (Alley et al., 2014).

Online coaching provide personal contact between client and expert, similar to traditional face-to-face interaction and is typically delivered through private messages (e-mail, SMS), real time instant messaging (chat) and group forums (Alley et al., 2014).

Although the effectiveness of online coaching is well established (Soetens et al., 2014), it has a much higher cost then computer-tailored advice, so Internet-based PA interventions rarely included online coaching (Joseph et al., 2013).

In spite a modest positive effect on PA level generated by Internet-based PA interventions (de Vries, Kremers, Smeets, Brug, & Eijmael, 2008; Lustria et. al., 2011; Neville, O'Hara, & Milat, 2009), there are severe engagement and retention problems, with reported dropouts that reach up to 40–50% (Bennett & Glasgow, 2009). As the amount of exposure to the intervention content is strongly linked to behavioral outcomes, low participant retention and engagement may limit the effectiveness of Internet-based PA interventions (Alley et al., 2014).

Despite the above mentioned potentialities of website-delivered interventions for PA behavioral change, the evaluation and the optimization of those interventions is yet little investigated (Joseph et al., 2013).

2. Online Social Networks and Physical Activity

Online Social Networking refers to activities, performances and behaviors between communities of people who gather online to share information, knowledge, and opinions using conversational media (Safko & Brake, 2009). They can be categorized as blogging and microblogging (eg, Twitter), media sharing (eg, YouTube) or image sharing (e.g. Pinterest, Instagram) and SN (eg, Facebook; Google Plus, LinkedIn) (Thackeray, Crookston, & West, 2013), that comprehend forums and message boards, review and opinion sites, including image and media sharing.

Opposite to online information seeking, SN allow users to generate, distribute, and share information independent of any organization and people engage in different forms of participation, from consuming to creating content (Thackeray et al., 2013). SN provides new opportunities for people to connect, collaborate, create, circulate, and disseminate contents (Gabarron et al., 2013).

SN offers potential for delivery of public health campaigns, since they can reach large audiences, messages can be delivered via existing contacts and SN typically achieves high levels of user engagement and retention (Maher et al., 2014).

Considering that social support is a well-established correlate of greater PA, a growing number of web-based health interventions have employed SN (online bulletin board services, group chats) to increase PA (Cavallo et al., 2012).

Another significant aspect of SN is online recommendations - platforms that advice products or services and provide information from experienced users (Vandelanotte et al., 2007). This can be especially important when considering recommendations on PA, where the influences of friends/family are particularly important (Anderson-Bill, Winett, & Wojcik, 2011).

Nowadays people have embraced social networks focused on PA, such as Fitocracy, Spark People, and Run Keeper, which currently have an estimated 1 million, 15 million, and 23 million users, respectively (Nakhasi, Shen, Passarella, Appel, & Anderson, 2014).Others similar SN such Dailymile, Traineo, Mapmyfitness, Mbodyment, PumpUp can also be found and used to exchange PA experiences.

Concerning the effect of SN on PA, YouTube (with over 100 million videos) has become a valuable resource to disseminate PA education messages, but videos found can range from high quality to sales propaganda or pseudo-scientific scams (Gabarron et al., 2013).

SN influence on PA patterns is yet sparsely investigated and given their promising features and potential) reach, efforts to further understand how SN can be used in health promotion should be pursued (Cavallo et al., 2012). Maher et al. (2014) consider that there are many uncertainties about how SN might be harnessed to improve health and question whether people even desire to use SN to engage in health behavior change.

3. New Technology to Become Active

Technologic devices have been used as motivational tools to promote exercise adherence. The most important of those devises are pedometers, accelerometers, and heart-rate monitors, since they evaluate parameters to the exercise control. Pedometer-based walking increases PA level upon 27% over baseline levels (Barrera, Glasgow, Mckay, Boles, & Feil, 2002).

Newer technologies and approaches being used to promote PA include global positioning system (GPS), geographic information systems (GIS) and interactive video games (Heyward & Gibson, 2014). Mobile fitness apps and the online fitness networks (like RunKeeper, Endomondo, Strava, Mapmyrun), that present a steady increase in users in recent years (Stragier, Mechant, & De Marez, 2013).

GIS provides information about location and the near environment, stored in computer programs, enabling people to choose the best options to outdoor exercise.

Although interactive video games as Wii-Sports, Wii-Fit and Microsoft Kinect designed to increase fun and engaging game play, may produce positive health benefits (Jacobs et al., 2011). Many fitness centers, schools, and senior centers are now offering interactive games to promote PA (Heyward & Gibson, 2014).

E-Marketer (2014) expects smartphone users worldwide will reach 1.75 billion in 2014. Fanning, Mullen, & McAuley (2012) refer that smartphones characteristics present several potentialities for PA promotion, allowing to: collect objective and self-report measures of activity in real time; provide feedback and support at the point of decision; provide interactive, immersive, and individualized content that is automatically generated; and deliver materials on a device that is already carried by the individual. In May 2013, the iTunes and Google Play stores contained 23,490 and 17,756 smartphone applications (apps) categorized as Health and Fitness, respectively (Middelweerd, Mollee, van der Wal, Brug, & Te Velde, 2014).

Mobile fitness apps and the online fitness networks have a great potential to promote PA since an increasing number of smartphone applications enable people to track fitness workouts and share these with online peers. This sharing adds a new dimension to PA (Stragier et al., 2013), and the effect of this recent technologic innovation on PA patterns are yet to be studied (Fanning et al, 2012). The social engagement of exercise achievements with online peers could create a motivation SN that promotes exercise adherence.

The new technologic devices, aggregated to active mobile, are a new field of research for both healthy and unhealthy people and mobile apps specially designed to promote and control PA on healthy with different pathologies (diabetes, autism, cardiovascular diseases, hypertension, among others) should be developed (Bort-Roig, Gilson, Puig-Ribera, Contreras, & Trost, 2014).

4. PA Information Quality on the Internet and in Online Social Networks

There has been expressed concern about the quality of health information available online and as there is a quick growth of health sources on the Internet (Goetzinger, Park, Lee, & Widdows, 2007) the problem tends to grow. The main issues with online information are: information overload, disorganization, searching difficulties, inaccessible or overly technical language, lack of user friendliness and lack of performance (inconsistent updating, sites disappear, etc.) (Cline & Haynes, 2001). This lack of information quality raises problems, as health professionals has to spent time dealing with clients who base their actions on wrong information, increasing costs and health risks as they assume wrong behaviors (Edejer, 2000). Some dangers considering the PA information seeking on the Internet, referring that the majority of the exercise information on the Web does not meet the high standards of quality requested (Chalmers, 2005). Adams (2010) considers the problem of blending advertising with informative content, considering commercial interest behind information as a major impairment to reliability of web-based information.

Most of Internet applications that provide information have a static mode of delivery, with little interactivity and maintenance, compared to those with commercial background. This may lead to a bigger problem: "serious" information is much less appealing that commercial one (Brouwer et al., 2009).

Leslie et al. (2005) reinforce this idea, referring that websites with PA information may be more 'passive' than has been previously assumed and defend the need to discuss with web designers the necessity to make websites more dynamic, to update website material regularly and to make them more appealing and useful to users.

Solutions and Recommendations

Given the technological boom that has been happening in recent years, the promotion of PA will increasingly involve the use of new communication technologies.

Strategies of e-intervention to promote PA are needed, whenever it is based only Internet sites that intend to provide adequate PA information or involving more specific and integrative solutions that engage a large population, interactive interfaces and provide personalized advices.

In the first case, innovate and re-design of classic Internet web sites should be considered, so they could become more attractive and interactive, capable of provide adequate PA information.

In the second case, programs and interventions to promote PA should provide personalized advice (in opposition to generic information), social contacts (to individual share their experience and interact with others) and expert support, that gives fitness advices and motivational tips. This kind of interventions, particularly if requiring expert advices, may import costs, what may be a challenge: are customers ready to pay for this kind of service? This is a future research important topic.

Other pertinent problem is the efficacy of e-interventions to promote PA. In order to evaluate the real-time effect of e-interventions on PA the use of sensors (e.g., integrated accelerometer and GPS devices) should be empathized. If integrated in smartphone technology, those sensors may evaluate PA level combined with geographic information, allowing for a more detailed examination of the environmental context (Stragier et al., 2013) and the response to the intervention solicitations. This feedback is essential to optimize e-intervention, towards the behavior changes desired.

Not only immediate, but also the long time effect of e-interventions on PA is a controversial issue. Do those interventions achieve long-term behavioral change with an increase PA level?. Joseph et al. (2013) defend that future studies should incorporate delayed post intervention follow-up assessments as they provide a method to evaluate the longer-term impacts of the Internet-based PA interventions.

In spite of most people around the world use the Internet, when considering promoting PA, two aspects should be considered: the minor e-skills reported for older and low educated people and the differences found on Internet penetration among countries. So, the worldwide policy for PA promotion must combine new (Internet sites, mobile apps, specific e-interventions, social groups) and traditional (face-to-face, newspapers/magazines; TV/Radio/school education/medical personal advices) ways of delivery.

Information quality is also a problem of concern. To improve the information quality, websites should be thought taking into account include web information quality, web interaction quality and site design quality (Shchiglik & Barnes, 2004). Web sites can attempt to make their health-related information more credible, observing the code of conduct, implementing a quality label and a user guidance system, filtering tools or third-party accreditation (Wilson & Risk, 2002).

Health and fitness apps, together with exercise technologic devices, should be able to measure several exercise indicators, in order to provide real time personalized information. Apps that not only promote but also control exercise patterns, even with expert intervention should be develop, creating a virtual, low cost, all time accessible personal trainer.

FUTURE RESEARCH DIRECTIONS

Literature refers that health information seeking related to wellbeing often includes looking for PA information. Future investigation is necessary, not only to evaluate the effect (immediate and long term) of e-interventions to promote PA but also to develop new ways of using technology among physical activities.

1. The evaluation of Internet based interventions has been researched, but the optimization of those interventions is still an important research field.
   a. Mobile Apps are relatively new tools in PA interventions and only very little research has been published on the content and the effectiveness on PA level (Middelweerd et al., 2014).
2. New technologic devices, aggregated to mobile apps specially designed to promote and control PA on healthy individuals and considering different pathologies (diabetes, autism, cardiovascular diseases, hypertension, among others) should be developed.

3. Develop technology to promote and control exercise in context of "Mobile Cities", whereas walking around the city is an activity simultaneously touristic, cultural and healthy, where personalized exercise tips are presented on smartphones along city pathways.

4. Develop mechanism that may guarantee e-health (in this case PA) information, in order to provide users with accurate and adequate exercise information.

CONCLUSION

Internet is the biggest medical library in the world and is likely to play an important role both in future healthcare related communication (Dumitru et al., 2007) and in health/PA interventions (Bennett & Glasgow, 2009).

The considerable benefits of PA on health, the high prevalence of physical inactivity among worldwide population and the extraordinary development of communication technology in recent years make the Internet and the SN an important way of PA promotion and an important PA information source.

PA seekers can find in the Internet and SN high standard information mixed with myths, scams and erroneous facts, what may impair information quality and source reliability.

The effects of e-interventions and active mobile apps to promote PA are not completely understood, since they are part of a new technological, communicational and relational paradigm.

REFERENCES

Adams, S. A. (2010). Revisiting the online health information reliability debate in the wake of "web 2.0": An inter-disciplinary literature and website review. *International Journal of Medical Informatics*, *79*(6), 391–400. doi:10.1016/j.ijmedinf.2010.01.006 PMID:20188623

Alley, S., Jennings, C., Plotnikoff, R. C., & Vandelanotte, C. (2014). My Activity Coach-Using video-coaching to assist a web-based computer-tailored physical activity intervention: A randomised controlled trial protocol. *BMC Public Health*, *14*(1), 738. doi:10.1186/1471-2458-14-738 PMID:25047900

Anderson-Bill, E. S., Winett, R. A., & Wojcik, J. R. (2011). Social cognitive determinants of nutrition and physical activity among web-health users enrolling in an online intervention: The influence of social support, self-efficacy, outcome expectations, and self-regulation. *Journal of Medical Internet Research*, *13*(1), e28. doi:10.2196/jmir.1551 PMID:21441100

Atkin, C. K. (1973). Instrumental utilities and information seeking. In P. Clarke (Ed.), *New models for communication research* (pp. 205–242). Beverly Hills, CA: Sage.

Atkinson, N. L., Saperstein, S. L., & Pleis, J. (2009). Using the Internet for Health-Related Activities: Findings From a National Probability Sample. *Journal of Medical Internet Research*, *11*(1), e4. doi:10.2196/jmir.1035 PMID:19275980

Barrera, M. Jr, Glasgow, R. E., Mckay, H. G., Boles, S. M., & Feil, E. G. (2002). Do Internet-based support interventions change perceptions of social support?: An experimental trial of approaches for supporting diabetes self-management. *American Journal of Community Psychology*, *30*(5), 637–654. doi:10.1023/A:1016369114780 PMID:12188054

Bennett, G. G., & Glasgow, R. E. (2009). The delivery of public health interventions via the Internet: Actualizing their potential. *Annual Review of Public Health*, *30*(1), 273–292. doi:10.1146/annurev. publhealth.031308.100235 PMID:19296777

Bort-Roig, J., Gilson, N. D., Puig-Ribera, A., Contreras, R. S., & Trost, S. G. (2014). Measuring and influencing physical activity with smartphone technology: A systematic review. *Sports Medicine (Auckland, N.Z.)*, *44*(5), 671–686. doi:10.1007/s40279-014-0142-5 PMID:24497157

Brouwer, W., Oenema, A., Crutzen, R., de Nooijer, J., de Vries, N. K., & Brug, J. (2009). What makes people decide to visit and use an Internet-delivered behavior-change intervention?: A qualitative study among adults. *Health Education*, *109*(6), 460–473. doi:10.1108/09654280911001149

Cavallo, D. N., Tate, D. F., Ries, A. V., Brown, J. D., DeVellis, R. F., & Ammerman, A. S. (2012). A social media–based physical activity intervention: A randomized controlled trial. *American Journal of Preventive Medicine*, *43*(5), 527–532. doi:10.1016/j.amepre.2012.07.019 PMID:23079176

Chalmers, G. R. (2005). Exercise information resources on the World Wide Web. *Medical Reference Services Quarterly*, *24*(4), 79–88. doi:10.1300/J115v24n04_06 PMID:16203703

Cline, R., & Haynes, K. (2001). Consumer health information seeking on the Internet: The state of the art. *Health Education Research*, *16*(6), 671–692. doi:10.1093/her/16.6.671 PMID:11780707

de Vries, H., Kremers, S. P., Smeets, T., Brug, J., & Eijmael, K. (2008). The effectiveness of tailored feedback and action plans in an intervention addressing multiple health behaviors. *American Journal of Health Promotion*, *22*(6), 417–425. doi:10.4278/ajhp.22.6.417 PMID:18677882

Dumitru, R. C., Bürkle, T., Potapov, S., Lausen, B., Wiese, B., & Prokosch, H. U. (2007). Use and perception of Internet for health related purposes in Germany: Results of a national survey. *International Journal of Public Health*, *52*(5), 275–285. doi:10.1007/s00038-007-6067-0 PMID:18030943

E-Marketer. (2014). *Smartphone users worldwide will total 1.75 billions in 2014*. Retrieved September 3, 2014, from http://www.emarketer.com/Article/Smartphone-Users-Worldwide-Will-Total-175-Billion-2014/1010536#sthash.kkEU1QoB.dpuf

Edejer, T. T. (2000). Disseminating health information in developing countries: The role of the Internet. *British Medical Journal*, *321*(7264), 797–800. doi:10.1136/bmj.321.7264.797 PMID:11009519

Fanning, J., Mullen, S. P., & McAuley, E. (2012). Increasing physical activity with mobile devices: A meta-analysis. *Journal of Medical Internet Research*, *14*(6), e161. doi:10.2196/jmir.2171 PMID:23171838

Fox, S., & Jones, S. (2009). *The social life of health information*. Washington, DC: Pew Internet & American Life Project.

Gabarron, E., Fernandez-Luque, L., Armayones, M., & Lau, A. Y. (2013). Identifying measures used for assessing quality of YouTube videos with patient health information: A review of current literature. *Interactive Journal of Medical Research*, *2*(1), e6. doi:10.2196/ijmr.2465 PMID:23612432

Goetzinger, L., Park, J., Lee, Y. J., & Widdows, R. (2007). Value-driven consumer e-health information search behavior. *International Journal of Pharmaceutical and Healthcare Marketing*, *1*(2), 128–142. doi:10.1108/17506120710762988

Griffin, R. J., Dunwoody, S., & Neuwirth, K. (1999). Proposed model of the relationship of risk information seeking and processing to the development of preventive behaviors. *Environmental Research, 80*(2), S230–S245. doi:10.1006/enrs.1998.3940 PMID:10092438

Heyward, V. H., & Gibson, A. (2014). *Advanced Fitness Assessment and Exercise Prescription (7th ed.).* Champaign, IL: Human Kinetics.

Hirvonen, N., Huotari, M. L., Niemelä, R., & Korpelainen, R. (2012). Information behavior in stages of exercise behavior change. *Journal of the American Society for Information Science and Technology, 63*(9), 1804–1819. doi:10.1002/asi.22704

Jacobs, K., Zhu, L., Dawes, M., Franco, J., Huggins, A., Igari, C., & Umez-Eronini, A. (2011). Wii health: A preliminary study of the health and wellness benefits of Wii Fit on university students. *British Journal of Occupational Therapy, 74*(6), 262–268. doi:10.4276/030802211X13074383957823

Johnson, J. D., & Case, D. O. (2012). *Health information seeking.* New York, NY: Peter Lang.

Jones, S., & Fox, S. (2009). *Generations online in 2009.* Washington, DC: Pew Internet & American Life Project.

Joseph, R. P., Durant, N. H., Benitez, T. J., & Pekmezi, D. W. (2013). Internet-based physical activity interventions. *American Journal of Lifestyle Medicine, 8*(1), 42–68. doi:10.1177/1559827613498059 PMID:25045343

Klavestrand, J., & Vingård, E. (2009). Retracted: The relationship between physical activity and health-related quality of life: a systematic review of current evidence. *Scandinavian Journal of Medicine & Science in Sports, 19*(3), 300–312. doi:10.1111/j.1600-0838.2009.00939.x PMID:19895380

Lambert, S. D., & Loiselle, C. G. (2007). Health information—seeking behavior. *Qualitative Health Research, 17*(8), 1006–1019. doi:10.1177/1049732307305199 PMID:17928475

Leslie, E., Marshall, A. L., Owen, N., & Bauman, A. (2005). Engagement and retention of participants in a physical activity website. *Preventive Medicine, 40*(1), 54–59. doi:10.1016/j.ypmed.2004.05.002 PMID:15530581

Lustria, M. L. A., Smith, S. A., & Hinnant, C. C. (2011). Exploring digital divides: An examination of eHealth technology use in health information seeking, communication and personal health information management in the USA. *Health Informatics Journal, 17*(3), 224–243. doi:10.1177/1460458211414843 PMID:21937464

Maher, C. A., Lewis, L. K., Ferrar, K., Marshall, S., De Bourdeaudhuij, I., & Vandelanotte, C. (2014). Are health behavior change interventions that use online social networks effective? A systematic review. *Journal of Medical Internet Research, 16*(2), e40. doi:10.2196/jmir.2952 PMID:24550083

Maibach, E. (2007). The influence of the media environment on physical activity: Looking for the big picture. *American Journal of Health Promotion, 21*(4s), 353–362. doi:10.4278/0890-1171-21.4s.353 PMID:17465181

Marcus, B. H., Lewis, B. A., Williams, D. M., Dunsiger, S., Jakicic, J. M., Whiteley, J. A., & Parisi, A. F. (2007). A comparison of Internet and print-based physical activity interventions. *Archives of Internal Medicine, 167*(9), 944–949. doi:10.1001/archinte.167.9.944 PMID:17502536

McCully, S. N., Don, B. P., & Updegraff, J. A. (2013). Using the Internet to Help With Diet, Weight, and Physical Activity: Results From the Health Information National Trends Survey (HINTS). *Journal of Medical Internet Research, 15*(8), e148. doi:10.2196/jmir.2612 PMID:23906945

Middelweerd, A., Mollee, J. S., van der Wal, C., Brug, J., & Te Velde, S. J. (2014). Apps to promote physical activity among adults: A review and content analysis. *The International Journal of Behavioral Nutrition and Physical Activity, 11*(1), 97. PMID:25059981

Nakhasi, A., Shen, A. X., Passarella, R. J., Appel, L. J., & Anderson, C. A. (2014). Online Social Networks That Connect Users to Physical Activity Partners: A Review and Descriptive Analysis. *Journal of Medical Internet Research, 16*(6), e153. doi:10.2196/jmir.2674 PMID:24936569

Neville, L. M., O'Hara, B., & Milat, A. (2009). Computer-tailored physical activity behavior change interventions targeting adults: A systematic review. *The International Journal of Behavioral Nutrition and Physical Activity, 6*(1), 30. doi:10.1186/1479-5868-6-30 PMID:19490649

Pinheiro, P., Esteves, D., & Brás, R. (2011). Evaluation of New Information Technologies Exposure on Knowledge Retention Regarding Benefits of Physical Activity on Health Status. *Electronic Journal of Information Systems Evaluation, 14*(1), 122–133.

Safko, L., & Brake, D. K. (2009). *The Social Media Bible–Tactics. Tools & for Business Success.* Hoboken, NJ: Wiley.

Shchiglik, C., & Barnes, S. (2004). Evaluating website quality in the airline industry. *Journal of Computer Information Systems, 44*(3), 17–25.

Soetens, K. C., Vandelanotte, C., de Vries, H., & Mummery, K. W. (2014). Using Online Computer Tailoring to Promote Physical Activity: A Randomized Trial of Text, Video, and Combined Intervention Delivery Modes. *Journal of Health Communication, 19*(12), 1377–1392. doi:10.1080/10810730.2014 .894597 PMID:24749983

Steele, R. M., Mummery, W. K., & Dwyer, T. (2007). Examination of program exposure across intervention delivery modes: Face-to-face versus Internet. *The International Journal of Behavioral Nutrition and Physical Activity, 4*(1), 7. doi:10.1186/1479-5868-4-7 PMID:17352817

Stragier, J., Mechant, P., & De Marez, L. (2013). Studying Physical Activity Using Social Media: An Analysis of the Added Value of RunKeeper Tweets. *International Journal of Interactive Communication Systems and Technologies, 3*(2), 16–28. doi:10.4018/ijicst.2013070102

Thackeray, R., Crookston, B. T., & West, J. H. (2013). Correlates of health-related social media use among adults. *Journal of Medical Internet Research, 15*(1), e21. doi:10.2196/jmir.2297 PMID:23367505

Vandelanotte, C., Spathonis, K. M., Eakin, E. G., & Owen, N. (2007). Website-delivered physical activity interventions: A review of the literature. *American Journal of Preventive Medicine, 33*(1), 54–64. doi:10.1016/j.amepre.2007.02.041 PMID:17572313

Weaver, J. B. III, Mays, D., Weaver, S. S., Hopkins, G. L., Eroğlu, D., & Bernhardt, J. M. (2010). Health information–seeking behaviors, health indicators, and health risks. *American Journal of Public Health, 100*(8), 1520–1525. doi:10.2105/AJPH.2009.180521 PMID:20558794

Webb, T., Joseph, J., Yardley, L., & Michie, S. (2010). Using the Internet to promote health behavior change: A systematic review and meta-analysis of the impact of theoretical basis, use of behavior change techniques, and mode of delivery on efficacy. *Journal of Medical Internet Research*, *12*(1), e4. doi:10.2196/jmir.1376 PMID:20164043

Wilson, P., & Risk, A. (2002). How to find the good and avoid the bad or ugly: a short guide to tools for rating quality of health information on the internet Commentary: On the way to quality. *British Medical Journal*, *324*(7337), 598–602. doi:10.1136/bmj.324.7337.598 PMID:11884329

KEY TERMS AND DEFINITIONS

Accelerometers: Technology for body acceleration record, providing detailed information about the frequency, duration, intensity and patterns of movement.

Health and Fitness Smartphone Applications (Apps): Software programs designed specifically to run on mobile devices, included in "health and fitness" category in Apple's App-Store that aim to improve health status and/or exercise behavior.

Internet Based Interventions to Promote Physical Activity: Also called e-intervention to promote PA are organized (usually by a research team or by exercise and health professionals), population restricted, usually free of charges interventions designed to promote PA using the Internet (exclusively or with other delivery modes like telephone, face-to-face or text messages).

Moderate-Intensity Physical Activity: PA performed with a moderate amount of the effort and noticeably accelerates heart-rate. Examples: walking briskly, dancing, gardening, housework, recreational sports games, moving moderate loads.

Pedometer: Device that count the number of steps taken throughout the day.

Physical Activity Online Social Networks: Communities of people who gather online to share information, knowledge, and opinions focused on physical activity.

Physical Activity Information Seeking: Action considered as a sub-level of health information seeking by Pew Surveys. Regarding health information seeking literature considers two groups: one more related to illness and other related with wellbeing (intend to retrieve exercise and diet information).

Wellbeing: A phenomenological expression by the individual about the quality of his/her life. Emotional, self-concept, bodily state, global perceptions, health and life satisfactions are considered the main domains of wellbeing.

ISO/IEEE11073 Family of Standards:
Trends and Applications on E-Health Monitoring

Ignacio Martínez Ruiz
University of Zaragoza (UZ), Spain

David Sancho Cohen
University of Zaragoza (UZ), Spain

Álvaro Marco Marco
University of Zaragoza (UZ), Spain

INTRODUCTION

Throughout the last two decades, healthcare applications have gradually experienced a substantial progress. This is mainly due to advances in Information and Communication Technology (ICT) resources and the evolution of Medical Devices (MDs) into Personal Health Devices (PHDs) focusing in user e-Health services. These devices use wireless technologies and portable computing devices in order to report signals and events for remote supervision.

Nevertheless, device manufacturers usually provide not only single devices but also optional hardware and software resources to improve their functionalities and the system overall performance. Making them work flawlessly is usually achieved by making the devices and the other components communicate conforming to a protocol with specific features using proprietary models and data formats. This lack of interoperability constitutes the main obstacle to the mainstream development of e-Health services (Martínez I. et al, 2010). Finally, the end user is forced to use a unique brand of devices, regardless of their specifications such as reliability, security, usability, price, etc. As a result of that, other devices with similar or even better specifications are disregarded, and updates or changes missed because they use different communication protocols than the implemented by the system developer.

In this context, a standardization effort has been strongly remarked to solve this problem and, as result, the ISO/IEEE11073 family of standards is proposed as the international recommended norm for interoperability of medical devices and personal health devices in e-Health services. In this chapter for "Encyclopedia of e-Health and Telemedicine", a complete review of ISO/IEEE11073 family of standards for interoperable communication of devices (MDs and PHDs) is proposed.

INTEROPERABILITY AND E-HEALTH SOLUTIONS: ISO/IEEE11073

Interoperability in the healthcare domain can be compared with the nervous system of the human body, wherein standardized information is conveyed back and forth for seamless understanding, analysis and effective information sharing (Perficient, 2014). The concept behind this is to accept basic electronic communication standards such as controlled vocabularies, code-data set, etc. that will enable stakeholders to uniformly transmit, store, manage and interpret data (Walker et al., 2005).

DOI: 10.4018/978-1-4666-9978-6.ch050

E

While the development of a design for an individual medical device itself is so complex, the concept of plug-and-play increases the design complexity, and a manufacturer may choose not to implement interoperability features for his stand-alone instruments. On the other hand, traditional barriers such as time, resources, cost, space, power consumption or system resources, can be solved with strategies to simplify adoption of standardization and interoperability features, being proposed to health devices companies to encourage adoption with their products (Leone, 2011; Jacob, 2012).

In addition, there is increasing evidence supporting the value of e-Health monitoring for individuals with chronic conditions, including: 35-56% reduction in mortality, 47% reduction in risk of hospitalization, 6 days average reduction in length of hospital admission, 65% reduction in office visits, 40-64% reduction in physician time for checks and 63% reduction in transport costs (Willmitch B. et al., 2012). These advances towards interoperability play a key role in e-Health monitoring, as they are the way to guarantee transparent end-to-end integration (with new medical use cases) promoting the auto-control and follow-up of the own health through newest e-Health monitoring solutions (Trigo J.D. et al., 2010).

E-HEALTH APPLICATION DOMAINS

A wide-adopted segmentation of the e-Health solutions and health devices market is done in three large domains: health and wellness (including fitness, sport activities, among other topics), living independently longer (including Ambient Assisted Living (AAL), Active Healthy Ageing (AHA) and home monitoring of elderly people, among other topics), and chronic conditions management (including diabetes, heart failure, patients who have undergone surgery, urgencies and emergencies, etc.) (Haux, R., 2010; Hovenga, E. J. S., 2010).

These application domains present a similar topology (see Figure 1) that includes the health devices associated to every health scenario, a gateway or information manager, and a third care provider to man-

Figure 1. General topology for three wide-adopted e-health application domains (health and wellness, living independently longer and chronic conditions management), including health devices, services and providers

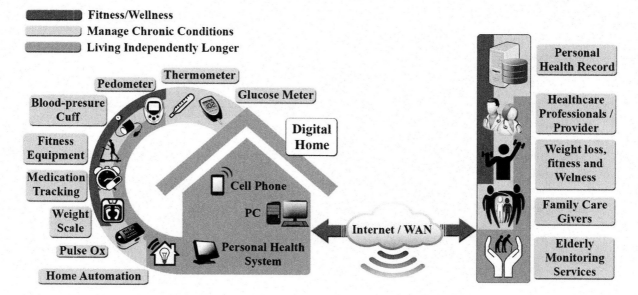

age all data gathered through the Health Information System (HIS). Moreover, these domains can be schematized, as it is shown in Figure 1, in a comparative way regarding their associated health devices, services and providers.

ISO/IEEE11073: FROM POINT-OF-CARE TOWARDS PERSONAL HEALTH DEVICES

Introduction to ISO/IEEE11073

The ISO/IEEE11073 family of standards was born on 2004 (as their first documents were appeared) and it was proposed in 2006 (to be approved in 2008) by the Special Working Group for Personal Health Devices (PHDWG). This group was composed by the Institute of Electrical and Electronics Engineers (IEEE), the International Organization for Standardization (ISO) and the Committee European Normalization (CEN) (CEN PHDWG, 2015).

Since then, ISO/IEEE11073 is the internationally recommended standard for interoperability of medical devices in e-Health environments. The specification proposes a solution for the communication problem among different devices, acting as *agents*, and a centralized element, acting as *manager*. This manager is nowadays called Aggregation Manager, and it gathers all the medical data provided by the agents in a Personal Area Network (PAN) standardizing the format of this information. Then, it transfers this information, usually over wireless technologies (WiFi, 2G, 3G & 4G), to a Telehealth Service Center and exposes it to other Health Information Systems (such as the health records of the users), through both a Wide Area Network (WAN) and a Health Record Network interfaces, as it is shown in Figure 2.

Figure 2. General scheme of interoperability from personal health devices to health records
Source: Continua Health Alliance.

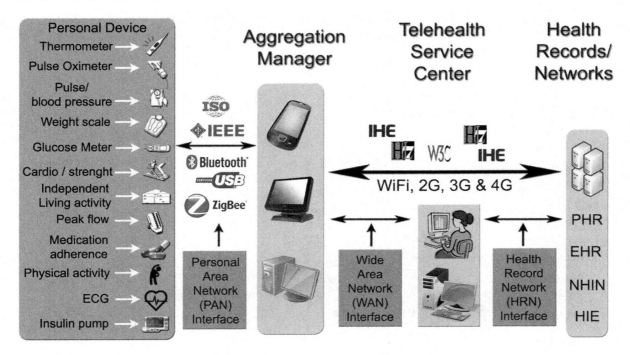

Thus, the information gathered by any health device can be post-processed later in a Personal Health Record (PHR) or Electronic Health Record (EHR) systems, which can correlate it for providing enhanced monitoring using clinical decision algorithms, or it can be integrated directly into the hospital workflow through the Nationwide Health Information Network (NHIN) and be exchanged across organizations within a region, community or hospital system through Health Information Exchange (HIE) (Continua, 2015).

ISO/IEEE11073 Point-of-Care (X73PoC)

The first version of ISO/IEEE11073 was initially designed to address Intensive Care Unit (ICU) scenarios focused on covering medical devices interoperable communication at the Point-of-Care (PoC) or near the site of patient care: X73PoC (IEEE 11073-20101, 2004). The X73PoC protocol architecture was designed by absorbing three previous standards to compose a 7-layers stack for the communication scheme:

- A standard for vital signs information representation (ENV13734 or VITAL (IEEE VITAL, 2004)), which comprises the upper layers (related to the user application and specific features of medical devices).
- A standard for interoperability of patient connected medical device (ENV13735 or INTERMED (IEEE INTERMED, 2004)), which comprises the intermediate layers (related to the intercommunication process).
- A standard for the Medical Information Bus (MIB/IEEE1073 (Kennelly & Gardner, 1997)), which comprises the lower layers (related to the connection technologies).

By combining the three of them, a complete and complex communication stack could be created, which provides the required base for an interoperable information exchange framework. An outline of the documents that compose the stack is shown in Table 1. Following, the upper most relevant layers of the standard protocol stack are described and detailed. Lower levels of X73PoC stack include wired (RS-232) and wireless (IrDA) transport technologies.

Medical Device Data Language (MDDL)

This layer has two objectives. First, to define a set of vocabulary terms and its semantic descriptions upon which the rest of the standard is based and the medical data is mapped, which will be the *Common Nomenclature*. The content of this name library is considerably large as medical vocabulary from several different fields needs to be adopted. Far from completed, the addition of new device specializations which are considered suitable for the standard use will bring new terms to the collection.

Secondly, in a lower level, the MDDL is the responsible part for designing an *object-oriented* modeling of the medical device logical structure which will contain both the configuration and specifications of the device. This first abstract device model is called Domain Information Model (DIM), and it will be used to model several device specializations. The DIM includes the Static Model (which provided an object orient model for representing any medical device following the standardized definitions) and the Dynamic Model (which provided a communication model based on the ISO concept of agent-manager with a 'Device Communication Controller' (DCC) and a 'Bedside Communication Controller' (BCC), respectively).

Basically, the device will be replaced by a hierarchical structure composed by:

Table 1. Scheme of the X73PoC protocol stack

ISO Level	ISO/IEEE# 11073	Contents (Sources Related)	
7	1xxxx	MDDL — Medical Device Data Language (related Vital-Intermed/IS017109)	
	10101	MDDL — Common Nomenclature (vital+intermed)	
	10201	MDDL — Domain Information Model (DIM)	
	103xx	Virtual Medical Device (VMD) specializations: withdrawn	
		3.1 – Infusion device	3.9 – Airflow
		3.2 – Vital signs monitor	3.10 – Cardiac output
		3.3 – Ventilator	3.11 – Capnometer
		3.4 – Pulse oximeter	3.12 – Hemodynamic
		3.5 – Defibrillator	3.13 – Pulmonary
		3.6 – ECG	3.14 – Respirator
		3.7 – Blood Pressure	3.15 – Weighting scale
		3.8 – Temperature	
7-5	2xxxx	MDAP - Medical Device Application Profiles (related Intermed/10B2/CEN1427)	
	20101	MDAP - Base Standard	
	20102	MDAP - WB elements	
	20201	MDAP - polling Mode profile	
	20202	MDAP - Baseline Profile	
	20301	MDAP - Optional Package, remote control	
	20302	MDAP - Optional Package, symmetric communications	
4-1	3xxxx	TPP - Transport & Physical Profiles (common)	
	30100	TPP - Connection Mode (3.1a-Amendment 1)	
	30200	TPP - IrDA cable based connected (3.2a- Amendment 1)	
	30300	TPP - Infrared wireless	
1	4xxxx	Physical Layer Interface Profiles	
3	5xxxx	Internetworking Support	
4	6xxxx	Application Gateways (related HL7 messages)	
4	9xxxx	Related - NCCLS POCT - 1A	

- A Virtual Medical Object (VMO) *class*. This is an abstract class not instantiable, used as the base class from the rest of object classes in the Medical Package.
- A Virtual Medical Device (VMD) and a Medical Device System (MDS) *object classes*. These are the upper-most components of the tree, which define the specification of the device and the configuration, like working mode, Identifier (ID), battery, manufacturer, etc.
- A Channel Object. This merges measurements related to the same metric, such as blood pressure.
- Several measurement object classes and related information containers: *numeric, sample array, real-time sample array, enumeration,* and *persistent metric.*

Medical Device Application Profiles (MDAP)

The purpose of these profiles is to provide with different alternative mechanisms to perform connection management (*establishing, holding* and *releasing* a logical communication channel) and information exchange procedures (*requesting* and *acknowledging* data packets). Data will be transferred from the X73PoC agent to the X73PoC manager following either a *baseline* or *polling* retrieving schema, operating upon a Finite-State Machine (FSM) designed to provide a connection status flow. Once a packet is ready for sending, the abstract values, protocol fields and Application Protocol Data Units (APDUs) described in Abstract Syntax Notation One (ASN.1) need to be mapped into Presentation Protocol Data Units (PPDUs). For this, new Medical Device Encoding Rules (MDER) are preferred, although other options such as XML Encoding Rules (XER) or Basic Encoding Rules (BER) are also accepted.

As mentioned, X73PoC was specifically designed to address ICU scenarios covering medical devices interoperable communication at the Point-of-Care of the patient, considering the specific features of those devices and their application development. That involved meeting strong security and reliability constraints. However, X73PoC, which was based upon other existing specifications and thus fragmenting the content into various documents, was considered far too complex to be adopted by manufacturers of medical devices. Furthermore, with the emerging of new transport technologies (such as USB, Bluetooth or ZigBee) and the increasing popularity of personal and patient-oriented health devices and applications, X73PoC was considered obsolete in some aspects, which led to the development of a more lightweight version for PHDs: X73PHD (IEEE 11073-20601, 2008).

ISO/IEEE11073 Personal Health Devices (X73PHD)

The previous X73PoC standard was not meant to be applied to medical devices with restrictive configuration such as lower computational power and requirements, smaller and portable. Also, neither the transmission techniques nor the protocol overhead were optimized for that purpose. Meanwhile, enhanced telemonitoring and telecare use cases are willing to adopt a new generation of devices which meet this new e-Health paradigm.

Within this situation, the above mentioned PHDWG decided to shift the development on the X73PoC work to release a standard for Personal Health Devices. Although the content of the new standard leverages aspects from X73PoC, the new X73PHD is adapted and optimized for personal health environments and allows adopting technology enhancements. With this evolution, X73PoC maintains its relevance in ICU and hospital environments and X73PHD evolves to personal, mobile and ubiquitous healthcare solutions (Trigo J.D. et al., 2010; Martínez I. et al, 2010).

The main architecture of X73PHD, which evolves by thoroughly simplifying the X73PoC model, is divided into the following three models (see Figure 3):

- **Domain Information Model (DIM):** This typifies the information inside the agent by describing an abstract model composed of a set of object classes which are instanced and can be referenced in an X73PHD-based communication. Each object class has one or more attributes which describe measurement data that are sent to the manager and elements that control the behavior of the agent. The DIM includes the methods and actions that can be executed on each of the attributes and elements. It covers also the definition of the MDS object (root object in the PHD modelling), scanner objects (for health device data reporting), different metrics (numeric, real time sample array and enumeration objects) and Persistent Metric (PM) store and segments (for data storing).
- **Service Model:** This provides methods to access data that are used by agent and manager to establish the interchange of the DIM data. Thus, it defines the means by which the manager can interact with the agent and distinguishes two different types of services: association and object access. Association services provide methods to negotiate and agree upon a common configuration

Figure 3. Evolution of the protocol stack and architecture from X73PoC to X73PHD

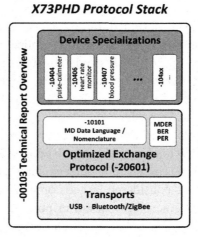

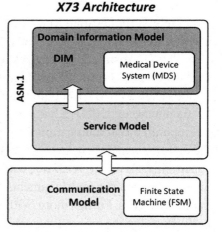

(association request and response), release associations and abort connections. Object access services provide methods that allow for a manager to interact with an agent by, remotely, executing actions and allowing access object attributes, through the link established. These services include *event reports* (often implemented by scanner objects and the MDS) that are initiated by the agent and used to send its configuration (during the association procedure) or medical or personal health data (once the association has been established), get and set methods that allow for the manager to access object attributes, and actions that allow for the manager to execute Remote Procedure Calls (RPCs) over the agent's objects. While event reports are initiated by the agent objects, *get*, *set* and *action* reports are executed over them and initiated by the manager.

- **Communication Model:** This describes the network architecture in which one or more agents communicate with a single manager via point-to-point connections. Thus, it defines an FSM (for both agent and manager) that controls the link state and transport mechanisms. All the transitions in the FSM are well defined and they involve the execution of some actions internally in the agent or the manager, the reception or the sending of a message, etc. The FSM determines the sequence diagrams in any X73PHD-based communication and an important key point is that it is transport-independent, which means that implementations of the stack can be shared among different transport technologies. It also defines different Encoding Rules (ER), Service Elements (SE) and the algorithms responsible for transforming the abstract model given by the DIM into a stream of bytes through a protocol.

This main architecture implies a translation in a protocol stack for the intercommunication between agents and manager. The protocol stack has been simplified in X73PHD evolving from X73PoC with a new stack that is divided into three levels (see Figure 3):

- **Device Specializations:** Similarly as in the previous X73PoC, the Device Specializations are a DIM configuration modeling a specific device, adopting the hierarchy of elements based on the information and behavior of the device. This is a set of model descriptions which gathers the total of objects and attributes related to the DIM, such as an overall system configuration (MDS), PM-Store and Segments or Metric Specifications. For instance, a blood pressure monitor has up to four numeric elements implemented (which correspond to: *Systolic Component, Diastolic Component, Average Component and Heart Rate*), but more complex devices, such as electrocardiographic (ECG) signal monitor, will implement objects such as Real-Time Sample Array (IEEE 11073-20601, 2008). At the time of this writing, a release of X73PHD along with 15 different associated device specifications (indexed as 11073-104xx) have been already published by IEEE (13 of them with standard category –10 of them by the ISO as well and 2 of them are considered as Final Draft International Standard (FDIS) by ISO– while 2 more are in drafting process), as it is shown in Table 2.

- **20601 Optimized Exchange Protocol:** The main part of the standard consists of a medical and technical terminology framework (Domain Information Model, DIM) which will be encapsulated inside the APDUs. This protocol corresponds to both models: Communication and Service. Firstly, the Communication Model describes a point-to-point connection based on the agent-manager architecture through the FSM. The X73PoC defined these concepts in its Part1 as MDDL (including the DIM) and in its Part 2 as MDAP for the X73 communication model. Secondly, the Service Model defines a set of messages and instructions to retrieve data from the agent, based on the DIM. These messages have to be coded for this further implementation using ASN.1. In addition to this, it provides a data conversion from the ASN.1 notation to transfer syntax, using optimized MDER, as well as standard BER and Packet ER (PER) support. Furthermore, X73PHD maintains the SE from the X73PoC. These are: Remote Operation (ROSE, optimized for MDER) between

Table 2. IEEE11073-104xx specializations for medical devices and personal health devices

Active Versions of the Standard Specializations	Medical/Personal Health Device
ISO/IEEE 11073-10404-2010 IEEE 11073-10404-2008	Pulse oximeter
IEEE 11073-10406-2011 (ISO/IEEE 11073-10406: 2012)	Basic electrocardiograph (1 to 3 lead ECG)
ISO/IEEE 11073-10407-2010 IEEE 11073-10407-2008	Blood pressure monitor
ISO/IEEE 11073-10408-2010 IEEE 11073-10408-2008	Thermometer
ISO/IEEE 11073-10415-2010 IEEE 11073-10415-2008	Weighing scale
IEEE 11073-10417-2011 (ISO/IEEE 11073-10417: 2014) IEEE 11073-10417-2010	Glucose meter
IEEE 11073-10418-2011 (ISO/IEEE 11073-10418: 2014)	International Normalized Ratio (INR) monitor
IEEE 11073-10420-2010 (ISO/IEEE 11073-10420: 2012)	Body composition analyzer
IEEE 11073-10421-2010 (ISO/IEEE 11073-10421: 2012)	Peak expiratory flow monitor (peak flow)
(draft) IEEE 11073-10424-2014	Sleep Apnea Breathing Therapy Equipment (SABTE)
(draft) IEEE 11073-10425-2014	Continuous Glucose Monitor (CGM)
(FDIS/ISO) IEEE 11073-10441-2013	Cardio fitness and activity monitor
(FDIS/ISO) IEEE 11073-10442-2008	Strength fitness equipment
IEEE 11073-10471-2010 IEEE 11073-10471-2008	Independent living activity hub
IEEE 11073-10472-2010 (ISO/IEEE 11073-10472: 2012)	Medication monitor

call requests and responses, Association Control (ACSE) and Common Management Information (CMISE). Thus, it includes algorithms for the encapsulation of the messages generated by the DIM in order to transform the abstract model into the corresponding PDUs of X73PHD.

- **Transport Technologies:** In this layer resides one of the most notable improvements within the X73PHD, compared to the X73PoC. The transport layer has to meet some security and quality conditions in order to be adopted by the standard. Thus, transport and lower layers' specifications are out of the current scope of X73PHD; although other SIGs are working towards providing new profile definitions for both wired (RJ-45 and USB) and wireless technologies (Bluetooth and ZigBee) not included inX73PoC (that only adopted IrDA and RS-232 interfaces). X73PHD defines the concept of "type of communication profile" to classify different features offered by available transport technologies. These types are:
  - ○ **Type 1:** Profiles that offer both "reliable" and "best-effort" transport services, where there shall be one or more virtual channels of reliable transport services and zero or more virtual channels of best-effort transport services.
  - ○ **Type 2:** Profiles that contain only a unidirectional transport service.
  - ○ **Type 3:** Profiles that contain only a best-effort transport service, where there shall be one or more virtual channels of best-effort transport services.

Transport Technologies

The lower levels (layers 1-4 in the OSI model) adopt the transport technologies that are outside the scope of X73PHD, although three of them have recently received a specialized medical profile for X73PHD: Universal Serial Bus Personal Health Device Class (USB PHDC), Bluetooth Personal Health Device (BT HDP) and ZigBee Health Care Profile (ZHC).

Universal Serial Bus Personal Health Device Class (USB PHDC)

USB was the first technology to publish a X73PHD-compatible profile in April 2007. Before that, USB-based health devices were forced to implement their own proprietary protocols to exchange information. This USB PHDC specification describes the full architecture that a health device and a host must support, as it is shown in Figure 4.

The specification is composed of descriptors (data structure which contains information about the device) and commands to exchange medical data. The USB PHDC profile defines a hierarchy of descriptors which can be classified into standard, class specification and optional. Within the hierarchy, endpoints are defined as a logical entity within the device to establish a connection with the host by setting logical channels (pipes). Each one has its own Quality of Service (PHDC QoS) descriptor to describe latency and reliability (Low Good, Medium Good, Medium Better, Medium Best, High Best and Very High Best) and an optional meta-data descriptor (PHDC meta-data). In addition, USB PHDC defines a set of additional endpoints implementing the above-mentioned QoS requirements: *Control endpoint* (mandatory, default bidirectional control pipe), *Bulk Out endpoint* (mandatory, path from the host to the device), *Bulk In endpoint* (mandatory, path from the device to the host) and *Interrupt In endpoint* (optional, path to the host when sending data in constant mode is necessary). The communication procedure is as follows: when a device connects to the USB bus, the host initiates the enumeration process, reads the device descriptor, and assigns a unique number (from 0 to 127) to the device. If supported, the

Figure 4. X73PHD protocol stack over USB PHDC (a), BT HDP (b) and ZHC (c)

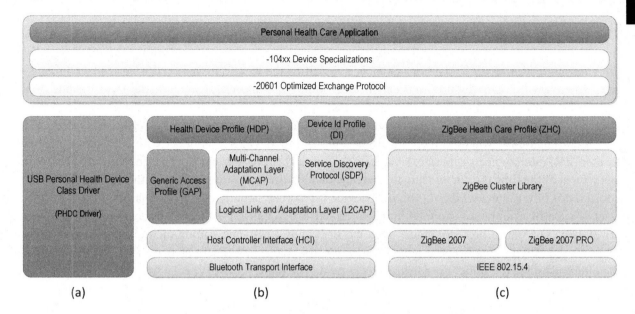

proper communication drivers will be loaded depending on which class the device belongs to. Exchanged frames can contain raw data and must not exceed 63 Kbytes.

Bluetooth Health Device Profile (BT HDP)

Typically, BT-based health devices used to be built using proprietary formats over the Serial Port Profile (SPP). To enhance homogeneity, the Bluetooth Special Interest Group (SIG) created in 2006 a Medical Working Group (MedWG) to design a specific profile for PHD. As the result of this work, the Bluetooth Health Device Profile (BT HDP) was published in June 2008 along with a new specific protocol called the Multi-Channel Adaptation Protocol (MCAP) that manages the creation of a control channel and one or more data channels. Moreover, the BT HDP includes other protocols enabling several functions, as shown in Figure 4.

Logical Link Control and Adaptation Protocol (L2CAP) define multiplexing of all higher protocols, flow control, QoS, retransmission, segmentation and reassembly of all packages. Service Discovery Protocol (SDP) manages the discovery of other BT devices and services. Generic Access Profile (GAP) defines common processes for all profiles, such as authentication and encryption. Host Controller Interface (HCI) describes commands and events which are compatible with all hardware implementations of a BT module. In BT HDP, the X73PHD terms of agent and manager are replaced by source and sink, respectively. Noteworthy features are: Enhanced Retransmission Mode (ERTM), Frame Check Sequence (FCS), reliable-type by using L2CAP ERTM mode, stream-type by using L2CAP Streaming Mode (SM), optimized reconnection (avoids redundancy) and an optional Clock Synchronization Protocol (CSP). The communication procedure begins with one of the two devices (source or sink) establishing a control channel. This channel is used only for MCAP traffic, and both devices can use it to coordinate the creation of one or more data channels to carry X73PHD traffic. Finally, one end terminates the connection, either by closing the first data channels and then the control channel, or directly closing the control channel.

ZigBee Health Care Profile (ZHC)

The ZigBee Alliance Board of Directors approved the ZHC profile in 2010, which provides a description of the device clusters containing a set of attributes that represent the state of the device along with the communication commands. For instance, it specifies the location where a device is placed using a predefined set of codes (bathroom, kitchen, bedroom, etc.), allows for manufacturers to include non-standard features using specific clusters and enables devices to send voice through the use of Voice over ZigBee Cluster. Within a ZigBee network there may be up to three types of devices: ZigBee Coordinator (ZC) controls the network and the paths to be followed by devices to connect with each other, ZigBee Router (ZR) interconnects separate devices on the network topology, and ZigBee End Device (ZED) can sleep most of the time thus increasing the average battery-life and communicate with its parent node (the coordinator or a router) while not to other devices. To create a data tunnel compatible with X73PHD, a set of specific commands grouped in the so-called 11073 Cluster Tunnel Protocol Library have been developed. The entire protocol stack is shown in Figure 4 (c). The communication procedure begins when two X73PHD tunnels are established. In one, the manager behaves as the server and the agent as the client, while in the other, the roles are reciprocal. The manager then checks whether an agent has set a X73PHD profile and generates a connection request. The agent will respond with a connected status notification from which they can exchange X73PHD frames. The fact that all profiles are defined using clusters of the ZigBee Cluster Library (ZCL) allows reusing clusters used by multiple profiles.

TRENDS AND CHALLENGES OF E-HEALTH INTEROPERABILITY

Throughout the last two decades, the focus about trends and challenges of e-Health is not only on basic issues related to healthcare such as universal access and equity, but also on quality of care and progressive delivery concepts such as people-centered care. With the increase in affordability among a large section of the population, there is an increased demand for care to be delivered and monitored in a technologically enabled environment. With the most recent advances in e-Health, this need has led to a sharp growth in manufacturing from multinational medical device companies. With a greater number of healthcare providers embracing technology in their care delivery process, this growth is estimated to only increase in the near future. However, extensive use of such medical devices has their own set of challenges, with interoperability leading the chart because it does not brings only about standardization of the care delivery and monitoring processes, but also paves the way for equitable healthcare. In addition to these, adoption of interoperability standards would provide a chance for medical devices manufacturers to take their products onto the international market, thereby driving revenues through exports (Rodrigues, R., 2008).

However, the issue of interoperability is missing from the agenda of the industry and the policy makers alike. This is the reason why the efforts for several years on promoting standardization from international initiatives, organizations, research groups and institutions such as Health Level Seven International (HL7), Integrating the Healthcare Enterprise (IHE), National Institute of Standards and Technology (NIST), Healthcare Information and Management Systems Society (HIMSS) and Continua Health Alliance, among others as ISO, IEEE and CEN, have been decisive to overcome the interoperability problem and promote a homogeneous e-Health ecosystem (Jean J.H. et al., 2013).

HL7 has over 2300 members including 500 corporate members covering more than 90% of information system providers in the healthcare sector. They provide all-embracing frameworks and standards for digital exchange of information between healthcare systems. HL7 strives to improve knowledge transfer between healthcare providers, government agencies, the vendor community, fellow SDOs and patients.

IHE has its main aim to make quality, efficiency and safety of clinical care better by making relevant health care information easily available to both providers and patients. One of the main reasons for its existence is to profile HL7 messages and trim down the range of implementation possibilities allowed by HL7, making IHE compliment systems more predictable in content and form.

NIST collaborates with IHE on testing compatibility of HL7 messages to IHE Patient Care Device (PCD) domain profiles and works with ISO/IEEE11073 committees (ISO, IEEE, CEN and PHDWG), and also with the IHE PCD Point-of-care Integration Work Group and the Continua Health Alliance on producing software tools for constructing models of device capabilities.

Continua Health Alliance is a consortium comprising over 200 companies dedicated mainly to ensure interoperability of personal connected health solutions for better patient care. The principle is to extend and to apply these connected solutions for enabling independence and empowering individuals to better manage their health and wellness needs in a home based setting. Their core domain is in establishing design guidelines for manufacturing home networks, health and wellness services and tele-health platforms. They also certify products, allowing them for including their logo after the certification, what enables recognizing of interoperability of such devices. It also collaborates with government regulatory agencies and leaders in healthcare industry.

HIMSS is a non-profit organization focused on providing global leadership for the optimal use of information technology (IT) and management systems for the betterment of healthcare. HIMSS represents nearly 50.000 individual members, of which more than two-thirds work in healthcare provider, governmental and non-profit organizations. HIMSS frames and leads healthcare practices and public policy through its content expertise, professional development, research initiatives and media vehicles, which are designed to promote information and management systems' contributions for improving the quality, safety, access and cost-effectiveness of patient care.

Recently, Continua Health Alliance, HIMSS and the m-Health Summit (the largest event of m-Health that convenes a diverse international delegation to explore the limits of mobile and connected health, including technology, business, research and policy for mobile, wireless, digital, wearable, telehealth, gaming, connected health and consumer engagement) have founded Personal Connected Health Alliance (PCHA). PCHA is a global non-profit group focused on personalized connected health solutions to offer a unique perspective and expertise: combining to create a holistic view and approach for promoting the advancement of healthcare technologies that focus on the person. Their aim is joining together healthcare providers, device makers, technology providers, governments and consumers to create a global framework for healthcare, in which the individuals play a central role in managing their health.

With all these premises, the trends for next decades of e-Health monitoring is clear that will be focused on bringing the health and wellness paradigm in today society, driving advancements in mobile and communications technologies, and on the growing use of new devices, health trackers and apps by consumers and healthcare providers. Thanks to readily-available consumer technologies (such as smart, wearables and health devices), people are taking charge of their health and wellness, accessing their personal health data, receiving targeted health and wellness education, consulting with healthcare providers and gaining support from friends and family to improve their health (Matysiewicz, J., 2009).

There is the need for generating greater awareness, availability and access to plug-and-play, consumer-friendly personal health technologies to empower individuals to better manage their health and wellness, anywhere at any time. And e-Health monitoring technologies face some challenges to ensure that they are user-friendly, secure and can easily collect, display and relay personal health data. Thus, these new perspectives will put "consumer first" at the center of focus and will promote the global adoption, standardization and appropriate regulation of newest health devices and systems to empower people to self-manage their health. Besides, they will create stronger links between not only healthcare providers, consumers and their social networks but regulators, government agencies and industry to create the technology ecosystem required to deliver on the promise of personal, connected and interoperable e-Health paradigm (Hardiker, N., 2011).

CONCLUSION

This chapter accomplishes a complete review of the ISO/IEEE11073 family of standards for interoperable communication of Medical Devices and Personal Health Devices.

The first version was proposed to address communication on Intensive Care Unit (ICU) scenarios focused on the Point-of-Care of the patient, leading to X73PoC. But, along with other handicaps, this standard was considered too complex, therefore it was not adopted by the industry.

The emerging of new transport technologies (such as USB, Bluetooth or ZigBee) and the increasing popularity of personal and patient-oriented health devices and applications led to the development of a more lightweight version for Personal Health Devices: X73PHD, based on X73PoC but simpler, and delegating some of the security and quality transport constraints to lower layers, outside of the scope of X73PHD.

Indeed, some of the transport technologies on which X73PHD would be based have defined specific profiles for medical devices, such as the Universal Serial Bus Personal Health Device Class, the Bluetooth Personal Health Device and the ZigBee Health Care Profile.

The main challenge for the next years is still on the interoperability, and a number of international organizations and institutions like Health Level Seven International (HL7), Integrating the Healthcare Enterprise (IHE), National Institute of Standards and Technology (NIST), Healthcare Information and Management Systems Society (HIMSS) and Continua Health Alliance are committing efforts to overcome the interoperability problem and promote an homogeneous e-Health ecosystem.

And with all these premises, the trends for next decades of e-Health monitoring is clear that will be focused on bringing the health and wellness paradigm in today society, driving advancements in mobile and communications technologies, and on the growing use of new devices, health trackers and apps by consumers and healthcare providers.

REFERENCES

BT HDP. (2008). *Bluetooth Health Device Profile version 1.0.* BT HDP (retrieved from http://www.bluetooth.com/Research%20and%20White%20Papers/HDP_Implementation_WP_V10.pdf)

CEN PHDWG. (2015). *Comiteé European Normalisation. Technical Comiteé CEN/TC251. Personal Health Devices Working Group.* CEN PHDWG. Retrieved from http://www.cen.eu

Continua. (2015). *Continua Health Alliance* (retrieved from http://www.continuaalliance.org/home)

Hardiker, N., & Grant, M. (2011). Factors that influence public engagement with eHealth: A literature review. *International Journal of Medical Informatics*, *80*(1), 1–12. doi:10.1016/j.ijmedinf.2010.10.017 PMID:21112244

Haux, R. (2010). Medical informatics: Past, present, future. *International Journal of Medical Informatics*, *79*(9), 599–610. doi:10.1016/j.ijmedinf.2010.06.003 PMID:20615752

Hovenga, E. J. S., Kidd, M. R., Garde, S., & Cossio, C. H. L. (2010). *Health Informatics: An Overview*. Amsterdam, The Netherlands: IOS Press.

IEEE 11073-20101. (2004). *IEEE Standard for Health Informatics - Point-Of-Care Medical Device Communication - Part 20101: Application Profile - Base Standard*. IEEE. Retrieved from http://standards.ieee.org/findstds/standard/11073-20101-2004.html

IEEE 11073-20601. (2008). *ISO/IEC/IEEE Health informatics - Personal health device communication - Part 20601: Application profile - Optimized exchange protocol*. IEEE. Retrieved from http:// standards.ieee.org/ findstds/ standard/11073-20601-2008.html

IEEE INTERMED. (2004). *IEEE Standard for Health Informatics - Interoperability of patient connected medical devices - ENV13735 - CEN/TC251*. INTERMED. IEEE. Retrieved from http://standards.ieee.org/ findstds/ standard/1073.2.1.1-2004.html

IEEE VITAL. (2004). *IEEE Standard for Health Informatics - Vital signs information Representation*. IEEE. Retrieved from http://standards.ieee.org/findstds/standard/1073.1.1.1-2004.html

Jacob, J. M. (2012, April). *Develop Medical Devices with Real Interoperability to Any Application, Any Device, Any Where*. Paper presented at the Interconnected Health 2012 Conference, Rosemont, IL.

Jean, J. H. (2013). Performance Analysis of Smart Healthcare System Based on ISO/IEEE 11073 and HL7. *LNCS*, *235*, 1045–1053.

Kennelly, R. J., & Gardner, R. M. (1997). Perspectives on development of IEEE 1073: The Medical Information Bus (MIB) standard. *International Journal of Clinical Monitoring and Computing*, *14*(3), 143–149. doi:10.1023/A:1016930319825 PMID:9387003

Leone, A. (2011, January 28). An embedded solution for medical device interoperability. *EE Times*. Retrieved from http://www.eetimes.com/document.asp?doc_id=1278537

Martínez, I. (2010). Seamless Integration of ISO/IEEE11073 Personal Health Devices and ISO/EN13606 Electronic Health Records into an End-to-End Interoperable Solution. *Telemedicine Journal and e-Health*, *16*(10), 993–1004. doi:10.1089/tmj.2010.0087 PMID:21087123

Matysiewicz, J., & Smyczek, S. (2009). *Consumer Trust - Challenge for E-healthcare. Fourth International Conference on Cooperation and Promotion of Information Resources in Science and Technology (COINFO 2009)*. doi:10.1109/COINFO.2009.40

Perficient. (2014). *System Interoperability for Healthcare*. Retrieved from: https://www.perficient.com/Industries/Healthcare/System-Interoperability

Rodrigues, R. (2008). *Compelling issues for adoption of e-health*. The Commonwealth Health Ministers Reference Book. Retrieved from http://www.ehealthstrategies.com/files/Commonwealth_MOH_Apr08.pdf

Trigo, J. D., Chiarugi, F., Alesanco, Á., Martínez-Espronceda, M., Serrano, L., Chronaki, C. E., & García, J. et al. (2010). Interoperability in Digital Electrocardiology: Harmonization of ISO/IEEE x73-PHD and SCP-ECG. *IEEE Transactions on Information Technology in Biomedicine, 14*(6), 1303–1317. doi:10.1109/TITB.2010.2064330 PMID:20699215

USB PHDC. (2007). *Implementers Forum, Inc. Universal Serial Bus Device Class Definition for Personal Healthcare Devices version 1.0*. USB PHDC. Retrieved from http://www.usb.org

Walker, J., Pan, E., Johnston, D., Adler-Milstein, J., Bates, D.W. & Middleton, B., (2005, January). *The value of health care information exchange and interoperability*. Boston, MA: Center for Information Technology Leadership.

Willmitch, B., Golembeski, S., Kim, S. S., Nelson, L. D., & Gidel, L. (2012, February). Clinical outcomes after telemedicine intensive care unit implementation. *Critical Care Medicine, 40*(2), 450–454. doi:10.1097/CCM.0b013e318232d694 PMID:22020235

ZHC. (2010). *ZigBee Health Care Profile specification version 1.0*. ZHC. Retrieved from http://www.zigbee.org

Lative Logic Accomodating the WHO Family of International Classifications

E

Patrik Eklund
Umeå University, Sweden

INTRODUCTION

Traditional logic is informal about the production of terms and sentences, and even worse, often avoids to clearly describe how terms latively appear in sentences, i.e., how sentences proceed from terms, and are in fact constructed using terms. Continuing that lativity towards entailment and provability, it is clear that sentences appear in provability, but provability as a statement should not be seen as a sentence. This creates self-referentiality which leads to peculiar situations, both theoretically as well as in WHO's classifications on health.

Logic, as a structure, contains signatures, terms, sentences, theoremata (as structured sets of sentences, or 'structured premises'), entailments, algebras, satisfactions, axioms, theories and proof calculi. This chapter also shows how the notion of signature often needs to be expanded to levels of signatures, in particular when dealing with type constructors. Lative logic produces a huge potential of applications using terminology, nomenclature and ontology in particular in social and health care. WHO classifications are logically lative. The reference classifications ICD and ICF then appear in structured relation with each other. Similar transformations can be made for the derived classifications as well as for the related classifications ICPC-2, ICECI, ISO9999, ATC/DDD and ICNP.

Formal mappings, e.g., between ICD and ICF are rare, and this is mostly due to a lack of understanding terminology and nomenclature as terms in a logic. ATC/DDD for drugs embraces 'dose' but not 'intervention', which means that drug-drug interactions are possible to describe whereas drug-condition is more complicated. IHTSDO's SNOMED CT subdivides 'concepts' within its hierarchy consisting e.g. of clinical findings disorders, body structure, pharmaceutical/biologic product, social context, staging and scales, and qualifier values, but has been developed only with intuitive connections with WHO classifications. Further, SNOMED's assumption that "health ontology" needs the same or a similar underlying logic as "web ontology", is a fatal mistake not promoting the "dialogue and interrelation of classifications and nomenclature" in useful application oriented directions.

The pillars and underlying observations of the chapter are the following:

- Modern type theory is not formal enough to recognize the need to arrange type constructors in a level of signatures.
- This provides tools to establish generalized relations as formal concepts, and also as substitution theory required to manage nomenclature and ontology in health care.
- Signatures and terms for nomenclatures and terms are in turn building blocks used in sentences that appear in guidelines and recommendations in social and health care.
- WHO and other international organizations as well as national authorities do not embrace a formal logic that is required in particular to develop relations and mapping between nomenclatures.

DOI: 10.4018/978-1-4666-9978-6.ch051

There are lots of "Yes, we can!" claims within authorities and industry about such nomenclatures and their intertwining, and this chapter very clearly shows "No, you cannot!, unless we first properly clean the logic mess appearing around nomenclatures in health.

The lack of regional strategies together with scattered and unstructured guidelines for prevention, detection and intervention related to older persons decline in cognitive and functional capabilities is the most serious threats against a sustainable development of supportive environments for the older persons. Further, the lack of well-structured guidelines and well-organized utility of assessment and, in particular, rigorous assessment based decision-making and care provisioning, leads to overlaps and inefficiency, and even worse, to subjective decision-making and care processes that cannot be measured nor evaluated. Socio-economic modelling of the social welfare effect due to demographic change is therefore of utmost importance, on the one hand, for municipality resource planning and objective decision making, and on the other hand, for enabling required accuracy of business models as used by public and private actors in the social sector.

This chapter is structured as follows. We first provide some examples and nomenclature detail related to fall risk and fall injuries. These descriptions are not intended to be complete from the viewpoint of the whole spectrum of fall risk factor, but rather serve to provide a few examples of terminology related to risk factures and fall related injuries. We then proceed to discuss the "osteoporosis fractures dogma", which is a debate to what extent fractures for older persons is more or less related to weak bone. This also includes an example of ICD encoding of a particular type of fracture. This reveals some logical problems involved when countries develop their own extensions to the core ICD nomenclature. Functioning is thereafter discussed in detail for the ICF nomenclature where the generic scale as related to kind of an uncertainty attachment is important. A brief survey of typing and lativity in logic concludes the chapter.

FALL AND FALL INJURIES

Fall prevention and fall risk is largely treated in the literature, but it is surprising that the traditional definition of fall is very shallow. This is very critical since cohorts and studies dealing with target groups and populations need to adapt to more specific definitions. This then often means that studies are not comparable. The literature does provide logically strict definitions of falls [Lach et al 1991], which prevents the use of those data in potentially comparable studies. Therefore, the operational definition of a fall is highly important. However, even if there are many different types of falls definitions, this does not necessarily mean we should aim at a simplified version of a definition. The definition of fall is very important to understand as the definition used in studies determines when observations for risk factors are registered and how falls and non-falls are discriminated.[1]

Although there is still no universally accepted definition or consensus as to what a fall should be, some definitions are more popular than others. In 1987 the Kellogg International Working Group on the prevention of falls in the elderly defined a fall as "an unintentionally coming to the ground or some lower level as a consequence of sustaining a violent blow, loss of consciousness, sudden onset of paralysis as in stroke or an epileptic seizure". Since then, many researchers have used this or very similar definitions of a fall. Depending on the focus of study, however, some researchers have used a broader definition of falls to include those that occur as a result of dizziness and syncope. The Kellogg definition is appropriate for studies aimed at identifying factors that impair sensorimotor function and balance control, whereas the broader definition is appropriate for studies that also address cardiovascular causes of falls such as postural hypotension and transient ischaemic attacks. WHO defines falls more broadly as "an unexpected event in which the participant comes to rest on the ground, floor or lower level", and indeed without excluding particular events as in Kellogg's definition. The NICE (2004) definition is similar to WHO, defining fall as "an event whereby an individual comes to rest on the ground or another lower level with or without loss of consciousness". In summary, a fall could be defined as an unintentionally coming to the ground or some lower level from standing, sitting or horizontal position with or without loss of consciousness and with or without injury, excluding intentional change in position to rest in furniture, wall or other objects.

It is important to point out the distinction between fall and consequence of fall, where a fall injury is an example of such a consequence. This distinction separates falls from injuries caused by falls, so that selections of data records for more general-purpose analysis is done based on well-founded definitions of falls without too specific relations to injuries resulting from falls. As an example, injury types related to drop attacks are expected to be different from injury types caused by fall due to dysequilibrium.

As the definition of fall is hard to provide, the definition of previous falls is even harder, as these data are usually collected from different sources like medical records, various care providers, or from patients themselves and family members. The definition of falls among these sources is obviously not unique, and e.g. the number of previous falls is often really hard to estimate. Interventions must focus on the cause of the fall, not the precipitation of it.

Precipitations lead to findings related to causes, and thereby to suggestions of interventions. The effect of interventions targets the cause but is often measured at precipitation. It is further important to realize that fall risk assessment is embraced by more general assessment of function and cognition, in turn embedded in the overall scope and content of medical and social data, so we must not isolate risk factors of fall and risk assessments of fall from more general assessments of function and cognition. The structure of general assessments is in some sense easier as there is a larger consensus about general assessments scales [Burns et al 2009]. Concerning fall risk assessment the situation has not reached the same level of consensus.

Severity degree of injury and degree of harm can be view in the context of the conceptual framework for the *International Classification for Patient Safety* (ICPS), where the degree of harm is defined as follows:

- **None:** Patient outcome is not symptomatic or no symptoms detected and no treatment is required.
- **Mild:** Patient outcome is symptomatic, symptoms are mild, loss of function or harm is minimal or intermediate but short term, and no or minimal intervention (e.g., extra observation, investigation, review or minor treatment) is required.

Figure 1. Distinction between cause and precipitation of falls

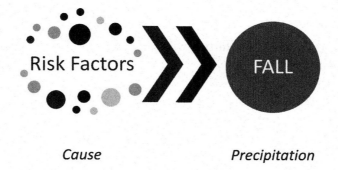

Cause   Precipitation

- **Moderate:** Patient outcome is symptomatic, requiring intervention (e.g., additional operative procedure; additional therapeutic treatment), an increased length of stay, or causing permanent or long term harm or loss of function.
- **Severe:** Patient outcome is symptomatic, requiring life-saving intervention or major surgical/ medical intervention, shortening life expectancy or causing major permanent or long term harm or loss of function
- **Death:** On balance of probabilities, death was caused or brought forward in the short term by the incident.

The important logical aspect here is the invocation of uncertainty considerations.

FALL RISK AND RISK ASSESSMENT

Systematic considerations of fall risk factors were initiated in 1960 [Sheldon 1960]. There are many well-known contributions [Downton 1993, Lord et al 2007, Tinetti et al 1986] to descriptions of fall risk, but there is no harmonized nomenclature. Further, the hierarchical structure of such nomenclatures cannot be claimed to be unique. However, in order to enable different levels of granularity in various structures of datasets for falls, the structure of fall risk factors indeed needs to be hierarchical rather than 'flat'. The hierarchical structure, however, does not in itself suffice to provide a correct and complete ontology structure of risk factors. In fact, the hierarchical listing is even inappropriate as, on the one hand, it doesn't explicitly reveal overlaps, and, on the other hand, it does not come with any typing or terminology whatsoever of the risk factors. The latter means that there is no distinction made e.g. between risk factors and clusters and groups of risk factors.

Examples of items in a hierarchical listing in this chapter shows pieces of a summary [Eklund 2012] of risk factors extracted from the relevant literature on risk factors for falls. Listing of risk factors should aim at being fairly broad and reasonably covering, and in fact kind of a *consensus listing* from fall risk factor ontology point of view.

Fall risk assessment need to be seen as part of or complementary to a more broad geriatric assessment [Eklund 2009]. A set of assessment scales usually comprises of some ADL (Activities of Daily Living) scales combined with suitable cognitive scales like MMSE. Combination scales, like the CDR (Clinical Dementia Rating) for ADL/DEMENTIA, are also widely used in particular in connection with assessments related to dementia syndromes. Non-cognitive signs are captured e.g. by NPI (Neuropsychiatric Inventory), CMAI (Cohen-Mansfield Agitation Inventory) and BEHAVE-AD. Depression is usually captured in its own right as a non-cognitive aspect of dementia, where e.g GDS (Geriatric Depression Scale) is widely used in home care. Depression is known to correlate with fear of fall, and depression also accelerates cognitive decline. Nutrition scales are important, as are the scales for social conditions, and so on and so forth.

Concerning risk factors for falls, and starting with postural control, part of a hierarchical description could be as in the following:

- Impaired postural stability (including standing, leaning, stepping, perturbation).
- Gait pattern of limb movement and gait characteristics:
  - Level walking (including gait velocity, variability in cadence, step length).
  - Stair walking.

Figure 2. The Observe-Assess-Decide (OAD) scope of geriatric and fall risk assessment

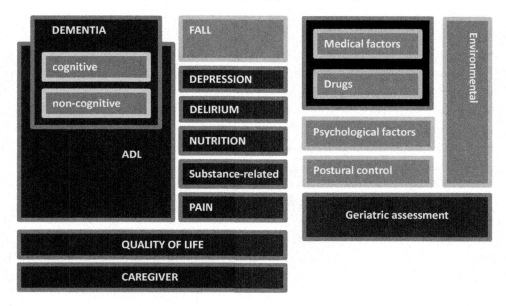

- ○ Tripping and slipping.
- ○ Stepping over and obstacle avoiding.
- Muscle functions (ICF b730-b749):
  - ○ Muscle power functions (b730):
    - ▪ Power of isolated muscles and muscle groups (b7300).
    - ▪ …
  - ○ Muscle tone functions (b735).
  - ○ Muscle endurance functions (b740).
  - ○ …

As a further example in these respects, near tandem standing (standing with one foot in front of the other) [Lord et al 1999], unipedal standing (standing on one foot) [Vellas et al 1997], and forward leaning ability [Duncan et al 1992] have all been shown to clearly discriminate between fallers and non-fallers.

The effect of drugs of falls, and in a multifactorial setting, has been extensively studied. Psychotropics, opiates and potent anticholinergics have been identified as fall-risk-increasing drugs (FRIDs) in a sub-analysis [Salonoja et al 2012] of a randomized, controlled multifactorial fall prevention study. These studies are very detailed about use of particular FRIDs. The psychotropics included were antidepressives (N06A, N06CA01), antipsychotics (N05A), BZDs/BZDRDs (A03CA, N03AE01, N05BA, N05CD, N05CF, N06CA01, R06AE53, M09AA72) and others (N05BE01). Opioids (N02A) and potent anticholinergic drugs (A03CA02, A03CA05, C01BA01, G04BD04, G04BD07 G04BD08, G04BD09, M03BC51, N04AA02, N05BB01, R01BA52) were additionally seen as possible FRIDs.

Part of a hierarchical view of drug related risk factors are then as follows:

- C cardiovascular system:
  - ○ C01 cardiac therapy:
    - ▪ C01A cardiac glycosides -> C01AA digitalis glycosides -> C01AA05 digoxin
  - ○ C02 antihypertensives.

- ○ C03 diuretics:
  - ▪ C03A thiazide diuretics -> C03AA thiazides -> C03AA01 bendroflumethiazide.
- N nervous system:
  - ○ N02 analgesics.
  - ○ N05 psycholeptics:
    - ▪ N05A antipsychotics.
    - ▪ N05B anxiolytics -> N05BA benzodiazepine derivatives -> N05BA01 diazepam, long-acting drug for insomnia.
    - ▪ N05C hypnotics and sedatives -> N05CD benzodiazepine derivatives -> N05CD02 nitrazepam, long-acting drug for insomnia.
    - ▪ N05C hypnotics and sedatives -> N05CF benzodiazepine related drugs -> N05CF02 zolpidem, short-acting drug for insomnia.
  - ○ N06 psychoanaleptics.

Medical factors include vision (glaucoma, cataracts, macular degeneration) and neurological problems (stroke, Parkinson's disease, vestibular pathologies like Benign Paroxysmal Positional, Menières disease and vestibular neuronitis). Neural failure of postural control in turn is related to syncope, which in turn is due to cardiovascular problems like ventricular tachycardia, orthostatic hypotension or transient ischaemic attack.

For fall risk assessment we need to be careful when we distinguish between individual risk factors and factors as they appear in risk assessment scales. A value or estimation for risk factor is different from a value or estimation for risk assessment scale. *Impaired postural stability* is a risk factor or a risk factor group, whereas the *Berg Balance Scale* (BBS) is and risk assessment scale. Items in a scale, like 'foot on stool' may relate to risk factors chosen e.g. under the group *impaired postural stability*. Use of drugs like *sedatives* is a fall risk factor in itself, but appears also as an item e.g. in Downton's Fall Risk Index (DFRI). This is an interesting situation where DFRI uses 'sedatives' as a notion on ATC level 3, without making any distinction between FRIDs as described on ATC levels 4 and 5. A more formal modelling of data and information requires being quite precise and logical about data types. The use of "sedatives" in DFRI is of type no/yes, and the granularity is therefore very coarse. It doesn't e.g. provide any difference between long-acting and short-acting benzodiazepine derivatives, knowing that psychotropic drugs are targeted in revisions of pharmacologic treatments, and are in some cases subject to consideration of withdrawal. MMSE as an assessment scale for cognitive decline appears by its value as an item in many risk assessment scales. These are just some examples showing how risk assessments are not at all harmonized with respect to the items used in respective scales and questionnaires. Similar and more examples could be provided for such "abuse" of logical language related to the utility of assessment scales and questionnaires.

There is indeed a wide range of fall risk assessment scales and screening tools. Here's a short (and incomplete) list:

- Fall Risk Assessment and Screening Tools:
  - ○ Downton Fall Risk Index.
  - ○ Falls Risk for Older People in the Community (FROP-COM).
  - ○ Falls Risk Assessment Tool (FRAT).
- Fall Risk Factor Assessment and Screening Tools:
  - ○ Timed Up-and-Go test (TUGT).

○ Performance Oriented Balance and Mobility Assessment (POMA).
○ Berg Balance Scale (BBS).
○ Alternate Step Test (AST).
○ Sit-to-Stand test with five repetitions (STS5).
○ Functional Reach Test.
○ Physiological Profile Assessment (PPA).

BONE MINERAL DENSITY AND FRACTURES

It is indeed very important to distinguish between "fall risk" and "fall injury risk", the latter being related to bone mineral density (BMD) and fractures. There is a further distinction to be made between osteoporosis and osteopenia, the former being defined as BMD of two and a half standard deviations, the so called T-score, from normal bone mass, and the latter refers to a condition where BMD is lower than normal but not as low as being classified as osteoporosis.

The osteoporotic focus mainly claims that fractures among older person are mainly caused by bone fragility, and therefore lowering risk of fractures concentrates on bone-targeted pharmacotherapy. Strontium ranelates and alendronates are typically prescribed, where strontium ranelates have been seen to have better effect on improving BMD, but recent recommendations point out the higher risk of myocardial infarction when using strontium ranelates. Alendronates may on the other hand cause severe bone, muscle and joint pain, which obviously is counterproductive to exercising.

The antithetic focus says that falling, not osteoporosis, is the most important factor for fractures among older persons, and therefore lowering risk of fractures is most suitably done by lowering risk of fall.

This chapter suggests to adopt a focus a fall risk factors regardless of the debate between two fall injury risk dogmatic views. This then also means that we explicitly say that we cannot lean on and comply only with the FRAX® view related to drug treatment of osteopenia. Strontium ranelates and alendronates are typically prescribed, where strontium ranelates have been seen to have better effect on improving BMD, but recent recommendations point out the higher risk of myocardial infarction when using strontium ranelates. Alendronates may on the other hand cause severe bone, muscle and joint pain, which obviously is counterproductive to exercising.

The antithetic focus as compared with the 'osteoporotic fractures' dogma says that falling, not osteoporosis, is the most important factor for fractures among older persons, and therefore lowering risk of fractures is most suitably done by lowering risk of fall. This deliverable has a focus a fall risk factors regardless of the debate between these two fall injury risk dogmatic views. Clearly, in this deliverable we lean more on the view that falling is the most important reason for fractures, since otherwise this deliverable would be basically obsolete.

From datasets and information structures point of view, the encoding of fractures involves some subtleties which need to be recognized before discussing the potential of international databases. Encoding builds upon common ICD-10 diagnosis encoding, but also in presence of national modifications. In the following we use the Australian, German, Swedish and US modifications as examples.

If we look at fractures of the forearm, in ICD-10 we have

S52: Fracture of forearm.
S52.5: Fracture of lower end of radius.

and ICD-10 doesn't go deeper than that in these specific codes. The ICD-10-CM adopted in the US goes further in direction of

S52.53: Colles' fracture of radius.
S52.532: Colles' fracture of left radius.
S52.532D: Colles' fracture of left radius, subsequent encounter for closed fracture with routine healing.

where "3" for 'Colles' means dorsal displacement, "2" after "53" means 'left arm', and "D" means subsequent encounter for closed fracture with routine healing.

The underlying logic for encoding ICD and in particular as involving fractures is now not trivial, since we first need to decide about some informal format for statements like "... fell, because..." and "... fracture of type..., with healing...". An encoding favouring the latter statement may exclude the possibility to support the former, and indeed would not support the unification of encoding related both to "fall risk" as well as "fall injury risk".

A logically somewhat dubious adaptation is the ICD-10

M84: Disorders of continuity of bone.
M84.4: Pathological fracture, not elsewhere classified, where "not elsewhere classified" almost says "where no injury types apply", corresponding to ICF's "8" in its generic scale of quantifiers. Strangely enough, the CM version also has:
M84.40XD: subsequent encounter for fracture with routine healing where, however, the 'open/closed' is not present. Therefore,
S52.53-G: Colles' fracture of radius, subsequent encounter for closed fracture with delayed healing without specifying left or right arm, appears to be logically "quite equivalent" to

[S52.53 Colles' fracture of radius]

AND

[M84.40XD subsequent encounter for fracture with routine healing]

or to

[S52.53 Colles' fracture of radius]

WITH

[M84.40XD subsequent encounter for fracture with routine healing]

Here obviously the latter WITH is a candidate logical operator, and it is obviously not all that unique. The CM version further says "M84.40XD is a billable ICD-10-CM code that can be used to specify a diagnosis", so economy enters a clinical setting. This mixture of concept is logically quite *ad hoc*, and it is hard to syntactically separate the codes without a logically more formal approach for this reference classification. From fall risk and fall injury risk point of view, encoding e.g. involving ICD, ICF and ATC is therefore clearly very important.

CLASSIFICATION OF FUNCTIONING

ICF is quite specific concerning typing and also uncertainties related to truth values. In ICF, there is a 5-scale, so that e.g. "Power of muscles of all limbs (b7304)" is not just a matter of yes/no. In ICF, the set of logical truth degrees are shown in Table 1.

This means e.g. that an environmental risk factor like 'obstructed walkway' could use the ICF logical truth degrees in order to express presence of that risk factor e.g. in terms of 'mildly obstructed walkway' or 'severely obstructed walkway'.

The degrees xxx.0 to xxx.4 can be seen as an ordered set of truth degrees including five points, where it is tempting to say that 'xxx.0' is logically 'false' and 'xxx.4' is logically 'true'. However, this binding should not be done at a syntax level, but may be considered on a semantic level. Note that there is, from implementation point of view, an important distinction to be made between 'xxx.8 not specified' and 'xxx.9 not applicable', the former basically saying that a truth degree has yet not been provided, and the latter basically saying that the typing of the factor is not applicable. Note also that 'xxx.8 not specified' is not split into the meanings of "deliberately not specified" in the sense of "possibly never to be specified (even if applicable)" and "not yet specified" in the sense "not yet, but most probably later".

In [Eklund et al 2014] we presented theoretical benefits of using quantales as the algebraic structure for representing such generic scales. The main advantage is that logical terms can be formally constructed over a categorical domain that integrates uncertainty models within that underlying domain. That domain n turn builds upon underlying signatures (sorts and operators). This logic consideration goes far beyond much simpler logical adaptations e.g. of description logic as an underlying logic for health ontology, as appearing in SNOMED.

If 'not specified' is represented by the unital 'e' in an underlying quantale with 5-valued set {F, a, b, c, T} of truth values, corresponding to the ICF valuations, then a first observation is that the unital can appear in different relations with respect to the other values.

A further observation is that a non-commutative situation may be adopted for combining values in that generic scale. The example involving AND and WITH in connection with fracture codes clearly suggests that AND is commutative, but WITH is non-commutative. Assessment scales ignore this situation completely as item values are converted to numbers, and a typical approach is simply to add those numbers. Addition is commutative, so non-commutative phenomena will never be made explicit.

As an example of providing terminology for muscle function related fall risk, we may use e.g. ICF's neuromusculoskeletal and movement-related functions, including functions of the joints and bones (ICF b710-b729), *muscle functions* (ICF b730-b749), and movement functions (b750-b789). Muscle functions in turn subdivide in ICF e.g. into *muscle power functions* (b730), muscle tone functions (b735) and muscle

Table 1.

xxx.0 NO problem	(none, absent, negligible,…)	0-4%
xxx.1 MILD problem	(slight, low,…)	5-24%
xxx.2 MODERATE problem	(medium, fair,…)	25-49%
xxx.3 SEVERE problem	(high, extreme, …)	50-95%
xxx.4 COMPLETE problem	(total,…)	96-100%
xxx.8 not specified		
xxx.9 not applicable		

Figure 3. The unital as 'not specififed' in the quantale for ICF's generic scale

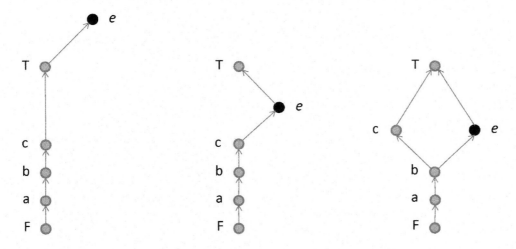

endurance functions (b740). Muscle power functions subdivides further, e.g. with *power of muscles of all limbs* (b7304) being a specific muscle power function for which no further subdivision is provided within ICF. Power of muscles of all limbs related to *the force generated by the contraction of muscles and muscle groups of all four limbs*, and inclusions are impairments such as *tetraparesis* and *tetraplegia*.

LATIVE LOGIC

Lativity in logic, aiming to be careful about self-referentiality, is two-fold. On the one hand, metalanguage and object language should not be mixed. On other hand, within a language we indeed have a lativity between words and sentences, and so on, and for logic languages, also between truth and provability, the latter building upon proof rules. In logic, we should indeed be lative, respectively, when dealing with the ingredients of logic.

The role of signatures, i.e., sorts and operators, is fundamental for sortedness aspects. For ATC codes, respective levels also need to be typed. According to the three-level arrangement of signatures [Eklund et al 2014], with the second level involving type constructors, we may define a typing on level two as

1st, 2nd, 3rd, 4th, 5th: -> type

and on signature level three we would include

PharmacologicIntervention: -> P(3rd)

indicating that PharmacologicIntervention is a set of pharmacological subgroup items (on ATC level 3). We may further specify

DrugPrescriptions: -> P(5th)

indicating that DrugPrescriptions is a set of 5th level ATC items, i.e., a set of drugs. The operator P appear as a powertype constructor on the level two

P: type -> type

of the three-level arrangement of signatures. Further, we need specifications like

hypnotics_and_sedatives: -> 3rd

benzodiazepine_derivatives: -> 4th

nitrazepam: -> 5th

and additionally, which is often overlooked, we need transformations between the ATC levels.

5to4: 5th -> 4th

4to3: 4th -> 3rd

5to3: 5th -> 3rd

This then makes a clear distinction between nitrazepam as a term of type 5th and 5to3(nitrazepam) as a sedative of type 3rd. Further, for a variable drug of type 5th, we can make a substitution with nitrazepam, because the types match, but we cannot substitute with hypnotics_and_sedatives. For

Downton's DFRI the consequence is that 5to3(nitrazepam) may appear as a value in the scale, but not drug. This is also important in considerations of uncertainty. A relative to a patient may be fairly sure about hypnotics_and_sedatives, but not all that certain about that sedative being a benzodiazepine_derivatives. Additional operators is required to capture the notion of uncertainty being carried over between ATC levels.

Similar specifications can be done for ICD and ICF, where again the powerset type constructor becomes important, and even other type constructor when we need a richer structure than that enabled by relations only. Relations can be described by mappings to powersets, so enriching relations with more algebraic structure means that we need to specify corresponding richer versions of powerset type constructors. This would be a key method also for enriching the description logic based ontology of SNOMED, but nothing in this direction has been observed or desired. This is a huge disadvantage of SNOMED.

Basically what we say is that generality and universality of language is not enough. We need lativity, both internally and externally. Internal lativity is what we respect concerning the ingredients of logic, as we have pointed out concerning the underlying category of sorts, and terms being integrated into sentences. External lativity relates to the relation between metalanguage and object language. In universality we start from something smaller and concrete, and then we provide abstraction.

REFERENCES

Burns, A., Lawlor, B., & Craig, S. (2009). *Assessment Scales in Old Age Psychiatry* (2nd ed.). Informa Healthcare.

Downton, J. H. (1993). *Falls in the Elderly*. Edward Arnold.

Duncan, P. W., Studenski, S., Chandler, J., & Prescott, B. (1992). Functional reach: Predictive validity in a sample of elderly male veterans. *Journal of Gerontology*, *47*(3), M93–M98. doi:10.1093/geronj/47.3.M93 PMID:1573190

Eklund. (2012). *Risk factors for falls*, Deliverable 1.1, AAL Call 4 project AiB (Ageing in Balance), May 2012.

Eklund, P. (n.d.). Assessment scales and consensus guidelines encoded in formal logic. *Journal of Nutrition, Health and Aging, 13*(Suppl 1), S558-S559.

Eklund, P., Galán, M. A., Helgesson, R., & Kortelainen, J. (2014). Fuzzy terms. *Fuzzy Sets and Systems*, *256*, 211–235. doi:10.1016/j.fss.2013.02.012

Hauer, K., Lamb, S. E., Jorstad, E. C., Todd, C., & Becker, C. (2006). Systematic review of definitions and methods of measuring falls in randomised controlled fall prevention trials. *Age and Ageing*, *35*(1), 5–10. doi:10.1093/ageing/afi218 PMID:16364930

Lach, H. W., Reed, A. T., Arfken, C. L., Miller, J. P., Paige, G. D., Birge, S. J., & Peck, W. A. (1991). Falls in the elderly: Reliability of a classification system. *Journal of the American Geriatrics Society*, *39*(2), 197–202. doi:10.1111/j.1532-5415.1991.tb01626.x PMID:1991951

Lord, S., Sherrington, C., Menz, H., & Close, J. (2007). *Falls in Older People*. Cambridge University Press. doi:10.1017/CBO9780511722233

Lord, S. R., Rogers, M. W., Howland, A., & Fitzpatrick, R. (1999). Lateral stability, sensorimotor function and falls in older people. *Journal of the American Geriatrics Society*, *47*(9), 1077–1081. doi:10.1111/j.1532-5415.1999.tb05230.x PMID:10484249

Salonoja, M., Salminen, M., Vahlberg, T., Aarnio, P., & Kivelä, S.-L. (2012). Withdrawal of psychotropic drugs decreases the risk of falls requiring treatment. *Archives of Gerontology and Geriatrics*, *54*(1), 160–167. doi:10.1016/j.archger.2011.02.015 PMID:21420744

Sheldon, J. (1960). On the natural history of falls in old age. *British Medical Journal*, *2*(5214), 1685–1690. doi:10.1136/bmj.2.5214.1685 PMID:20789006

Tinetti, M. E., Williams, T. F., & Mayewski, R. (1986). Fall Risk Index for elderly patients based on number of chronic disabilities. *The American Journal of Medicine*, *80*(3), 429–434. doi:10.1016/0002-9343(86)90717-5 PMID:3953620

Vellas, B. J., Wayne, S. J., Romero, L., Baumgartner, R. N., Rubenstein, L. Z., & Garry, P. J. (1997). One-leg balance is an important predictor of injurious falls in older persons. *Journal of the American Geriatrics Society*, *45*(6), 735–738. doi:10.1111/j.1532-5415.1997.tb01479.x PMID:9180669

KEY TERMS AND DEFINITIONS

Ageing: Ageing and older persons refers here to individuals already in at least a mild stage of cognitive and function decline.

Assessment Scales: Assessment scales are typically questionnaires or scales where the challenge is how to provide overall assessments given particular information in these areas, and finally, to provide decision-making on care levels and interventions based on these assessments.

Classification: Classification refers mainly to WHO's reference classifications.

Fall Prevention: Fall preventions refers to guidelines and procedures adapted in order to identify person at risk of fall, and to provide preventive measures in order to reduce fall risk and thereby also to reduce falls and fall related injuries.

ENDNOTE

[1]   This is pointed out very significantly also within EIP AHA's (European Innovation Partnership on Active and Healthy Ageing) working group on fall prevention.

Learning ICT–Mediated Communication through Computer–Based Simulations

Paula Poikela
Lapland University of Applied Sciences, Finland

Hanna Vuojärvi
University of Lapland, Finland

INTRODUCTION

Working life practices in healthcare and social work have undergone significant changes in recent years. Among other things, employees are required to contribute to multi-professional teamwork, make urgent decisions under pressure, attend to their clients' safety as well as their own, and make clients aware of their rights and the conditions of the services. All these challenges require careful communication (Bradley, 2006; Fryer, 2013; Milligan, 2007), which nowadays is often supported and mediated by information and communication technologies (ICTs). In Finland, the use of State Security Networks Ltd. (called the VIRVE network in Finland) and TErrestrial Trunked RAdio (TETRA) phones is recommended in all health and social care routine communication processes and emergency-rescue situations. This is due to Finland's geographical location and sparse population.

The VIRVE network is a digital network built specifically for the use of authorities. It was established at the beginning of 2000 according to the pan-European TETRA standards and is currently used in everyday practice and in crises by the armed forces, rescue services, border guards, police, health and social services, as well as some private and government companies that operate closely with the authorities. The Ministry of Transport and Communications provides permits for the use of the VIRVE network. Similar networks are also used in other countries, for example, RAKEL (*RAdioKommunikation för Effektiv Ledning*) in Sweden, *The Airwave Network* in Britain, and Astrid (*All-round Semi-cellular Trunked Radio communication network with Integrated Dispatching*) in Belgium. Even though the TETRA network is mostly used in Europe, it is also spreading rapidly into regions of Asia, the Middle East, and South America. In Finland, the VIRVE network covers the entire Finnish global system for mobile (GSM) communication networks (Fryer, 2013; Poikela, Ruokamo, & Keskitalo, 2013) and assures flawless communication even when the distribution of electricity is interrupted.

The TETRA phone that was used in the study described in this article resembles a traditional GSM phone and actually affords common GSM functionalities, such as phone calls and SMS messages. Its appearance and technology are designed to endure water splashes and cold, and it can be accessed even with gloves on, for example, by firemen. The phone includes basic number buttons, and an additional emergency button and a tangent button that enable fast communication with several recipients simultaneously.

TETRA phones are widely used by authorities due to several benefits they have in communication processes. For example, in healthcare, they can be used for communication in emergency situations and daily working processes, where they enable the flow of patient information among professionals. Both the VIRVE network and TETRA phones have a high level of data security, which enables users to send

DOI: 10.4018/978-1-4666-9978-6.ch052

and receive even confidential information, such as patient information. Wide use of the TETRA technology is also useful for work involving multi-professional teams that use a shared tool for communication. In disaster situations, such as large traffic accidents or rescue situations, TETRA and VIRVE together enable effective and fast communication. The VIRVE network and TETRA phones work even in situations where GSM fails.

Despite the recent development in technologies, there are some gaps that need to be addressed to make communication more fluent and efficient and to establish the wider use of phones in areas of healthcare and social work. Often, these gaps are not so much about technological questions—that is, what types of devices would be most useful—but more about developing human processes and working practices.

The need to develop communication skills has also been acknowledged in healthcare education, which has transformed teaching and learning methods, especially over the past two decades. In particular, it has led to the development of simulation pedagogy, through which it is possible to teach not only individual skills but also multi-professional teamwork and care processes (Gaba, 2004; Milligan, 2007; Rall & Dieckmann, 2005; Rall, van Gessel, & Staender, 2011) that involve several professionals and can take place in several phases and places—for example, from a car accident site to a helicopter or an ambulance, and from an emergency room to surgery and finally to an intensive care unit. The simulation-based methods increase large-scale know-how and respond to the educational needs of the younger generation that is currently studying to be healthcare professionals (Poikela, Ruokamo, & Keskitalo, 2013).

The study presented here focuses on computer-based simulations. The research activities were a part of the MediPro research project (2012–2014) that investigated technology-supported service processes, especially the use of the TETRA telephone, in the social work and healthcare sectors. The aim of the project was to develop pedagogical models to support teaching and learning processes and technology using simulation-based learning. The objective of this study was to examine students' perceptions of how meaningful learning themes—concrete, personal, social, liable, content-based, and metacognitive (Poikela & Ruokamo, 2014)—occur in computer-based simulation that focused on learning ICT-mediated communication via TETRA phones. Quantitative data (N = 124) were collected over 11 simulation training sessions and analyzed statistically. The results of this study will contribute to developing computer-based simulation training, both in terms of pedagogical practices and technical devices.

In the following section, the concept of simulation pedagogy is presented and discussed, with a focus on the pedagogical models developed for computer-based simulation training and how the results of quantitative analysis support the themes of meaningful learning. Later, the study and its results are presented and discussed.

BACKGROUND

Simulation Pedagogy

Simulations have been used as a teaching method for several decades in many fields of expertise (Rosen, 2008). Since the late 1990s, their use has also become common in healthcare education, and there is vast potential for using simulations in teaching and learning processes with or without the support of different types of ICTs. There is a wide range of simulation modalities available, and they can be categorized as:

1. Task trainers,
2. Low fidelity simulations,

3. High fidelity simulations,
4. Standardized patient simulations,
5. Gaming simulations,
6. Virtual reality simulations, and
7. In-situ simulations (Holtschneider, 2007).

Sokolowski and Banks (2011) categorized simulations from the users' perspective into

1. Live simulations using real people in simulations,
2. Virtual simulations using virtual simulated equipment in learning, and
3. Constructive simulations using an immersive virtual environment.

The use of simulations is closely related to the advancements in ICTs. With regard to computer-based simulations in particular, it has been acknowledged that their use provides healthcare students with the opportunity to explore content-related problems and to learn to make decisions (Eldabi, Paul, & Taylor, 1999). They enable concrete drilling practices at both the individual and collaborative level. It has also been discovered that simulations are closely connected to emotionality in both teachers and students (Bong, Lightdale, & Fredette, 2010).

Developing computer-based simulation software is, however, a challenging task. Developers and researchers need to create a balance between developing simulations that serve the learning goals on one hand and the expectations of users on the other. The challenge usually is that computer-based simulation software has been developed for practical experience and does not consider pedagogical premises. The following section presents the developmental process for a pedagogical model that can be used as a practical tool for creating computer-based simulation training. The process aims to provide information for both educators and software developers to diminish the gap between tools and pedagogies.

Developing Pedagogical Models for Computer-Based Simulations

The pedagogical models used here are based on those described by Joyce and Weil (1980), as general plans that can be used to shape curricula, design materials for instruction, and guide instructors' work. In this paper, computer-based simulations are discussed using the framework of the ISSD (*Introduction, Simulation, Scenario, Debriefing*) pedagogical model that was designed for TETRA phone user training (Poikela, Ruokamo, & Keskitalo, 2013) (Figure 1).

The ISSD model was developed in keeping with the principles of the Design-Based Research (DBR) (Barab & Squire, 2004; Design-Based Research Collective, 2003), which is generally considered to be a series of approaches designed to improve educational practices through iterative stages of design, implementation, analysis, and refinement. Its intrinsic character is the close connection between theory and practice, which is significant in developing computer-based simulation training. In practice, this is reflected by the close collaboration between researchers and practitioners, which is the basis for all activities in DBR studies (Barab & Squire, 2004; Wang & Hannafin, 2005).

The close connection between research and practice is the basis of the dual goal of DBR. First, it aims to produce new theories, artifacts, and practices that may have an impact on learning (Collins, Joseph, & Bielaczyc, 2004; Edelson, 2002). Second, it assesses these theories and investigates the changes they suggest at a local level. In the study presented here, this meant considering computer-based simulations as a tool for learning how to use TETRA phones in communication. Students participated in the process

Figure 1. The initial ISSD pedagogical model for computer-based simulations

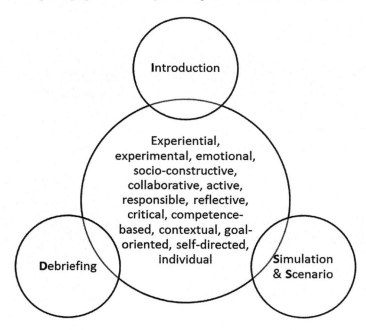

as co-designers by providing information about their experiences using the computer-based simulation software TETRAsim in learning and making their views known through data collection. This dual goal makes DBR the kind of learning that takes place in real-life, naturalistic settings (Barab & Squire, 2004).

The DBR process during which the ISSD pedagogical model was developed is presented in Figure 2.

The first version of the ISSD model (Poikela et al., 2013) was created on the basis of theoretical knowledge on simulation pedagogy and previously developed evidence-based simulation learning models (Dieckmann, 2009), in particular the FTL (*Facilitating, Training, Learning*) pedagogical model (Keskitalo, Ruokamo, & Väisänen, 2010). The FTL model's simulation-based learning processes are characterized by 14 meaningful learning characteristics: experimental, experiential, emotional, social, constructive, collaborative, active, responsible, reflective, competence-based, contextual, goal-oriented, self-directed, and individual.

The first time this model was implemented, it was to determine which of these meaningful learning characteristics appeared in computer-based simulation training according to students and which were missing (Hakkarainen, Saarelainen, & Ruokamo, 2007; Poikela et al., 2013). As a result of the analyzed

Figure 2. The design-based research process of developing the ISSD pedagogical model

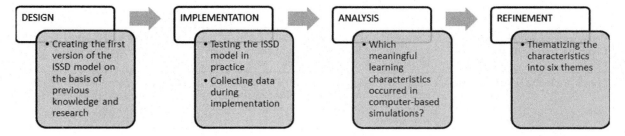

data collected during the first implementation, the ISSD model was refined and the 14 characteristics of the initial model were organized under the following six themes: concrete, personal, social, liable, content-based, and metacognitive (Table 1) (Poikela, Ruokamo, & Keskitalo, 2014).

Although the close involvement between teaching and research can be perceived as a strength of DBR, it can also be viewed as a threat to the validity of the research (Barab & Squire, 2004). It is acknowledged, however, that DBR works with, through, and alongside the contexts, which are never neutral or without agency. Researchers are expected to intervene when required (Cobb et al., 2003). In this case, this meant that researchers were actively present in the simulation training sessions during which data were collected. They did not take part in the training sessions as students, but rather acted as facilitators or observers, by discussing and making field notes.

The next phase of the DBR process tested the refined pedagogical model to find out how strongly students saw the six themes occurring in computer-based simulation training. This phase was conducted as a series of simulation days and data collections. The details of this process and the related results, discussions, and suggestions are discussed in the following section.

DEVELOPING THE ISSD MODEL FURTHER

Research Design

The research question of this study was: *How do the themes of meaningful learning appear in computer-based simulation learning processes from a student perspective?*

The study was structured as a series of 11 simulation days that were arranged between spring 2013 and spring 2014 at the University of Applied Sciences, Rovaniemi, Finland. The aim of these simulation days was to test the use of the computer-based simulator TETRAsim that was used to teach how to use TETRA phones in communication and also to find out how meaningful learning themes occurred during simulations, according to students. The structure of the simulation days is presented in Figure 3.

Table 1. Meaningful learning themes for, in, and on reflection

Themes of Meaningful Learning	Description	Concrete Simulation Experience
Experimental = Concrete	Practicing nursing skills, trying many times, establishing role clarity, communicating effectively, knowing the environment	Reflection In Action (during action)
Emotional, Individual = Personal	Facial expression, gestures, confusion, happiness, joy, mobilization of resources	
Socio Constructive, Collaborative = Social	Finding a solution together, discussing, using cognitive aids, designating leadership roles	
Active, Self-directed, Responsible = Liable	Eagerness to learn even though others students are passive	
Competence-based, Goal-oriented, Contextual, Experiential = Content-based	Goal-oriented action combined with previous knowledge and skills, ability to integrate all available information, ability to distribute the workload	Reflection for/in/on Action (before/during/after action)
Critical, Reflective = Metacognitive	Ability to critically examine one's own actions and reflect on one's own thinking, common skills and knowledge, wise allocation of attention, anticipation and planning	Reflective Observation In/On Action (during/after action)

Poikela & Ruokamo, 2014.

Figure 3. Structure of the computer-based simulation training based on the ISSD model

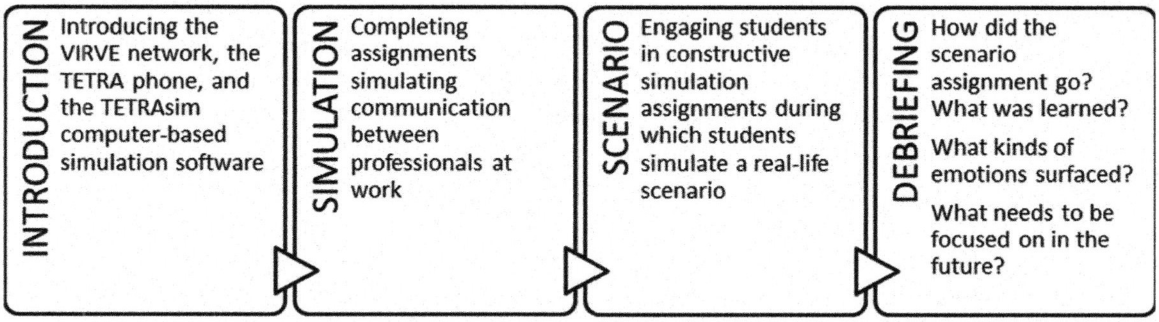

INTRODUCTION	SIMULATION	SCENARIO	DEBRIEFING
Introducing the VIRVE network, the TETRA phone, and the TETRAsim computer-based simulation software	Completing assignments simulating communication between professionals at work	Engaging students in constructive simulation assignments during which students simulate a real-life scenario	How did the scenario assignment go? What was learned? What kinds of emotions surfaced? What needs to be focused on in the future?

To start the training according to the ISSD model, the introduction (I) phase presented the course, the central concepts, the VIRVE network, and the usage of TETRA phones in Finland. Students also received information about the basics of simulation-based learning, and their learning objectives were formulated. Second, during the simulation (S) phase, the computer-based simulation software TETRA-sim was introduced to the students. They were trained on the basic functions of TETRA phones through computer-based simulations, and they also performed some basic interaction activities guided by the simulation software. Additionally, students were provided four TETRA phones that they could hold in their hands and try out while completing the simulation tasks on their computers. The first two phases lasted for about three hours.

Third, during the scenario (S) phase, students participated in a training session that included a task related to the content (for example, how to diagnose a cardiac arrest and resuscitate a patient), during which they were required to communicate via TETRA radio. The scenario was based on the pedagogical learning objectives set during the introduction phase. The fourth and last phase, debriefing (D), consisted of discussing the scenario immediately after it occurred and giving feedback. This last phase can be conducted with or without the instructor; in this case, there were two instructors present during the debriefing. The researchers were present on all simulation days, and they observed all the phases and activities, made notes, and collected data.

Data Collection

Several types of data were collected during the simulation days. This article reports the results based on survey data that were collected after the introduction (I) and simulation (S) phases. The data were collected by means of an online questionnaire that was created by using the Webropol tool. At the beginning of the simulation day, the students were given an informed consent form that introduced the study, the MediPro project, and the researchers involved in it, and explained the purpose of the collected information. Students were also informed about their right to gain information about the study, and that they were free to resign from the study at any point.

There were a total of 143 participants who attended the computer-based simulation training, among whom 124 agreed to participate in the study. Their email addresses were collected, and they were sent an email message containing a personal link to the questionnaire. The questionnaire included four items related to the students' demographic variables—gender, age, work experience in years, and the year of study. Twenty-nine items focused on the themes of the ISSD pedagogical model. Students were asked to assess the items on a Likert scale of 1–5 (1 = disagree, 2 = moderately disagree, 3 = neither agree nor disagree, 4 = moderately agree, 5 = agree) how strongly they thought the themes appeared during the computer-based simulation training. The same Likert scale was used for all the 22 items querying the students' emotions during the computer-based simulation training. At the end of the questionnaire, there were also two open-ended questions about the students' opinions on how training based on computer-based simulation could be developed and the difficulties they encountered during the training.

All the 124 students who agreed to participate in the study responded to the questionnaire. Of the respondents, 79.8% were female and 20.2% were male. The majority, 52%, were between the ages of 20 and 25 years. They only had little work experience: 70% of the participants had worked for one year or less. Thirty-six respondents were first-year nursing students, 58 were second-year nursing students, and 24 were adult nursing students (they already had an occupation, but not necessarily in healthcare). Moreover, six of the participants were professional social workers. The social workers were in different phases of their education process and had different know-how and knowledge backgrounds, but their experience with simulation-based training and with using the TETRA phone was at the same level as the rest of the participants, and they also aimed to learn how to use TETRA phones in professional communication processes, so their responses were included in the data analysis.

Analysis

All data was analyzed quantitatively using *SPSS Version 21.0*. Twenty-five preselected items were subjected to factor analysis (principal component analysis, varimax rotation) to sort out the items that best describe the themes of meaningful learning. Altogether, seven themes with eigenvalues above 1 emerged from the data (Table 2), with a Kaiser-Meyer-Olkin measure of sampling adequacy value of .809.

Individual questionnaire items, grouped by factor analysis, were used to create seven scales. The internal consistency of the created scales was tested by calculating Cronbach's alpha (Cronbach, 1951). Cronbach's alpha assumes values from 0 (indicating no correlation) to 1 (indicating identical results), and an alpha value of 0.7 or above is considered as evidence of acceptable internal consistency (Nunnally, 1978). The alpha value was above 0.7 for four scales. However, the alpha value did not exceed 0.7 for three scales: "Technical", "Personal" and "Theory driven" (Cronbach's alpha values were .646, .625 and .521, respectively). These three scales were therefore excluded from further analysis. It is possible that the formulation of the questions was unsatisfactory and that the content of these three themes needs to be addressed in further studies as the ISSD model is developed further.

To sort out the items that describe students' emotions when learning with TETRAsim, 20 pre-selected items were subjected to factor analysis (principal component analysis, varimax rotation) to sort out the items that best describe the themes of meaningful learning (Table 3).

Four themes with eigenvalues over 1 emerged from the data with a Kaiser-Meyer-Olkin measure of sampling adequacy value of .841. Individual questionnaire items, grouped by factor analysis, were used to create four scales. All the scales had an alpha value above 0.7, expect for "Comfortable" (alpha = .549), which was excluded from further analysis.

Results

The study presented here aimed to find out how the themes of meaningful learning appear in computer-based simulation learning processes from a student perspective. To start, the frequencies were calculated from the final four themes: "Transferable," "Liable," "Social," and "Metacognitive." The results are presented in Table 4.

Table 2. Results of the factor and reliability analysis

	1	2	3	4	5	6	7
"Transferable" (α =.820)							
TETRAsim helped me to understand different perspectives related to what was learned.	.472						
I can utilize what I learned in other contexts.	.724						
Competencies needed in working life were developed through practice with TETRAsim.	.656						
Instructors' activities supported my learning.	.545						
TETRAsim approached learning tasks from multiple perspectives.	.442						
It is possible to apply the learning results directly to work life.	.643						
"Liable" (α =.801)							
Learning with TETRAsim improved my problem-solving skills.		.802					
Learning with TETRAsim improved my critical thinking skills.		.760					
Learning with TETRAsim improved my managing skills.		.659					
Learning with TETRAsim improved my skills for acquiring and assessing information.		.618					
"Social" (α =.796)							
TETRAsim enabled collaborative learning.			.822				
Collaborative learning was successful.			.680				
Learning with TETRAsim improved my collaboration and interaction skills.			.720				
"Metacognitive" (α =.796)							
It was possible to integrate what was learnt with my earlier experiences.				.831			
I aimed to apply my own practical experiences when using TETRAsim.				.826			
TETRAsim deepened my understanding of what I had learned before.				.584			
It was possible to use my own experiences as starting points for learning.				.767			
"Technical" (α =.646)							
TETRAsim included technical hindrances to learning.					.567		
I was responsible for learning the results alone.					.787		
I spent my time learning how to use TETRAsim.					.814		
"Personal" (α =.625)							
I was able to affect the level of difficulty in TETRAsim						.736	
It was possible to learn in my individual way, in a way that is suitable for me.						.560	
I was able to assess my learning when using TETRAsim.						.690	
"Theory Driven" (α =.521)							
TETRAsim made it possible to reach my personal goals.							.545
The practical examples in TETRAsim were considered in a theoretical framework.							.641
Extraction Method: Principal Component Analysis. **Rotation Method:** Varimax rotation with Kaiser normalization.[a]							

[a]Rotation converged in seven iterations.

Table 3. Results of factor and reliability analysis of items describing emotions

	1	2	3	4
"Unease" (α =.883)				
Frustrated	.651			
Concerned	.639			
Disappointed	.785			
Stressed	.559			
Irritated	.743			
Deflated	.675			
Deficient	.682			
Ashamed	.553			
Bored	.627			
"Eager" (α =.815)				
Confident		.598		
Excited		.749		
Joyful		.664		
Interested		.723		
Satisfied		.719		
"Tense" (α =.90)				
Challenged			.697	
Nervous			.709	
Relaxed			-.565	
Uncertain			.569	
"Comfortable" (α =.549)				
Relieved				.714
Community				.728
Extraction Method: Principal Component Analysis. **Rotation Method:** Varimax rotation with Kaiser Normalization.				

[a]Rotation converged in 13 iterations.

Table 4. Frequencies of the themes of the ISSD pedagogical model

		Transferable	Liable	Social	Metacognitive
N	Valid	120	122	123	122
	Missing	4	2	1	2
Mean		3.8	3.3	4.2	3.4
Median		3.8	3.3	4.3	3.4
Std. Deviation		0.60	0.77	0.70	0.84

The analysis indicates that students appreciated the collaborative tasks of TETRAsim and found their learning to be social. They also saw that the learning contents were applicable in other contexts, for example, in work places. Students' perceptions were quite neutral concerning the liability and meta-cognitivity of their learning.

It seems that students perceive the use of TETRAsim quite positively and are eager to learn. It can be considered a positive finding that feelings of unease and tension were not common among the students (Table 5).

Finally, the presence of a correlation between the experienced emotions and the appearance of meaningful learning themes was analyzed. The results are presented in Table 6.

The analysis revealed that feeling eager correlates positively with how transferable ($r = .639$, $p = 0.01$), liable ($r = .501$, $p = 0.01$) or social ($r = .558$, $p = 0.01$) the learning experience is perceived to be. This confirms earlier results according to which emotional factors have an influence on learning and on the creation of community (Jones & Issroff, 2005). This can also be perceived the other way around: gaining the experience that the learned content is also applicable in other contexts, and that the feeling of being in charge of one's own learning in a safe community and staying positive during learning can be challenging at times.

Table 5. Frequencies of students' emotions

		Uneasy	Eager	Tense
N	Valid	121	121	122
	Missing	3	3	2
Mean		1.9	3.9	2.9
Median		2	4	3
Std. Deviation		0.72	0.63	0.50

Table 6. Correlations between emotions and meaningful learning themes

		Transferable	Liable	Social	Metacognitive
Unease	Pearson Correlation	-.342**	-.139	-.392**	-.153
	Sig. (2-tailed)	.000	.131	.000	.096
	N	117	119	120	119
Eager	Pearson Correlation	**.639****	**.501****	**.558****	.164
	Sig. (2-tailed)	.000	.000	.000	.073
	N	118	120	120	120
Tense	Pearson Correlation	.116	.157	.156	-.034
	Sig. (2-tailed)	.212	.086	.088	.710
	N	118	120	121	120

**Correlation is significant at the 0.01 level (2-tailed).
*Correlation is significant at the 0.05 level (2-tailed).

DISCUSSION AND RECOMMENDATIONS

As can be seen from Figure 3, the facilitators were involved in the introduction phase, but after this phase, the students completed the computer-based simulation tasks by themselves. The facilitators' involvement in the computer-based simulations is something that could be taken into consideration when developing the ISSD model and computer-based simulation training further. The themes of the ISSD model might have been stronger if the facilitator were involved in the process.

It would also be beneficial to take a closer look at the structure of the simulation tasks in the TETRAsim computer-based simulation software: whether or not it is designed carefully enough to support meaningful simulation-based learning. Nevertheless, it seems that including collaborative tasks in computer-based simulations is a good strategy than focusing merely on drilling practices to learn the functionalities of TETRA phones. Collaborative tasks could be developed further also by making them more complex so that they require decision-making skills. This could also enhance the metacognitivity of learning (Rutten, van Joolingen, & van der Veen, 2012).

Design experiments, such as the one presented here, have some fundamental limitations that make the conclusions uncertain and that need to be considered. A large number of variables affect the success of the design, many of which cannot be controlled. Effective pedagogical practices are developed through subsequent refining and testing, and it needs to be noted that this was only the second implementation of the ISSD model. Moreover, the analysis is based on quantitative data alone. The analysis could also be strengthened by comparing results across designs or across contexts to gain more varied information regarding the content, as well as the design of the training (Collins et al., 2004). Nonetheless, the findings indicate that collaboration between researchers, content experts, and computer scientists is a workable method to design computer-based simulation software.

FUTURE RESEARCH DIRECTIONS

Computer-based simulation training can be regarded as beneficial but also challenging for working professionals. The challenges are not so much related to the content of the training, but rather to the practical arrangements (Curtin et al., 2011). The ISSD model entails a training concept in which the participants are present at the same time and at the same place. If we use a team of social workers or the staff of emergency units as an example, it is rather impossible for them to participate together in a training program at the same time during working hours. It may therefore be useful to direct the research and development towards designing and testing mobile applications for simulation-based training. It would be interesting to find out, for example, if a facilitator actually needs to be physically present or not.

Hence, it might be useful in the future to take a closer look at the possibilities that mobile technologies provide for simulation pedagogy. Decentralized simulations combine the ideas of mobile learning with simulation pedagogy, and they have the potential to support the participation of individual students and the virtual presence of facilitators in trainings. This type of development could potentially enhance the 'personal' theme of the ISSD model. Moreover, developing computer-based simulations in the direction of more game-based activities would support more engaging and personal learning processes while at the same time enable student creativity and promote their motivation and problem-solving skills.

REFERENCES

Barab, S., & Squire, K. (2004). Design-based research: Putting a stake in the ground. *Journal of the Learning Sciences*, *13*(1), 1–14. doi:10.1207/s15327809jls1301_1

Bong, C., Lightdale, J., Fredette, M., & Weinstock, P. (2010). Effects of simulation versus traditional tutorial-based training on physiologic stress levels among clinicians: A pilot study. *Simulation in Healthcare*, *5*(5), 272–278. doi:10.1097/SIH.0b013e3181e98b29 PMID:21330809

Bradley, P. (2006). The history of simulation in medical education and possible future directions. *Medical Education*, *40*(3), 254–262. doi:10.1111/j.1365-2929.2006.02394.x PMID:16483328

Collins, A., Joseph, D., & Bielaczyc, K. (2004). Design research: Theoretical and methodological issues. *Journal of the Learning Sciences*, *13*(1), 15–42. doi:10.1207/s15327809jls1301_2

Cronbach, L. J. (1951). Coefficient alpha and the internal structure of tests. *Psychometrika*, *16*(3), 297–334. doi:10.1007/BF02310555

Curtin, L. B., Finn, L. A., Czosnowski, Q. A., Whitman, C. B., & Cawley, M. J. (2011). Computer-based simulation training to improve learning outcomes in mannequin-based simulation exercises. *American Journal of Pharmaceutical Education*, *75*(6), 113. doi:10.5688/ajpe756113 PMID:21931451

Dieckmann, P. (2009). Simulation settings for learning in acute medical care. In P. Dieckmann (Ed.), Using simulation for education, training and research (pp. 40-51). Lengerich, Germany: Pabst Science Publisher.

Edelson, D. (2002). Design research: What we learn when we engage in design. *Journal of the Learning Sciences*, *11*(1), 105–121. doi:10.1207/S15327809JLS1101_4

Eldabi, T., Paul, R. J., & Taylor, S. J. E. (1999). Computer simulation in healthcare decision making. *Computers & Industrial Engineering*, *37*(1–2), 235–238. doi:10.1016/S0360-8352(99)00063-7

Fryer, L. A. (2013). Human factors in nursing: The time is now. *The Australian Journal of Advanced Nursing*, *30*(2), 56–65.

Gaba, D. M. (2004). The future vision of simulation in health care. *Quality & Safety in Health Care*, *13*(suppl. 1), i2–i10. doi:10.1136/qshc.2004.009878 PMID:15465951

Hakkarainen, P., Saarelainen, T., & Ruokamo, H. (2007). Towards meaningful learning through digital video-supported case-based teaching. *Australasian Journal of Educational Technology*, *23*(1), 87–109.

Holtschneider, M. (2007). Better communication, better care through high-fidelity simulation. *Nursing Management*, *38*(5), 55–57. PMID:17486016

Jones, A., & Issroff, K. (2005). Learning technologies: Affective and social issues in computer-supported collaborative learning. *Computers & Education*, *44*(4), 395–408. doi:10.1016/j.compedu.2004.04.004

Joyce, B., Calhoun, E., & Hopkins, D. (2002). *Models of learning—Tools for teaching*. Buckingham: Open University Press.

Keskitalo, T., Ruokamo, H., & Gaba, D. (2014). Towards meaningful simulation-based learning with medical students and junior physicians. *Medical Teacher*, *36*(3), 230–239. doi:10.3109/0142159X.2013.853116 PMID:24261916

Keskitalo, T., Ruokamo, H., & Väisänen, O. (2010). How does the facilitating, training and learning model support characteristics of meaningful learning in a simulation-based learning environment from facilitators` and students` perspectives? In *Proceedings of World Conference on Educational Multimedia, Hypermedia and Telecommunications 2010* (pp. 1736–1746). Chesapeake, VA: AACE.

Milligan, F. J. (2007). Establishing a culture for patient safety—the role of education. *Nurse Education Today*, *27*(2), 95–102. doi:10.1016/j.nedt.2006.03.003 PMID:16713030

Nunnally, J. C. (1978). *Psychometric theory*. New York: McGraw-Hill.

Poikela, P., & Ruokamo, H. (2014). *Comparison of meaningful learning characteristics in simulated nursing practice after traditional versus computer-based simulation method: A qualitative videography study*. Manuscript in process.

Poikela, P., Ruokamo, H., & Keskitalo, T. (2013). A computer-based simulation to enhance official communication in the health care process—How does it promote the facilitating and learning processes? In T. Bastiaens, & G. Marks (Eds.), *Proceedings of World Conference on E-Learning in Corporate, Government, Healthcare, and Higher Education 2013* (pp. 2051–2060). Chesapeake, VA: AACE.

Poikela, P., Ruokamo, H., & Keskitalo, T. (2014). Does teaching method affect learning and how meaningful learning is from student perspectives? In *Proceedings of World Conference on Educational Multimedia, Hypermedia and Telecommunications 2014* (pp. 1684–1692). Chesapeake, VA: AACE.

Rall, M., & Dieckmann, P. (2005). Simulation and patient safety: The use of simulation to enhance patient safety on a systems level. *Current Anaesthesia and Critical Care*, *16*(5), 273–281. doi:10.1016/j.cacc.2005.11.007

Rall, M., van Gessel, E., & Staender, S. (2011). Education, teaching & training in patient safety. *Best Practice & Research. Clinical Anaesthesiology*, *25*(2), 251–262. doi:10.1016/j.bpa.2011.02.013 PMID:21550549

Rosen, K. R. (2008). The history of medical simulation. *Journal of Critical Care*, *23*(2), 157–166. doi:10.1016/j.jcrc.2007.12.004 PMID:18538206

Rutten, N., van Joolingen, W. R., & van der Veen, J. T. (2012). The learning effects of computer simulations in science education. *Computers & Education*, *58*(1), 136–153. doi:10.1016/j.compedu.2011.07.017

Sokolowski, J. A., & Banks, C. M. (2011). *Modeling and simulation in the medical and health sciences*. Hoboken, NJ, USA: Wiley. doi:10.1002/9781118003206

State Security Networks Ltd. (2013). *Homepage*. Retrieved from http://www.erillisverkot.fi/en/erillisverkot/home_page/

Terrestrial Trunked Radio. (2013). Retrieved from http://www.ascom.com/ws/en/tetra-article.pdf

Wang, F., & Hannafin, M. (2005). Design-based research and technology-enhanced learning environments. *Educational Technology Research and Development*, *53*(4), 5–23. doi:10.1007/BF02504682

KEY TERMS AND DEFINITIONS

Design-Based Research: A practice-oriented research approach that aims to yield theoretical knowledge and practical implications.

ICT-Mediated Communication: Communication between two persons or within a team mediated through one or several digital tools.

ISSD Model: A pedagogical model designed for training that combines different kinds of simulations with computer-based simulation training.

Meaningful Learning: A learning process characterized by certain process characteristics.

Mediated Communication: Communication between two persons or within a team mediated through a tool that can be symbolic (e.g., language) or physical (e.g., phone).

Pedagogical Model: A general pedagogical plan that can be used to shape curricula, design teaching materials, and guide instructors' work in the classroom and other settings.

Simulation Environment: Either a physical space or an online environment where healthcare workers' skills or processes can be simulated.

Simulation Pedagogy: A developing field of theoretical and pedagogical foundation that guides teaching and learning processes.

Multi–Agent Systems for E–Health and Telemedicine

Federico Bergenti
University of Parma, Italy

Agostino Poggi
University of Parma, Italy

Michele Tomaiuolo
University of Parma, Italy

INTRODUCTION

Health care is characterized by high degree of distributed, labor-intensive works, mobility, and information access to large set of dynamic and unstructured information, distributed over a large number of information systems. The advent of Internet and the evolution of information technologies promote the development of Internet based applications that try to facilitate the remote interaction between health-care providers and their patients and among health-care providers and to automatize the acquisition, exchange and manipulating of information distributed in a large number of (heterogeneous) information systems.

Multi-agent systems represent the most promising information technology for coping with a class of problems (i.e., remote and heterogeneous software applications integration, distributed tasks execution coordination, and remote monitoring and assistance) which are typical problems of the large part of Internet based health care applications (see, e.g., Jennings et al., 1995; Muller, 1998; Bordini et al., 2005). In particular, applications for healthcare can take outstanding advantage of the intrinsic characteristics of multi-agent systems because usually they are composed of loosely coupled (complex) systems, are realized in terms of heterogeneous components and legacy systems, manage distributed data and resources; and are accessed by remote users in (synchronous) collaboration (Moreno & Nealon, 2003; Annicchiarico et al., 2008).

The goal of this chapter is to describe the main reasons why multi-agent systems are considered one of the most interesting technologies for the development of applications for health care. It provides some guidelines intended to help identifying the kinds of applications that can truly take advantage of the features of multi-agent systems, and it presents some of the most important international projects that used multi-agent systems in the healthcare and social services domain.

BACKGROUND

Although there are several definitions of agent (see, e.g., Russell & Norvig, 2003; Wooldridge & Jennings, 1995; Genesereth & Ketchpel, 1994), all the definitions agree that an agent is essentially an autonomous software entity that should at least be designed to operate continuously in dynamic and uncertain environments, reacting to events while showing an intelligent behavior to pursue its own objectives. An agent usually provides interoperable interfaces for interacting with other agents, either concurrently or

DOI: 10.4018/978-1-4666-9978-6.ch053

cooperatively, exchanging messages formulated according to some syntax, semantics and pragmatics. Since an agent behaves proactively, it requires some degree of trust by its user, and it can receive delegations from either human users or other agents in the form of required actions or desired goals, matched with permissions to access necessary resources. Additionally, an agent may also be able to perform complex reasoning at run-time and can also learn and change their behavior over time, to improve its performance. Finally, it is even able to move for one computational node to another, to follow its own user or to exploit some local resource more efficiently.

Agent-based systems are often realized by loosely coupling various agents, i.e. autonomous software entities, thus modelling a proper multi-agent system, characterized by a higher level of modularity and a richer descriptive model, if compared with a solitary agent working within its environment – either with the presence of users or not. Multi-agent systems can be also considered as abstractions capable of capturing the essence of many software systems at different levels of detail, rather than a single technology supporting the realization of distributed intelligent systems. In particular, agents and multi-agent systems are often considered the highest system level (Newel, 1982; Jennings, 2000) that we can access today and they are meant to provide a truly novel level of abstraction in the analysis, design and implementation of complex software systems (Bergenti & Huhns, 2004).

MULTI-AGENT SYSTEMS AND E-HEALTH

Sociality is one of the main distinguishing characteristic of multi-agent systems. In particular, multi-agent systems allow the delegation of goals and tasks as a mean to realize emerging social behaviors. Multi-agent systems are generally considered an appropriate abstraction for modelling complex, distributed systems, even if such a multiplicity naturally introduces the possibility of having different agents with potentially conflicting goals. Agents may decide to cooperate for mutual benefit, or they may compete to serve their own interests. Agents take advantage of their social ability to exhibit flexible coordination behaviors that make them able to both cooperate in the achievement of shared goals or to compete on the acquisition of resources and tasks. Agents have the ability of coordinating their behaviors into coherent global actions.

This characteristic fit quite well the new environment where health care and social services are being provided. In fact, significant societal changes are the mark of these years, including ageing of population, growing value attributed to personal care, preference for living at home also when needing assistance, interconnection and integration of diverse services.

Care provision is usually based either on the effort of relatives, or on hospitals and care centers. In recent years, both those approaches are being questioned and the situation is changing. In fact, the support of relatives is becoming less and less viable, as family members are frequently occupied with work. On the other side, the relocation of patients, elders and people needing social care, outside of their communities is not desirable for their own wellness; in many cases, it is not even necessary, as they preserve enough strength and capabilities to stay at home. Moreover, rooms in hospitals and care centers are in a limited number and the trend is toward their reduction, in spite of a growing number of elders. Consequently, the traditional approach to provide cares and social services in hospitals and institutional centers is being paralleled with a growing tendency to provide cares in the community, directly. In this kind of "community care" or "domiciled care", services to assisted people are provided directly in their home or in their habitual environment, allowing them to continue to live as much independently as they can. The range of services varies from the delivery of meals and other goods to domestic help, from generic home monitoring and assistance to nursing and medical care. In some cases, thanks to the diffusion of computer networks and computing devices, those activities allow some degree of automation.

Usually, those services are supplied by a number of organizations and agencies, which act largely in an independent way, with different responsibilities and goals. An important fact which is not always emphasized enough, is the large support provided by family, community members and other informal caretakers who can be paradoxically excluded from the rest of the community care. However, all those agencies and informal caretakers need to coordinate their actions, in order to avoid serious service inefficiencies, and so they need the availability of systems to share information about the assisted, without breaching the official confidentiality requirements. The coordination of these autonomous bodies and of single professionals is a challenging problem, that could result in misunderstandings among the involved professionals, ignorance of important notions about the assisted, fragmentation of care, overlapping and duplication of assessments.

Involving autonomous entities, the communication process aimed at reaching a mutually accepted agreement on the overall care management is necessarily a negotiation process. This kind of process is exactly one of the scenarios where multi-agent systems can be applied more conveniently (Jennings, 2001). According to the different goals of the agents involved, which in general are to be considered autonomous, negotiation can be either competitive or cooperative. In particular, contracting is a common negotiation mechanism used to assign a desired task to the most appropriate agent among those available. In this mechanism, agents can take on two roles, i.e., manager and contractor, in a decentralized market structure; a manager have some task to assign, while a contractors can propose itself as the most appropriate executor (Smith & Davis, 1980).

In multi-agent systems, managing and monitoring the distributed execution of the tasks needed to implement the desired functionalities is often based on organizational structuring techniques, together with contracting and multi-agent planning. While contracting solves the problems of searching and selecting the agents that can perform the set of tasks necessary to achieve a goal, it does not give any help in defining the way, i.e., the new plan, in which they are executed to achieve it. Instead, multi-agent planning techniques enable agents to elaborate plans guiding them towards their common/individual goals preventing any possible interference among the actions of different agents (Durfee, 1999; Tonino et al., 2002). In order to avoid inconsistent or conflicting actions and interactions, agents build a multi-agent plan that details all the future actions and interactions required to achieve their goals, and they interleave execution of such a plan with needed planning and re-planning.

The current tendency is to manage the provision of cares in complex systems, based on the interaction of a number of different entities, including neighborhood and institutional care centers, day centers and social security institutions, each of them involving people with various roles e.g. health care professionals, social care assistants, assisted people and their relatives. It is not a tendency mainly driven by technology, but technology will play a fundamental role in the realization of the underlying information systems, for the overall care management. Computer networks and innovative software tools, in fact, are able to support the realization of integrated systems that greatly ease the collaboration among the various involved agencies and persons, driving the evolution of those systems towards so-called "virtual organizations", where the various involved humans operate as part of a virtual community (Franchi et al., 2013).

In general, organizational structuring is a coordination technique that allows the definition of the organization that governs the interaction among the agents of a system, i.e., the organization that defines the information, communication, and control relationships among the agents of the system (Horling &

Lesser, 2005). In the context of integrated care systems, multi-agent systems represent quite a natural solution, as they intrinsically represent autonomous entities and overall "virtual organizations", as those concerning the case of health and social services.

Agent technology, and in particular mobile agents, provide a means by which effective co-operation (information sharing and communication between autonomous information systems) can take place without compromising the security of the assisted and the agencies involved, particularly in the highly volatile environment of community care. Since each agent is completely autonomous it can respond according to the rules of the organization it represents, providing an effective and assured guardian that is totally under that organization's control. No other architectural framework for distributed information systems gives this capability without serious reliability problems.

An important issue that most e-health services address regards the possibility of jointly supporting professionals in their highly specialized work. Computer-Supported Cooperative Work (CSCW) is already common practice in tele-surgery and tele-assistance and it seems an important ingredient of next-generation e-health services. Notably, the inherent cooperative nature of agents and the very fact that many CSCW technologies are already based on agents is another important contribution of multi-agent systems to e-health.

Since simplified user interaction and communication among users are central to e-health and similar systems, this immediately promotes multi-agent systems as ideal candidates to support next-generation e-health services and social applications. Similarly, the central venue that security and privacy-awareness have in multi-agent systems again stresses their importance of them with respect to e-health. In the agent realm, the issues of privacy-awareness are treated under the umbrella of the more expressive notion of trust (Poggi et al., 2003; Poggi et al., 2005; Tomaiuolo, 2013). Likewise, social services strongly remark the importance of preserving confidentiality and guaranteeing a high level of security for classified information about patients.

Moreover, technological changes intertwine into this scenario, with widespread adoption of various types of computing devices, ranging from laptop and lighter mobile devices to mobile phones, accompanying users through different locations and different countries. Accordingly, e-health deals naturally with mobile users, e.g., in tele-assistance scenarios, and it is common understanding that e-health should transparently accommodate fixed and mobile users. So-called m-health services should be accessible to anyone, anywhere, anytime, anyhow. In mobile scenarios, various devices can be used to collect, transmit and process vital patients' data, e.g., heart rate and blood pressure, in real time (De Mola et al., 2006). Such systems are especially important in applications that remotely monitor patients with chronic ailments or in homecare.

Broadly speaking, such systems are designed to access medical information in a mobile and ubiquitous setting. This access may be either

1. The retrieval of relevant medical information for use of healthcare practitioners, e.g., a hospital doctor on his/her ward round; or
2. The acquisition of patient-generated medical information, e.g., tele-monitoring the patient's health state outside the hospital.

In both cases, it is extremely important to ensure that the person retrieving or generating information could interact with a ubiquitous and pervasive e-health system without any obstruction or adaptation of the normal workflow or style of working. In particular, fault-tolerance, reliability, security and privacy-awareness are necessary in order to accommodate the strict requirements of all healthcare applications.

Moreover, such applications require a smoothly integration of context and location awareness, i.e., the access and the visualization of health-related information should always depend on the overall contexts of the patient and of the user (Bricon-Souf & Newman, 2007). Finally, such applications should take advantage of effective mobile devices to provide access to relevant health-related information independently of the current physical location and physical condition of the user; and of unobtrusive sensor technology to enable the gathering of physiological information from the patient without hampering his/her daily life.

All mentioned requirements immediately recall the characterizing features of multi-agent systems and it comes with no surprise that many ubiquitous and pervasive e-health systems are developed using multi-agent abstractions and technologies. In particular, the JADE framework and its lightweight version JADE-LEAP (Bergenti et al., 2001) do take special care of transparently and dynamically allocating users and agents on heterogeneous network of different types of devices.

An important issue in e-health is about supporting the interoperability of (legacy) medical information systems in order to enable the integrated provision of services for accessing information from different, remote sources. The dream of a single, universally accepted middleware supporting the development of new services together with the renewal of legacy services was quickly abandoned. Nowadays recent technologies, that were originally intended to support the (semantic) interoperation between heterogeneous services, are commonly adopted in practice. This, again, emphasizes the role of multi-agent systems for providing important contributions to e-health, because of the inherent semantics-awareness of the interaction between agents, which make them ready to deliver semantic interoperability.

A lot of work has been done in the last decade for spreading the use of multi-agent systems for the realization of software applications and services, with particular attention to interoperability among agent platforms and with other systems. Several technological specifications are the results of such work. Among them, the two main results to date are:

1. FIPA specifications (Poslad & Charlton, 2001), a set of specifications intended to support the interoperability between heterogeneous agent-based systems; and
2. An agent development framework, called JADE (Bellifemine et al., 2008), that implements FIPA specifications and that supports interoperability between agents using consolidated technologies, e.g., Java and CORBA.

E-HEALTH MULTI-AGENT SYSTEMS

As is described above, multi-agent systems can become a key ingredient of the next-generation e-health services and applications, however, in the last ten years they have been already used for realizing e-health applications and, in particular, for realizing assistive living, diagnostic, physiological tele-monitoring, smart hospital and smart emergency applications.

Nowadays both professionals and patients prefer the provision of health and social services directly in the community of the assisted people. In this sense, the integration of smart-home automation is an essential aspect of assisted living, above all for chronically ill patients, elderly, impaired, psychologically or socially diseased people (Mynatt et al, 2000; Liffick, 2003, Mann, 2005). All projects in this domain are notably challenging because they should naturally accommodate many, if not all, the challenging aspects of the kinds of applications mentioned above. Elderly people tend to suffer from at least one chronic disease, which requires tele-monitoring. Additional age impairments make independent living at home difficult and therefore assistance for daily activities is required. Moreover, the additional context information provided by a smart-home environment enhances a better interpretation of physiological sensor information, e.g., whether the patient is running or sleeping has significant influence on the blood pressure (Lee et al., 2012; Pustišek et al. 2013). Overall, multi-agent systems are the common denominator of the kinds of uses that we listed above and this is the reason why we believe that they are a key factor for the coherent and successful development of assistive living applications. Four of the most interesting projects are CASIS (Jih et al., 2006), K4CARE (Campana et al., 2008), PRiDE (Turcu & Turcu, 2013) and SESA (Bielskis et al., 2015).

Tele-monitoring is becoming an extremely important application domain in the context of e-health, mainly because of the progression of chronic ailments in the aging society (Meystre, 2005). First, such applications enable healthcare institutions to manage and monitor the therapies of their patients. Second, they serve as instrument for performing large-scale medical researches and studies. Third, they support the timely activation of emergency services in case of severe health conditions. Due to the nature of such applications, that are continuously monitoring physiological signals, unobtrusiveness and mobility of the patient are key requirements. Moreover, these applications can offer additional comfort services, like assistive services, information services and communication services, which leads us naturally to the adoption of multi-agent systems for the realization of physiological tele-monitoring applications (Rialle et al., 2003). Six of the most interesting projects that use multi-agent systems are: MobiHealth (Van Halteren et al., 2004), U-R-SAFE (Castanie et al., 2005), AID-N (Gao et al., 2007), MyHeart (Amft & Habetha, 2007), SAPHIRE (Laleci et al., 2008) and MADIP (Su & Wu, 2011).

When located at caregiver's site, e-health applications are often known as smart-hospital applications. Such applications try to improve the daily activities of doctors and nurses. This is commonly done by providing tools to access patient records or, more generally, clinical information systems, as well as to schedule and track patients and hospital resources in a wireless, mobile, and context-aware manner. It is worth noting that recent projects introduce the use of RFID technology for further improving these applications, as exemplified in the Jacobi case study (Fuhrer & Guinard, 2006). Another case of e-health at the caregiver's site regards emergency management by means of mobile devices. Emergency physicians are able to access the records of their patients in advance while they are still in the ambulance car approaching the location of the patient. If we also consider the triggering of emergencies and access of current physiological signals, these applications spans the bridge between the caretaker and patient's site. Three of the most interesting projects that use multi-agent systems are: ERMA (Mabry et al., 2004), Akogrimo (Racz et al., 2007) and CASCOM (Schumacher et al., 2008).

FUTURE RESEARCH DIRECTIONS

The applications for modern healthcare and social services are distributed and complex by their nature. In this kind of scenarios, multi-agent systems have been proved as one of the most convenient paradigms. In particular, multi-agent systems should be considered as a model that provides a novel level of abstraction, rather than a single technology. The approach based on multi-agent systems is concretized into different technologies depending on the concrete needs of various advanced applications. This allows describing various projects and applications that concretely use diverse technologies in terms of agents and multi-agent systems, and, in particular, the paradigm fits quite well the e-health and social services scenarios, too. In fact, the overall management of cares in vast open environments requires shared and distributed decision-making processes, which are based on the communication and coordination of complex and diverse forms of information between involved organizations and people. Therefore, the coupling of multi-agent systems and social cares is quite natural: multi-agent systems have the suitable features for modelling and realizing current and future applications in the health and social fields; by converse, multi-agent systems are offered the suitable requirements for experimenting at best their applicability and, so, for receiving a great contribution to their own evolution and success.

Nevertheless, to provide valuable contribution to healthcare, ICT solutions have to face important challenges. Among the open issues, some are identifiable in any application domain, such as user expectations and acceptance, and lack of centralized control; others are typical of the healthcare domain, such as legal and ethical issues like privacy, integrity and authentication in the exchange of patient information between agents. In general, the adoption of advanced ICT solutions is not happening at the rapid pace fostered by the early optimism. Problems originate from the inherent difficulties of having ICT accepted in healthcare and social services from the technical, social, ethical, political, legal and economical points of view. This is a well-discussed topic in the literature and interested readers can refer to some notable works (Barnes & Uncapher, 2000; Jadad et al., 2000; Laxminarayan & Stamm, 2002; Wilson et al., 2004; Kvedar et al., 2014). The distance between the actual research and the real status of the health and social system poses several problems to a wide adoption of ICT. Another obstacle, for the widespread adoption of advanced ICT solutions in healthcare and social services, is the lack of data and methodology for the economic evaluation of the impact of new technologies (e.g. the reimbursement for provided services is not well defined). Finally, interoperability is another important barrier to adoption of telemedicine (Helal et al., 2011; Gaynor, 2015). In fact, interoperability is necessary for making possible and simplifying the exchange of data between the devices of the patients and data storage providers. To cope with such problem, a help can be given by Continua Health Alliance (Carroll et al, 2007), an industry consortium involving worldwide companies whose goal is the definition of standardized protocol specifications addressing data collection and storage. Moreover, as discussed above, multi-agent systems have always considered a suitable means for supporting systems interoperability and so they will be a possible solution for the implementation of the software layer providing an interoperable data exchange between patient's devices and data storage providers

CONCLUSION

In conclusion, the application of a multi-agent approach to e-health and social services does not imply that all those problems are definitely solved. However, most of those problems are intrinsic to the application scenario, and the solid theoretical model of multi-agent systems only provide a better ground to identify and trace them. Real programs built on the multi-agent paradigm are still evolving towards a complete maturity, and the variety and complexity of the e-health scenario make it one of most interesting application fields, able of verifying the advantages of their use and of conditioning their evolution.

According to Altman (Altman, 1999), one of the most important challenges, in the field of Artificial Intelligence, regards having medical records "based on semantically clean knowledge representation techniques." Most models of autonomous software agents provide semantic communication as a basic feature. Moreover, thanks to their intrinsically distributed nature and their autonomy, agents provide a clean way to make such records available anywhere, at any time. Agents will improve healthcare organizations, by supporting doctors and caregivers. However, the use of agent technology will mean quite a radical and general change in how healthcare and assistance will be provided, with a large impact on patients, too. Finally, agent technology can be a key component for realizing the envisioned "smart use of computation" (Annicchiarico et al., 2007). In all these senses, multi-agent systems will greatly benefit from the current work on their integration with Web services (Nguyen, 2005; Poggi et al., 2007), the Semantic Web (Hendler, 2001; Bergenti et al., 2005) and workflows (Negri et al., 2006). In fact, such technologies already and/or will be fundamental components of healthcare and social services (Bicer et al., 2005).

REFERENCES

Altman, R. B. (1999). AI in medicine: The spectrum of challenges from managed care to molecular medicine. *AI Magazine, 20*(3), 67.

Amft, O., & Habetha, J. (2007). The MyHeart Project. In L. Langenhove (Ed.), *Smart textiles for medicine and healthcare* (pp. 275–297). Cambridge, UK: Woodhead Publishing. doi:10.1533/9781845692933.2.275

Annicchiarico, R., Cortés, U., & Urdiales, C. (2008). *Agent Technology and e-Health*. Babel, Switzerland: Birkhäuser Verlag. doi:10.1007/978-3-7643-8547-7

Barnes, G. A., & Uncapher, M. (2000). *Getting to e-Health: The Opportunities for Using IT in the Health Care Industry*. Arlington, VA: Information Technology Association of America.

Bellifemine, F., Caire, G., Poggi, A., & Rimassa, G. (2008). JADE: A Software Framework for Developing Multi-Agent Applications. Lessons Learned. *Information and Software Technology Journal, 50*(1-2), 10–21. doi:10.1016/j.infsof.2007.10.008

Bergenti, F., & Huhns, M. N. (2004). On the use of agents as components of software systems. In F. Bergenti, M. P. Gleizes, & F. Zambonelli (Eds.), *Methodologies and Software Engineering for Agent Systems* (pp. 19–31). New York, NY: Kluwer. doi:10.1007/1-4020-8058-1_3

Bergenti, F., & Poggi, A. (2002). LEAP: A FIPA platform for handheld and mobile devices. In *Intelligent Agents VIII* (pp. 436–446). Berlin, Germany: Springer. doi:10.1007/3-540-45448-9_33

Bergenti, F., Poggi, A., Tomaiuolo, M., & Turci, P. (2005). An Ontology Support for Semantic Aware Agents. In *Seventh International Workshop on Agent-Oriented Information Systems (AOIS-2005)*.

Bicer, V., Kilic, O., Dogac, A., & Laleci, G. B. (2005). Archetype-Based Semantic Interoperability of Web Service Messages in the Health Care Domain. *International Journal on Semantic Web and Information Systems, 1*(4), 1–23. doi:10.4018/jswis.2005100101

Bielskis, A. A., Andziulis, A., Ramasauskas, O., Guseinoviene, E., Dzemydiene, D., & Gricius, G. (2015). Multi-Agent Based E-Social Care Support System for Inhabitancies of a Smart Eco-Social Apartment. *Elektronika ir Elektrotechnika, 107*(1), 11-14.

Bordini, R. H., Dastani, M., Dix, J., & El Fallah Seghrouchni, A. (2005). *Multi-Agent Programming: Languages, Platforms and Applications*. Berlin, Germany: Springer.

Bricon-Souf, N., & Newman, C. (2007). Context awareness in health care: A review. *International Journal of Medical Informatics, 76*(1), 2–12. doi:10.1016/j.ijmedinf.2006.01.003 PMID:16488663

Campana, F., Moreno, A., Riano, D., & Varga, L. Z. (2008). K4care: Knowledge-based homecare e-services for an ageing europe. In *Agent Technology and e-Health* (pp. 95–115). Babel, Switzerland: Birkhäuser Verlag. doi:10.1007/978-3-7643-8547-7_6

Carroll, R., Cnossen, R., Schnell, M., & Simons, D. (2007). Continua: An interoperable personal healthcare ecosystem. *Pervasive Computing, IEEE, 6*(4), 90–94. doi:10.1109/MPRV.2007.72

Castanie, F., Mailhes, C., & Henrion, S. (2005). End-to-end signal processing from the embedded body sensor to the medical end user through QoS-less public communication channels: The UR-SAFE experience. *Studies in Health Technology and Informatics, 117*, 172–179. PMID:16282667

De Mola, F., Cabri, G., Muratori, N., Quitadamo, R., & Zambonelli, F. (2006). The UbiMedic Framework to Support Medical Emergencies by Ubiquitous Computing. *International Transactions on Systems Science and Applications, 1*(1), 15–26.

Durfee, E. H. (1999). Distributed problem solving and planning. In G. Weiss (Ed.), *Multiagent Systems: A Modern Approach To Distributed Artificial intelligence* (pp. 121–164). Cambridge, MA: MIT Press.

Franchi, E., Poggi, A., & Tomaiuolo, M. (2013). Open Social Networking for Online Collaboration. [IJeC]. *International Journal of e-Collaboration, 9*(3), 50–68. doi:10.4018/jec.2013070104

Fuhrer, J. P., & Guinard, D. (2006) Building a Smart Hospital Using RFID Technologies. In *Proc. of the First European Conference on eHealth (ECEH06)*, (pp. 131-142).

Gao, T., Massey, T., Selavo, L., Crawford, D., Chen, B. R., Lorincz, K., & Welsh, M. et al. (2007). The Advanced Health and Disaster Aid Network: A Light-weight Wireless Medical System for Triage. *IEEE Transactions on Biomedical Circuits and Systems, 1*(3), 203–216. doi:10.1109/TBCAS.2007.910901 PMID:23852414

Gaynor, M. G. (2015). *Evaluation of Patient to Provider Oriented Telemedicine in Hospitals and Physician Practices*. Retrieved June 27, 2015 from http://digitalcommons.usm.maine.edu/cgi/viewcontent.cgi?article=1101&context=muskie_capstones

Genesereth, M. R., & Ketchpel, S. P. (2004). Software agents. *Communications of the ACM, 37*(7), 48–53, ff. doi:10.1145/176789.176794

Helal, S., Bose, R., Chen, C., Smith, A., De Deugd, S., & Cook, D. (2011). STEPSTONE: An intelligent integration architecture for personal tele-health. *Journal of Computing Science and Engineering, 5*(3), 269–281. doi:10.5626/JCSE.2011.5.3.269

Hendler, J. (2001). Agents and the Semantic Web. *IEEE Intelligent Systems, 16*(2), 30–37. doi:10.1109/5254.920597

Horling, B., & Lesser, V. (2005). A Survey of Multi-Agent Organizational Paradigms. *The Knowledge Engineering Review, 19*(4), 281–316. doi:10.1017/S0269888905000317

Jadad, A. R., Goel, V., Rizo, C., Hohenadel, J., & Cortinois, A. (2000). The Global e-Health Innovation Network - Building a Vehicle for the Transformation of the Health System in the Information Age. In *Business Briefing: Next Generation Healthcare*, (pp. 48-54). Academic Press.

Jennings, N. R. (2000). On Agent-Based Software Engineering. *Artificial Intelligence, 117*(2), 277–296. doi:10.1016/S0004-3702(99)00107-1

Jennings, N. R., Corera, J. M., & Laresgoiti, I. (1995). Developing Industrial Multiagent Systems. In *Proc. of the First International Conference on Multiagent Systems*, (pp. 423-430). Menlo Park, CA: AAAI Press.

Jennings, N. R., Faratin, P., Lomuscio, A. R., Parsons, S., Sierra, C., & Wooldridge, M. (2001). Automated negotiation: Prospects, methods and challenges. *Group Decision and Negotiation, 10*(2), 199–215. doi:10.1023/A:1008746126376

Jih, W., Hsu, J. Y., & Tsai, T. (2006) Context-aware service integration for elderly care in a smart environment. In *2006 AAAI Workshop on Modeling and Retrieval of Context Retrieval of Context*, (pp. 44-48). Menlo Park, CA: AAAI Press.

Kvedar, J., Coye, M. J., & Everett, W. (2014). Connected health: A review of technologies and strategies to improve patient care with telemedicine and telehealth. *Health Affairs, 33*(2), 194–199. doi:10.1377/hlthaff.2013.0992 PMID:24493760

Laleci, G. B., Dogac, A., Olduz, M., Tasyurt, I., Yuksel, M., & Okcan, A. (2008). SAPHIRE: A Multi-Agent System for Remote Healthcare Monitoring through Computerized Clinical Guidelines. In *Agent Technology and e-Health* (pp. 25–44). Babel, Switzerland: Birkhäuser Verlag. doi:10.1007/978-3-7643-8547-7_3

Laxminarayan, S., & Stamm, B. H. (2002). Technology, Telemedicine and Telehealth. In *Business Briefing: Global Healthcare* (Vol. 3, pp. 93–96). London, UK: World Medical Association.

Lee, D., Helal, S., Anton, S., De Deugd, S., & Smith, A. (2012). Participatory and persuasive telehealth. *Gerontology, 58*(3), 269–281. doi:10.1159/000329892 PMID:21893945

Liffick, B. W. (2003). Assistive technology in computer science. In *Proc. of the First international Symposium on information and Communication Technologies*, (pp. 46-51).

Mabry, S. L., Hug, C. R., & Roundy, R. C. (2004). Clinical decision support with IM-agents and ERMA multi-agents. In *Proc. of the 17th IEEE Symposium on Computer-Based Medical Systems (CBMS 2004)*, (pp. 242-247). doi:10.1109/CBMS.2004.1311722

Mann, W. C. (2005). *Smart Technology for Aging, Disability, and Independence: The State of the Science*. Hoboken, NJ: John Wiley & Sons. doi:10.1002/0471743941

Meystre, S. (2005). The Current State of Telemonitoring: A Comment on the Literature. *Telemedicine Journal and e-Health, 11*(1), 63–69. doi:10.1089/tmj.2005.11.63 PMID:15785222

Moreno, A., & Nealon, J. (Eds.). (2003). *Applications of Software Agents Technology in the Health Care Domain. Whitestein Series in Software Agent Technology*. Babel, Switzerland: Birkhäuser Verlag. doi:10.1007/978-3-0348-7976-7

Muller, J. P. (1998). Architectures and applications of intelligent agents: A survey. *The Knowledge Engineering Review, 13*(4), 353–380. doi:10.1017/S0269888998004020

Mynatt, E. D., Essa, I., & Rogers, W. (2000). Increasing the opportunities for aging in place. In *Proc. of the 2000 Conference on Universal Usability*, (pp. 65-71). doi:10.1145/355460.355475

Negri, A., Poggi, A., Tomaiuolo, M., & Turci, P. (2006). Agents for e-Business Applications, In *Proc. of the 5th International Joint Conference on Autonomous Agents and Multi Agent Systems*, (pp. 907-914).

Newell, A. (1982). The Knowledge Level. *Artificial Intelligence, 18*(1), 87–127. doi:10.1016/0004-3702(82)90012-1

Nguyen, X. T. (2005). Demonstration of WS2JADE. In *Proc. of the Fourth International Joint Conference on Autonomous Agents and Multi Agent Systems*, (pp. 135-136). doi:10.1145/1082473.1082820

Poggi, A., Tomaiuolo, M., & Turci, P. (2007). An Agent-Based Service Oriented Architecture. In WOA 2007: Dagli Oggetti agli Agenti.

Poggi, A., Tomaiuolo, M., & Vitaglione, G. (2003). Security and Trust in Agent-Oriented Middleware. Lecture Notes in Computer Science, 2889, 989-1003. doi:10.1007/978-3-540-39962-9_95

Poggi, A., Tomaiuolo, M., & Vitaglione, G. (2005). A Security Infrastructure for Trust Management in Multi-agent Systems. Lecture Notes in Computer Science, 3577, 162-179. doi:10.1007/11532095_10

Poslad, S., & Charlton, P. (2001). Standardizing agent interoperability: The FIPA approach. In *Multi-Agent Systems and Applications* (pp. 98–117). Berlin, Germany: Springer. doi:10.1007/3-540-47745-4_5

Pustišek, M., Stojmenova, E., Zebec, L., & Kervina, D. (2013). *Bringing health telemonitoring into IPTV based AMI environment*. Other Publications of the AMEA Association. Retrieved June 27, 2015 from http://www.ambientmediaassociation.org/Journal/index.php/previous/article/viewFile/28/26

Racz, P., Burgos, J. E., Inacio, N., Morariu, C., Olmedo, V., Villagra, V.,... Stiller, B. (2007). Mobility and QoS Support for a Commercial Mobile Grid in Akogrimo. In Mobile and Wireless Communications Summit, (pp. 1-5). doi:10.1109/ISTMWC.2007.4299247

Rialle, V., Lamy, J., Noury, N., & Bajolle, L. (2003). Telemonitoring of patients at home: A software agent approach. *Computer Methods and Programs in Biomedicine*, 72(3), 257–268. doi:10.1016/S0169-2607(02)00161-X PMID:14554139

Russell, S. J., & Norvig, S. J. (2003). *Artificial Intelligence: A Modern Approach*. Upper Saddle River, NJ: Pearson Education.

Schumacher, M., Helin, H., & Schuldt, H. (2008). *CASCOM: Intelligent Service Coordination in the Semantic Web: Intelligent Service Coordination in the Semantic Web*. Berlin, Germany: Springer. doi:10.1007/978-3-7643-8575-0

Smith, R., & Davis, R. (1980). The contract Net protocol: High level communication and control in a distributed problem solver. *IEEE Transactions on Computers*, 29(12), 1104–1113. doi:10.1109/TC.1980.1675516

Su, C. J., & Wu, C. Y. (2011). JADE implemented mobile multi-agent based, distributed information platform for pervasive health care monitoring. *Applied Soft Computing*, 11(1), 315–325. doi:10.1016/j.asoc.2009.11.022

Tomaiuolo, M. (2013). dDelega: Trust Management for Web Services. *International Journal of Information Security and Privacy*, 7(3), 53–67. doi:10.4018/jisp.2013070104

Tonino, H., Bos, A., de Weerdt, M., & Witteveen, C. (2002). Plan coordination by revision in collective agent based systems. *Artificial Intelligence*, 142(2), 121–145. doi:10.1016/S0004-3702(02)00273-4

Turcu, C. E., & Turcu, C. O. (2013). Internet of things as key enabler for sustainable healthcare delivery. *Procedia: Social and Behavioral Sciences*, 73, 251–256. doi:10.1016/j.sbspro.2013.02.049

Van Halteren, A., Bults, R., Wac, K., Dokovsky, N., Koprinkov, G., Widya, I., & Herzog, R. et al. (2004). Wireless body area networks for healthcare: The MobiHealth project. *Studies in Health Technology and Informatics*, *108*, 181–193. PMID:15718645

Wilson, P., Leitner, C., & Moussalli, A. (2004). Mapping the Potential of eHealth: Empowering the Citizen through eHealth Tools and Services. In *Proc. of E-Health Conference 2004*.

Wooldridge, M. J., & Jennings, N. R. (1995). Intelligent Agents: Theory and Practice. *The Knowledge Engineering Review*, *10*(2), 115–152. doi:10.1017/S0269888900008122

KEY TERMS AND DEFINITIONS

Contracting: A process where agents can assume the role of manager and contractor and where managers try to assign tasks to the most appropriate contractors.

Coordination: Coordination is a process in which a group of agents engages in order to ensure that each of them acts in a coherent manner.

Multi-Agent Planning: A process that can involve agents plan for a common goal, agents coordinating the plan of others, or agents refining their own plans while negotiating over tasks or resources.

Multi-Agent System: A multi-agent system (MAS) is a loosely coupled network of software agents that interact to solve problems that are beyond the individual capacities or knowledge of each software agent.

Negotiation: A process by which a group of agents come to a mutually acceptable agreement on some matter.

Organizational Structuring: A process for defining the organizational structure of a multi-agent system, i.e., the information, communication, and control relationships among the agents of the system.

Social Service: A service usually provided by a public organization for improving the quality of life of persons.

Software Agent: A software agent is a computer program that is situated in some environment and capable of autonomous action in order to meet its design objectives.

Neuropsychological Assessment from Traditional to ICT–Based Instruments

Isabel Almeida
Centro de Reabilitação Profissional de Gaia, Portugal

Artemisa Rocha Dores
Polytechnic Institute of Porto, Portugal

Paula Pinto
Centro de Reabilitação Profissional de Gaia, Portugal

Sandra Guerreiro
Centro de Reabilitação Profissional de Gaia, Portugal

Fernando Barbosa
Universidade do Porto, Portugal

INTRODUCTION

Achieving effective neuropsychological assessment is a major challenge for professionals in the field. The objective is to understand the interaction of cognitive, emotional and behavioral changes experienced by people who have sustained brain injuries. After acquired brain injury, neuropsychological assessment may be needed to determine the extent of their losses due to injury, if the person can benefit from rehabilitation and for planning interventions addressed to address individual needs. It is thought that improved focus of interventions will improve rehabilitation outcomes. Therefore, it assists clinicians to understand their patients' cognitive weaknesses and strengths. Nevertheless assessment of some cognitive functions, such as executive functions, is particularly demanding and difficult. Not only due to the complexity of the functions themselves but also due to the limitations of the available tools. A growing number of studies provide evidence that patients with executive dysfunctions can show good performances in conventional neuropsychological testing but at the same time, have problems successfully achieving simple daily activities. This questions the reliability of using only psychometric instruments for evaluation. Some limitations of psychometric tests documented in literature can clarify this phenomenon: situations are not really presented, but merely verbally described; decisions are only invoked, not performed; exercises fail in event sequencing (action-reaction); action is temporally concentrated; and evaluation procedures often occur in highly structured situations and therefore distant to the real life scenario of daily life activities. In order to overcome the limitations of traditional tools, information and communication technologies (ICT) tools are increasingly used in this area. A growing number of scientific publications evidence the role of ICT in the development of more ecological instruments for neuropsychological assessment. This literature review presents advantages and disadvantages of traditional and ICT based neuropsychological assessment instruments for evaluating cognitive functions.

DOI: 10.4018/978-1-4666-9978-6.ch054

BACKGROUND

Historical Perspective on Neuropsychological Assessment

Clinical Neuropsychology can be defined as the field of knowledge dedicated to the study of brain (dys) function in its relations to cognition, emotion and behavior. The development of this applied field is associated with the recognition, from several areas of knowledge, that people's behaviors and reactions are dependent on brain structures (Stringer, Cooley, & Christensen, 2002). This idea had been present in medical practice for several epochs, but it has gradually diminished its presence under the influence of other beliefs. World War II prompted the growth of neuropsychology as a scientific discipline, and revival of interest in brain-behavior understanding (Camargo, Bolognani, & Zuccolo, 2008). The necessity to evaluate, diagnose and rehabilitate cognitive, emotional and behavioral disorders presented by brain injured soldiers constituted a crucial moment for clinical neuropsychological practices. It created large-scale demands for neuropsychological evaluations and rehabilitation programs, promoting the development of observational and experimental studies about brain (dys)functions, and refined examination and intervention methods. In the last decades, with the development of advanced neuroimaging techniques, the knowledge of biological and biochemical basis of brain structures has progressed the understanding of mechanisms underpinning our behaviors and thoughts. These techniques have been widely diffused and used for the detection and localization of brain damage areas (Buckner, Wheeler, & Sheridan, 2001). As a consequence neuropsychological assessment had to change it's primarily goal and focus of interest away from an emphasis on helping to identify hypothesized lesion locations. It must now assist clinicians in understanding the extension and impact of cognitive, behavioral and socio-emotional consequences of brain injury on people's life in an integrated basis with current advances (Camargo et al., 2008).

Neuropsychological Assessment after Acquired Brain Injury

Acquired Brain injury (ABI) can be defined as a damage to the brain, which occurs after birth and is not related to a congenital or a degenerative disease. The deficits can be temporary or permanent and cause partial or functional disability or psychosocial maladjustment.

Neuropsychological assessment can be defined as a performance-based method used to examine the cognitive, behavioral and emotional consequences of damage to brain structures (Harvey, 2012). Damage of a brain area can affect the whole neuropsychological system and therefore evaluation must be comprehensive and investigate several domains: sensory and perceptual systems, motor functions, executive function, attention, memory, language skills, emotional state and behavior.

Assessment provides a comprehensive idea of a patients' global functioning; evaluates their actual competencies and the potential to benefit from rehabilitation programs. It also ought to help clinicians to understand the way in which a patients' central nervous system functioning is interacting with their unique psychosocial environment (Teeter & Semrud-Clikeman, 2007).

Neuropsychological assessment addresses a variety of questions, and neuropsychologists must be aware of both neurological and psychological aspects of the patient's capacities and handicaps (Lezak, Howieson, & Loring, 2004). This imposes constant challenges to examiners during the process, they are constantly balancing the need to respond to the actual purpose of the examination and at the same time to evaluate patients at levels that are suitable for their capacities and limitations.

Lezak, Howieson, and Loring (2004) argued that neuropsychological assessments may serve different objectives:

1. **Diagnosis:** Although its use as a diagnostic tool has diminished, it can still be very useful to discriminate between neurological and psychiatric symptoms, to screen mental functioning, to identify the nature of residual behavioral strengths and deficits, and to document mental (dis)abilities that may be inconsistent with anatomic lesions;

2. **Patient Care and Planning:** Comprehensive neuropsychological assessment, including patients history and background, qualitative and quantitative observations and test scores can help to provide realistic information, to patients, professionals and caregivers about patients (dis)abilities, the degree of adjustment to the deficits, the best compensation strategies that can be used, and the benefits of rehabilitation;

3. **Treatment Planning and Remediation:** Neuropsychological assessment is necessary for determining the more suitable intervention for each patient after brain injury; to achieve this goal, evaluations have to be sensitive, accurate, and include various areas of functioning so they can be helpful to define problematic areas and estimate the patients' strength competences and potential for rehabilitation;

4. **Treatment Evaluation:** The growing need of evidenced-based services, has put into rehabilitation the pressure to measure the cost-benefits of interventions and to provide evidence of their value; neuropsychological assessments can help to understand the psychological and social value of the changes that rehabilitation programs are promoting;

5. **Research:** The study of brain structures and functions, and its correlation with behaviors was, and still is, supported by neuropsychological assessment; with a strong exchange between research and clinical practice.

6. **Medico-Legal Neuropsychology:** Neuropsychological assessments for legal procedures are often conducted in order to assist decisions about monetary compensation of brain injured people, their potential for rehabilitation, and the extension and type of future care they will need in their lives.

The main role of neuropsychological assessments has changed. Its field of intervention has evolved from diagnostic and lesion location proposes to treatment decisions guidance, identification of patients' strengths, weaknesses and needs, and assistance of treatments' effectiveness and interventions evaluation and monitoring (Lezak et al., 2004; Root, D'Amato, & Reynolds, 2005). It must assist on the identification of interventions that are able to improve patient's autonomy, functionality and quality of life (Witsken, D'Amato & Hartlage, 2008). Clinicians have nowadays to, based on tests results, elaborate considerations about functional performances in natural settings, responding to questions regarding abilities to competently perform tasks as living independently or returning to previous jobs (Troster, 2000).

FROM TRADITIONAL TO ICT BASED INSTRUMENTS

Issues, Controversies, Problems

Traditional Based Instruments

Usually neuropsychological assessment is undertaken through the application of paper-and-pencil batteries that include tests of several areas of the cognitive and emotional functioning, being essentially performance-based. The compendium of commonly used tests can be standardized or targeted for the individual who's being assessed. Tests used are designed to require individuals to demonstrate their skills in the presence of an examiner. Based on tests results, clinicians are often required to provide appropriate recommendations for interventions and to describe how the deficits and strengths of cognitive and emotional functioning will impact upon performance in real-life situations. Many studies can be found in literature referring to psychometric proprieties of these instruments, their normative data, reliability and sensitivity, strengthening traditional tests capability for detecting deficits after brain injuries. Some examples of commonly used traditional neuropsychological batteries are presented in Table 1.

Despite the published claims of test utility, criticisms of this approach include:

1. Extensive time needed to perform the assessment,
2. Expensiveness of administration,
3. Limited accessibility of evaluation services;
4. The presence of practice effects and the limited existence of alternative test forms;
5. Poor ecological validity.

There are several explanations why standard measures frequently demonstrate poor ecological validity: test tasks are different from real-world scenarios, because they do not reproduce the multiplicity of stimuli that are experienced in real contexts and are differently affected by effort and motivation; scenarios are not really presented, but merely verbally described; decisions are only invoked, not performed; exercises fail in event sequencing (action-reaction); action is temporally concentrated; and the fact that evaluation procedures often occur in highly structured situations and therefore distant to the real life scenario of daily life activities. In addition, the assessment of functional outcomes is essential not only for planning treatment but also to deduce the impact of deficits on long-term functionality (Newman, Heaton, & Lehamn, 1978), and traditional instruments often neglect this evaluation. While several studies support the predictive value of standard neuropsychological measures (Dikmen, Machamer, Powell, & Temkin, 2003; Newman et al., 1978), there are rising questions about the capability of these instruments to accurately predict real-life performance because of their poor ecological validity.

Table 1. Most used traditional neuropsychological batteries

Function	Tests
General cognitive function	Intelligence Test (e.g. Wechsler Adult Intelligence tests)
Psychomotor Speed	Finger Tapping, Grooved Pegboard, Continuous Performance Tasks (reaction time)
Attention/Executive Function	• Trail Making test A & B • Coding tasks (e.g. symbol digit substitution) • Letter-number sequencing (working memory) • Stroop color-word tasks • Wisconsin Card Sorting Test
Learning & Memory	• Wechsler memory scales • Auditory Verbal Learning Tasks • Rey-Osterreith Complex Figure memory
Language	• Boston Diagnostic Aphasia Exam • Verbal Fluency Tests • Token Test
Visuoperceptual abilities	Complex figure tasks, Block design tasks
Depression symptoms	Beck Depression Inventory

The Question of Ecological Validity in Neuropsychological Assessment

The ecological validity of traditional test results beyond the structured clinic context is a critical concept in neuropsychological assessment. Ecological validity can be defined as the "functional and predictive relationship between the patient's performance on a set of neuropsychological tests and the patient's behavior in a variety of real world settings" (Sbordone, 1996, p.16). Ecological validity refers to the extension in which the test is a reliably measure of the function it claims to measure and the degree of assistance in making valid predictions of patients' functionality within various contexts. Franzen and Wilhelm (1996) identified two common approaches to establish ecological validity: verisimilitude and veridicality. Verisimilitude refers to the resemblance between the assessment tasks and everyday demands. Tests designed according to this approach contain everyday cognitive tasks allowing the neuropsychologist to make reliable inferences about the patients' capacity to perform similar tasks in daily life (Spooner & Pachana, 2006), overcoming some of the limitations encountered by other traditional tools. Some traditional standardized tests with adequate verisimilitude have already been developed such as The Test of Everyday Attention (Roberston, Ward, Ridgeway, & Nimmo-Smith, 1994), the Behavioral Assessment of the Dysexecutive Syndrome (Wilson, Alderman, Burgess, Emslie, & Evans, 1996), the Rivermead Behavioral Memory Test (Wilson, Cockburn, & Baddeley, 1985), and the Cambridge Test of Prospective Memory (Wilson et al., 2004). The other approach, veridicality, refers to the degree in which results of the assessment are related to scores on other measures that predict performance in real-world tasks. It uses statistical methods to determine the strength of the relationship between performance in traditional tools and measures of everyday functioning, such as employment status, clinician's ratings, and behavioral observations. There have been several critics to this approach, since the relation between the demands required on traditional tests and functional performance is not always obvious (Wilson, 1993).

A study, carried out by Chaytor and Schmitter-Edgecombe (2003), investigated the comparative effectiveness of these two approaches at predicting everyday cognitive abilities. They pointed out the existence of some support for the superiority of the verisimilitude approach, as there was a tendency for the results of these tests to be more highly and consistently related to everyday cognitive performance. Higginson, Arnett, and Voss (2000), in a single study examining attention test, also found that verisimilitudinous tests were better predictors of general functional outcome than traditional tests.

Regarding these findings the conceptualization behind the design of most tests has not yet reflected the shifting focus that neuropsychological assessment has made. Many older tests face limitations on their efficiency and ability to make predictions about patients' real world functioning. To produce inferences about performance in everyday life neuropsychologists still rely on the face validity of the tests and on their clinical experience, which is of concern.

SOLUTIONS AND RECOMMENDATIONS

Computerized Neuropsychological Assessment

Given the challenges of ecological validity and administration costs of traditional instruments, innovation is needed. Clinicians have reconsidered and developed assessment procedures in ways that help them to make inferences about patients' performance on their life contexts and therefore supply more accurate information for providing more efficient and effective treatments (Traughber & D'Amato, 2005). ICT can be an answer to this problem, as computerized assessment tools are being developed rapidly, and increasingly being used in this area. Computerized neuropsychological testing devices can be defined as "any instrument that utilizes a computer, digital tablet, handheld device, or other digital interface instead of a human examiner to administer, score, or interpret tests of brain function and related factors relevant to questions of neurological health and illness" (Bauer et al., 2012, p.363). Historically this movement started by computerizing traditional paper-and-pencil neuropsychological tests, such as Wechsler Adult Intelligence Scale or Wisconsin Card Sorting Test, among others. Although researchers have, in most of the cases, demonstrated that psychometric proprieties of traditional and computerized versions of the same tests were equivalent, psychometric proprieties of the computerized versions were questioned. The growing interest in the development of new tests using ICT technology, has led to the definition of criteria for their use and standardization (Bauer et al, 2012). Some batteries, such as Integrated Visual and Auditory Continuous Performance Test (Sandford & Turner, 2004) and Test of Variables of Attention (Dupuy & Cenedela, 2000), were especially developed for computerized assessment and standardized according to APA criteria. In sport-related concussion assessment computorized tools such as CogSport (CogState, 1999) or Immediate Post Concussion Assessment and Cognitive Testing (Lovell, Collins, Podell, Powell, & Maroon, 2000) are widely used and have proved to be of great assistance to assess even minor changes to indivuduals' baseline performance of and to rapidly and unexpensively assess a large number of atheletes. Computerized assessment batteries and tests have been proliferating (Table 2 for some examples) and may assume a dominant place in the neuropsychological assessment repertory.

Among potential advantages of using computerized tests we can point out the ability to:

1. Capture and engage patients' interest;
2. Rapidly test a large number of patients;
3. Measure more accurately performance on time-sensitive tasks (e.g. reaction time); (iv) potentially reduce time of assessment;
4. Reduce costs of test administration and scoring;
5. Facilitate data collection and exportation for research purposes;

Table 2. Computerized batteries and tests

Batteries and Tests	Functions
CogState™	Reaction time, attention, executive function, working memory, learning
Testing Attentional Performance – TAP	Reaction time, attention, executive function
Cambridge Neuropsychological Test Battery – CNTB	Planning, visuo-spatial memory, working memory, attention
Computerized Test Battery – CNTB	Reaction time, executive functions, visual memory, episodic memory, learning, language
Swinburne University Computerized Cognitive Assessment Battery – SUCCAB	Reaction time, episodic memory, working memory, attention
CNS Vital Signs	Executive functions, reaction time, visual memory, verbal memory, working memory
Automated Neuropsychologic Assessment Metrics – ANAM	Reaction time, executive functions, spatial memory
MicroCog	Spatial memory, reaction time
Computerized Memory Battery Test – CMBT	Episodic memory, verbal memory
Computerized test of spatial memory and reaction time	Attention, spatial memory, working memory, reaction time.

6. Enlarge accessibility of assessment for patients that cannot access existing neuropsychological services;
7. Design tasks more verisimilar to real world demands.

Some drawbacks are:

1. Less flexibility for changes in assessment,
2. Interference in performance of patients less familiar with computers,
3. Loss of rich information that can be obtained by observation of spontaneous behavior.

Literature in this domain indicates that virtual reality (VR) technology can be of great assistance in reducing these limitations, when performing assessment of complex and integrated cognitive functions such as executive functions, or memory. By allowing the user to interact and/or immerse in a computer-generated environment that simulates a real world milieu, VR can be a way of bringing together assessment instruments and the ability to understand how patients do perform in their natural contexts. The fact that scenarios created by a VR computer system can have data information displayed in all sensory modalities allows fully immersion and experience of the setting by the patient. These technologies also have the capacity to provide a consistent environment where endless repetitions of the same assessment task can be made, while preserving the flexibility to alter sensory presentations, task complexity, and response requirements (Thompson, Barett, Patterson, & Craig, 2012). The easy manipulation and realism of the stimuli and the higher ecological validity of task demands are among the advantages of using VR in neuropsychological assessment, especially of complex cognitive functions such as executive functioning, memory or attention. Assessment tools that use VR technology can bring to assessment several benefits that will help clinicians understand the impact of brain injury on daily life functioning:

1. The provision of a more realistic environment, with its distractions and stressors allowing patients to forget that they are being tested and neuropsychologists to assess behaviors closer to those occurring in patients' life;
2. Increased users participation, as interactivity and immersion in scenarios can enhance motivation for performing tasks;
3. Enhanced flexibility and capacity for self-initiation and structuring of behavior;
4. Better reliability and control of assessments enabling specialists to better tailor evaluation by defining stimulus presentation and measure of responses accordingly to clinicians' specifications and patients' abilities and needs;
5. Possibility to safely assess dangerous situations like driving;
6. Increase standardization of assessment protocols.

Studies analyzing the efficiency of VR environments on testing cognitive functions have found a strong correlation between real-world performance and test performance measured with a virtual environment (Brooks, Rose, Potter, Jayawardena, & Morling, 2004; Buckwalter & Rizzo, 1997; Zhang et al., 2001, 2003). Using VR evaluation protocols neuropsychologists can have instruments that support objective measurement of behaviors in ecologically valid, secure, and controllable milieus (Schultheis & Rizzo, 2001). Computerized assessment tools do not replace the role of neuropsychologists, but do give the possibility to conduct more ecological assessments, helping clinicians to better understand the impact of the deficits in daily situations. The clinical knowledge remains necessary to integrate the information received from the different data, in order to formulate clinical judgments.

FUTURE RESEARCH DIRECTIONS

The current amount of research and evidence produced about ICT based assessment instruments is important and should be taken into consideration by neuropsychologists. There is evidence supporting potential efficiency in providing ecological validity in evaluations. The introduction of ICT in the field of neuropsychological assessment may lead to more innovative practices, allowing more patients to be assessed at lower costs (e.g. online, self assessment devices), the opportunity for patients to access to services that otherwise would be excluded and the possibility to provide a more dynamic and motivating approach for patients (vis a vis, 'gamification' trends http://www.newscientist.com/article/mg20927940.300-game-on-when-work-becomes-play.html). Neuropsychologists are progressively integrating these instruments in their regular practices and the difficulties remaining in their use in clinical practice should be better understood (e.g. technology adjustment in cases of severe cognitive impairment). Researchers should aim to better understand why the integration of these tools in clinical practice is not growing as fast as their development. More accessible ICT tools for neuropsychological assessment are being developed, both in utilization and cost, and are also providing more evidences of their effectiveness in larger samples, with several neurological populations. But the challenge is far from being resolved and research still needs to focus in create more flexible, accessible and affordable computerized assessments instruments that will enable examiner to also access information about the processes that patients employed in performance.

CONCLUSION

There is an increasing need to go beyond traditional tests, and develop assessment tools that are more ecological and verisimilar to real context. Despite the growing presence and development of computerized assessment instruments, their integration in practice and research is still at the beginning. Changes in theories and views on assessment-based issues in neuropsychology can take some time to be fully integrated and accepted. The growing appreciation of neuropsychologists about the value of ecological assessments is helping the validation of ICT tools for clinical practice. The belief that traditional tests are ecologically valid, the degree of familiarity with the administration, scoring and interpretation of traditional assessment measures, the perception that computerized tests do not have psychometric norms and studies of validity, and the idea that natural behavior can be determined upon results of specific and concrete domains of function, may delay the systematic use of ICT tools in neuropsychological assessment.

Traditional neuropsychological assessment instruments play an important role in measuring performance across a broad range of cognitive functions, often with the benefit of good reliability, validity, and comprehensive normative data, but clinicians are realizing that they are insufficient to assist on the task of making inferences about patients' performance in the real-world. Thus both approaches, traditional and computerized, can co-exist in neuropsychological assessment equipping neuropsychologists better to respond to the complex questions about performance, potential of rehabilitation, best rehabilitation strategies, and prediction of long-term impacts of impairments.

REFERENCES

Bauer, R. S., Iverson, G. L., Cernich, A. N., Binder, L. M., Ruff, R. M., & Naugle, R. I. (2012). Computerized Neuropsychological Assessment Devices: Joint Position Paper of the American Academy of Clinical Neuropsychology and the National Academy of Neuropsychology. *Archives of Clinical Neuropsychology*, *27*(3), 362–373. doi:10.1093/arclin/acs027 PMID:22382386

Brooks, B. M., Rose, F. D., Potter, J., Jayawardena, S., & Morling, A. (2004). Assessing Stroke Patients´ Prospective Memory Using Virtual Reality. *Brain Injury: [BI]*, *18*(4), 391–401. doi:10.1080/0269905 0310001619855 PMID:14742152

Buckner, R. L., Wheeler, M. E., & Sheridan, M. (2001). Encoding processes during retrieval tasks. *Journal of Cognitive Neuroscience*, *13*, 406–415. PMID:11371316

Buckwalter, J. G., & Rizzo, A. A. (1997). Virtual reality and the neuropsychological assessment of persons with neurologically based cognitive impairments. *Studies in Health Technology and Informatics*, *39*, 17–21. PMID:10168914

Camargo, C. H. P., Bolognani, S. A. P., & Zuccolo, P. F. (2008), O exame neuropsicológico e os diferentes contextos de aplicação. In M. – D. Fuentes, C. Camargo, & Collegues (Eds.), Neuropsicologia: teoria e prática. Porto Alegre, RS: Artmed.

Chaytor, N., & Schmitter-Edgecombe, M. (2003). The ecological validity of neuropsychological tests: A review of the literature on everyday cognitive skills. *Neuropsychology Review*, *13*(4), 181–197. doi:10.1023/B:NERV.0000009483.91468.fb PMID:15000225

CogState. (1999). *CogSport*. Parkville, Australia: Cogstate, Ltd.

Dikmen, S. S., Machamer, J. E., Powell, J. M., & Temkin, N. R. (2003). Outcome 3 to 5 years after moderate to severe traumatic brain injury. *Archives of Physical Medicine and Rehabilitation*, *84*(10), 1449–1457. doi:10.1016/S0003-9993(03)00287-9 PMID:14586911

Dupuy, T., & Cenedela, M. (2000). *Test of Variables of Attention: User's guide*. Los Alamitos, CA: Universal Attention Disorders.

Franzen, M. D., & Wilhelm, K. L. (1996). Conceptual foundations of ecological validity in neuropsychological assessment. In R. J. Sbordone & C. J. Long (Eds.), *Ecological validity of neuropsychological testing* (pp. 91–112). Boca Raton, FL: St Lucie Press.

Harvey, P. D. (2012). Clinical applications of neuropsychological assessment. *Dialogues in Clinical Neuroscience*, *14*(1), 91–99. PMID:22577308

Higginson, C. I., Arnett, P. A., & Voss, W. D. (2000). The ecological validity of clinical tests of memory and attention in multiple sclerosis. *Archives of Clinical Neuropsychology*, *96*(3), 185–204. doi:10.1093/arclin/15.3.185 PMID:14590548

Lezak, M. D., Howienson, D. B., & Loring, D. W. (2004). *Neuropsychological assessment* (4th ed.). New York: Oxford University Press.

E

Lovell, M. R., Collins, M. W., Podell, K., Powell, J., & Maroon, J. (2000). *ImPACT: Immediate Post-Concussion Assessment and Cognitive Testing.* Pittsburgh, PA: NeuroHealth Systems, LLC.

Newman, O. S., Heaton, R. K., & Lehamn, R. A. (1978). Neuropsychological and MMPI correlates of patients future employment characteristics. *Perceptual and Motor Skills, 46*(2), 635–642. doi:10.2466/pms.1978.46.2.635 PMID:662567

Roberston, I. H., Ward, T., Ridgeway, V., & Nimmo-Smith, I. (1994). *The Test of Everyday Attention (TEA).* Bury St. Edmunds, UK: Thames Valley Test Company.

Root, K. A., D'Amato, R. C., & Reynolds, C. R. (2005). Providing neurodevelopmental, collaborative, consultative, and crisis intervention school neuropsychological services. In R. C. D'Amato, E. Fletcher, & C. R. Reynolds (Eds.), *Handbook of school neuropsychology* (pp. 15–40). Hoboken, NJ: Wiley.

Sandford, J. A., & Turner, A. (2004). *Iva + Plus ™: Integrated Visual and Auditory Continuous Performance Test administration manual.* Richmond, VA: Brain Train, Inc.

Sbordone, R. J. (1996). Ecological validity: Some critical issues for the neuropsychologist. In R. J. Sbordone & C. J. Long (Eds.), *Ecological validity of neuropsychological testing* (pp. 15–41). Boca Raton, FL: St Lucie Press.

Schultheis, M. T., & Rizzo, A. A. (2001). The application of virtual reality technology in rehabilitation. *Rehabilitation Psychology, 46*(3), 296–311. doi:10.1037/0090-5550.46.3.296

Spooner, D. M., & Pachana, N. A. (2006). Ecological validity in neuropsychological assessment: A case for greater consideration in research with neurological intact populations. *Archives of Clinical Neuropsychology, 21*(4), 327–337. doi:10.1016/j.acn.2006.04.004 PMID:16769198

Stringer, A. Y., Cooley, E. L., & Christensen, A.-L. (2002). *Pathways to prominence in neuropsychology. Reflections of twentieth century pioneers.* New York: Psychology Press.

Teeter, P. A., & Semrud-Clikeman, M. (2007). *Child neuropsychology: Assessment and intervention for neurodevelopment disorders* (2nd ed.). New York: Springer Publishing.

Thompson, O., Baret, S., Patterson, C., & Craig, D. (2012). Examining the Neurocognitive Validity of Commercially Available, Smart-Based Puzzle Games. *Psychology (Savannah, Ga.), 3*(7), 525–526.

Traughber, M. C., & D'Amato, R. C. (2005). Integrating evidence-based neuropsychological services into school settings: Issues and challenges for the future. In R. C. D' Amato, E. Fletcher-Janzen, & C. R. Reynolds (Eds.), *Handbook of school neuropsychology* (pp. 827–857). Hoboken, NJ: Wiley.

Troster, A. I. (2000). Clinical neuropsychology, functional neurosurgery, and restorative neurology in the next millennium: Beyond secondary outcome measures. *Brain and Cognition, 42*(1), 117–119. doi:10.1006/brcg.1999.1178 PMID:10739615

Wilson, B. A. (1993). Ecological validity of neuropsychological assessment: Do neuropsychological indexes predict performance in everyday activities? *Applied & Preventive Psychology, 2*(4), 209–2015. doi:10.1016/S0962-1849(05)80091-5

Wilson, B. A., Alderman, N., Burgess, P. W., Emslie, H., & Evans, J. J. (1996). *Behavioral Assessment of the Dysexecutive Syndrome.* Bury St. Edmunds, UK: Thames Valley Test Company.

Wilson, B. A., Cockburn, J. M., & Baddeley, A. D. (1985). *The Rivermead Behavioral Memory Test.* Thames Valley Test Company/National Rehabilitation Services.

Wilson, B. A., Shiel, A., Foley, J., Emslie, H., Groot, Y., Hawkins, K., & Watson, P. (2004). *Cambridge test of Prospective memory.* Bury St. Edmunds, UK: Thames Valley Test Company.

Witsken, D. E., D'Amato, R. C., & Hartlage, L. C. (2008). Understanding the Past, Present, and Future of Clinical Neuropsychology. In R. C. D'Amato & L. C. Hartlage (Eds.), *Essentials of neuropsychological assessment – Treatment Planning for Rehabilitation* (pp. 3–29). Springer Publishing Company.

Zhang, L., Abreu, B. C., Masel, B., Scheibel, R. S., Christiansen, C. H., Huddleston, N., & Ottenbacher, K. J. (2001). Virtual reality in the assessment of selected cognitive function after brain injury. *American Journal of Physical Medicine & Rehabilitation*, *80*(8), 597–604. doi:10.1097/00002060-200108000-00010 PMID:11475481

Zhang, L., Abreu, B. C., Seale, G. S., Masel, B., Christiansen, C. H., & Otterbacker, K. J. (2003). A virtual reality environment for evaluation of daily living skills in brain injury rehabilitation: Reliability and validity. *American Journal of Physical Medicine & Rehabilitation*, *84*, 1118–1124. doi:10.1016/S0003-9993(03)00203-X PMID:12917848

KEY TERMS AND DEFINITIONS

Acquired Brain Injury: Any damage to the brain occurred after birth that can cause total or partial functional impairment or psychosocial maladjustment.

Clinical Neuropsychology: The field of knowledge that studies the relation between neural mechanisms, cognitive functions and behavior.

Computerized Neuropsychological Assessment: An assessment procedure that utilizes a computer interface instead of a human examiner for the administration and scoring of neuropsychological tests.

Ecological Validity: The functional and predictive relationship between patients' performance on a set of neuropsychological tests and its behavior in a variety of real world settings.

Neuropsychological Assessment: Performance-based method used to assess various cognitive skills, such as attention, memory, language, processing speed, spatial orientation, and executive functioning, in order to understand the impact of brain damage in cognitive, emotional and social performance.

Non-Intrusive Health-Monitoring Devices

Yujun Fu
The Hong Kong Polytechnic University, Hong Kong

Hong Va Leong
The Hong Kong Polytechnic University, Hong Kong

Grace Ngai
The Hong Kong Polytechnic University, Hong Kong

Stephen Chan
The Hong Kong Polytechnic University, Hong Kong

INTRODUCTION

Technological advancements in medical and health-care areas have brought about the longevity of human beings. The World Health Organization recognizes that "the world population is rapidly ageing" and that it is necessary to "reinvent our assumptions of old age" to promote healthy living (WHO, n.d.). The subsequent increase in health-related expenses has imposed significant financial burdens on many governments and individuals. The US government has had to push for a reform in the country's medical system in order for it to stay sustainable in the future. Monitoring well-being, early disease detection and preventive health-care are becoming increasingly important in reducing the high cost of treatment and recovery from illness. This can be alleviated through the realization of e-health, by computerizing the whole process and analyzing data on a continuous basis. There are many facets of e-health. In the large scale, it involves the complete workflow of acquiring, storing and retrieving medical records, controlling accessibility and access privileges to those records, and managing the security and privacy issues that arise, for instance, the Cardiovascular Health Informatics and Multi-modal E-record (CHIME) (Zhang, Poon, & MacPherson, 2009). Monitoring and analysis on the health condition could also be performed over the cloud, riding on recent advancement of efficient and high bandwidth communication infrastructure (Li, Guo, & Guo, 2014). It has been demonstrated that the continually acquired heart-beat rate and blood pressure time series could be very useful in monitoring patient progress and predicting patient survival rate via machine learning approaches (Lehman et al., 2015). In the context of health monitoring, a major focus is on the efficient acquisition of medical information for storage and analysis. Advances in health monitoring technologies have also blurred the distinction between health and disease to make it a continuum, with a paradigm shift towards prevention, prediction, personalized treatment and participatory medicine (Andreu-Perez, Leff, Ip, & Yang, 2015). In this chapter, the preventive stage of health problem, along the venue of effective health monitoring, is studied.

Many contemporary health-monitoring technologies are more or less based on *intrusive* devices, which impose certain burdens on users and demand that they adapt to the presence of those devices. Even though this is rather accepted for a patient, this is not quite desirable for a normal person, since it will inevitably affect his/her daily life and work, especially when continual monitoring is in place. In this chapter, contemporary health-monitoring technologies are revisited, with an emphasis being paid

DOI: 10.4018/978-1-4666-9978-6.ch055

on health-monitoring devices and non-intrusive approaches. The design of a novel physiological mouse that measures the heart-beat rate and respiratory rate of a user is presented, based on the processing of photoplethysmographic signals. A prototype is built with diodes and light sensors, conveying the measured light intensities for further processing upon a conventional mouse. Finally, experiments are conducted to validate the physiological mouse design, demonstrating its usability and good accuracy.

HEALTH MONITORING AND NON-INTRUSIVE TECHNOLOGY

Health monitoring has long been an important issue, and affordability and demand have always been important aspects for consideration. The former comes as a positive influence as technology advances and smaller and smarter devices become available at lower cost. The latter is induced by the changing demographics of an aging society in which more people need to rely on the technology for ensuring their health. According to (Celler & Sparks, 2015), there are currently over 40 major international manufacturers of tele-monitoring systems, and yet far more products to monitor health for vital signals. However, most contemporary health-monitoring devices are expensive, or intrusive. For instance, one cannot expect everybody to own an ECG (electrocardiogram) device at home. It is also very tedious and intrusive to attach the many needed electrodes to a human. Though such sophisticated devices are in general capable of returning a lot of sensing data, they also create heavy demand on the computation power for processing. Another example is the health chair (Anttonen & Surakka, 2005; Griffiths, Saponas, & Brush, 2014). Though not as intrusive as the ECG devices and many other similar devices, these chairs are often fairly expensive with a good number of sensors attached and they cannot often follow the users to move from places to places freely. The processing overhead or computational demand is also non-negligible.

To enhance usage and to reduce cost, this chapter focuses on *wearable health-monitoring devices* created in recent years, as they are devices that possess the potential to help ordinary users to monitor their health at home or perhaps at work. The evolution of pervasive health monitoring devices and technologies is summarized in (Andreu-Perez et al., 2015) from episodic monitoring to continuous sensing and integrated care, stepping into the era of exciting and yet demanding big data processing context. Processing and communication mechanism, security and privacy, data fusion and prediction, and other relevant issues need to be studied in this new context. Common contemporary health-monitoring devices range from simple temperature monitors, pulse monitors, to slightly more complex respiration monitors, $SpO2$ (oxygen saturation in blood) monitors, activity monitors, and so on. To make this health monitoring paradigm more effective, remote health monitoring over the internet is advocated. The advantages of this approach include cost-effectiveness through reducing the reliance on expensive medical personnel, and automatic recording and processing of data streams, alerting remote medical officers when there is a need based on prescribed rules representing domain knowledge. The ratio of medical doctors to patients can be increased drastically to satisfy the increasing medical demand. This has even a more far reaching effect in developing countries, where the supply for doctors is usually in severe shortage. For instance, the authors have conducted community services in the countryside of Cambodia and in Rwanda in providing health-related services mainly to kids. Some apps are developed that would be able to perform screening before enlisting a medical doctor to help. Going one step further, the communication media between devices and associated systems can become wireless. The applications for those wireless sensors, often biosensors, in the e-health domain can be classified into five major categories (Waluyo, Yeoh, Pek, Yong, & Chen, 2010), with health monitoring being the focal point in this chapter.

More recently, multiple ubiquitous wearable devices have converged to support a more comprehensive monitoring paradigm. A common approach is to deploy a body area network (BAN) to sense, process and report on the wearer's health-related attributes (Jurik & Weaver, 2008). Normally a BAN will go wireless (WBAN) to interconnect tiny nodes with sensor (usually biosensor) or actuator capabilities in, on, or around a human body. The collected information can be routed back to a local or central server for processing, and possibly visualization by medical experts granted access to the central server. Nevertheless, it can be conceived that the BAN is still quite bulky, exerting much burden on the wearer. For instance, the WVSM (Wireless Vital Signs Monitor) is capable of measuring NIBP, SpO2 and lead II ECG (mini-Medic, n.d.) and is worn by a patient on the upper arm, being an improved product over previous mini-Medic with electrodes attached to the human body. Bioharness3 (n.d.) is a belt worn around the chest of the user. The former is quite intrusive to the user and the latter would still exert impact on the user as the belt must be placed around the heart, being obstructive to normal dressing. BP@Home system (Kusk et al., 2013) relies on an A&D blood pressure sensor that must be worn by the user. The MobiSense system (Waluyo et al., 2010) is capable of returning heart-beat and activity information to a server based on accelerometer and ECG sensor information, but it still suffers from the intrusion problem. The comprehensive PSYCHE system (Lanata, Valenza, Nardelli, Gentili, & Scilingo, 2015), taking the form of a T-shirt with embedded textile electrodes, piezoresistive sensors and accelerometers, is developed to measure the heart-beat, respiration and patient activity (Castano & Flatau, 2014) for clinical decision to improve the diagnosis and management of psychiatric disorder. Nevertheless, the T-shirt still causes some nuisance to the wearer.

Addressing the device intrusion problem, an innovative way is proposed to monitor the health of human beings in a *non-intrusive manner*, through the use of handy electronic gadgets. There are several technical approaches to achieve non-intrusiveness (Zheng et al., 2014), of which the analysis of reflected light captured by a sensor, i.e., the photoplethysmographic approach adopted in this work, is quite common. Wearable sensors are produced in the form of wrist bands or earpieces (Poh, Kim, Goessling, Swenson, & Picard, 2009), which are capable of measuring the heart-beat rate and respiratory rate for the wearer. WatchMe (Ransiri & Nanayakkara, 2012) is designed to monitor the health of elderlies. Some wrist band devices such as Smartband (n.d.) are designed to track body movement and sleep patterns. Most others are designed for the huge fitness market. In general, these devices do not demand very accurate measurement results. The long sought-after Apple iWatch is designed to keep track of the user's daily activities, via built-in sensors, classified into movement, exercise, and standing. It can be geared towards daily fitness goal, for instance, amount of distance travelled, amount of calories burnt and pace of exercise. It is also equipped with a heart-beat rate sensor. Another type of devices known as biofeedback devices, such as StressEraser (n.d.), is capable of detecting and advising the user to regulate their breathing pattern to attain better physiological functions. A recent commercial small biofeedback device is the AliveCor (n.d.), which is a small attachment to a compatible smartphone to convert the latter into an ECG device, capable of recording ECG signals to alert user about some anomaly, upon the installation of an app. Among recent research works, a contactless and thus completely non-intrusive approach has been proposed and prototyped to identify sleep apnea, by programming smartphones to emit sonar waves and analyze the reflected waves captured by microphone to detect minute chest and abdomen movements caused by breathing (Nandakumar, Gollakota, & Watson, 2015).

Along a similar research direction, the innovative *physiological mouse*, an otherwise conventional mouse equipped with purpose-designed add-on electronics, is proposed and designed. It is supplemented with tailor-made signal processing software. This physiological mouse is capable of capturing raw data in order to indirectly measure the heart-beat rate and respiratory rate of a user using the mouse while accessing the computer. There are at least three advantages of this physiological mouse. First, the cost of such a mouse is very low, compared with other specially built devices. Second, good accuracy has been achieved even with the relatively simple prototype. Third, due to the ubiquitous nature of mouse usage, the continuous stream of physiological data can be stored and analyzed for the well-being of the users, especially when tracked over a period of time.

THE PHYSIOLOGICAL MOUSE

In this section, the design and implementation of a *prototype* of the physiological mouse is presented, by augmenting a regular mouse with a small optical component for capturing user photoplethysmographic (PPG) signal. The prototype is depicted in Figure 1(a). A small light sensor is attached to the left side of the mouse (green box), touching the thumb of the user. The light sensor is a photodiode. The LED emitting infrared light (yellow circle) is attached next to the sensor. The sensor picks up and relays the intensity of the infrared light reflected by the thumb when the user is holding the mouse, as depicted in Figure 1(b) via an Arduino board to the PC through a thin wire. Modeling clay and tape are used to fix the little gadget together. Though it is not very nice-looking in the current prototype, users in general do not report discomfort when using it in the experiments.

The research approach is geared towards the monochromatic infrared signal reflected by the human finger. This assumption simplifies the hardware design, as well as data processing procedure, since it is no longer necessary to consider the combined RGB signals as in some related research works based on a web camera. The light sensor used can measure variation of the reflected light intensity. The peak sensitivity for this sensor is about 940nm, so it can detect the infrared. The sensor can fit on almost any human finger, but it is placed near the thumb for the sake of general human habit in using a mouse and experimental results are in support of this placement. A 5V power supply is required for normal operation of the LED and the light sensor. The original signal coming from the sensor is weak and noisy, with a maximum output voltage of only 40mV. An amplifier circuit is utilized to amplify the signal to a maximum of 2V. The outputs are sampled at a rate of 200 per second and scaled to 1024 levels intensity for further processing. Currently, signal processing is performed at an ordinary computer in order to serve as a proof-of-concept approach. In fact, once the idea of physiological mouse becomes well-accepted, it is not hard for product engineers to design a hardware solution that moves the whole gadget onboard the mouse. It could come in the form of a light sensor and light source attached to the side, in addition to the conventional pair at the bottom of an optical mouse.

A Fast Fourier Transform has been applied on the input PPG signal after performing some smoothing steps such as those shown in Figure 2(a). After cleansing the signal, it is possible to identify the heartbeat rate by applying a band-pass filter for the designated frequency band. An example of the extracted

Figure 1. The physiological mouse: (a) the mouse; (b) mouse in use

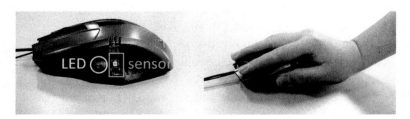

Figure 2. Signal processing: (a) smoothened signal; (b) heart-beat frequency

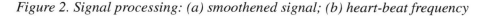

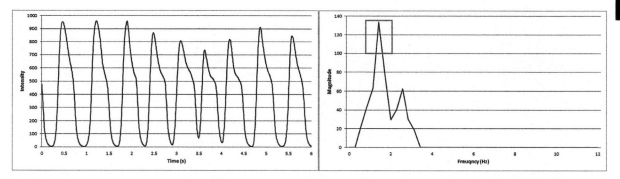

heart-beat rate, in terms of Hz, is shown in Figure 2(b) in which the dominating frequency is extracted representing the heart-beat rate.

Unlike heart-beat, respiration does not directly manifest itself in the periodic PPG signal, but corresponds closely to the high frequency component of the signal variation (Brown, Beightolm, Koh, & Eckberg, 1993). Thus, it is important to study the heart-beat rate variability, in the form of the timing difference between successive heart-beats and identify a very useful parameter called the inter-heart-beat-interval. Processing this second order signal on the timing difference gives a clue in computing the respiratory rate through spatial analysis. An example of extracting the respiratory rate based on a histogram technique on the potential dominating second order signal is illustrated in Figure 3, where the peak frequency in the normalized histogram corresponds to the respiratory rate.

The processed data will be stored on the computer, and can be analyzed online or offline. When anomalies are detected in the physiological signals, the computer can alert both the user and if situation is acute, also the family physician or even a medical doctor. The family physician or medical doctor could follow up with the case, either via tele-medical conversation thanks to advances in information and communication technologies, or paying a physical visit. The harvested physiological data would be

Figure 3. Respiratory rate identification

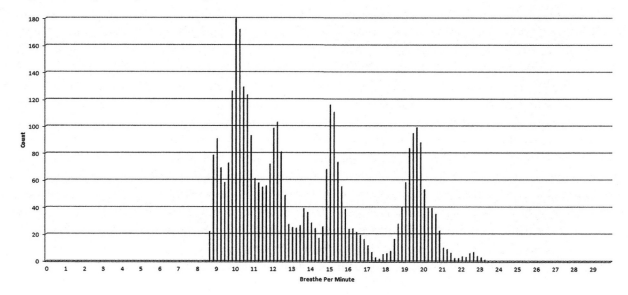

valuable towards making a good diagnosis. Subject to privacy agreement, the data could be archived in a suitable form for long-term health monitoring, forming part of the personal medical record.

In general, the mission of producing a non-intrusive mouse which is capable of measuring the physiological signals of a user has largely been fulfilled in this research. Since computer use is becoming ubiquitous and users often use a mouse with the computer, this generates a continuous, constantly updated source of signals. With sufficient amount of accumulated data, machine learning approaches could be adopted to extract useful rules and patterns to pinpoint and to predict interesting user information and behaviors. Based on the detected human behaviors, which form one important piece of contextual information that is not available based on current technologies, computers can also respond better to human requests and intents.

Considering potential applications with the physiological mouse, it can be noticed that when a human becomes motivated, or becomes angry, his/her heart-beat rate will increase. A bored person displays a relatively low respiratory rate. Slow respiration can be regarded as indicative of a relaxed state, while irregular rhythm and quick variations correspond to anger or fear. These physiological signals are often controlled through subconscious inner-body mechanisms, for example, a rise in the level of adrenaline. As a result, the innovative gadget could be adapted to monitoring the stress level of the user at work, thereby helping to maintain human mental health, in addition to physiological health. The mouse would also be useful in other applications, for instance, e-learning applications. When the mouse detects that a student becomes nervous, displaying increasing heart-beat rate when answering questions, the questions may be shown at a slower pace, or with additional tutorial materials provided. This piece of research work will likely provide a good starting point for designing future emotion-aware devices, as well as building interesting application towards emotion-adaptive applications, an approach recently shown to be viable (Wac & Tsiourti, 2014).

VALIDATION

The accuracy of the physiological signals obtained when users are playing around with the physiological mouse prototype is evaluated. Twelve students have been invited as subjects to participate in the experiments in using the mouse. To measure the heart-beat rate, the iHealth Pulse Oximeter (iHealth, n.d.) is used as the gold standard against which the accuracy of the physiological mouse is measured. Each subject has the equipment clipped onto his/her finger to measure the heart-beat, which is logged to the computer. In the experiments, the heart-beat rates of the twelve subjects are measured by the iHealth equipment, providing an average of 80.0, with individual rates ranging from 66 to 104, whereas the physiological mouse returns an average rate of 78.2, individual rates ranging from 62 to 101. Even though the heart-beat rates of the subjects vary quite a bit, up to 57% (104 versus 66), the difference between measurements returned by the two devices is only about 2.3%, ranging from a minimum of 0.3% to a maximum of 6.6% for the subjects. This demonstrates the effectiveness and accuracy of the non-intrusive physiological mouse in measuring heart-beat rates. The full set of heart-beat rates for the twelve subjects and their corresponding errors can be found in Figure 4, where the left *y*-axis represents the heart-beat rate and the right *y*-axis represents the error (in red-colored line).

The accuracy of detecting respiratory rates is the next target of study. The same twelve subjects are requested to breathe according to the preset target rates of 10, 12, 14 and 16 per minute, via a metronome. A simple metronome is implemented by displaying an inhale and exhale indicators and the subjects are requested to follow the rhythm. The returned light intensity signals are processed into heart-beat sig-

Figure 4. Heart-beat rate performance

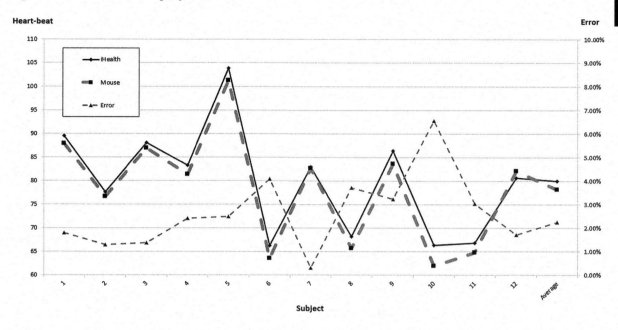

nal, then inter-heart-beat-interval signal and finally the estimated respiratory rate. The four individual respiratory rates for the twelve subjects are first considered, and then compared with the standard rates of 10, 12, 14 and 16. The measurements indicate 10.1, 12.1, 14.2 and 15.9 respectively for the four metronome respiratory rates, corresponding to error rates ranging from 0.6% to 1.2%, averaging at 0.8%. It is further noticed that there is a higher variation at a higher respiratory rate. The individual respiratory rates for each subject are considered next, being averaged over the four respiratory patterns. Across the twelve subjects, the error rates are shown to range from 1.7% to 5.5%, which is higher than the global average of 0.8%. Nevertheless, the resultant accuracy is still good enough to be of use. The individual results are depicted in Figure 5(a), where the measured rates stay close to the four reference rates, and the blue curve (rate of 16) exhibits a higher fluctuation over other curves, for instance, the very nice green curve (rate of 12).

Figure 5. Respiratory rate performance: (a) controlled breathing; (b) natural breathing

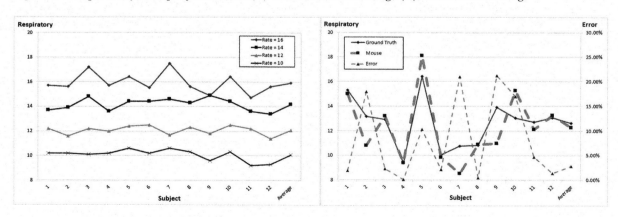

Furthermore, the control factor in the respiratory experiment is lifted, with the twelve subjects being requested to breathe naturally without following the metronome, with their respiratory rates being counted and compared with those returned by the physiological mouse. To be precise, the breathing of subjects is video-taped and counted manually the actual respiratory rates from the video to form the ground truth for comparison and future validation. In general, the natural respiratory rates for the subjects range from 9.4 to 16.4, representing a variation of 75%, which is higher than the 57% variation in heart-beat rate, whereas our mouse returns rates ranging from 8.5 to 18.1, implying a variation of 112%. It is discovered that the breathing patterns for a few subjects are not quite satisfactory, yielding relatively high error rates of around 20%, whereas most other subjects only suffer from error rates of 10% or below. When the error between the average rates of the twelve subjects is measured, the resultant error is found to be only 2.8%. This means that though the individual error may be high, the general error is still acceptable. The individual results and their corresponding errors are depicted in Figure 5(b), where the left *y*-axis represents the respiratory rate and the right *y*-axis represents the error (in red-colored line).

Additional pilot experiments have also been conducted through requesting the subjects to play games, for which the variation of heart-beat rates has been observed, especially when the player is facing a particularly challenging scenario or facing the prospect of beating the boss by a narrow margin and winning the game. This is anticipated, since the human body reacts to anxiety and excitement by increasing the secretion of adrenaline, which leads to an increase in heart-beat rate in preparation for addressing a severe situation. The authors believe that when the physiological signals are used in conjunction of other modalities, for instance, simple video analysis via a webcam, there is a strong potential in determining the human health status more accurately.

CONCLUSION

In this chapter, a survey has been conducted on contemporary health-monitoring technologies, with a focus targeted upon technologies with wearable devices. Narrowing down from wearable health-monitoring technology, devices that are non-intrusive have been advocated as the most appropriate and promising ones. This idea for a non-intrusive health-monitoring device is demonstrated through the design and implementation of a novel physiological mouse, by augmenting a regular mouse with a small optical component for capturing user PPG signal in order to derive human physiological measurements. Experimental results demonstrate the good accuracy of this novel non-intrusive physiological mouse in measuring two main human physiological signals, namely, heart-beat rate and respiratory rate. Some potential applications for the mouse have been highlighted, both in the e-health domain, and more interestingly, in the upcoming affective computing domain (Wac & Tsiourti, 2014).

REFERENCES

AliveCor. (n.d.). Retrieved from http://www.alivecor.com/

Andreu-Perez, J., Leff, D. R., Ip, H. M. D., & Yang, G. (2015). From wearable sensors to smart implants - towards pervasive and personalised healthcare. *IEEE Transactions on Bio-Medical Engineering, 62*(12), 2750–2762. doi:10.1109/TBME.2015.2422751 PMID:25879838

Anttonen, J., & Surakka, V. (2005). Emotions and heart rate while sitting on a chair. In *Proceeding of the SIGCHI Conference* (pp. 491-499). doi:10.1145/1054972.1055040

BioHarness3. (n.d.). Retrieved from http://zephyranywhere.com/products/bioharness-3/

Brown, T. E., Beightolm, L. A., Koh, J., & Eckberg, D. L. (1993). Important influence of respiration on human RR interval power spectra is largely ignored. *Journal of Applied Physiology, 75*(5), 2310–2317. PMID:8307890

Castano, L. M., & Flatau, A. B. (2014). Smart fabric sensors and e-textile technologies: A review. *Smart Materials and Structures, 23*(1), 1–27.

Celler, B. G., & Sparks, R. S. (2015). Home telemonitoring of vital signs - Technical challenges and future directions. *IEEE Journal of Biomedical and Health Informatics, 19*(1), 82–91. doi:10.1109/JBHI.2014.2351413 PMID:25163076

Griffiths, E., Saponas, T. S., & Brush, A. J. B. (2014). Health chair: Implicitly sensing heart and respiratory rate. In *Proceedings of ACM International Joint Conference on Pervasive and Ubiquitous Computing* (pp. 661-671). doi:10.1145/2632048.2632099

iHealth. (n.d.). *iHealth Pulse Oximeter*. Retrieved from http://www.ihealthlabs.com/fitness-devices/wireless-pulse-oximeter/

Jurik, A. D., & Weaver, A. C. (2008). Remote Medical Monitoring. *IEEE Computer, 41*(4), 95–98. doi:10.1109/MC.2008.133

Kusk, K., Nielsen, D. B., Thylstrup, T., Rasmussen, N. H., Jørvang, J., Pedersen, C. F., & Wagner, S. (2013). Feasibility of using a lightweight context-aware system for facilitating reliable home blood pressure self-measurements. In *Proceedings of International Conference on Pervasive Computing Technologies for Healthcare* (pp. 236-239). doi:10.4108/icst.pervasivehealth.2013.252107

Lanata, A., Valenza, G., Nardelli, M., Gentili, C., & Scilingo, E. P. (2015). Complexity index from a personalized wearable monitoring system for assessing remission in mental health. *IEEE Journal of Biomedical and Health Informatics, 19*(1), 132–139. doi:10.1109/JBHI.2014.2360711 PMID:25291802

Lehman, L. H., Adams, R. P., Mayaud, L., Moody, G. B., Malhotra, A., Mark, R. G., & Nemati, S. (2015). A Physiological Time Series Dynamics-Based Approach to Patient Monitoring and Outcome Prediction. *IEEE Journal of Biomedical and Health Informatics, 19*(3), 1068–1076. PMID:25014976

Li, Y., Guo, L., & Guo, Y. (2014). Enabling health monitoring as a service in the cloud. In *Proceedings of IEEE/ACM International Conference on Utility and Cloud Computing* (pp. 127-136). IEEE. doi:10.1109/UCC.2014.21

mini-Medic. (n.d.). Retrieved from http://www.athenagtx.com/

Nandakumar, R., Gollakota, S., & Watson, N. (2015). Contactless sleep apnea detection on smartphones. In *Proceedings of International Conference on Mobile Systems, Applications, and Services* (pp. 45-57). ACM. doi:10.1145/2742647.2742674

Poh, M. Z., Kim, K., Goessling, A., Swenson, N., & Picard, R. (2009). Sensor earphones and mobile application for non-obtrusive health monitoring. In *Proceedings of IEEE International Symposium on Wearable Computers*. doi:10.1109/ISWC.2009.35

Ransiri, S., & Nanayakkara, S. (2012). WatchMe: wrist-worn interface that makes remote monitoring seamless. In *Proceedings of ACM SIGACCESS Conference on Computers and Accessibility* (pp. 243-244). doi:10.1145/2384916.2384974

Shimokakimoto, T., & Suzuki, K. (2011). A chair-type interface for long-term and ambient vital sensing. In *Proceedings of Annual International Conference of Engineering in Medicine and Biology Society* (pp. 1173-1176). IEEE. doi:10.1109/IEMBS.2011.6090275

SmartBand. (n.d.). Retrieved from http://www.sonymobile.com/global-en/products/smartwear/smartband-swr10/

StressEraser. (n.d.). Retrieved from http://www.stress.org/certified-product-stress-eraser/

Wac, K., & Tsiourti, C. (2014). *Ambulatory assessment of affect: survey of sensor systems for monitoring of autonomous nervous system's activation in emotion. IEEE Transactions on Affective Computing.*

Waluyo, A. B., Yeoh, W.-S., Pek, I., Yong, Y., & Chen, X. (2010). MobiSense: Mobile body sensor network for ambulatory monitoring. *ACM Transactions on Embedded Computing Systems*, *10*(1), 13–42. doi:10.1145/1814539.1814552

WHO. (n.d.). *10 Facts on Ageing and the Life Course*. Retrieved from http://www.who.int/features/factfiles/ageing/ageing_facts/en/

Zhang, Y. T., Poon, C. C. Y., & MacPherson, E. (2009). Editorial note on health informatics. *IEEE Transactions on Information Technology in Biomedicine*, *13*(3), 281–283. doi:10.1109/TITB.2009.2021443 PMID:19423427

Zheng, Y., Ding, X., Poon, C. C. Y., Lo, B. P. L., Zhang, H., Zhou, X., & Zhang, Y. et al. (2014). Unobtrusive sensing and wearable devices for health informatics. *IEEE Transactions on Bio-Medical Engineering*, *61*(5), 1538–1554. doi:10.1109/TBME.2014.2309951 PMID:24759283

KEY TERMS AND DEFINITIONS

Affective Computing: The study and development of systems and devices that can recognize, interpret, process, and simulate human affects (emotions). It was derived from human computer interaction and has since grown into an interdisciplinary field spanning computer science, psychology, and cognitive science.

Body Area Network: Previously known as a body sensor network, extending from the sensor network to a network of wearable sensors located on/with/in the body of a human being that cooperate for the benefit of the human, normally returning readings concerning the human. The network is mostly deployed to the support of m-health (mobile health) and even u-health (ubiquitous health).

E-Health: Systems and supporting technology for health-care, carried out with the help of information technology, in terms of data acquisition, data storage, data retrieval, data maintenance, and data dissemination. It can be considered as the electronic version of a more conventional health-care system.

Health Monitoring: Techniques and devices associated with the capturing of important parameters about the health of a person, oftentimes, a patient. Communication and alert mechanisms should also be included so that a proper authority or party can be notified in case of emergency or anomaly.

Intrusive and Non-Intrusive Measurement: Intrusive measurement refers to the use of devices or measurement procedures that affect the normal situation of the person, bringing a significant impact on

E

the mobility or comfort of the person involved, e.g., a person wearing a headmount device with electrodes attached. Non-intrusive measurement refers to the use of devices or measurement procedures that induce minimal impact on the person involved. In an extreme case, the person being monitored would not even notice the existence of the device or procedure, e.g., a user being watched by a webcam that collects changes in his/her facial skin tone.

Physiological Signals: Readings or measurements that are produced by the physiological process of human beings, e.g., heart-beat rate (electrocardiogram or ECG/EKG signal), respiratory rate and content (capnogram), skin conductance (electrodermal activity or EDA signal), muscle current (electromyography or EMG signal), brain electrical activity (electroencephalography or EEG signal).

Sensors and Biosensors: A sensor is capable of making some measurement about its target, e.g., a thermometer. A sensor that is designed to measure biological phenomenon or a sensor that is combined with a biological component is called a biosensor, e.g., thermometer measuring the body temperature of a human under the ear or measurement of glucose concentration in blood.

Online Resources, Support, and E–Health for Families of Children with Disabilities:
A Review of Empirical Evidence Regarding Attitudes, Use, and Efficacy

Cristin M. Hall
The Pennsylvania State University, USA

Erica D. Culler
The Pennsylvania State University, USA

Anne Frank-Webb
The Pennsylvania State University, USA

INTRODUCTION

In the last 10 years, web-based support and information for parents of children with disabilities has grown exponentially (Jones et al., 2013; Pagliari et al., 2005). Researchers, practitioners, and educators who serve these children and their families have increasingly turned to technology to find innovative ways to increase parent engagement, expand the reach of empirically-based interventions, and collect data on usability, acceptability, and efficacy. Although access to the internet, web-based applications, social media, mobile devices, real-time video calls, and other technology have great potential to increase support and access for families, important questions remain about their actual impact.

The quintessential questions around the use of internet-based tools involve four key issues. First, there is the question of the *digital divide* (Graham, Hale, & Stephens, 2012). While access to the internet has increased across socioeconomic boundaries (U.S. Census Bureau, 2010), there are still reservations regarding whether or not those that could most benefit from internet-based services (such as those living in remote or underserved areas) actually have the requisite access to a reliable network and associated technical support, hardware, and software to utilize the tools. Second, even if families can consistently access a network, there are issues related to the *acceptability divide* or the degree to which parents find these services helpful, credible, or engaging compared to other modalities. Third, ethical considerations based on maintaining privacy and confidentiality, ensuring parents are informed consumers, and verifying the quality of online information and resources continue to plague the emergence and widespread adoption of remote delivery models for professionals and researchers alike (Self-Brown & Whitaker, 2008). Finally, rigorous study of the actual impact of online information, support, and interventions is still in its infancy and thus, many questions remain regarding when, how, and for whom these tools are most beneficial.

Although a critical review of all four of these areas is beyond the scope of this chapter, the present review seeks to specifically address how the current literature base elucidates feasibility, acceptability, and empirical support for impact of internet technology for parents of children with developmental,

DOI: 10.4018/978-1-4666-9978-6.ch056

learning, and social-emotional disabilities. Specifically, this chapter examines the current literature on internet-based support, online learning, and information-seeking for parents, and family-centered interventions for families of children with developmental and related disabilities.

BACKGROUND

The term "disability" can encompass a number of conditions including cognitive, physical, psychological, acquired or congenital conditions. The Individuals with Disabilities Education Improvement Act (IDEA, 2004) recognizes 13 distinct disability categories for eligibility for special education services. For the purposes of this chapter we focus on those disabilities that include significant behavioral, psychological, and cognitive impact, specifically, neurodevelopmental disorders. Although focusing on a specific diagnostic category (e.g., traumatic brain injury [TBI] or intellectual disability) may make for clearer diagnosis-to-treatment conclusions, many of the disorders for which parents seek assistance include overlapping symptom profiles and comorbid diagnoses. Neurodevelopmental disorders (ND) characterize a number of developmental disabilities including Intellectual Disabilities (ID), communication disorders, Autism Spectrum Disorders (ASD), attention deficit hyperactivity disorder (ADHD), neurodevelopmental motor disorders, and Specific Learning Disorders (SLD) (American Psychiatric Association [APA], 2013a). Symptoms range widely, but generally involve one or more impairments related to personal, social, academic, or occupational functioning that generally manifest before a child enters grade school (American Psychiatric Association [APA], 2013a). Although not categorized as such in the Diagnostic and Statistical Manual of Mental Disorders (5th ed.; DSM-5; APA, 2013b), Neurobehavioral Disorder Associated with Prenatal Alcohol Exposure, otherwise known as Fetal Alcohol Spectrum Disorder (FASD), is considered an extension of ND given the neurological basis and the similarities in functional impairments (Di Pietro, Whiteley, Mizgalewicz, & Illes, 2013).

Millions of children nationwide are diagnosed with ND, FASD, and TBI. It is estimated that 5% of children by first grade have a speech or language impairment (National Institute on Deafness and Other Communication Disorders, 2014); ASD and ID effect about 1% of children; SLD estimates range between 5-15% of all children; and ADHD affects around 5% of children (APA, 2013a). Despite improved diagnostic and treatment options, schools and professionals struggle to provide adequate services due to lack of funding, resources, and trained professionals to deliver evidence-based interventions consistently and with fidelity. Without professional services or guidance, parents and caregivers must search for, and determine the credibility of, information on their own. Advances in technology can connect parents to professionals and other caregivers for information, support, and treatment, but the research in this area is relatively young. Identification of factors associated with reliable and valid sources of online information and the utility and efficacy of remote service delivery is needed.

PRESENT REVIEW METHODOLOGY

The present review includes a comprehensive and systematic review of the literature related to how internet technology (including information seeking, support, e-Learning, and *e-Health*) may assist families of children with neurodevelopmental, learning, or behavioral/ mental health disorders. The study was guided by two primary aims. First, the study aimed to understand the breadth of research available on information and services for parents available online. Specifically, only one diagnostic category was not selected (e.g., autism-only) because it was hypothesized that the research on internet applications for parents of children of a particular disability would not yield many results. Relatedly, given that many of the kinds of information seeking, social support, and services that parents may want for one disability type (such as autism) may greatly overlap with the nature of services and information sought for other disorders (such as ADHD, TBI, or FASD), it would be difficult to identify supports that are undoubtedly specific to one given disability. Second, the study aimed to understand the current state of the evidence by examining the methods, measures, and techniques used to study internet use and parents of children with disabilities.

Method

In order to conduct such a comprehensive review, a systematic literature search approach with snowballing and hand-inspection was used. On the search engines ERIC, PubMed, and PsychINFO were searched using the terms *parent* or *parents*. These terms were then cross referenced with the following terms:

1. *Online support, social media, discussion boards, massive open online courses, web-based learning, online learning, parent intervention, parent advocacy, e-Health, telemedicine, telehealth;* and
2. *Rare disorders, traumatic brain injury, special education, developmental disorders, autism, autism spectrum disorders, Asperger's, intellectual disability, mental retardation, specific learning disability, emotional and behavioral disorders, emotional disturbance, behavioral disorders, mental health disorders*

This search yielded a total of 773 articles. To further cross-verify our search, snowball sampling, specifically the examination of the references of included studies and a check of Web of Science to include subsequent publications that utilized the target article in the references were used. Hand examination and cataloguing of the studies included specific inclusion criteria for the present review. Inclusion criteria were that studies must be: 1) published in English, 2) published in a peer reviewed journal or a published dissertation, 3) related to a behavioral, emotional, or neurodevelopmental disability (including ASD, ID, mental health disorders, TBI, SLD, other developmental or learning condition), and 4) included a specific tool for use by parents (e.g., parent support, parent training, parent learning). Excluded from this review were medical conditions such as asthma, allergies, or diabetes. The final inclusion count of studies was 47.

In order to better represent the breadth of studies found in the present systematic search please see Table 1. Citations are listed alphabetically and have indicators for the target population, technology characteristics, and measurement characteristics in the study. Target populations included are neurodevelopmental disorders (57%), traumatic brain injury (13%), fetal alcohol spectrum disorder (2%), other mental health conditions (15%), and multiple disability types (4%). In four instances, studies were included even when a specific disability type was not included as part of the study. These studies were retained because they included reviews or studies of information online that could be applicable to parents of children with disabilities and provided unique contributions to the review (Mitchell, Godoy, Shabazz, & Horn, 2014; Nieuwboer, Fukkink, & Hermanns, 2013; Oermann, Lowery, & Thornley, 2003; Stroever, Mackert, McAlister, & Hoelscher, 2011).

Technology types were coded using five categories according to the following descriptive subtypes. First, information-seeking only included those studies where online information seeking, web-searching behavior or web content was examined. A second category included studies that utilized interactive

Table 1. Summary of characteristics of reviewed articles

Citation	Target Population*	Technology Characteristics+					Measurement**						
		IO	IW	SP	RP	SM	US	SA	AU	KA	OPC	OCC	SR
Barahav & Reiser, 2010	ND				X		X	X					
Bennett, Pourmand, Shokoohi, Shesser, Sanches, & Joyce, 2014	MH					X						X	
Black & Baker, 2011	M			X			X						
Carey, Wade, & Wolfe, 2008	TBI		X		X		X						X
Chowdhury, Drummond, Fleming, & Neitfeld, 2002	ND	X					X			X			
Clifford & Minnes, 2013	ND			X				X	X				X
Comer et al., 2013	MH		X		X		X	X					X
Curtin, 2010	MH	X		X			X						X
Di Pietro, Whiteley, Mizgalewicz, & Illes, 2013	ND	X					X			X			
Enebrink, Högström, Forster, & Ghaderi, 2012	MH		X		X								X
Fain, 2009	ND	X						X					
Ferdig, Amberg, Elder, Donaldson, Valcante, & Bendixen, 2009	ND	X					X						
Fleischmann, 2004	ND			X				X					
Fleishmann, 2005	ND	X		X				X					
Garbe, 2008	ND			X				X	X				X
Gibbs & Toth-Cohen, 2011	ND				X			X				X	
Gooding, Klaas, Yager, & Kanchanaraksa, 2013	M		X				X		X				
Heitzman-Powell, Buzhardt, Ruskino, & Miller, 2014	ND		X		X		X			X	X		
Jang, Dixon, Tarbox, Grenpeesheh, Kornack, & de Nocker, 2012	ND		X							X			
Kable, Coles, Strickland, & Taddeo, 2012	FASD		X							X			X
Kaiser, 2011	ND		X		X								
Kelso, Fiechtl, Olsen, & Rule, 2009	ND				X		X	X					
Kirby, Edwards, & Hughes, 2008	ND			X			X						
Kobak, Stone, Wallace, Warren, Swanson, & Robson, 2011	ND		X					X		X			
Kolb, 2007	ND		X		X						X		
Mast, Antonini, Raj, Oberjohn, Cassedy, Makoroff, & Wade, 2014	TBI		X		X						X	X	
Mitchell, Godoy, Shabazz, & Horn, 2014	-	X					X	X					
Miyahara, Buston, Cutfield, & Clarkson, 2009	ND			X			X	X				X	
Nelson, Barnard, & Cain, 2006	MH		X										X

continued on following page

Table 1. Continued

Citation	Target Population*	Technology Characteristics+					Measurement**						
		IO	IW	SP	RP	SM	US	SA	AU	KA	OPC	OCC	SR
Nieuwboer, Fukkink, & Hermanns, 2013	-			X				X					
Oermann, Lowery, & Thornley, 2003	-	X					X						
Ossebaard, van Gemert-Pijnen, Sorbi, & Seydel, 2010	ND	X							X	X			
Powell & McCauley, 2012	ND	X											
Reichow, Naples, Steinhoff, Halpern, & Volkmar, 2012	ND	X					X			X			
Scharer, 2005	MH			X					X				
Sharer, Colon, Moneyham, Hussey, Tavakoli, & Shugart, 2009	MH			X									X
Stephenson, Carter, & Kemp, 2012	ND	X					X			X			
Stroever, Mackert, McAlister, & Hoelscher, 2011	-					X	X						
Suess et al., 2014	ND			X							X	X	
Vismara, McCormick, Young, Nadhan, & Monlux, 2013	ND		X		X						X	X	
Vismara, Young, & Rogers, 2012	ND		X		X						X	X	
Wade, Oberjohn, Conaway, Osinska, & Bangert, 2011	TBI		X		X		X	X					
Wade, Wolfe, Brown, & Pestian, 2005a	TBI		X		X			X					X
Wade, Wolfe, Brown, & Pestian, 2005b	TBI		X		X		X						X
Wade, Wolfe, & Pestian, 2004	TBI		X		X			X					X
Wainer & Ingersoll, 2013	ND		X						X	X	X	X	
Zeman, Swanke, & Doktor, 2011	ND			X				X					

* *Note.* ND = Neurodevelopmental Disorder, FASD = Fetal Alcohol Spectrum Disorder, TBI = Traumatic Brain Injury, MH = Child Mental Health Problems (not classified as a ND), M = Multiple Disorders.

+*Note.* IO = Information-Only on Internet, IW = Interactive Web-Based Materials, SP = Supportive Platforms, RP = Relationship with Professional/ Supporting Contact (includes VTC), SM = Social Media.

***Note.* US = Usability, SA = Satisfaction, AU = Actual Use, KA = Knowledge Acquisition, OPC = Observed Parent Change, OCC = Observed Child Changes, SR = Self-Report.

web-based materials (such as e-Learning, interactive video and audio, or massive open online courses [MOOCs]). Third, a support platform category included those articles that studied platforms such as dedicated online support groups, listservs, and the analysis of discussion boards that are not part of other social media platforms, such as Facebook, Twitter, or other commercial platforms. Separate from support platform, social media could be coded for those studies that looked at parent use of broader commercial social media outlets for support or information including Facebook or other media. Finally, studies could be coded as including a relationship with a professional or supportive contact (such as face-to-face sessions, *synchronous communication*, or other contact such as phone calls). Some studies did include more than one technology feature being studied. Studies that included dedicated or center-based telemedicine were not included, but studies that used the term "telemedicine" or "telehealth" that were using internet-based (or e-Health) services were included (e.g., Gibbs & Toth-Cohen, 2011).

Studies were also coded based upon the types of measurement used to demonstrate changes. Studies found in the search were categorized by any and all of the measurement types used in the study. Usability comprised those studies that examined feasibility, cost or value-added components, readability, or accessibility by parents. Studies that examined the content of online resources were coded as measuring usability and knowledge (e.g., Di Pietro et al., 2013). Satisfaction included studies that examined the satisfaction of parents or professionals in the use of the application. Qualitative studies of parent experiences were coded as satisfaction studies (e.g., Fain, 2009). Studies that included measures of the uptake or typical use of internet technology were coded as including actual use measures. Knowledge application was included for those studies that measured parent knowledge of disability-related issues or technology-related issues. Studies that utilized observation or direct study of parent outcomes (separate from self-report) were coded as observed parent change and similarly studies that directly observed child behavior or symptom change (other than relying on parent report only) were coded as observed child change. Studies that utilized self-report of behavior or symptom change were coded as self-report which was distinct from those measures of knowledge or satisfaction subsumed in the other categories. The results of the review will be described in sections including support for parents, online learning and information, and online consultation, information, and training for parents.

INTERNET-BASED SUPPORT FOR PARENTS

Supportive Platform

Parents utilize online sources for assistance based on two platforms: support and advocacy. The *supportive platform* allows parents to establish online connections that provide encouragement, advice, and first-hand knowledge related to raising a child with a disability. The supportive platform includes access to websites and support groups that are dedicated to a particular diagnosis or related disability groups (often co-morbid disorders) of concern. Popular examples range from simple, *asynchronous communication* (not in real-time) on discussion boards on society websites (e.g., *Autism Speaks),* to multifaceted parent-generated sites that consist of blogs, background information, and links to related resources in addition to a *moderated discussion board* (e.g., *RecoveringKids.com)*. Another way that parents use supportive platforms has come from the outgrowth of existing social media tools such as participation in Facebook groups, writing or following blogs, watching or creating YouTube videos, following or maintaining a Pinterest page, and interacting via Twitter handles and hashtags related to various disabilities. The use of pre-existing social media platforms may broaden the networking opportunities for parents in a convenient way given that they may already utilize some of these tools for reasons not related to their child's disability (e.g., Facebook).

Systematic study of the impact of supportive platform tools is limited. Although blogs have been suggested as a way to build family-school or family-professional relationships (Powell & McCauley, 2012), there is little research on whether they actually engage families in therapeutic processes or reduce parental stress. There are some small studies, including dissertation work, that have focused on both qualitative and quantitative examination of the use of online parent support groups for ASDs (Clifford & Mines, 2013; Garbe, 2008) and children with emotional problems (Curtin, 2010; Scharer et al., 2009). The largest review included an examination of published studies of online support groups from 1998 to 2010 (Nieuwboer et al., 2013). This study included a review of studies of both professional peer support and parent support. The authors found positive outcomes for parent support; however, the study focused on broader parenting topics and thus may not specifically represent the current impact and use of parent support for children with developmental disabilities.

Research on parent blogs are largely qualitative and descriptive in nature. Studies to date offer an important insight into how blogs are used by parents to come to a sense of empowerment or acceptance about their child's condition. For example, studies by Fleischmann (2004, 2005) demonstrated that parents showed themes of preparing themselves for action and used their posts as a way to reach out to others and reduce feelings of isolation in helping their child. More recently, Zeman, Swanke, and Doktor (2011) outlined how mothers came to understand areas of risks and successes of their children, and their perspectives on the current state of the field of services. Quantitative examinations of online posts and message boards explored how often parents were sharing with others in the areas of specific learning disability (Kirby, Edwards, & Hughes, 2008) and children with mental health conditions (Scharer, 2005).

Social media may be used in another way, specifically, as a way to get information about their children's individual symptoms and risk. A case study reviewed by Bennett and colleagues (2014) detailed an instance where a female patient's friends informed her parents regarding concerning posts on Facebook indicating that she was at-risk for self-harm. This notification and the content of the Facebook posts and photographs shared were used as part of the evaluation and admissions process for this girl to receive proper psychiatric treatment. Although parents are routinely cautioned about monitoring their child's behavior online, professionals and parents alike are coming to grapple with the implications of how such posts and communications should be monitored and used for evaluating risk and symptomology.

Advocacy Platform

The second way that parents can utilize the internet for support is by capitalizing on the reach of the internet across geographical and other boundaries to become leaders themselves in advocacy. In the context of the *advocate platform,* parents share their personal experiences to inform or encourage others through blogging, and they create grass-roots efforts to improve the quality of care for their own families. In many ways the internet has been touted as the "great equalizer" allowing for the kind of visibility and access that at one time required limited distribution via University libraries, professional marketing skills, paper newsletters, or cold-calling. Questions abound regarding whether or not low-income, non-English speaking, high-risk, or low-literacy families will utilize either the supportive or advocate platforms available via the internet. Furthermore, there is continued concern about self-appointed advocates that may cause (unintended) harm by dissemination of inaccurate information (such as the anti-vaccine movement related to ASD).

No literature at the time of this writing specifically examined how parents were using online tools for advocacy, fundraising, or other grassroots efforts. However, an illustrative case from the United Kingdom described how parent advocates used the internet and social media to create the International Dravet syndrome Epilepsy Action (IDEA) League (Black & Baker, 2011). Currently, the IDEA League is a world leader in outreach, support for research, and collaboration for professionals dealing with Dravet syndrome and other related disorders. This particular case study, although related more to epilepsy than a rare neurological disorder, demonstrates how parents and patients have effectively utilized online tools to bridge important partnerships and gain community awareness and support.

Recently, a grassroots campaign, *The Ice Bucket Challenge*, garnered national and international attention for raising awareness and donation levels for Amyotrophic Lateral Sclerosis (ALS). The campaign, which targeted social media outlets and challenged "nominated" individuals to 1) donate $100 to the ALS association and/ or 2) dump a bucket of ice water over their own head, led to a significant increase in funding for the ASL association (94.3 million dollars donated between July 29 and August 27 of 2014 compared to 2.7 million dollars between July 29 and August 27 of 2013; Munk, 2014). There are vast opportunities for similar grassroots campaigns to highlight awareness and funding of neurodevelopmental disorders to provide additional support for parents and families.

Limitations and Problems

Clearly, online tools have the potential for unprecedented access to parent support. Nevertheless, important limitations exist. First, the existing literature base for both the supportive and advocacy platforms lack methodological rigor or more substantial sampling to better understand: the actual use of online support and advocacy, the degree to which parents find such resources helpful, and the degree to which they actually have a positive impact on parent stress and other proximal outcomes for children and families. Second, the problem of the digital divide continues to plague issues of online use for parents. Specifically, the digital divide may be thought of not only as a matter of access to the network (e.g., wifi, cellular, or broadband access that is affordable and reliable) but also a matter of barriers related to literacy and trust of the resources found. Finally, there is important work to be done related to how the use of internet-only support may compare to the use of the internet as a supplement to other forms of face-to-face (F2F) support. Studies of the use of online support for new parents has found mixed results (Bartholomew, Schoppe-Sullivan, Glassman, Kamp Duch, & Sullivan, 2012) and specifically indicated that social media use in particular leads to better outcomes for those that have adequate F2F social support as well.

Recommendations and Future Directions

Parent advocacy and support groups can and should continue to utilize the existing technology and reach of social media outlets (e.g., Facebook) and the ever-increasing ease of creating websites without programming knowledge (e.g., Weebly, WordPress). However, questions remain around how professionals make recommendations to parents about which online groups to join and how to most effectively utilize additional online support options (e.g., blogs, social media, parent-generated websites). Researchers across disciplines, such as those interested in parent stress, special education, various disability areas, and translational research, are in a good position to begin to understand the principles, which will improve the online support and advocacy experiences of parents with specific needs. For example, parents of children with rare developmental disorders may only have web-based options to connect with other parents facing similar challenges from a shared diagnosis. Given the lack of alternatives, it is essential to determine which aspects of online support are most beneficial to enhance the parents' experience. In other instances where web-based resources for support or advocacy are available, researchers need to understand what the requisite characteristics are of the user (e.g., parent), the web-interface, and the nature of the community's communication (synchronicity, frequency, quality) that encourage consumers to utilize the online option.

ONLINE LEARNING AND INFORMATION-SEEKING FOR PARENTS

Information regarding developmental disorders is readily available online. As of this writing (June, 2015), a search of the term "autism" on Google resulted in over 68 million websites. Given the vast number of hits for just a single term such as autism, it is not surprising that the internet has become the most commonly used method for parents to find information on ASDs and other developmental disorders (Chowdhury, Drummond, Fleming, & Neitfeld, 2002; Mackintosh, Myers, & Goin-Kochel, 2005). Use of the internet for information can broadly be described as initial searches, confirmatory or disconfirmation searches, and massive open online courses (MOOCs), each of which will be reviewed in turn. Concerns abound related to the accuracy, relevance, and availability of quality information on the internet for parents. We will discuss below the current literature about online sources of information and their limitations.

A qualitative study found that when a child was initially diagnosed with an ASD, parents urgently conducted a concentrated internet search on diagnoses, causes, symptoms, and potential services and treatments (Fain, 2009). Although parents are regularly using the internet for information that could help their child, there are few quality control systems to ensure that online information is reliable, accurate, or even updated. Therefore, parents are tasked with completing an appropriate search with the correct key words to obtain relevant information and determining which of the multitude of search options is the most credible source. Unfortunately, vetting the quality, accuracy, and accessibility of all the potentially relevant online resources is an insurmountable task for professionals, researchers, or parent advocates given the exponential growth and change of internet resources despite the best efforts of organizations (such as the Health On the Net Foundation)..

Locating Available Resources

The initial challenge is related to the location of publically available resources. Although over 68 million websites are identified through Google's search engine, there is evidence that individuals generally only scan the first few search results (Eysenbach & Köhler, 2002). Parents further scrutinize websites based on professional appearance and apparent sponsorship (Fain, 2009). Although parents may feel this process is the best option given the lack of additional vetting criteria, it is difficult to ignore the likelihood that for-profit companies are more apt to develop expensive, professional-looking websites to endorse their own products and interventions, which may further decrease parents' ability to locate objective, evidence-based information.

An additional complication to locating appropriate resources is the role of the specific search engine. Each search engine utilizes a different algorithm to obtain search results; therefore, lists are often inconsistent (Bar-Ilan, 2005; McCracken, 2011). An evaluation across search engines found that when searching for "autism" on Google, Yahoo, and Bing, only 21 sites were identified in the top 100 hits for all three search engines, indicating that users are likely to experience different results depending on their preferred search engine (Reichow, Naples, Steinhoff, Halpern, & Volkmar, 2012).

Readability: The Acceptability and Other Divides

The second challenge involves the readability of the content. The Flesch-Kincaid readability formula measures reading level, with scores ranging from 0 (Very Difficult) to 100 (Very Easy). Scores between 60 and 69 are *Standard* and are considered appropriate for the average adult with a reading level between 5th and 8th grade. An evaluation of three ASD parent advocacy websites found the average readability score was 38 (Di Pietro et al., 2013). Sadly, content written specifically to encourage parents to advocate for their children with ASD is written at a level that may be too difficult for many parents to comprehend. This finding is consistent across other online health-related information (Di Pietro et al., 2013; Oermann et al., 2003).

Quality vs. Quantity: Informed Consumers of Online Information

Another challenge involves a lack of evidence-based information. The first result from Google searches for "autism" conducted in 2009, 2010, and 2011 was Wikipedia (Reichow et al., 2012). Although the consistency is encouraging, Wikipedia is a free encyclopedia that anyone with Internet access can edit with no process to ensure accuracy. Despite the questionable use of Wikipedia as a valid resource, a survey found that 72% of consumers using the internet for health information reported all or most of the information presented online was believable and only a quarter of respondents verified information obtained online (Fox & Raine, 2002).

Parents who recognize the need for more reliable information may search for disability category-specific websites, including tailored organization associations, with the belief that associations specific to a disorder would provide current, accurate information. However, association websites demonstrate a clear need for more effective communication regarding efficacy of interventions (Stephenson, Carter, & Kemp, 2012). Stephenson and colleagues (2012) identified 29 interventions within the autism literature, rated each based upon their varying levels of supporting evidence and compared the list with those interventions listed on eight autism-specific websites. The authors found that across association websites, the listed ASD interventions were not consistent. Further, sites did not prioritize interventions with strong support and those with more support were not highlighted or described differently than those with weak support. Worse, descriptions of each intervention did not align with scientific information. Only two interventions were described as "negative," and one of those was Applied Behavior Analysis (ABA) Discrete Trials, which has strong scientific support with no evidence of iatrogenic effect. Clearly, parents are looking for sound advice and are potentially being misled due to bias from organizations or a lack of knowledge of the field. In these situations, bad advice appears to be worse than no advice at all.

Accurate information was also limited on advocacy sites for parents (Di Pietro et al., 2013). Three high-traffic advocacy websites for each of three neurodevelopmental disorders (ASD, cerebral palsy [CP], and FASD) were evaluated for evidence of safety and efficacy for treatment information described on the sites. Across all three disorders, advocacy websites made unsubstantiated claims about safety and efficacy, background information, and allusion to scientific studies (61%, 41%, and 50% of all treatments identified, respectively; Di Pietro et al., 2013). To further complicate matters for parents, even when references were provided, 52% required institutional subscriptions to medical journals or costly payments for access (Di Pietro et al., 2013), further inhibiting parents from obtaining evidence-based information to support their children.

MOOCs: Another Mode of Information Seeking

Another option for dissemination that may appear more credible to families involves web-based trainings. Kobak, Stone, Wallace, Warren, Swanson, and Robson (2011) developed and evaluated a web-based parent training for parents of children with Autism. Results were encouraging. Parents who completed the tutorial demonstrated a significant increase in content knowledge and provided positive ratings for user satisfaction and system usability (Kobak et al., 2011). However, evidence-based trainings will only be effective if they are marketed well and are easily accessible.

MOOCs increase the access of evidence-based trainings to the general population by offering courses developed by content experts free of cost and with no restrictions on registration, substantially decreasing the burden on individuals to obtain training that was previously only available to students enrolled in higher education institutes (Hoy, 2014). Despite the possibility for more trustworthy information through MOOCs if presented by professionals, MOOCs offered by lay persons or well-intended but less well-informed authors may fall victim to similar concerns with quality of information. However, studies have repeatedly demonstrated that attrition is a significant issue for MOOC participants (Gooding, Klaas, Yager, & Kanchanaraksa, 2013; Liyanagunawardena, Adams, & Williams, 2013; Ossebaard, van Gemert-Pijnen, Sorbi, & Seydel, 2010). Specifically, fewer than 10% of individuals who enroll in a MOOC complete it (Liyanagunawardena et al., 2013). However, given the adversity parents of children with ASDs face and the difficulty associated with independently locating reliable, evidence-based information, parents struggling to understand and assist their children diagnosed with an ASD may possess stronger internal motivation to complete web-based trainings.

In an attempt to increase availability of evidence-based information, health experts have begun to search for more effective routes of dissemination, including use of mobile technology. A study evaluating the impact of mobile technology to communicate with parents regarding health information found that while a sample of urban, African American parents used mobile technology for social interactions, they were less likely to use it for obtaining health information (Mitchell et al., 2014). Further, an attempt to utilize social media outlets to communicate child health information to low-income, predominantly Hispanic families was ineffective as parents reported concerns about credibility of information obtained through social media (Stroever et al., 2011). As the internet and mobile technology continue to grow in their capability to be *de facto* libraries, issues related to acceptability and reliability of information must continue to be challenged and studied.

Recommendations and Future Directions

Parents of children with disabilities appear to have embraced the opportunity to learn more about a particular diagnosis, associated symptoms and behaviors, trajectories for the future, and appropriate treatments and interventions within a web-based setting. However, many parents are not equipped to vet the available resource to determine the most appropriate and accurate information. Some organizations have attempted to provide guidance to families. For example, the Health On the Net Foundation (HON, 2013), a non-profit, non-government organization, has developed a coding system to assist families identify "reliable and trustworthy medical websites" that meet minimum standards to ensure users are aware of the source and purpose of the information they are reading, with an annual reassessment. However, even this vetting option does not seek to rate the accuracy, validity, or appropriateness of the information itself (Health On the Net Foundation [HON], 2013). Although it is helpful to provide some guidance, these efforts may not be as clearly beneficial for families. Unfortunately, it may not be feasible to vet disability-specific information on websites given the vast costs (i.e., time, money, personnel) required and the ever-increasing options available online.

Instead, researchers and practitioners should develop their own repositories of websites and online information to share with parents that they have carefully reviewed for accuracy of facts, research evidence to support recommendations, functionality of the site, and accessibility to parents. Further, an annual update of one's repository is essential to ensure recommended sources of information remain updated and in working condition. Finally, it is recommended that practitioners consistently reach out to parents and family members to determine what resources they are finding on their own. Discussion should center on helping parents weigh the merits of each site and the information found, with an ultimate goal of assisting parents in becoming savvy consumers of web-based information, leading to fewer misconceptions and less time in spent within the professional setting attempting to correct inaccurate or ineffective information.

ONLINE PARENT TRAINING, CONSULTATION, AND INTERVENTIONS

Parents and caregivers of children with developmental disabilities or other conditions may not always have access to skilled service providers or other professional resources. Families without skilled services are left without direct intervention, coaching in intervening with their children, or support in learning to help their children. The kinds of technology-assisted services that may be available to parents in remote locations (or in underserved areas) may include parent education, consultation, or family-centered or family-delivered interventions (Hall & Bierman, 2015). These three modalities can be used individually (e.g., online learning alone) or in combination to create more comprehensive programming, such as online learning modules, online consultation, and provision of intervention services.

Remote service delivery models for parents of children with disabilities have been most widely utilized and studied in the areas of TBI (e.g., Carey, Wade, & Wolfe, 2008), ASD (e.g., Vismara, Young, & Rogers, 2012), and in early intervention (e.g., Kelso, Fiechtl, Olsen, & Rule, 2009). Most models that attempt to provide parent training or other parent or family-centered intervention have utilized either a telemedicine approach or a home-based e-Health approach. A *telemedicine* approach for the purposes of this chapter involves services delivered to families in dedicated telemedicine suites that are hosted in a regional center or clinic. Telemedicine approaches have been studied in a variety of ways including the reliability of their use for diagnosis (Reese et al., 2013), parent satisfaction compared with F2F delivery, and cost-benefit analysis of the services compared to home-visits or clinic-based services (Kelso et al., 2009). *Home-based e-health services* (hereafter home-based e-health) are those in which parents participate in parent training, consultative, or intervention services using online learning materials, and synchronous (i.e., real-time) online coaching through Skype or similar applications. To evaluate the fidelity of service delivery and to provide coaching to parents, some models require parents to submit digital video recordings to intervention staff.

Interventions for Families

Autism Spectrum Disorders

Remote services for families of children on the autism spectrum comprise the most often published research studies related to e-health interventions. Broadly, the majority of these studies include those that examine the adaptation of existing, empirically-based, F2F interventions and online self-directed learning programs. The adaptations typically utilize several delivery components such as synchronous consultation, interactive online learning course materials, and knowledge quizzes or other checks for understanding. Other studies have examined the utility of remote service models for assessment of symptomology and parent satisfaction with e-health approaches. Wainer and Ingersoll (2013) created an online learning program for families and professionals. Wainer and Ingersoll's study utilized a rigorous multiple baseline experimental design and demonstrated that observed parent and child skills improved after utilizing the training materials.

Of those existing models adapted for remote delivery, the most widely studied include Early Start Denver Model (EDSM; Vismara, McCormick, Young, Nadhan, & Monlux, 2013; Vismara et al., 2012), ABA (Heitzman-Powell, Buzhardt, Rusinko, & Miller, 2014; Jang et al., 2012), and functional communication training (FCT; Suess et al., 2014) for remote delivery. All studies reported positive findings including increases in social behavior and joint attention in children (Vismara et al., 2012; Vismara et al., 2013) and increased parent knowledge and fidelity of implementation (Jang et al., 2012; Heitzman-

Powell et al., 2014). There is other literature regarding the delivery of online learning materials and consultation for parents that is not tied to an existing F2F framework, including professionals that developed original intervention frameworks for remote delivery instead of adapting existing F2F interventions (Ferdig et al., 2009; Kolb, 2007). Other studies examine how online sessions or coaching can supplement F2F services such as occupational therapy (Gibbs & Toth-Cohen, 2011) and speech therapy (Baharav & Reiser, 2010) for parents of children with autism. A pilot study of an e-health program in Colorado was showcased as a promising undertaking (Kaiser, 2011), but the published article did not outline the methodology, measurement, or results of the pilot. All studies of remotely delivered, evidence-based models demonstrated increased parent knowledge and parent satisfaction.

Traumatic Brain Injury

One research group dominates the research on providing e-Health delivery of parent training and behavior intervention for families with children diagnosed with a TBI. Wade and colleagues have systematically studied their delivery model starting in 2007. Their intervention, called the *Family Problem Solving* (FPS) model, has been evaluated in several trials that included initial feasibility studies (Wade, Wolfe, & Pestian, 2004; Wade, Wolfe, Brown, & Pestian, 2005a, 2005b) and randomized trials that compared online services to internet resource provision (Carey et al., 2008; Mast et al., 2014). FPS has demonstrated promise in that parents reported satisfaction with the services and it appeared to reduce antisocial behavior in children and parent depression. The FPS group has also contributed a number of important papers that outlined technical, ethical, and other logistical issues with e-health delivery for parents. Further, the FPS group has attempted to minimize the potential confound between parent comfort with and knowledge of technology and the effect of the program. A later iteration of their online intervention, called I-InTERACT (Internet-Based Interacting Together Everyday, Recovery After Childhood TBI) has demonstrated strong therapeutic alliance between parents and therapists, and high satisfaction for parents and therapists even with limited computer skills (Wade, Oberjohn, Conaway, Osinska, & Bangert, 2011).

Internalizing and Externalizing Mental Health Disorders

Study of interventions delivered by e-health for parents of children with social-emotional and mental health disorders include the study of programs designed for both internalizing and externalizing disorders. Primary trends emerge including study of the remote delivery of parent management training for children with attention deficit-hyperactivity disorder (ADHD) (Enebrink, Högström, Forster, & Ghaderi, 2012), cognitive behavior therapy delivered for parents (jointly with children receiving services as well) for internalizing disorders such as depression (Comer et al., 2013; Nelson, Barnard, & Cain, 2006), and obsessive compulsive disorder (OCD) (Corner et al., 2013). Study of adapted, existing interventions includes the Communication Method (Comer et al., 2013; Enebrink et al., 2012). For interventions for internalizing disorders, the intervention for depression, when compared to a face-to-face intervention demonstrated similar rates of symptom remission (Nelson et al., 2006). The cognitive behavior therapy intervention for OCD is still in its early feasibility stage of development and shows promise by showing improvement in symptom levels, although in a very small sample (n=5; Comer et al., 2013).

Early Intervention and Other Developmental Disorders

Smaller studies of e-health interventions for early intervention efforts and other developmental disorders are limited. Studies demonstrate mixed findings (Kable, Coles, Strickland, & Taddeo, 2012; Miyahara, Buston, Cutfield, & Clarkson, 2009) for disorders such as fetal alcohol spectrum disorder and developmental coordination disorders. Overall, these projects were small in size and had some significant methodological limitations such as non-experimental designs (Miyahara et al., 2009) and attrition (Kable et al., 2012).

Limitations and Problems

Current models for e-health and other services provided to families online have several limitations. First, many programs are currently in their infancy and have not gone to scale for the general public, thus leaving families without services unless they are recruited for research participation. Second, some of the programs have had significant problems with attrition rendering the intervention, regardless of how theoretically sound, ineffective due to lack of engagement. It is not clear whether these attrition issues are related to comfort with, or knowledge of, technology use by the parents, design of the online learning materials, or needs of the families. Third, some of the current studies are plagued with methodological problems such as sampling problems and comparing the use of their program to a waitlist control rather than a comparable condition (i.e., access to other learning materials or a F2F intervention). Finally, as professionals embark on adapting existing interventions for remote delivery, issues around technology infrastructure, access, and best practices in e-health need to be continually examined as we attempt to keep up with the rapid changes in the tools available to our field. This is especially challenging due to the constantly changing information technology infrastructure "baseline".

Recommendations and Future Directions

As researchers and professionals navigate the empirical questions around remote service delivery, several trends will likely emerge and several recommended next steps are apparent. It is likely that more adaptations of evidence-based programs will surface and be adapted for online delivery. In this process, it will become necessary for allied behavioral services professionals to have a collaborative relationship with professionals in instructional design, digital marketing, and information technology. As new relationships and perspectives are merged it will also be important for trials to be designed that utilize cutting-edge designs to include such techniques as the multiphase optimization strategy (MOST; Collins, Murphy, & Strecher, 2007) that unpacks multi-component interventions to understand those components that optimally impact outcomes of interest. If technology-assisted delivery is to ever become effective and fiscally feasible, a broader understanding must exist about the appropriate interplay between F2F components, communication capability, online social support, and online learning tools that have the greatest impact on family outcomes.

FUTURE RESEARCH DIRECTIONS

Researchers in special education, school psychology, and related disciplines may ask, "How can we possibly research something that changes every day? The technology becomes obsolete faster than we can study it." It is true that with the continued march of Moore's Law or the exponential growth of computing technology (Moore, 1998), researchers interested in application or use of technology likely will never keep pace.

Future study of web-based and mobile technologies may do well to center around three key themes. First, researchers should focus on the capability and utility of the tool in question, such as synchronous versus asynchronous communication, rather than focusing on specific software or gadgets. Second, researchers should focus their attention on the user characteristics that may have moderating effects on outcomes such as SES, reading level, technology experience and comfort level, cultural factors, or other factors. Our review has demonstrated that there are some important findings, though sometimes conflicting, about attrition, engagement, and user characteristics that may well inform the design and use of technology-assisted delivery models or adaptations of interventions. Finally, the internet itself has evolved from a static environment (Web 1.0) to a collaborative and user-connected space (Web 2.0) and continues to evolve into a "smart" (e.g., searches engines anticipating user needs based on aggregated data and sophisticated programming), portable (use of smart phones), and livestreaming environment (Web 3.0; "Web 1.0 vs Web 2.0 vs Web 3.0", 2011). Researchers will need to evolve with the technology and its use in order to best capitalize on connecting with families, educators, practitioners, and key stakeholders. Whereas once having a static website was enough to promote a message, now messages need to interface with social media and the user directly.

CONCLUSION

For parents of children with special needs, the internet has likely become one of the most important means of obtaining information and seeking support. Yet, parents' search for information is greatly influenced by the information accuracy and reliability available on the internet. Supportive and advocacy platforms, such as social media sites, blogs, and discussion boards, provide parents with access to networking and support services, though questions remain about how parents use these tools. According to recent study by the Pew Foundation (Fox, 2011), one in five adults have gone online to find other adults like themselves which would likely hold true for parents of children with special needs. Opportunities for parents to find support and community online are indisputable tools for parents to reduce feelings of loneliness and isolation.

Online information seeking provides a vast sea of information for parents to gain knowledge that used to be limited to library access and advanced research skills. Several limitations exist for online information seeking including trustworthiness of websites and reliable access to the internet. It is encouraging that some organizations have attempted to set minimum standards for identification of reliable websites and online resources (e.g., HON), yet there remains to be a current system that vets accuracy, research-base, functionality, and accessibility. Because of the veritable insurmountable task of monitoring and vetting all internet resources, quality control issues remain clear concerns for parents and professionals. Despite these limitations, promising support for parents exists in form of free training provided by professionals through MOOCs, information from professional organizations, and researchers beginning to take on the problem of vetting online resources (Crangle & Kart, 2015; Gooding et al., 2013; HON, 2013).

E-health approaches have been utilized for parent training and family-based interventions (e.g., Vismara et al., 2012). These interventions include adaptations of existing, empirically-based interventions for a range of disorders, and results have been positive and promising. However, limitations and barriers in remote delivery exist, including programs not yet being publicly available, high parent attrition rates, methodological issues in existing studies, and technological infrastructure concerns. It will also be important to develop and maintain interdisciplinary partnerships between the health and technology fields to provide the necessary online support to parents and to adapt programs that will optimally service families of children with special needs in remote areas.

Researchers and practitioners alike can benefit from the present literature base regarding online resources for parents of children with disabilities. Researchers may advance the current field by studying online resource options utilizing more rigorous designs, examining user characteristics and implementation concerns, and gain further knowledge regarding for whom internet resources benefit the most and what technological features best benefit parents and children. Practitioners may gain from the present literature base primarily by understanding the importance of taking charge of online resources, vetting them for parent use, engaging in open discussion with parents regarding their online resource use (and steering them toward high quality resources), and thinking creatively about how Web 2.0 applications may facilitate their current treatment practice with parents and children.

REFERENCES

American Psychiatric Association (APA). (2013a). Neurodevelopmental disorders. In Diagnostic and statistical manual of mental disorders (5th ed.). doi:10.1176/appi.books.9780890425596.514988

American Psychiatric Association (APA). (2013b). Conditions for further study. In Diagnostic and statistical manual of mental disorders (5th ed.). doi:10.1176/appi.books.9780890425596.773234

Baharav, E., & Reiser, C. (2010). Using Telepractice in Parent Training in Early Autism. *Telemedicine Journal and e-Health*, *16*(6), 727–731. doi:10.1089/tmj.2010.0029 PMID:20583950

Bar-Ilan, J. (2005). Comparing rankings of search results on the web. *Information Processing & Management*, *41*(6), 1511–1519. doi:10.1016/j.ipm.2005.03.008

Bartholomew, M. K., Schoppe-Sullivan, S. J., Glassman, M., Kamp Duch, C. M., & Sullivan, J. M. (2012). New parent's Facebook use at the transition to parenthood. *Family Relations*, *61*(3), 455–469. doi:10.1111/j.1741-3729.2012.00708.x PMID:23671354

Bennett, A., Pourmand, A., Shokoohi, H., Shesser, R., Sanches, J., & Joyce, J. (2014). Impacts of social networking sites on patient care in the emergency department. *Telemedicine Journal and e-Health*, *20*(1), 94–96. doi:10.1089/tmj.2013.0055 PMID:24160899

Black, A. P., & Baker, M. (2011). The impact of parent advocacy groups, the Internet and social networking on rare diseases: The IDEA League and IDEA League United Kingdom example. *Epilepsia*, *52*, 102–104. doi:10.1111/j.1528-1167.2011.03013.x PMID:21463291

Carey, J. C., Wade, S. L., & Wolfe, C. R. (2008). Lessons learned: The effect of prior technology use on web-based interventions. *Cyberpsychology & Behavior*, *11*(2), 188–195. doi:10.1089/cpb.2007.0025 PMID:18422412

Chowdhury, J., Drummond, J., Fleming, D., & Neitfeld, S. (2002). Content analysis of online autism specific sites. *Journal on Developmental Disabilities*, *9*(2), 157–165. Retrieved from http://www.oadd.org/

Clifford, T., & Minnes, P. (2013). Logging on: Evaluating an online support group for parents of children with autism spectrum disorders. *Journal of Autism and Developmental Disorders*, *43*(7), 1662–1675. doi:10.1007/s10803-012-1714-6 PMID:23143075

Collins, L. M., Murphy, S. A., & Strecher, V. (2007). The Multiphase Optimization Strategy (MOST) and the Sequential Multiple Assignment Randomized Trial (SMART): New methods for more potent ehealth interventions. *American Journal of Preventive Medicine*, *32*(5), S112–S118. doi:10.1016/j.amepre.2007.01.022 PMID:17466815

Comer, J. S., Furr, J. M., Cooper-Vince, C. E., Kerns, C. E., Chan, P. T., Edson, A. L., & Freeman, J. B. et al. (2013). Internet-delivered, family-based treatment for early-onset OCD: A preliminary case series. *Journal of Clinical Child and Adolescent Psychology*, *43*(1), 74–87. doi:10.1080/15374416.2013.855 127 PMID:24295036

Crangle, C. E., & Kart, J. B. (2015). A questions-based investigation of consumer mental-health information. *PeerJ*, e867. https://dx.doi.org/10.7717/peerj.867

Curtin, M. E. (2010). *Internet advocacy support for families of children with emotional difficulties* (Doctoral dissertation). Retrieved from ProQuest Dissertation Abstracts International. (DAI No. AAI3433132)

Di Pietro, N. C., Whiteley, L., Mizgalewicz, A., & Illes, J. (2013). Treatments for neurodevelopmental disorders: Evidence, advocacy and the internet. *Journal of Autism and Developmental Disorders*, *43*(1), 122–133. doi:10.1007/s10803-012-1551-7 PMID:22592952

Enebrink, P., Högström, J., Forster, M., & Ghaderi, A. (2012). Internet-based parent management training: A randomized controlled study. *Behaviour Research and Therapy*, *50*(4), 240–249. doi:10.1016/j.brat.2012.01.006 PMID:22398153

Eysenbach, G., & Köhler, C. (2002). How do consumers search for and appraise health information on the world wide web? Qualitative study using focus groups, usability tests, and in-depth interviews. *British Medical Journal*, *324*(7337), 573–577. http://www.bmj.com/ doi:10.1136/bmj.324.7337.573 PMID:11884321

Fain, N. (2009). *Internet use among parents of children with autism spectrum disorder*. (Doctoral dissertation). Retrieved from ProQuest Dissertation Abstracts International. (DAI No. AAI3367475)

Ferdig, R. E., Amberg, H. G., Elder, J. H., Donaldson, S. A., Valcante, G., & Bendixen, R. (2009). Autism and family interventions through technology: A description of a web-based tool to educate fathers of children with autism. *International Journal of Web-Based Learning and Teaching Technologies*, *4*(3), 55–69. doi:10.4018/jwbltt.2009090804

Fleischmann, A. (2004). Narratives published on the internet by parents of children with autism: What do they reveal and why is it so important? *Focus on Autism and Other Developmental Disabilities*, *19*(1), 35–43. doi:10.1177/10883576040190010501

Fleischmann, A. (2005). The hero's story and autism: Grounded theory study of websites for parents of children with autism. *Autism*, *9*(3), 299–316. doi:10.1177/1362361305054410 PMID:15937044

Fox, S. (2011). Peer-to-peer health care. *Pew Research Center*. Retrieved from http://www.pewinternet.org/2011/02/28/peer-to-peer-health-care-2/

Fox, S., & Raine, L. (2002). Vital decisions: How internet users decide what information to trust when they or their loved ones are sick. *Pew Research Center.* Retrieved from http://www.pewinternet.org/2002/05/22/vital-decisions-a-pew-internet-health-report/

Garbe, E. K. (2008). *Online support groups and maternal stress for mothers of children with autistic spectrum disorder* (Doctoral dissertation). Retrieved from ProQuest Dissertation Abstracts International. (DAI No. AAI3312812)

Gibbs, V., & Toth-Cohen, S. (2011). Family-centered occupational therapy and telerehabilitation for children with autism spectrum disorders. *Occupational Therapy in Health Care, 25*(4), 298–314. doi:10.3109/07380577.2011.606460 PMID:23899082

Gooding, I., Klaas, B., Yager, J. D., & Kanchanaraksa, S. (2013). Massive open online courses in public health. *Frontiers in Public Health, 1,* 1–8. doi:10.3389/fpubh.2013.00059 PMID:24350228

Graham, M., Hale, S., & Stephens, M. (2012). Digital divide: The geography of internet access. *Environment & Planning, 44*(5), 1009–1010. doi:10.1068/a44497

Hall, C. M., & Bierman, K. L. (2015). Technology-assisted interventions for parents of young children: Emerging practices, current research, and future directions. *Early Childhood Research Quarterly, 2015,* 21–32. doi:10.1016/j.ecresq.2015.05.003

Health On the Net Foundation. (2013). *Methodology.* Retrieved from http://www.hon.ch/HONcode/Patients/method.html

Heitzman-Powell, L. S., Buzhardt, J., Rusinko, L. C., & Miller, T. M. (2014). Formative evaluation of an ABA outreach training program for parents of children with autism in remote areas. *Focus on Autism and Other Developmental Disabilities, 1*(1), 23–38. doi:10.1177/1088357613504992

Hoy, M. B. (2014). MOOCs 101: An introduction to massive open online courses. *Medical Reference Services Quarterly, 33*(1), 85–91. doi:10.1080/02763869.2014.866490 PMID:24528267

Individuals With Disabilities Education Act, 20 U.S.C. §1400 (2004).

Jang, J., Dixon, D. R., Tarbox, J., Granpeesheh, D., Kornack, J., & de Nocker, Y. (2012). Randomized trial of an eLearning program for training family members of children with autism in the principles and procedures of applied behavior analysis. *Research in Autism Spectrum Disorders, 6*(2), 852–856. doi:10.1016/j.rasd.2011.11.004

Jones, D. J., Forehand, R., Cuellar, J., Kincaid, C., Parent, J., Fenton, N., & Goodrum, N. (2013). Harnessing innovative technologies to advance children's mental health: Behavioral parent training as an example. *Clinical Psychology Review, 33*(2), 241–252. doi:10.1016/j.cpr.2012.11.003 PMID:23313761

Kable, J. A., Coles, C. D., Strickland, D., & Taddeo, E. (2012). Comparing the effectiveness of on-line versus in-person caregiver education and training for behavioral regulation in families of children with FASD. *International Journal of Mental Health and Addiction, 10*(6), 791–803. doi:10.1007/s11469-012-9376-3

Kaiser, K. (2011). Telehealth: Families finding ways to connect in rural Colorado. *Exceptional Parent, 41*(4), 18–19. Retrieved from http://www.eparent.com/

Kelso, G. L., Fiechtl, B. J., Olsen, S. T., & Rule, S. (2009). The feasibility of virtual home visits to provide early intervention: A pilot study. *Infants and Young Children, 22*(4), 332–340. doi:10.1097/IYC.0b013e3181b9873c

Kirby, A., Edwards, L., & Hughes, A. (2008). Parents' concerns about children with specific learning difficulties: Insights gained from an online message centre. *Support for Learning, 23*(4), 193–200. doi:10.1111/j.1467-9604.2008.00393.x

Kobak, K. A., Stone, W. L., Wallace, E., Warren, Z., Swanson, A., & Robson, K. (2011). A web-based tutorial for parents of young children with autism: Results from a pilot study. *Telemedicine Journal and e-Health, 17*(10), 804–808. doi:10.1089/tmj.2011.0060 PMID:22011005

Kolb, M. J. (2007). *An online training program for parents of children with autism.* (Doctoral dissertation). Retrieved from ProQuest Dissertation Abstracts International. (DAI No. AAI3316404)

Liyanagunawardena, T. R., Adams, A. A., & Williams, S. A. (2013). MOOCs: A systematic study of the published literature 2008-2012. *International Review of Research in Open and Distance Learning, 14.* Retrieved from http://www.irrodl.org/index.php/irrodl/article/view/1455/2531

Mackintosh, V. H., Myers, B. J., & Goin-Kochel, R. P. (2005). Sources of information and support used by parents of children with autism spectrum disorders. *Journal on Developmental Disabilities, 12,* 41–52. Retrieved from http://oadd.org/Journal_14.html

Mast, J. E., Antonini, T. N., Raj, S. P., Oberjohn, K. S., Cassedy, A., Makoroff, K. L., & Wade, S. L. (2014). Web-based parenting skills to reduce behavior problems following abusive head trauma: A pilot study. *Child Abuse & Neglect.* doi:10.1016/j.chiabu.2014.04.012 PMID:24844734

McCracken, H. (2011). Engine Overhaul: Google takes steps to downgrade shoddy content in search results. *Times International, 177*(10), 47.

Mitchell, S. J., Godoy, L., Shabazz, K., & Horn, I. (2014). Internet and mobile technology use among urban African American parents: Survey study of a clinical population. *Journal of Medical Internet Research, 16*(1), e9. doi:10.2196/jmir.2673 PMID:24418967

Miyahara, M., Buston, R., Cutfield, R., & Clarkson, J. E. (2009). A pilot study of family-focused tele-intervention for children with developmental coordination disorder: Development and lessons learned. *Telemedicine Journal and e-Health, 15*(7), 707–712. doi:10.1089/tmj.2009.0022 PMID:19694593

Moore, G. E. (1998). Cramming more components onto integrated circuits. *Proceedings of the IEEE, 86*(1), 82–85. doi:10.1109/JPROC.1998.658762

Munk, C. (2014, August 27). Ice Bucket Donations Continue to Rise: $94.3 Million Since July 29. *The ALS Association.* Retrieved from http://www.alsa.org/

National Institute on Deafness and Other Communication Disorders. (2014). *Statistics on voice, speech, and language.* Retrieved from http://www.nidcd.nih.gov/health/statistics/pages/vsl.aspx

Nelson, E.-L., Barnard, M., & Cain, S. (2006). Feasibility of telemedicine intervention for childhood depression. *Counselling & Psychotherapy Research, 6*(3), 191–195. doi:10.1080/14733140600862303

Nieuwboer, C. C., Fukkink, R. G., & Hermanns, J. M. (2013). Peer and professional parenting support on the internet: A systematic review. *Cyberpsychology, Behavior, and Social Networking, 16*(7), 518–528. doi:10.1089/cyber.2012.0547 PMID:23659725

Oermann, M. H., Lowery, N. F., & Thornley, J. (2003). Evaluation of web sites on management of pain in children. *Pain Management Nursing, 4*(3), 99–105. doi:10.1016/S1524-9042(03)00029-8 PMID:14566707

Ossebaard, H. C., van Gemert-Pijnen, J. E., Sorbi, M. J., & Seydel, E. R. (2010). A study of a Dutch online decision aid for parents of children with ADHD. *Journal of Telemedicine and Telecare, 16*(1), 15–19. doi:10.1258/jtt.2009.001006 PMID:20086262

Pagliari, C., Sloan, D., Gregor, P., Sullivan, F., Detmer, D., Kahan, J., & MacGillivray, S. et al. (2005). What is eHealth (4): A scoping exercise to map the field. *Journal of Medical Internet Research, 7*(1), e9. doi:10.2196/jmir.7.1.e9 PMID:15829481

Powell, G., & McCauley, A. W. (2012). Blogging as a way to promote family-professional partnerships. *Young Exceptional Children, 15*(2), 20–31. doi:10.1177/1096250611428491

Reese, R. M., Jamison, R., Wendland, M., Fleming, K., Braun, M. J., Schuttler, J. O., & Turek, J. (2013). Evaluating interactive videoconferencing for assessing symptoms of autism. *Telemedicine Journal and e-Health, 19*(9), 671–677. doi:10.1089/tmj.2012.0312 PMID:23870046

Reichow, B., Naples, A., Steinhoff, T., Halpern, J., & Volkmar, F. R. (2012). Brief report: Consistency of search engine rankings for autism websites. *Journal of Autism and Developmental Disorders, 42*(6), 1275–1279. doi:10.1007/s10803-012-1480-5 PMID:22350454

Scharer, K. (2005). An internet discussion board for parents of mentally ill young children. *Journal of Child and Adolescent Psychiatric Nursing, 18*(1), 17–25. doi:10.1111/j.1744-6171.2005.00006.x PMID:15701095

Scharer, K., Colon, E., Moneyham, L., Hussey, J., Tavakoli, A., & Shugart, M. (2009). A comparison of two types of social support for mothers of mentally ill children. *Journal of Child and Adolescent Psychiatric Nursing, 22*(2), 86–98. doi:10.1111/j.1744-6171.2009.00177.x PMID:19490279

Self-Brown, S., & Whitaker, D. J. (2008). Parent-focused child maltreatment prevention: Improving assessment, intervention, and dissemination with technology. *Child Maltreatment, 13*(4), 400–416. doi:10.1177/1077559508320059 PMID:18567847

Stephenson, J., Carter, M., & Kemp, C. (2012). Quality of the information on educational and therapy interventions provided on the web sites of national autism associations. *Research in Autism Spectrum Disorders, 6*(1), 11–18. doi:10.1016/j.rasd.2011.08.002

Stroever, S. J., Mackert, M. S., McAlister, A. L., & Hoelscher, D. M. (2011). Using social media to communicate child health information to low-income parents. *Preventing Chronic Disease: Public Health Research, Practice, and Policy, 8*(6), 1-4. Retrieved from www.cdc.gov/pcd/issues/2011/nov/11_0028.htm

Suess, A. N., Romani, P. W., Wacker, D. P., Dyson, S., Kuhle, J. L., Lee, J. F., & Waldron, D. B. et al. (2014). Evaluating the treatment fidelity of parents who conduct in-home functional communication training with coaching via telehealth. *Journal of Behavioral Education, 23*(1), 34–59. doi:10.1007/s10864-013-9183-3

U.S. Census Bureau. (2010). *Computer and internet use in the United States: 2010*. Retrieved from http://www.census.gov/hhes/computer/publications/2010.html

Vismara, L. A., McCormick, C., Young, S. G., Nadhan, A., & Monlux, K. (2013). Preliminary findings of a telehealth approach to parent training in autism. *Journal of Autism and Developmental Disorders*, *43*(12), 2953–2969. doi:10.1007/s10803-013-1841-8 PMID:23677382

Vismara, L. A., Young, G. S., & Rogers, S. J. (2012). Telehealth for expanding the reach of early autism training to parents. *Autism Research and Treatment, 2012*, 1–12. doi:10.1155/2012/121878 PMID:23227334

Wade, S. L., Oberjohn, K., Conaway, K., Osinska, P., & Bangert, L. (2011). Live coaching of parenting skills using the internet: Implications for clinical practice. *Professional Psychology, Research and Practice*, *42*(6), 487–493. doi:10.1037/a0025222

Wade, S. L., Wolfe, C., Brown, T. M., & Pestian, J. P. (2005a). Putting the pieces together: Preliminary efficacy of a web-based family intervention for children with traumatic brain injury. *Journal of Pediatric Psychology*, *30*(5), 437–442. doi:10.1093/jpepsy/jsi067 PMID:15944171

Wade, S. L., Wolfe, C. R., Brown, T. M., & Pestian, J. P. (2005b). Can a web-based family problem-solving intervention work for children with traumatic brain injury? *Rehabilitation Psychology*, *50*(4), 337–345. doi:10.1037/0090-5550.50.4.337

Wade, S. L., Wolfe, C. R., & Pestian, J. P. (2004). A web-based family problem-solving intervention for families of children with traumatic brain injury. *Behavior Research Methods, Instruments, & Computers*, *36*(2), 261–269. doi:10.3758/BF03195572 PMID:15354692

Wainer, A. L., & Ingersoll, B. R. (2013). Disseminating ASD interventions: A pilot study of a distance learning program for parents and professionals. *Journal of Autism and Developmental Disorders*, *43*(1), 11–24. doi:10.1007/s10803-012-1538-4 PMID:22547028

Web 1.0 vs Web 2.0 vs Web 3.0 vs Web 4.0: A bird's eye on the evolution and definition. (2011, August). *Flat World Business*. Retrieved from http://flatworldbusiness.wordpress.com/flat-education/previously/web-1-0-vs-web-2-0-vs-web-3-0-a-bird-eye-on-the-definition/

Zeman, L. D., Swanke, J., & Doktor, J. (2011). Measurable successes for children with ASD: Perspectives from mother's virtual journals. *School Social Work Journal*, *36*(1), 61–78.

KEY TERMS AND DEFINITIONS

Acceptability Divide: The acceptability divide describes the extent to which users may be able to access the internet to get information but may find that information not easy to read, unreliable, not trust-worthy, intimidating, or confusing.

Advocacy Platform: A way in which parents may use online environments to gather support from parents, policy-makers, professionals, or other stakeholders in order to raise awareness, funds, or increase dissemination of knowledge about issues effecting their children.

Asynchronous Communication: Communication on discussion boards, social media posts, or other online environments where individuals cannot "talk" to each other in real time though not immediately after those have been posted.

E

Digital Divide: The degree to which certain persons may have no, limited, or unreliable access to the network that limits their capacity to participate fully with online communities or other online tools.

E-Health: E-health services include those in which parents participate in parent training, consultative, or intervention services using online learning materials, and synchronous (i.e., real-time) online coaching through Skype or similar applications.

Moderated Discussion Board: Online discussion boards that are monitored by a group leader, community organizer, consultant, or professional who can comment on the community's discussion, monitor for abusive or inappropriate content, and ensure the sharing of quality information.

Supportive Platform: A way in which parents may use online environments to find other families who are facing similar challenges in order to gain emotional support, ideas that may help their child or family, and make friendships.

Synchronous Communication: Sometimes called "instant messaging" or "chatting," synchronous communication provides a way for persons to communicate with almost instantaneous delivery and receipt of messages allowing for more natural conversation. This can include text-only or video chat options.

Telemedicine: Services delivered to families in dedicated telemedicine suites that are hosted in a regional health care center or other clinics (e.g., mental health agencies, hospitals) that include real-time video and audio communication. The term is also used to refer to internet-based or e-Health services, however, this chapter makes a distinction between the two.

Telepsychiatry: Telemedicine services that are specifically geared for psychiatric services such as medication prescription or monitoring.

Web 2.0: Internet interfaces that include user participation by way of commenting, posting, uploading media and content, and other interactive features. Web 2.0 includes examples such as blogging, microblogging (e.g., Twitter), social media, and content sharing.

An Overview of Serious Games in Cognitive Rehabilitation

Jorge Brandão
University of Minho, Portugal

Pedro Cunha
Minho University, Portugal

Vitor Hugo Carvalho
University of Minho, Portugal & Polytechnic Institute of Cávado and Ave, Portugal

Filomena O. Soares
University of Minho, Portugal

INTRODUCTION

Serious Games (SG) are an emergent field of research focused on the use of games with other purposes than mere entertainment with applications in many diverse areas. Although the term SG is becoming more and more popular, there is no current definition of the concept. Zyda (2005) was the first author to give a definition of SGs as "a mental contest, played with a computer in accordance with specific rules, that uses entertainment to further government or corporate training, education, health, public policy, and strategic communication objectives" (p. 26). Michael & Chen (2006) define SGs as "games that do not have entertainment, enjoyment or fun as their primary purpose" (p. 21). The authors classify SGs into a number of markets: military games, government games, educational games, corporate games, healthcare games, and political, religious and art games. Susi et al. gave an overview of SGs (Susi, 2005). Despite such classifications, many games could belong to more than one category and nowadays this concept is largely used in respect to computer games. The use of SG in rehabilitation has increased substantially over the past decade. By taking advantage of game technology in order to create more attractive user experiences and increasing playability, the environments and tasks simulated in the SG can be used to teach or train users in various situations (Rego, 2012). In particular, games applied in the field of neurorehabilitation are helping to improve the process of motor learning and recovery from incidents of stroke, traumatic brain injury, and other neuromuscular impairment by increasing user motivation during training (Perry, 2011).

In this chapter we present a review of the state of the art and evolution of SG in cognitive rehabilitation, revealing how they can help in the process of rehabilitation, pointing several advantages of their use, presenting some relevant SG available, as well as technologies and platforms used to their development. Furthermore, it will be also addressed new ways of human interactions and several cases of success applied to cognitive rehabilitation in patients. Lastly, some research opportunities and open problems will be identified.

DOI: 10.4018/978-1-4666-9978-6.ch057

BACKGROUND

Rehabilitation could be defined as a dynamic process of planned adaptive changes in lifestyle, in response to unplanned changes, due to disease or traumatic incident (Gunasekera, 2005). Rehabilitation of a variety of deficits resulting from diseases or traumatic incidents is a long term process consuming massive training and social/financial resources (Fok, 2009). The success of a rehabilitation program depends on various factors: appropriate timing, patient selection, choice of rehabilitation program, continued medical management and appropriate discharge planning. This can be achieved in a multidisciplinary way (medical, nursery, social personnel) and with an appropriate equipped rehabilitation department where adequate therapy treatments (physical therapy, occupational therapy, speech and language therapy, clinical psychology and social work) are combined in a planned and coordinated way towards a common goal (Gunasekera, 2005). Traditional rehabilitation therapies are usually considered boring and uninteresting due to their repetitive nature which leads patients to neglect the prescribed exercises (Burdea, 2003). For example, many tests from rehabilitation programs show that patients' function improves with an intensive training oriented to a particular goal but divided in specific tasks. However, the problem with this task-specific treatment approach is the lack of patient interest in performing repetitive tasks and in ensuring that they finish the treatment program (Burke, 2009a). It is important to increase the motivation of these patients in the practicing of the exercises, because an intensive repetition of the exercises is essential for their recovery (Rego, 2012) and it has been used as a determining factor in the outcome of rehabilitation (Maclean, 2002). It has been showed that games contribute to increase the motivation in rehabilitation sessions (Leeb, 2007). Positive results with SG implementation have been reported in several areas, including rehabilitation (Ma, 2008). One of the most promising applications is in fact in this area, in part because the characteristics of this technology help to overcome the difficulties associated with the rehabilitation process, which is often long, slow, costly and demanding (Rego, 2012). The games are more motivating to the patients because they have a storyboard and a set of challenges. Games offer to the patients the possibility of being immersed in a different environment (a virtual situation) where they try to accomplish the proposed goals being distracted from their disability condition and from the fact that they are in a rehabilitation activity. Apart the serious goal of the patients' recovery, the game gives also: immersion, challenge, motivation, enjoyment, sensations that they could not feel in a traditional rehabilitation plan (Rego, 2012). Prensky (2001) elaborated twelve elements of why games engage individuals. Hence, patients remain engaged until the rehabilitation objectives are achieved. Additionally, games are becoming more accessible to people in general. Computer systems are becoming more disseminated and affordable to users in general, in the form of several devices: game consoles, portable personal computers, large display television sets, among others. At the same time, people tend to have more knowledge in information systems and computer technologies, and this promotes the accessibility to computer games. The proximity of the scenarios and activities to real-life environments helps to increase the potential for generalization of acquired skills and consequently to improve the participation of patients in various contexts of life (Rego, 2012). Other reasons that explain this growing interest in cognitive rehabilitation are the limited efficacy of current drug therapies, the plasticity of the human central nervous system and the discovery that during ageing the connections in the brain are not fixed but instead they retain the capacity to change with learning (Smith, 2009). Today, many studies show evidence of neuronal plasticity that support neurocognitive rehabilitation beyond the functional gains (Johansson, 2011). Interventions with computer games have emerged as a valuable tool to promote brain plasticity that positively affect cognitive skills such as memory, attention, perception or orientation. For instance, Space Fortress is a computer game developed as a cognitive tool for studying learning and training strategies by simulating real-world tasks, such as piloting a vehicle or air traffic control (Gevins, 1997).

Cases of Success in Cognitive Rehabilitation with Serious Games

The application of new technologies to health and rehabilitation has grown significantly in recent decades, with good potential as they motivate the patient to accomplish the defined goals designed for rehabilitation. Several SG designed to improve cognitive abilities in rehabilitation process have been reported in the literature. In this section we review pertinent cases of success developed in this area with regard to foremost causes of cognitive impairments. Acquired Brain Injury (ABI) is the leading cause of death and disability in adults and children (Coronado, 2009). Among the causes of death by brain injury are road traffic accidents (23%), suicide (17%), violence (11%) and falls (7%) (Sohlberg, 2005). One relevant SG developed in this area is the project of Dores *et. al.* (2011). They developed the *Virtual City* gameplay, algorithm and architecture, as part of the Computer-Assisted Rehabilitation Program – Virtual Reality (CARP-VR). This platform is an instance of SG, customized to the rehabilitation of executive functioning and related cognitive tasks, such as vision-spatial processing, attention and memory in adult patients with Acquired Brain Injury (ABI) (Dores, 2011). Caglio *et. al.* (2009) assessed the modifications occurring in cognitive functions, in particular spatial and verbal memory in a patient after 3D video game rehabilitation training. The video game was a driving simulator. During the training, the participant was requested to explore a complex virtual town from a ground-level perspective. Stroke is a leading cause of severe physical disability in the United Kingdom and the cause of a range of impairments, such as loss of balance, attention and concentration deficiencies, pain, weakness and paralysis. As a result of these impairments, stroke sufferers are often unable to independently perform day-to-day activities (Anderson, 1992). Literature has shown that technology has potential benefits to therapy process and it can be an interesting and effective way of providing rehabilitation to people with stroke (Rizzo, 2005). For example, Burke *et. al.* (2009b) from University of Ulster are developing two systems for upper limb stroke rehabilitation through the integration of 3D virtual environments and sensor and camera technology The first game, Rabbit Chase, is being developed for single arm rehabilitation (either right or left arm). The second game, Arrow Attack, is being developed for bimanual rehabilitation (both arms). The study has shown encouraging results and positive feedback with regard to the playability and usability of the games by both able-bodied users and people with varying degrees of impairment caused by stroke (Burke, 2009b). Cameirão *et. al.* (2009) developed the Rehabilitation Gaming System (RGS), a VR based system for the rehabilitation of patients suffering from stroke and TBI. The system uses a camera based motion capture system with gaming technologies to activate intact neuronal systems that provide direct stimulation to motor areas affected by brain lesions. The RGS is designed to engage the patients in task specific intensive training tuned to the patients' needs and with continuous monitoring (Cameirão, 2009; Cameirão, 2007). Prokopenko *et. al.* (2011) developed a course of neuropsychological computer programs training, with the purpose of estimate the efficiency of new methods of neurorehabilitation of impairments of cognitive functions with the use of computer programs of correction in post-stroke patients. The tasks included training of attention with use of the computer programs on the basis of Schulte's test, the task for training visual storing with a set of pictures and symbols, the switching test, correction optical and spatial gnosis with test of narrative images and the test of «arrangements of hands of the clock» with possibility of a feedback. Preliminary results have shown good effect concerning both clinical aspects and the Patient Global Impression Scale (Prokopenko, 2011). Alzheimer's disease (AD) is the most common form of dementia among older people. According to World Health Organization (2013) it is estimated that the prevalence will increase to 0.44% in 2015 and to 0.56% in 2030. AD is characterized by progressive loss of memory and other mental abilities; this loss results in atrophy of the affected regions. Nowadays, finding an effective therapy for AD is a social need. La Guia *et. al.* (2013) developed a SG specifically to AD, in order to enhance and stimulate the cognitive abilities of people suffering from Alzheimer and to counteract the progress of the disease. The interactive system is based on emerging technologies such as Near Field Communication (NFC) and distributed user interfaces and tangible interaction to conduct cognitive rehabilitation, where the main objective is to improve the person's performance in real-life situations and the associated enhancement in the person's well-being, self-esteem, mood and behaviour (Guia, 2013). The system is composed of two different tools, namely, *Co-Brain Training* and *AlzGame*. The first tool is based on collaborative game and its main objective is to improve the cognitive, emotional and psychosocial conditions of Alzheimer's patients. The user has only to interact and bring the mobile device closer to tangible interfaces. The second tool 'AlzGame' consists of games executed on a touch screen tablet which allows users to carry out more specific cognitive stimulation therapies. The new interaction style offered by the tools is simple and intuitive; its purpose is to eliminate the technological gap for the elderly. Conconi *et. al.* (2008) introduced *PlayMancer,* a platform for rapid development of SGs, with a special focus on therapeutic support games for behavioural and addictive disorders, i.e. eating disorders and pathological gambling. It is modular and combines techniques from multimodal interaction (speech, touch, biosensors and motion-tracking), 3D engines, virtual and augmented reality, speech recognition and natural language processing. The prototype to be adopted for chronic mental disorders treatment, introduces the player to an interactive scenario which aims to increase his general problem solving strategies, self-control skills and control over general impulsive behaviours. The 3D interactive environment is made up of different islands that will be used as scenario. Each island will permit access to one or several types of resources which will facilitate and improve the game characters, and hence the player's relaxation techniques and planning skills. The game encourages the player to learn and develop new confrontation strategies. Martins *et. al.* (2011) designed a SG – Total Challenge (in Portuguese *Desafio Total*) that aims to support people with mild or moderate intellectual disabilities, allowing to verify the progress of these people in relation to memory, to decision-making time and to observation, learning and applying knowledge skills. Preliminary tests carried out with the game showed that users were very motivated, focused and excited, presenting continued interest in repeating the game in an attempt to achieve better scores. RehaCom is a system widely used and tested in the area of cognitive rehabilitation. Its effectiveness has been demonstrated in a number of studies well referenced in the RehaCom Catalogue. This system is well established in various hospitals and clinics, with a great number of patients being treated in rehabilitation programs. It can be easily accessed and tested regarding efficiency. RehaCom is a computer-assisted modular system that requires an experienced therapist. The system concept was developed by Hans Regel in 1986 and since then it has been refined over 20 years in clinics, with input from experts in the area. Since 1996 it has been developed by Hasomed (Inc, Ltd). For a few years, it has been market leader in Europe and it is currently available in 15 languages. The system is composed of training procedures for training different skills: attention, memory, executive, field of view and visual-motors. Each training procedure consists of a specific task that the patient must accomplish. The game interface is very simple and it is only two-dimensional.

New Forms of Interaction of Serious Games Applied to Cognitive Rehabilitation

Interaction in any kind of computer game is a key aspect that affects the experience provided to the player. Therefore, this aspect has the ability for dictate its success or failure in the market and between players for who it was been created. When the purpose of the computer game is rehabilitation, in this particular case, cognitive rehabilitation, the interaction between the player (patient) and the computer game acquire more relevance in the SG development. Another key aspect that contributes for positive results is patients' motivation as SGs recently developed are becoming more motivating (Rego, 2012, p. 1189). Considering the importance of interaction and motivation of the patients using of SGs for rehabilitation, more natural interfaces have been developed creating new forms of inputs that change the traditional interaction paradigm of mouse and keyboard. This is possible due to the investment of large companies of game industry that developed accessible systems that allow new forms of interaction like the *Microsoft Kinect system* (Microsoft, 2014), the *Nintendo Wii system* (Nintendo, 2014) or the *Sony PlayStation Move system* (Sony, 2014). These relevant new forms of inputs are:

- Gestures;
- Force feedback;
- Balance feedback;
- Image recognition;
- Facial expression recognition;
- Voice recognition.

The main improvement that these new forms of interaction brought was to enabling the development of SGs that provide a more natural and free experience to the patient, which is important to enhance the efficiency and the quality of the rehabilitation process (Rego, 2012, p. 1189). Aware of the importance that the forms of interaction have on the application and results of SGs for rehabilitation, new research is being developed in SGs, focusing on the forms of interaction and results achieved in each case. In their work, Garcia Marin *et al.* (2011) gather recent research projects for stroke rehabilitation. They present some SGs developed by other researchers to apply in rehabilitation of the elderlies, where new forms of interaction were used, such as: hands movements with gloves (gestures and image recognition); image recognition without markers and touching screen. All researchers use a set of different games that allow the patient to diversify, keeping thus the motivation and contribute for a longer, but pleasant, period of therapy (Burke, 2009; Annet, 2009; Fasola, 2010). Rego *et. al.* (2012) in their work note that in most of the reviewed games the forms of interaction are the traditional ones with simple interfaces. The use of the most natural forms of interaction appears since the year 2008, but with weak results in terms of rehabilitation process (Alankus *et. al.,* 2010; Battocchi *et. al.,* 2008; Burke, 2009; Cameirão, 2009; Conconi, 2008; Ma, 2008; Ryan, 2009; Vanacken *et. al.,* 2009). Rego *et. al.* (2012) considers that interaction technology was an important criterion to reach a higher motivational purpose in rehabilitation therapy when SGs are used. Also, they believe "that the use of more natural interfaces in games can contribute to diminish the problem of poor motivation in the rehabilitation sessions, since it can enable the way the patients interact with the system" (p. 1204). These entire studies alert to the importance of new forms of interaction for increasing patient´s motivation as the easier the interaction, the greater the motivation. Accordingly, future developments of SGs should take into account the introduction of more natural and intuitive forms of interaction, so the patient´s motivation is always present, making the therapy a pleasant experience.

FUTURE RESEARCH DIRECTIONS

The expected outcome of neurorehabilitation training is to achieve clinically-relevant patients' improvements. Towards this goal, the game design should primarily target improving function through task-oriented objectives, and maximize patient adherence to training.

A necessary step in the successful implementation of games in mainstream rehabilitation programs is the development of an integrated rehabilitation software platform that supports existing systemic relationships and methodologies to the specific illness. An important point of future research is the development of compatible low-cost rehabilitation devices and interfaces also available to patients' treatment at home, where they have the opportunity to train at higher frequencies and durations. Another major research opportunity is the study of how the effectiveness of computer games for rehabilitation can be increased by the incorporation of a social dimension. There is not reported work for systems where collaboration or competitiveness performs a major role on the rehabilitation process. Collaboration and competition add a new dimension that could allow the patients to enjoy the interaction and found the motivation and encouragement from others playing the same game. Although many recent game-based interventions for rehabilitation have been reported in the literature, most of them have some limitations, such as small sample size, limited time invested in usability and acceptance testing, testing comprising healthy users; and lack of regard for the therapist who is one of the primary end-users of the technology, so more studies are needed.

CONCLUSION

In the diversely growing field of neurorehabilitation it is recognized that SGs represent a powerful tool to increase motivation and active participation during training programs once it is difficult to maintain patient's motivation and interest. They improve the cognitive skills and reinforce learning offering a powerful opportunity to explore. The authors conducted a survey of the most relevant work available in the literature and have considered that rehabilitation games have significant potential for growth thus they have not yet been fully explored. According to Prensky (2001), "players of computer and video games not only learn how to do things in terms of the conceptual procedures, but they also practice the skills until the learning is internalized and becomes second nature". In this way, a successful game design could significantly increase not only the acquisition of skills during rehabilitation therapy, but also long-term retention after therapy cessation. There have been many attempts to create low-cost solutions to rehabilitation, for example, exploring the rehabilitation potential of commonly available computer games such Nintendo® Wii Fit or Playstation EyeToy®. The new forms of interaction founded to the users, despite some difficulties, made the user experience more attractive and intuitive.

Nowadays, a major disparagement of existing gaming scenarios for rehabilitation is that they have been designed primarily by engineers or scientists whose intent is to build and test the overall functionality of specific research-based hardware, and often lack the qualities required to be motivational for long-term and they are therefore less engaging for the patients. On the other hand, popular games for recreational use have typically not been designed with the criteria for neurorehabilitation in mind, and thus often lack essential components for therapeutic effectiveness, so careful attention must be given in this way, as it is extremely important to keep the level of challenge optimal in order to stimulate intrinsic motivation. Moving forward, the continuing use of SG and technology advances benefits rehabilitation and will unlock several of new opportunities to meet stakeholders' needs and expectations.

REFERENCES

Alankus, G., Lazar, A., May, M., & Kelleher, C. (2010). *Towards customizable games for stroke rehabilitation.* Paper presented at the 28th International Conference on Human factors in Computing Systems, Atlanta, GA.

Anderson, R. (1992). *The Aftermath of Stroke: The Experience of Patients and Their Families.* Cambridge, UK: Cambridge University Press. doi:10.1017/CBO9780511983238

Annett, M., Anderson, F., Goertzen, D., Halton, J., Ranson, Q., Bischof, W. F., & Boulanger, P. (2009). Using a multi-touch tabletop for upper extremity motor rehabilitation. In *Proceedings of the 21st Annual Conference of the Australian Computer-Human Interaction Special Interest Group.* doi:10.1145/1738826.1738869

Battocchi, A., Gal, E., Ben Sasson, A., Painesi, F., Venuti, P., Zancanaro, M., & Weiss, P. L. (2008). *Collaborative puzzle game An interface for studying collaboration and social interaction for children who are typically developed or who have Autistic Spectrum Disorder.* Paper presented at the 7th International Conference Series on Disability, Virtual Reality and Associated Technologies (ICDVRAT), Maia, Portugal.

Burdea, G. (2003). Virtual rehabilitation-benefits and challenges. In *Methods of Information in Medicine* (Vol. 42, pp. 519–523). Methodik der Information in der Medizin.

Burke, J. W., McNeill, M. D., Charles, D., Morrow, P., Crosbie, J. H., & McDonough, S. M. (2009). Optimising engagement for stroke rehabilitation using SGs. *The Visual Computer*, *25*(12), 1085–1099. doi:10.1007/s00371-009-0387-4

Burke, J. W., McNeill, M. D. J., Charles, D. K., Morrow, P. J., McDonough, S. M., & Crosbie, J. H. (2009). SGs for upper limb rehabilitation following stroke. In IEEE Intl. Conf. in Games and Virtual Worlds for Serious Applications (VS Games '09), (pp. 103–110). IEEE.

Caglio, M., Latini-Corazzini, L., D'agata, F., Cauda, F., Sacco, K., Monteverdi, S., & Geminiani, G. et al. (2009). Video game play changes spatial and verbal memory: Rehabilitation of a single case with traumatic brain injury. *Journal of Cognitive Processing*, *10*(S2), S195–S197. doi:10.1007/s10339-009-0295-6 PMID:19693564

Cameirão, M. S., Badia, S., Zimmerli, B. L., Oller, E. D., & Verschure, P. F. M. J. (2007). A Virtual Reality System for Motor and Cognitive Neurorehabilitation. In *Proc. 9ᵗʰ European Conf. for the Advancement of Assistive Technology in Europe – AAATE 2007*, (pp. 3—5).

Cameirão, M. S., Badia, S., Zimmerli, B. L., Oller, E. D., & Verschure, P. F. M. J. (2009). The Rehabilitation Gaming System: a Review. Studies in Health Technology and Informatics, 145, 65—83.

Coronado, V. G., Thurman, D. J., Greenspan, A. I., & Weissman, B. M. (2009). Epidemiology. In J. Jallo & C. M. Loftus (Eds.), Neurotrauma and Critical Care: Brain (pp. 3–19). New York: Thieme.

de la Guia, E., Lozano, M.D., & Penichet, V.R. (2013). Cognitive rehabilitation based on collaborative and tangible computer games. In *Pervasive Computing Technologies for Healthcare (PervasiveHealth), 2013 7th International Conference on.*

Dores, A. R. (2011). *SGs Development and Applications. Serious* Games: Are They Part of the Solution in the Domain of Cognitive *Rehabilitation? Computer Science, 6944*, 95–105.

Elaklouk, M. A., Mat, Z. N. A. & Shapii, A. (2013). A Conceptual Framework for Designing Brain Injury Cognitive Rehabilitation Gaming System. *International Journal of Digital Content Technology and its Applications, 7*(15).

Fasola, J., & Mataric, M. J. (2010). Robot exercise instructor: A socially assistive robot system to monitor and encourage physical exercise for the elderly. In *RO-MAN, 2010* (pp. 416–421). IEEE. doi:10.1109/ROMAN.2010.5598658

Fok, S. (2009). Internet-enabled exercises and prosthesis for home-based cognitive rehabilitation. *International Journal of Biomedical Engineering and Technology, 2*(1), 29–43. doi:10.1504/IJBET.2009.021906

Garcia, M. J., Felix, N. K., & Lawrence, E. (2011). SGs to improve the physical health of the elderly: A categorization scheme. In *CENTRIC 2011, The Fourth International Conference on Advances in Human-oriented and Personalized Mechanisms, Technologies, and Services,* (pp. 64-71).

Gevins, A., Smith, M. E., McEvoy, L., & Yu, D. (1997). High-resolution EEG mapping of cortical activation related to working memory: Effects of task difficulty, type of processing, and practice. *Cereb Cortex, 7*(4), 374–385. doi:10.1093/cercor/7.4.374 PMID:9177767

Jiménez-Murcia. (2008). PlayMancer: A Serious Gaming 3D Environment. In *Int. Conf. on Automated Solutions for Cross Media Content and Multi-channel Distribution - AXMEDIS'08*. IEEE.

Gunasekera, W. S. L., & Bendall, J. (2005). Neurosurgery. In *Rehabilitation of Neurologically Injured Patients*. Springer.

Johansson, B. B. (2011). Current trends in stroke rehabilitation. A review with focus on brain plasticity. *Acta Neurologica Scandinavica, 123*, 147–159.

Leeb, R., Lee, F., Keinrath, C., Scherer, R., Bischof, H., & Pfurtscheller, G. (2007). Brain-computer communication: Motivation, aim, and impact of exploring a virtual apartment. *IEEE Transactions on Neural Systems and Rehabilitation Engineering, 15*(4), 473–482. doi:10.1109/TNSRE.2007.906956 PMID:18198704

Ma, M., & Bechkoum, K. (2008). *SGs for movement therapy after stroke*. IEEE Sys. Man. Cybern.

Maclean, N., Pound, P., Wolfe, C., & Rudd, A. (2002). The concept of patient motivation a qualitative analysis of stroke professionals' attitudes. *Stroke, 33*(2), 444–448. doi:10.1161/hs0202.102367 PMID:11823650

Martins, T., Carvalho, V., Soares, F., & Moreira, M. F. (2011). SG as a tool to intellectual disabilities therapy: Total challenge. In *Serious* Games *and Applications for Health (SeGAH), 2011 IEEE 1ˢᵗ International Conference on*. IEEE.

Michael, D., & Chen, S. (2006). *Serious Games: Games that educate, train, and inform*. Boston, MA: Thomson Course Technology.

Microsoft Kinect System. (2014). Available: http://www.microsoft.com/en-us/kinectforwindows/

Nintendo Wii System. (2014). Available: http://www.nintendo.com/wiiu

Perry, J. C. et al.. (2011). Effective Game use in Neurorehabilitation: User-Centered Perspectives. In P. Felicia (Ed.), *Handbook of Research on Improving Learning and Motivation through Educational Games: Multidisciplinary Approaches* (pp. 683–725). doi:10.4018/978-1-60960-495-0.ch032

Prensky, M. (2001). *The digital game-based learning revolution.* Digital Game-Based Learning.

Prokopenko, S. V. (2011). Neurorehabilitation of poststroke cognitive impairments with the use of computed programs. In *Virtual Rehabilitation (ICVR), 2011 International Conference on.* doi:10.1109/ICVR.2011.5971851

Rego, P. A., Moreira, P. M., & Reis, L. P. (2012). New Forms of Interaction in Serious Games for Rehabilitation. In M. Cruz-Cunha (Ed.), *Handbook of Research on SGs as Educational* (pp. 1188–1211). Business and Research Tools. doi:10.4018/978-1-4666-0149-9.ch062

RehaCom Catalogue. (2009). Available: http://www.hasomed.de/en/products/rehacom-cognitivetherapy.html

Rizzo, A., & Kim, G. J. (2005). A SWOT analysis of the field of virtual reality rehabilitation and therap. *Presence (Cambridge, Mass.), 14*(2), 119–146. doi:10.1162/1054746053967094

Ryan, M., Smith, S., Chung, B., Cossell, S., Jackman, N., & Kong, J. (2009). *Rehabilitation games: Designing computer games for balance rehabilitation in the elderly.* Retrieved from http://oscarmak.net/fdg09.pdf

Smith, G. E., Housen, P., Yaffe, K., Ruff, R., Kennison, R. F., Mahncke, H. W., & Zelinski, E. M. (2009). A cognitive training program based on principles of brain plasticity: Results from the Improvement in Memory with Plasticity-based Adaptive Cognitive Training (IMPACT) study. *Journal of the American Geriatrics Society, 57*(4), 594–603. doi:10.1111/j.1532-5415.2008.02167.x PMID:19220558

Sohlberg, M. M., Todis, B., Fickas, S., Hung, P.-F., & Lemoncello, R. (2005). A profile of community navigation in adults with chronic cognitive impairments. Brain Injury, 19, 1249-1259.

Sony Playstation Move System. (2014). Available: http://pt.playstation.com/psmove/

Susi, T., Johannesson, M., & Backlund, P. (2005). *SGs – An Overview.* Sweden: Tech. Rep.

Vanacken, L., Notelaers, S., Raymaekers, C., Luyten, K., Coninx, K., van den Hoogen, W., & Feys, P. (2009). *Game-based collaborative training for arm rehabilitation of MS patients: A proof-of-concept game.* Paper presented at the GameDays 2009.

World Health Organization (WHO). (2013). *World report on disability.* WHO.

Zyda, M. (2005). From visual simulation to virtual reality to games. IEEE Comput., 38, 30-34.

KEY TERMS AND DEFINITIONS

Cognitive Rehabilitation: A dynamic process with a set of treatments and programs directed to improve or recover the patient cognitive skills that have been diminished by disease or traumatic injury; this therapy focus on the patient's reacquisition of the most independent or highest level of functioning.

E

Cognitive Skills: A term referred to the exclusive human's ability to have brain superior functions or brain based skills such as memory, speech, logic, reasoning, auditory/visual processing and understanding of written material, processing thoughts and perceptions.

Interaction Technology: Refers to the techniques and tools developed and available to users to interact with the therapy devices, such as desktop monitors and head-mounted displays (HMDs), haptic interfaces, and real-time motion tracking devices.

Natural User Interfaces: A system by which users interact with the computer composed by input devices other than the traditional keyboard or mouse devices that do not use commands and that give the user the sense of an easier and intuitive interaction with the system, making him to learn more rapidly how to control the computer application.

Patients: Persons who need healthcare for a particular disease or condition or are under medical assistance.

Rehabilitation: A set of treatments or a plan designed to assist people on the process of recovery some or all of the patient's physical, sensory, and mental capabilities from injury, illness, or disease to as normal a condition as possible.

Serious Games: Games which the main purpose is not the entertainment, but instead, promote learning and behavior changes in various areas, such business, industry, marketing, education and healthcare; they are designed to solve problems in several areas and involve challenges and rewards, using the entertainment and engagement components provided when user is playing games.

Technology: Refers to the set of miscellaneous tools and technical, including equipments, modifications, arrangements and procedures developed and used by humans, in order to control and to adapt to their natural, social or inner environments.

Possibilities of a Body–Region Separately Weighing System in Healthcare

Noriko Kurata
Chuo University, Japan

Masakazu Ohashi
Chuo University, Japan

Hiroshi Ichikawa
Otsuma Women's University, Japan

Mayumi Hori
Hakuoh University, Japan

Sumiko Kurata
Tokyo Kasei-Gakuin University, Japan

Tadao Kurata
Niigata University of Pharmacy and Applied Life Sciences, Japan

INTRODUCTION

In this chapter, a newly developed system for regional weight measurement of the human body; "body-region separately weighing system" (BRSW-system); was shown to be potentially applicable for self-measurement of regional weights of own body to use the measurement data for personalized health management.

The BRSW-system is the world's first regional body weight measuring system devised by Kurata, and patented in Japan (JP Patent No.4290704, 2009), US (US Patent No.8540649, 2013), EU (EP Patent No.1985978, 2014), and other countries; however, it is not commercially available currently.

BACKGROUND

The human body consists of the following six main regions: the head, the upper extremities, the torso and the lower extremities. Each of these body regions has its own functions and consists of its own set of tissues, such as connective tissue and muscle tissue, needed to perform those functions. As the weight of the tissues forming the various body regions differ from one region to another, the weights of the body regions themselves also differ.

From a kinesiological perspective, the two hands, two lower extremities, trunk and head participate in various movements and thus can be broadly regarded as components of the musculoskeletal system. Knowing the weight (or the mass, to be exact) of each body region is very important when scientifically assessing the mechanical role of each body region during movement and their contribution to postural control. Studies that measured the weights of body regions, however, have all been based on data from

DOI: 10.4018/978-1-4666-9978-6.ch058

cadavers in which the weight of each body region was measured after it was dismembered from the body (Dempster & Gaughran, 1967; Mozumdar & Roy, 2004), and no reports on the weighing of body segments on living bodies could be found. Thus, while the current way of measuring body weight throughout the world is to stand on a scale to determine whole body weight, the weights of and weighing methods of one's separate body regions, which is more important information as far as body movements in everyday life are concerned, are at present largely unknown.

Meanwhile, the rate of aging is accelerating in Japan,, as shown in Table 1, and according to the Ministry of Internal Affairs and Communications, the number of people aged 65 years or older is 32.96 million as of September 2014, accounting for an unprecedented 25.9% of the total population, with one in eight people now aged 75 years or older.

The average life expectancy of a Japanese person is long; 79.55 years for men and 86.30 for women as of 2010 according to the Ministry of Health, Labour and Welfare. However, healthy life expectancy is estimated to be 70.42 years for men and 73.62 years for women. Healthy life expectancy is the period in which an individual lives without health problems, so men have approximately nine years of life with health problems and women have approximately 12 years. The reasons behind reduced independence, being bedridden, or the need for assistance or long-term care are musculoskeletal disorders (23%), cerebrovascular disorders (22%), cognitive impairment (15%), debility (14%), and other problems (26%) (Ministry of Health, Labour and Welfare, 2012), thereby revealing the importance of health of the musculoskeletal system. Maintaining a healthy musculoskeletal system therefore greatly contributes to prolonging healthy life expectancy.

The musculoskeletal system is composed of the bones, joints, muscles, nerves, etc., in the body regions such as the upper and lower extremities that are necessary in order to freely move the body. The various parts of the musculoskeletal system all work together, so if any one of them deteriorates, the entire body will not move well. Reduced locomotive function of the body due to musculoskeletal impairment is called "locomotive syndrome" (LS), which may lead to an increased risk for requiring long-term care if it progresses. In other words, LS is a condition in which one or several of the various musculoskeletal tissues such as muscles, bone, joints, cartilage and intervertebral discs are impaired, thereby disrupting gait or other activities of daily living, and is a concept that was proposed by the Japanese Orthopaedic Association in 2007 following projections for Japan's future with its aging society.

Simple methods of managing health are therefore needed at the individual level in order to extend healthy life expectancy and maintain health until individuals reach the average life expectancy. Moreover, a simple method of quantitatively assessing muscles is required, although a method has yet to be established.

Table 1. Changes in the elderly population in Japan

Year	Total Population	Aged People (Over 65 Years of Age)	Percentage of Aged People (%)
1970	103,720,000	7,330,000	7.1
1980	117,060,000	10,650,000	9.1
1990	123,610,000	14,930,000	12.1
2000	126,930,000	22,040,000	17.4
2010	128,060,000	29,480,000	23.0
2020	124,100,000	36,120,000	29.1
2030	116,620,000	36,850,000	31.6

Data source: Bureau of Statistics, Ministry of Internal Affairs and Communications, 2014.

Methods of measuring the progression of LS that are generally used include measuring the time required to climb a staircase of a certain height or measuring the length of one stride.

Further, methods used to quantitatively measure lower limb functions include muscle strength measurement with Cybex or handheld dynamometer (Van et al., 1996; Nishijima et al., 2004), stabilometry in a standing position (Tokita, 1986; Matsunaga,1986), and automatic measurement of pennation angle from three-dimensional ultrasound images of gastrocnemius muscle (Nawa et al., 2013).

However, these methods require expensive equipment and can be used only in medical institutions where ultrasound instruments are available. Simpler measurement methods, therefore, have been demanded.

An approach studied to address this was the use of a commercially available body weight scale or other readily accessible devices.

For example, there is a published study in this line, in which the ambulatory performance in the elderly and stroke hemiplegia patients was investigated using a body weight scale to measure the tread force applied to the scale by each leg in a sitting position (Murata S. & Miyazaki M., 2005; Murata S, Ota T, and Arima T, 2005).

However, lower limb load measurements in a sitting position have been pointed out to be prone to errors because body trunk movements while a subject treads the measuring board are not controlled and the body trunk weight can be added to the lower limb load due to anteflexion of the body (Murata J., Murata A. et al., 2007).

A method devised to control trunk movements to a certain extent was to evaluate lower limb functions in a bridge posture in a supine position, in which a subject bends the legs while supporting the trunk at the back (Madokoro K., et al., 2012).

In the bridge-posture measurement method, the loaded force was measured by letting a subject tread the weight scale on the sole as strongly as possible while maintaining the hip flexion position.

Since the pelvis was inclined posteriorly and the buttocks were lifted from the floor during the bridge action, the muscle activity of the erector spinae increased and overall trunk functions were suggested to be reflected in addition to lower limb functions.

More precise quantitative computation of the lower limb functions is possible with measurement methods in sitting and supine positions, if the body trunk and lower limbs can be weighed. Therefore, there has been an increasing need for a gravimetric method to measure individual body parts.

Meanwhile, it is not only aging but also obesity that can cause LS. The musculoskeletal system can deteriorate from excessive obesity, which may lead to difficulty walking, as well as an inability to get out of bed in some cases. These obesity-related problems are now considered problems worldwide.

For example, in a paper that investigated the relationship between LS and body mass index (BMI) in 245 Japanese individuals aged 40–64 years, those suspected of having LS had a significantly higher BMI than those not suspected of having LS ($p = 0.004$). Similar results were obtained for a group of individuals aged 65 years or older ($p < 0.001$; Kamohara et al., 2012). This clearly demonstrates that obesity can have an effect on LS, emphasizing the importance of weight control. Thus, the problem of LS is closely linked to weight management.

Obesity is a major issue globally, as exemplified by an obesity rate of more than 70% among males in US, for example.

Japan has set a 25% decrease of the metabolic syndrome population, including those likely to become one, by fiscal 2015 from the fiscal 2008 level as a national target on the prevention of lifestyle-related diseases.

Japanese guidelines for diagnosis of metabolic syndrome published in 2005 set diagnostic criteria for accumulated visceral fat, which is an essential item, as a waist circumference of 85 cm or more for

E

men and 90 cm or more for women in a standing position, and a visceral fat area of 100 cm2 equivalent for both men and women, add that visceral fat mass measurement with "computed tomography" (CT) scan or other means is advisable.

This series of diagnostic criteria is still valid as of 2015.

However, as CT scan is not a method that individuals can readily access for health management, development of a measurement method that helps estimate visceral fat mass in conjunction with measured waist circumference is awaited.

"Body mass index" (BMI) is also used widely around the world as a method for obesity assessment and some other purposes, with an abundance of reported examples. "Whole body weight in a standing position" (BW), which is readily measurable with a commercially available scale, is used in the BMI calculation formula. However, BMI and BW are practically useless in evaluation of body parts.

If body parts can be weighed individually, a weight change in the whole body can be understood as a combination of weight changes in individual body parts. Such measurement can be useful, for example, to determine whether a weight gain is due to an increased weight in the abdominal region, and can be used for daily evaluation of weight changes.

In this chapter, a newly proposed way of measuring the weights of separate body parts will be discussed. Kurata et al. (Kurata, S., & Kurata, T., 2009; Kurata, S., Kurata, N., & Kurata, T., 2009; Kurata, S., Kurata, N., & Kurata, T., 2011) revealed that the weights of six different body regions could be measured with the body in the supine position with a measurement system composed of six commercially available digital scales and a personal computer. Afterwards, Kurata et al. (Kurata, N., Kurata, S., & Kurata, T., 2012a, 2012b) improved the weighing system to measure the weights of seven different body regions, and named as body region separately weighing system (BRSW-System).

With the BRSW-System, the weight of the head, right arm, left arm, upper trunk, lower trunk, right leg and left leg (seven regions in total) can be measured almost simultaneously in the supine position, and, moreover, the system was found to have good reproducibility. As the BRSW-System uses commercially available scales combined with a computer for its measurements, expensive medical devices such as "magnetic resonance imaging" (MRI) or CT scanners are unnecessary. Furthermore, since measurements do not need to be performed in a hospital or specialized research facility, but rather are possible with a combination of commercially available devices, this method can be considered simpler.

BRSW-System was originally designed to measure six body parts, since the human body appearance is composed of six body segments. Using BRSW-System, it is now possible to calculate the balance between left and right legs from the weight of each leg, or composition ratios to the whole body weight.

However, the upper and lower parts of the trunk contain respiratory and digestive organs, respectively, and significantly differ in function. This fact prompted the measuring of the upper and lower segments of the trunk to be performed separately. Measuring seven body segments in total, the system can weigh the abdominal region as a means to evaluate visceral fat accumulation.

BRSW-System contributes to providing elements for precise calculation of existing quantitative evaluation methods in studies on locomotive syndrome and metabolic syndrome. Moreover, it facilitates easy gravimetric determination of a specific body site in health management of individuals.

METHODS

1. **Components of the BRSW-System:**
    a. **Measurement Devices:** The following devices are used in the BRSW-System:

i. **FG30KBM Digital Scale with RS232C Interface (A&D Engineering):** Weighing capacity: 30 kg, minimum display: 2–5 g, weighing pan: 300 mm × 380 mm, height: 118 mm, weight of scale: 9.7 kg.

ii. **FG150KBM Digital Scale with RS232C Interface (A&D Engineering):** Weighing capacity: 150 kg, minimum display: 10–20 g, weighing pan, height, and weight of scale: same as for FG30KBM.

iii. **Data Processing Unit (CPU):** Commercially available laptop computer.

b. **BRSW-System:** Figure 1 shows the outline of the BRSW-System. The BRSW-System consists of seven FG30KBM scales as measurement units for measuring the different body regions (U1–U7) and a CPU connected to these seven measurement units by RS232C cables through RS232C-USB converters.

With this, the weight of the head, right arm, left arm, upper trunk, lower trunk, right leg and left leg was measured. In effect, seven FG30KBM scales were used as measurement units supporting the body regions and one CPU was used as a system to measure the weights of the seven body regions. The FG150KBM scale was used to measure whole body weight (BW) in a standing position.

2. **Measurement Method:**

a. **Establishing a Level Measurement Plane:** After placing the measurement units on a flat surface with little vibration, the weighing pan of each unit was leveled by using the spirit level mounted on the unit and finely adjusting the heights of the four legs with their four knobs for height fine adjustments. The positions of each measurement unit were arranged and adjusted in accordance with the subject's body type to obtain the optimum measurements.

b. **Achieving Proper Positioning:** When the subject lay in the supine position on the measurement units, the units were arranged so that the approximate center of gravity of each body region lined up as closely as possible with the center of the weighing pan of its respective

Figure 1. A schematic top view of the body-region separately weighing system for the measurement of seven body-regions
Kurata, N., Kurata S., & Kurata, T., 2012b.

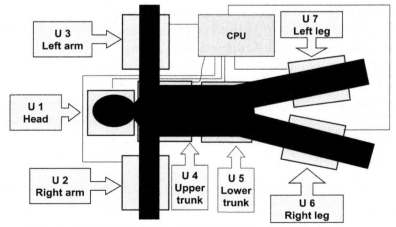

measurement unit. The upper extremities were positioned so that the middle of the forearm including the elbow was supported by the measurement surface of the scale, while the lower extremities were positioned so that the middle of the lower leg including the knee was supported in a similarly manner. A measurement unit was placed below the upper trunk region near the head in order to support the center of the upper back including the scapulae. Another measurement unit was placed below the lower trunk region near the legs in order to support the center of the lower back including the buttocks, pelvis and lumbar region.

c. **Measurement Procedure:** Figure 2 shows an outline of the measurement procedure, including collection, recording and assessment of measurement data. In general, it is preferable to carry out the measurement by two persons, namely a measurer and a subject, both for smooth positioning and for operation of the data processing system. However, it is also possible that a subject weighs own body parts alone, if the subject is familiar with the measurement procedure, etc. Details of the measurement procedure are as follows:

i. The subject lay in the supine position in a relaxed state with each body region placed atop a measurement unit. The investigators then adjusted the positions of the measurement units in accordance with the methods described above.

ii. Data collection from the measurement units was initiated with a command from the CPU and measurement data was transmitted to the CPU between six and ten times at fixed intervals of less than five seconds and recorded. The time required was less than a minute. WinCT-Plus, a free software supplied by A&D Engineering was used to collect data from the measurement units and send them to the CPU. Body region weight measurements were imported into Excel, where means and standard deviations were calculated.

iii. Dispersion of the body region weight measurements was checked to see if it was sufficiently low ($\delta i = 0.1 x i$), i.e. with a coefficient of variation of 10% or less. If the dispersion of measurements was too high, unintentional body movements that may have been due to the subject not relaxing enough or some other factor were identified, the leveling and positioning were adjusted as necessary and the measurements were repeated.

iv. When the dispersion of body segment weight measurements was sufficiently low, the mean value for each body region was assumed to be that region's weight and the difference between the sum of the regions' weights and BW was found.

v. In the event that the discrepancy obtained in step four between the sum of the regions' weights and BW was too large to ignore, dispersion of the body segment weight measurements was reexamined, leveling and positioning were adjusted as needed, and measurements were repeated after making the necessary corrections.

vi. If the discrepancy obtained in step four between the sum of the regions' weights and BW was suitably low ($\delta = 0.1 kg$), the mean value for each body region was then defined as that region's weight. The reason for setting $\delta = 0.1$ kg was that most commercially available scales have a minimum display value of 0.1 kg.

vii. The measurement session was concluded.

Figure 2. The body-region separately weighing flow with the body-region weight measuring unit (Ui)
Kurata, N., Kurata S., & Kurata, T., 2012b.

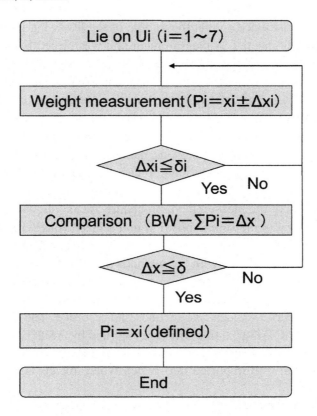

BW : body weight (in standing position)
Pi : weight of each body-region
X, xi : measured or calculated values
δ, δi : tolerance
Δx, Δxi : dispersion

RESULTS

Tables 2 and 3 shows the measurement results with the BRSW-System. Table 2 contains the results of 10 measurements for five Japanese men and women each. Table 3 contains the results for one subject who was measured repeatedly in order to check the reproducibility of each measurement. In effect, this particular subject underwent measurement, got up from the BRSW-System, and then underwent measurement again after the positioning procedure was performed anew. This was performed five times and the data summarized.

As shown in Table 2, the mean difference between the sum of the weights of the seven body regions and BW for the five subjects was favorable at ± 0.01 kg. Thus, body region measurements with sufficient reproducibility can be performed for healthy adults.

Table 2. Examples of the measurement of seven body-region weights of 5 Japanese adults using BRSW-system

Subject (BW*)	Head	Right Arm	Left Arm	Upper Trunk	Lower Trunk	Right Leg	Left Leg	Total*
A (50.92)	3.37±0.05	1.16±0.01	1.40±0.01	17.46±0.15	19.72±0.15	4.06±0.01	3.78±0.01	50.93±0.07
B (49.77)	3.92±0.11	1.18±0.01	1.07±0.01	12.46±0.17	22.19±0.14	4.37±0.01	4.58±0.01	49.78±0.03
C (66.21)	4.32±0.03	2.20±0.00	2.08±0.00	21.29±0.10	26.05±0.08	5.09±0.01	5.18±0.01	66.20±0.05
D (47.56)	3.89±0.01	1.39±0.01	1.39±0.01	12.58±0.17	19.92±0.16	4.25±0.01	4.12±0.01	47.55±0.05
E (52.78)	3.64±0.04	1.44±0.02	1.70±0.01	16.47±0.16	21.37±0.22	4.25±0.02	3.92±0.02	52.79±0.06

Adapted from Kurata, N., Kurata S., & Kurata, T., 2012b.
Measuring times: 10 times.
Body region weight: Average ± SD.
*BW: Body Weight in Standing Position.
*Total: Total of body-region weights.

Table 3. Reproducibility including the positioning adjustment in the measurement of seven body-region weights using BRSW-system

Subject (BW*)	Head	Right Arm	Left Arm	Upper Trunk	Lower Trunk	Right Leg	Left Leg	Total*
A (50.92)	3.47±0.08	1.09±0.07	1.32±0.07	17.56±0.17	19.57±0.24	4.06±0.06	3.85±0.06	50.93±0.02

Adapted from Kurata, N., Kurata S., & Kurata, T., 2012b.
Measuring times: 5 times.
Body region weight: Average ± SD.
*Total: Total of body-region weights.

Moreover, as shown in Table 3, standard deviations were less than 0.1 for all body regions apart from the trunk and coefficients of variation for all body regions including the upper and lower trunk were less than 10%, indicating very favorable results. Thus, it was confirmed that the measurement results from the BRSW-System had sufficient reliability.

FUTURE RESEARCH DIRECTIONS

In the above-mentioned process of measuring the weights of the seven body regions, the degree of variation in weight of the subject's upper and lower trunk regions was generally found to be considerably greater than that of the other body regions. Standard deviations for the upper and lower trunk regions were much greater than those for the other body regions, with some actual variations exceeding approximately 600 g.

On the other hand, the degree of variation of the whole trunk region, obtained by adding together the values for the upper and lower trunk regions, was much smaller. With many important organs such as the heart and the lungs contained within the trunk, it is highly likely that fluctuations in the center of gravity of the upper and lower trunk regions and so forth are caused by breathing associated with the expansion and contraction particularly of the thoracic cavity and lungs.

Measurements taken during ordinary breathing and when the breath was temporarily held were therefore examined.

When subjects were measured with their breaths held for 10 seconds, not only did the degree of variation in the weight of the upper and lower trunk regions decrease markedly, but degrees of variation in other body regions also decreased to a certain extent. Thus, it was strongly suggested that when measuring the weights of the seven separate body regions, taking the measurements with the breath held for a short period of time was effective in obtaining more accurate measurements.

As a result, it is possible that, unlike body weight measurements in a standing position, when measuring the weights of separate body regions in the supine position, breathing needs to be considered a factor influencing the measurement results. An investigation of this issue in further detail is planned.

CONCLUSION

As discussed above, the BRSW-System can be used to measure the weights of separate body regions. With this system, weights of the head, upper extremities, upper trunk, lower trunk and lower extremities—seven regions in all— can be measured. Since no studies that measured the weights of separate body regions in living persons could be found, this system can be regarded as offering a new and groundbreaking method of measurement.

This system also uses no specialized medical devices and requires no medical image analysis. It yields clear and easily understood values for each body region, so an individual can perform these measurements without having to visit a medical facility and manage the data obtained on his or her own.

For example, a stand-on scale can often be found in schools, nursing homes, or fitness facilities, and if the BRSW-System is added, anyone can easily measure the weight of each of his or her body regions at any time, save this as personal health management data, and thus track how much a given body region has gained or lost weight. Since the weights of each body region are measured simultaneously and recorded by a computer, saving the data is easy.

This system has been shown to provide highly reproducible measurement data if an individual gets up after taking measurements in the supine position and then lies down again for another measurement. Of course, the positioning of the body regions on the scales should be almost the same in each measurement. For example, an individual could visit a welfare facility once a week for BRSW-System measurements, keep track of his or her data on a computer, and plot in a graph the rises and falls in the weight of his or her different body regions.

Measuring the circumference of the leg or abdomen is another approach, but determining where on the abdomen to perform measurements is difficult due to respiration and the circumference changes no matter how one holds his or her breath. Comparing the obtained measurements in order to establish a balance is not easy. With the BRSW-System, by looking at the balance between the weight of each body region and whole body weight, one can clearly see what regions of the body are developing or declining at what rate compared with the development and decline of the whole body.

The ability to record the weights of one's own body regions in detail might lead to better self-control and enhanced self-efficacy in situations where one is tempted to ingest food, thereby preventing excessive food consumption.

Moreover, if this system were to become widely used and data on weights of separate body regions were to be collected from a large number of users, the distribution of weights could be calculated to indicate those at high risk of LS/obesity, might lead to a new quantitative assessment index for LS/obesity.

Thus, using this system might allow for health management related to particular region of body.

REFERENCES

Bureau of Statistics, Ministry of Internal Affairs and Communications. (2014). *Changes in the elderly population in Japan*. Retrieved from http://www.stat.go.jp/data/topics/topi721.htm

Dempster, W. T., & Gaughran, G. R. L. (1967). Properties of body segments based on size and weight. *The American Journal of Anatomy, 120*(1), 33–54. doi:10.1002/aja.1001200104

Kamohara, M., Shiomitsu, T., Hasegawa, T., Ohkuwa, Y., & Tsuruta, K. (2012). The Relationship of Locomotive Syndrome to Physical Fitness and Body Mass Index in Middle-Aged Adults. *The South Kyusyu Journal of Nursing, 10*(1), 29–36.

Kurata, N., Kurata, S., & Kurata, T. (2012a). A new body-region separately weighing system for individual health assessment-Especially, the weight measurement of the upper and lower trunk-. In *Proceedings of the 51st Annual Conference of Japanese Society for Medical and Biological Engineering* (p. 207) Fukuoka, Japan: Annual Conference of Japanese Society for Medical and Biological Engineering Association Press.

Kurata, N., Kurata, S., & Kurata, T. (2012b). Measurement method of seven body region weights by use of a body-region separately weighing system. *Transactions of Japanese Society for Medical and Biological Engineering, 50*(6), 637–644.

Kurata, S., Kurata, N., & Kurata, T. (2009). Body-region separately weighing system and its significance in health assessment. Annuals of Nutrition & Metabolism (vol. 55, p. 210). Basel, Switzerland: Karger Medical and Scientific Publishers.

Kurata, S., Kurata, N., & Kurata, T. (2011). A new body-region separately weighing system for individual health assessment. In *Proceedings of the 11th Asian Congress of Nutrition* (p. 175) Singapore: Singapore Nutrition and Dietetics Association.

Kurata, S., & Kurata, T. (2009). A Study on method for body-region weight measurement. *In Proceedings of the 63rd Japan Society of Nutrition and Food Science* (Vol. 1, p.212). Tokyo: Japan Society of Nutrition and Food Science Press.

Madokoro, K., Takei, K., Murata, S., Ihara, T., & Kai, Y. (2012). Reproducibility and validity of a bridging force measurement method using a scale. *Japanese Journal of Health Promotion and Physical Therapy, 2*(3), 97-100.

Matsunaga, R. (1986). Routine equilibrium function tests. *Heiko Shinkei Kagaku, 45*(4), 285–301. doi:10.3757/jser.45.285

Ministry of Health, Labour and Welfare. (2012). *From comprehensive survey of living conditions 2010: Graphical review of Japanese household*. Retrieved July 10, 2015, from http://www.mhlw.go.jp/toukei/list/dl/20-21-h22.pdf

Mozumdar, A., & Roy, S. K. (2004). Methods for estimating body weight in persons with lower-limb amputation and its implication for their nutritional assessment. *The American Journal of Clinical Nutrition, 80*, 868–875. PMID:15447892

Murata, J., Murata, A., & Kai, Y. (2007). Relationship between the Lower Limb Loading Force and Leg Muscle Activities. *Physical Therapy Science, 22*(2), 195-198.

Murata, S., & Miyazaki, M. (2005). Assessment of lower extremities function in elderly people with dysfunction -Measurement of lower limb supporting force with scales. *Physical Therapy Science, 20*(2), 111-114.

Murata, S., Ota, T., & Arima, T. (2005). Examination of the lower limb load force evaluation using a commercially available weight scale in stroke hemiplegia patient. *Physical Therapy Science Journal, 39*(12), 1101-1105.

Nawa, H., Watanabe, T., Fukuoka, D., Terabayashi, N., Hara, T., & Fujita, H. (2013). 3D image analysis of gastrocnemius muscle for quantitative evaluation of the Locomotive syndrome. In *Proceedings of IEICE Tech. Rep.,* (vol. 112, no. 411, pp. 69-72). The Institute of Electronics, Information and Communication Engineers Press.

Nishijima, T., Koyama, R., Naito, I., Hatakeyama, S., Yamasaki, H., & Oku, T. (2004). Relationship between knee extension muscle strength and walking ability in the elderly patients. *Physical Therapy Science., 19*(2), 95–99.

Tokita, R. (1986). Stabilometry. The Practical equilibrium function tests (126-133). Tokyo: Nanzando.

Van, M. W., Twisk, J., Molendijk, A., Blom, B., Snel, J., & Kemper, H. C. G. (1996). Subject-related risk factors for sports injuries: A 1-yr prospective study in young adults. *Medicine and Science in Sports and Exercise, 28*(9), 1171–1179. doi:10.1097/00005768-199609000-00014 PMID:8883006

KEY TERMS AND DEFINITIONS

Assessing Separate Weights of the Main Musculoskeletal Components: Assessing weights of the hands and feet, principal parts of the musculoskeletal apparatus, are needed in order to evaluate efficient or effective motor activities.

Body-Region Separately Weighing Method: A system that individually measures the weights of the body regions that form the human body. Note that the sum of the regional weights must always match the whole body weight measured in a standing position.

Health Management on an Individual Level: Individual people looking after their own exercise, diet, and body weight in order to maintain everyday health.

Healthy Life Expectancy: The period of living without any health problems. Specifically, the average period of life with no limitations to activities of daily living, or the average period in which people are aware that they are healthy.

LS. Abbreviation for Locomotive Syndrome: *Locomotive* should be taken to mean "pertaining to movement." Based on the idea that the musculoskeletal system provides a wide framework for an individual's health, the Japanese Orthopaedic Association coined this new expression to refer to the state of requiring long-term care (or the state of being at risk of requiring long-term care) due to a musculoskeletal disorder.

Seven Body Regions: Outwardly, the human body is made up of six regions: the head, the upper extremities, the trunk and the lower extremities. The torso, however, can be divided into upper and lower parts, giving an upper trunk region and a lower trunk region; thus, the six regions of the body become seven.

Weights of Separate Body Regions: This means the weight of each body region that make up the human body with respect to whole body weight.

Rare Diseases Internet Information Retrieval and Knowledge Discovery

E

José Miguel León Blanco
University of Seville, Spain

Pedro Luis González-R
University of Seville, Spain

Antonio M. Rabasco
University of Seville, Spain

María José Cózar-Bernal
University of Seville, Spain

Marcos Calle
University of Seville, Spain

María Luisa González-Rodríguez
University of Seville, Spain

Manuel Ojeda Casares
Fundación Mehuer, Spain

INTRODUCTION

A rare or orphan disease (RD) is that which affects only an insignificant percentage of population, so traditionally has not received the effort devoted to common diseases. In common diseases there are healing or palliative treatments while there are over 4000 RD without a known cure. In Europe, RD affect between 27 and 36 million people (Rodwell & Aymé, 2013). Any progress in this field has a great social impact that translates directly into an improved quality of life of those affected by RD (Dragusin et al., 2011). Therefore, any advance in knowledge generation in the context of RD is welcome. One of the most important developments has come from data mining (see (Groth, 1998), and (Tomar & Agarwal, 2013)). The reduced amount of data makes the application of data mining techniques not easy in the field of RDs. Although for one disease the number of patients and data is reduced, they are numerous as a whole. Several initiatives collect data from RD patients around the world using the power of Internet (Orphadata, 2015).

Given singularity of RDs, it is necessary to provide the information systems, the capacity to collect data and also promote cross-flow of information between the agents (patients and researchers). In this situation, it is interesting the development of projects like the one sponsored by the Avenzoar Chair (University of Seville, Spain), known as ER2.0 Project (see details in Rabasco et al. (2013a) and Rabasco et al. (2013b)). The underlying idea is to make it real to collaborate, share, and take decisions in a web 2.0 manner between patients and researchers in RDs.

This chapter contains, first, a review of the information networks associated with RD, highlighting the registry, typology, associations and consortia related as well as the existing relationships between

DOI: 10.4018/978-1-4666-9978-6.ch059

them. Next, follows a review of data mining techniques in the context of healthcare, especially of RDs. Later on, it is described the distinguishing aspects of a web tool for the collection and treatment of information provided by RD patients in the context of ER2.0 with the objective of being a starting point to apply data mining techniques to RD.

BACKGROUND

Information Networks Associated with Rare Diseases

There are recommendations from both the European Union and the United States about the importance of using information networks and databases on RD for systematic data collection with the participation of both patients and researchers (Mazzucato, Visonà Dalla Pozza, Manea, Minichiello, & Facchin, 2014). In Table 1 there is a summary of the main characteristics of RD information networks in RDs.

Table 1. Characteristics of RD information networks

Organization [Support]	Impact Google/Bing/Alexa	Network Soc./Inf.Flow/ Data	Partners
GARD [G,R]	79500/114000/215 (NIH,2015)	O/-/T,DB	NIH, NCATS
GRDR [G,PR]	5660/37/215 (NIH,2015)	O/P-P,E-E,P-E/T,L,DB	NIH/NCATS
ORDR [G,R]	84400/89500/215 (NIH,2015)	-/E-E/DB,T,L	NIH/NCATS, GRDR
RD Program (FDA) [G,PR]	2650/3450/4586 (FDA, 2015)	-/-/T,L	NIH/(NCATS)
RDRD (RD Repurposing Database) [G,PR]	1310/55/4586 (FDA, 2015)	-/-/T,DB,L	FDA
SpainRDR [G,R]	2020/130000/30052 (H. Inst. Carlos III, 2015)	-/-/T,BD,L	H. Inst. Carlos III, EUROPLAN, FEDER, IRDiRC
Orphanet [G,R]	1370000/707000/56070	-/E-E/DB,T,L	CARD, WHO, EuroP-Ean Commission, amongst others.
Patients Like Me [PA]	528000/164000/57444	S/P-E,E-E,P-P/DB,T, L	
CNMR [G,R]	317/33/100877	O,S/E-E,P-P,P-E/T,L	EUROPLAN
NORD [G,PA]	204000/90500/177751	S/P-E,E-E,P-P/L,T	EURORDIS, JPA, GARD
RareConnect [PA]	87600/32700/529546	S/P-P/T,L	EURORDIS, NORD
FEDER [G,PA]	52100/45100/600036	O/P-P,P-E,E-E/T,L	Mehuer, EURORDIS
EURORDIS [G,PA]	21400/12900/1051803	O/P-P/T,L	EUROPLAN, Black Swan F., FEDER, CARD, RD International
Findacure [R]	392/54/1337476	O,S/P-P,P-E,E-E/T,L	RE(ACT) Comm., Cures within Reach, EURORDIS, Rare Disease UK
EUROGENTEST [G,PR]	64600/38200/1523427	O/E-E/T,L	
JPA [PA]	64/52/2002261	O/-/T	EURORDIS
Fondation Maladies Rares [G,R]	8240/5310/3070126	O,S/P-P,P-E,E-E/-	RE(ACT) Community
IRDiRC [G,R]	2990/3000 –3821331	-/E-E/T,L	Orphanet, EuroP-Ean Comm, NIH
Rare Disease Dot Org [PA]	1190/3/4267630	S,O/P-P/T	

continued on following page

Table 1. Continued

Organization [Support]	Impact Google/Bing/Alexa	Network Soc./Inf.Flow/ Data	Partners
EUCERD [G]	2850/3210/4501141	-/E-E/-	
CORD [PA]	2920/5260/4808175	-/P-P/T,L	
Rarelink [G]	8/2/6245608	-/P-P/R	
RE(ACT) Community [PA]	5900/2900/6316815	O/P-P,P-E,E-E/T,L	Black Swan Foundation, EURORDIS, Assoc Enf. & Maladies Orphelines, E-Rare, Findacure
Black Swan Foundation [R]	4210/2680/6437082	O/-/-	EURORDIS, RE(ACT) Initiative, E-Rare
Mehuer [R]	190/63/9005787	O/-/-	FEDER
ERA-Net for Research Programmes on RD (E-Rare) [G,PR]	1060/1780/9094018	O/-/T	Orphanet, RE(ACT)
RD-Connect [G,PR]	15100/13000/10624267	-/-/L	EURORDIS, EURenOmics, RD-Neuromics, H. Inst. Carlos III, NIH-ORDR, Orphanet, Care4Rare
RD-Neuromics [GPR]	966/4410/10950884	-/-/-	RD-Connect, EURenOmics, IRDiRC
EPIRARE [G,PR]	333/63/11622256	S/E-E/T	Joint Research Centre, EURORDIS, H. Inst. Carlos III
Pro Rare Austria [PA]	1400/2320/12575327	O/P-P/T	EURORDIS
Rare Voices Australia [PA]	5790/3560/13110721	-/P-P/T,L	RareConnect, EURORDIS, NORD, NZORD, CORD, Rare Diseases International, Genetic Alliance
NZORD [PA]	2500/2320/18612243	O/P-P/L	
Phenomecentral [G,R]	945/24700/NA	S/E-E,P-E,P-P/DB,T	RD Connect, NIH/Undiagnosed Diseases Program
Eurenomics [G,PR]	3140/3090/NA	O/E-E/T,L	Neuromics, RD-Connect, IRDiRC
RareCareNet [G,PR]	1430/4170/NA	-/E-E/T,DB,L	
EUROPLAN [G,PR]	1260/2010/NA	-/E-E/-	EURORDIS, EUCERD, CNMR
CARD [PA]	1380/29/NA	O/-/-	EURORDIS, EUCERD, ORPHANET, EUROPLAN

The *Organization* is shown in the first column, whether governments have started and/or support the organization (G). Code (R) indicates research organizations, (PR) projects and (PA) patient associations. The link to the organization can be found in the reference section. It can be highlighted that Patient organizations are mainly non-governmental organizations and research organizations are mainly governmental. The vast majority of organizations are non-lucrative ones, and one exception is "Patients Like Me" (2015). Very few of them require a fee for the membership (e.g. CORD, RVA) as most of them obtain funds via anonymous donations or via partnership with private or public entities.

The *Impact* columns give an idea of the impact of the organization in the Internet via the number of pages returned by Google and by Bing when the complete name of the organization (e.g. EUCERD "European Union Committee of Experts on Rare Diseases") is searched. When there were no results, the name without quotes was used, and it is indicated between parentheses. It is also included the rank of the page in Alexa (Alexa, 2015), in order to give a measure of the visibility of the organization in the web. Most visited pages have a lower number in this classification (e.g. Google appears as number 1). It is important to remark that the highest rank is obtained by Orphanet (2015) independently, according to Alexa (2015), and GARD as a part of the web of a greater institution like FDA in U.S.. The results obtained by Google and Bing confirm this ranking. For sites with no ranking in Alexa, it is used the average returned pages by Google and Bing when it is greater than 500. The first page in the U.S., apart from those of National Health Service and Federal Drug Administration, is a private patient organization, "Patients Like Me" (2015) again confirmed by number of pages returned by the search engines. On the other hand, there are organizations that have not deployed a web site, like the Chinese RD Research Consortium.

The *Network Column* contains three parts:

- The *Social* Network in order to show which of the web sites include characteristics of social network websites. Many of them include their institutional profiles in Facebook, Twitter, Google+, LinkedIn or other social networks (coded with "O"). Some include the social network as a part of the site (coded with "S"). There is no code for organizations or projects that are part of higher institutions. These organizations refer to the site of their parent organization in social networks (e.g. EUCERD in European Commission or ORDR in FDA).
- The *Information Flow* column shows the direction of information between stakeholders provided by the site: Between patients (P-P), between patients and experts, clinicians or researchers, in the field of a RD (P-E) and experts with other experts (E-E). There is no code when the contact is limited to a form that is sent via e-mail.
- *Data* shows which of the organizations have made available data of RDs, not only serving as links to other points of information (L) or presenting a list of pathologies and their descriptions (R). These data may be in the form of or in databases following standardized languages (DB) or reports textual data (T). The vast majority of organizations provide at least a list of RDs and links to other sites with detailed information about the disease. This information of RDs comes in many cases from Orphanet information. Some of the websites reviewed are only a place to put information about the activities of the organization but with little added value. Few of the sites carry out the task of maintain a registry of RDs and make it available. Orphanet and Phenomecentral are references in this task.

It can be observed that there are few sites that provide an internal flow of information between all the actors. GRDR, Patients Like Me, or RE(ACT) community provide easy ways in their sites to put in contact patients with patients, patients with experts and experts with other experts in the different RDs. It has also been observed that many RD sites are devoted to only one or a few diseases (Eurenomics, 2015; RD-Genomics, 2015), focusing efforts but losing perspective and the possibility of finding similarities between diseases, their treatments and evolution.

Finally, the column *Partnership* lists organizations in the table related to the organization in first column. There are usually many other partners in each organization e.g. private corporations, governmental health organizations or universities. That's why some of them appear without partners.

Data Mining and Rare Diseases

Data mining is a collection of techniques based on the extraction of useful and understandable knowledge, previously unknown from large quantities of data stored in different formats (Witten & Frank, 2000). Some authors put data mining inside the process of knowledge discovery in databases (KDD) (Frawley, Piatetsky-Shapiro, and Mathews, 1992). Excellent reviews of these techniques in the field of healthcare can be found in Tomar & Agarwal (2013), Jacob & Ramani (2012), Yoo et al. (2012), Bellazzi & Zupan (2008), Perner (2006) and Koh & Tan (2005). Besides, there are several free and commercial data mining tools that let the researcher concentrate in data mining. Some free data mining tools were reviewed by Jovic, Brkic & Bogunovic (2014). Commercial tools were reviewed by Gheware, Kejkar & Tondare, (2014).

Tables 2 and 3 contain a summarized classification of these techniques in the field of healthcare. We omitted data-mining applications used in management of health companies. Table 2 include descriptive or supervised techniques and table 3 includes predictive or unsupervised techniques.

Both tables show the application of each technique, stressing if the technique is currently applied "A" in the field of RDs. If the technique is not currently applied but could be suitable to be used in RDs we ceded as "S". Finally, if not suitable in the RDs context we coded as "NS". In RDs, data are naturally not balanced, there are few positive cases and many negative, so methods will report high accuracy even when assigning all cases to the same category. Is the case of decision trees. The benchmark made by Jovic & Bogunovic (2011) help considering random forest as a suitable technique in RD diagnosis.

It can be observed that many mining techniques have been used in some areas of health care. It appears that, in most of the cases, the only barrier to applying these techniques on RDs is the availability of data to be exploited or not. In case of RDs, data preparation may help improve the characteristics of this technique like in Jovic & Bogunovic (2011) with random forests. Support vector machines is also receiving similar interest from the scientific community like neural networks.

Web Site Design for Gathering and Analysis of Information about RDs

The majority of reviewed sites devoted to RDs cover the collection of data of only one disease, and make an analysis of those data. The sites that gather data from several diseases, usually do not take advantage of the availability of such amount of data to apply data mining techniques, staying only in the stage of statistical processing. An exception to this rule is (PhenomeCentral, 2014).

Table 2. Summary of reviewed works in the field of descriptive data mining techniques and health care

Technique	Reference	Application	RD
Clustering (Expectation Maximization)	Jovic & Bogunovic (2011)	Heart diseases diagnosis	
	Cerrito et al (2002)	Patient classification	S
Partition based (K-means or K-medoids)	Jovic & Bogunovic (2011)	Heart diseases diagnosis	
Association techniques (Chi-square, association rules)	Brosette et al (1998)	Nosocomial infection pattern detection	S
	Paul, Groza, Hunter & Zankl (2012)	Risk factors in skeletal dysplasia	S
	Munson, Wrobel, Holmes, & Hanauer (2014)	Risk factors in Charcot foot	A

Table 3. Summary of reviewed works in the field of predictive data mining techniques and health care

Technique	Reference	Application	RD
Sequential pattern mining	Béchet et al (2012)	Relations between genes and RDs	S
Decision trees (e.g.: ID3, C4.5 or C5.0)	Jovic & Bogunovic (2011)	Heart diseases diagnosis	NS
	Bojarczuk, Lopes, Freitas & Michalkiewicz (2004)	Find classification rules in data sets	NS
Artificial neural networks	Jovic & Bogunovic (2011)	Heart diseases diagnosis	S
	Forsström, et al. (1991)	Diagnosis of Nephropatia epidemica	A
	Martínez et al. (2015)	Drug-disease reposition	A
Kernel methods (Support Vector Machines)	Ye et al (2008)	Alzheimer disease prediction	A
	Jovic & Bogunovic (2011)	Heart diseases diagnosis	S
	Asl, Setarehdan & Mohebbi (2008)	Heart diseases diagnosis	S
	Polat & Güneş (2007)	Heart diseases diagnosis	S
Bayesian methods (Naïve Bayesian Classifiers, Bayesian beliefs networks)	Jovic & Bogunovic (2011)	Heart diseases diagnosis	S
	Forsström, et al. (1991)	Diagnosis of Nephropatia epidemica	A
	Aussem, Rodrigues de Morais & Corbex (2012)	Identifying risk factors in nasopharyngeal carcinoma	S
Regression or Parametric statistical modelling	Batshaw et al (2014)	Diagnosis and effects of Urea Cycle Disorders	A
Logistic regression or Maximum Entropy (temporal data mining)	Patnaik et al (2011)	Temporal patterns in diseases	S
Ensemble methods (Random forests, bootstrap aggregating or bagging)	Jovic & Bogunovic (2011)	Heart diseases diagnosis	S

In this situation, takes sense the idea of a web site to gather and use information from data provided by patients of RD. The ideas that formed the basis for the implementation of the web site for information retrieval in RD have already been spread in several national and international conferences (Rabasco, A.M. et al., 2013a,b). The information retrieval system is centred in basic clinical data, avoiding the use of genomic data, aiming to make it easy for patients to insert data about their diseases in the system. Below follows a description of main areas of the site.

With the objective of promote communication P-P (patient to patient), the site includes a social network section apart from links to other social networks. The collaboration of patients as participants will lead to large sample sizes, which in turn will make possible the application of data mining techniques. It will also lead to updated data about the evolution of patients. The site also includes a forum, where those visitors that do not want to get involved in the social network can share experiences or look for some help.

Record subsection (Figure 1) has been included with the objective of promote communication P-E (patient to expert). The information requested avoids genomic data, as that kind of information is generally unknown by patients. This subsection will need to be adapted as patients detect its gaps. In sites devoted to only one RD, the design of this section is based in the opinion of healthcare providers and researchers (Johnson et al., 2013).

In addition to answer patients' questions when filling data in the record, another task of researchers in the site is to validate these data. Data is stored in a database that follows the Human Phenotype On-

Figure 1. Record subsection

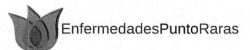

tology (HPO) (Robinson & Mundlos, 2010) as other web sites do (Bauer, Köhler, Schulz, & Robinson, 2012) in a way that it can be easily exported in the future to formats like the Ontology Web Language (OWL), more suitable to be analysed by data mining techniques.

The section "editing and research", captured in Figure 2, is included to promote the communication E-E (expert to expert). Experts in RD will act as editors, modifying contents, researchers, with access to anonymous information and statistics and head researchers, who will validate a new expert after having studied her background.

FUTURE RESEARCH DIRECTIONS

At the moment we have a very interesting potential for researchers and feel huge social impact.

Future research may come mainly from four parts:

1. **Use of Data:** It seems natural that the first thing to try is the use of data. For that we can study the relationships between phenotypes and genotypes. Paul et al. (2012) developed a probabilistic approach to compute probabilistic associations between sets of clinical features and disorders in patients of bone-dysplasia. They used Dempster-Shafter Theory and outperformed other machine

Figure 2. Editing and research subsection

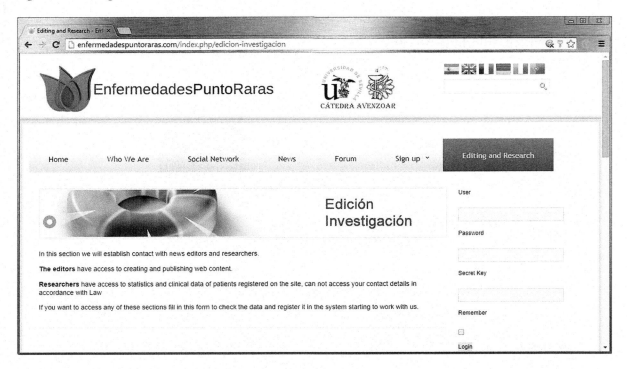

learning techniques and also the initial diagnostic made by a clinician in the database. Other research line could be in the direction of Groza, Hunter and Zankl (2013). They developed a technique they called biomedical named entity recognition (Bio-NER) under the project SKELETOME (2015) in order to make correlation analysis between phenotypes and genotypes or disorders related. They combined classifiers and aggregation techniques. In the same line, Taboada et al. (2012) found bidirectional relationships between phenotypes and genotypes by using OWL, which provides a machine understandable way to register patient data, SWRL to link phenotype descriptions and clinical data and SQWRL to query relations between phenotypes and genotypes. Girdea et al. (2013) developed a tool called PhenoTips. In this case, the tool stores phenotypic information following the HPO.

2. **Registry Evolution:** Other different research line is the search of relationships between RD registries. Santoro et al. (2015) published a data mining research of RD registries, looking for the interconnections between them. They found three typologies of registries: public health, clinical and genetic research, and treatment registries. Taruscio et al. (2014) proposed a normalization for RD registration in order to promote the use of common tools for the collection of comparable data.

3. **Development of Ontologies:** In aber-owl.net there are three registered ontologies related to RDs. DCO (Dispedia Core Ontology) HRDO (Disease Core Ontology applied to RDs) and ORDO (Orphanet RD Ontology). The three of them can be downloaded from the AberOWL Repository

4. **Web Mining:** The study of the behaviour of the stakeholders in the social network. There is an increasing interest in the use of this kind of systems to share disseminated knowledge about RDs. A review of web mining tools in healthcare was made by Kumar, V. & Ahmed, E. (2011). It may be necessary to make an effort of publishing the site, beginning with other RD associations in Spain and in Europe. Hilbert et al. (2012) expressed this burden when described the National Registry of DM and FSHD.

CONCLUSION

Although the implementation of the described site is still in an early state, it has served to learn the basics and relations between web sites, social networks, rare or orphan diseases and data mining. The first hurdle to overcome is related to the beginning of all kind of web sites. These information retrieval and sharing sites must be and look fresh and alive. This is a task for all of stakeholders but in the beginning for the research team, especially editors, because first time visitors are willing to find fresh information about their disease. In the beginning of the site, this information cannot be the result of processing data provided by patients. The initial research team must provide this information. Therefore, there will be a lapse of time while the information provided by patients reach a critical mass, and new researchers join the team, when the site requires a work of updating by the initial research team.

A second milestone will be reached when information sharing has produced a volume of data that makes sense to apply data mining techniques to extract knowledge. According to (Jegga, Zhu, & Aronow, 2012) a second hurdle to overcome in applying data mining techniques to RD research is the lack of a sufficient amount of data. The only way is to gather patients with the same disease from several countries. This is where web sites can act as attraction centres for patients.

REFERENCES

Aber-owl.net. (n.d.). Retrieved June 23, 2015 from http://aber-owl.net/

Alexa. (n.d.). *Actionable Analytics for the Web*. Retrieved June 23, 2015 from http://www.alexa.com

Asl, B. M., Setarehdan, S. K., & Mohebbi, M. (2008). Support vector machine-based arrhythmia classification using reduced features of heart rate variability signal. *Artificial Intelligence in Medicine*, *44*(1), 51–64. doi:10.1016/j.artmed.2008.04.007 PMID:18585905

Batshaw, M. L., Tuchman, M., Summar, M., & Seminara, J. (2014). A longitudinal study of urea cycle disorders. *Molecular Genetics and Metabolism*, *113*(1-2), 127–130. doi:10.1016/j.ymgme.2014.08.001 PMID:25135652

Bauer, S., Köhler, S., Schulz, M., & Robinson, P. (2012). Bayesian ontology querying for accurate and noise-tolerant semantic searches. *Bioinformatics (Oxford, England)*, *28*(19), 2502–2508. doi:10.1093/bioinformatics/bts471 PMID:22843981

Bechet, N., Cellier, P., Charnois, T., Cremilleux, B., & Jaulent, M.-C. (2012). Sequential pattern mining to discover relations between genes and rare diseases. *2012 25th IEEE International Symposium on Computer-Based Medical Systems (CBMS)*. IEEE.

Bellazzi, R., & Zupan, B. (2008). Predictive data mining in clinical medicine: Current issues and guidelines. *International Journal of Medical Informatics*, *77*(2), 81–97. doi:10.1016/j.ijmedinf.2006.11.006 PMID:17188928

Black Swan Foundation. (n.d.). Retrieved June 23, 2015 from http://www.blackswanfoundation.ch/

Bojarczuk, C. C., Lopes, H. S., Freitas, A. A., & Michalkiewicz, E. L. (2004). A constrained-syntax genetic programming system for discovering classification rules: Application to medical data sets. *Artificial Intelligence in Medicine*, *30*(1), 27–48. doi:10.1016/j.artmed.2003.06.001 PMID:14684263

Brosette, S. E., Spragre, A. P., Hardin, J. M., Waites, K. B., Jones, W. T., & Moser, S. A. (1998). Association Rules and Data Mining in Hospital Infection Control and Public Health Surveillance. *Journal of the American Medical Informatics Association*, *5*(4), 373–381. doi:10.1136/jamia.1998.0050373 PMID:9670134

CARD. (n.d.). Retrieved June 23, 2015 from http://raredisorderscyprus.com/

Cerrito, P. B., Cox, J. A., Mayes, M., & Thompson, W. (2002). Using text analysis to examine ICD-9 codes to determine uniformity in the reporting of MedPAR data. *Annual Symposium of the American Medical Informatics Association (AMIA) Proceedings*. CNMR, National Center for Rare Diseases. Retrieved June 23, 2015 from http://www.iss.it/cnmr

CORD. (n.d.). Retrieved June 23, 2015 from http://www.raredisorders.ca/

Dragusin, R., Petcu, P., Lioma, C., Larsen, B., Jørgensen, H., & Winther, O. (2011). Rare diseases diagnosis as an information retrieval task. In G. Amati & F. Crestani (Eds.), *Advances in Information Retrieval Theory* (Vol. 6931, pp. 356–359). Springer Berlin Heidelberg; doi:10.1007/978-3-642-23318-0_38

E-Rare. (n.d.). Retrieved June 23, 2015 from http://www.erare.eu/

ESDN. (n.d.). *European Skeletal Dysplasia Network*. Retrieved June 23, 2015 from http://www.esdn.org/

EUCERD. (n.d.). *European Union Committee of Experts on Rare Diseases*. Retrieved June 23, 2015 from http://www.eucerd.eu/

Eurenomics. (n.d.). Retrieved June 23, 2015 from http://eurenomics.eu/

Eurogentest. (n.d.). Retrieved June 23, 2015 from http://www.eurogentest.org/

European Commission expert group on rare diseases. (n.d.). Retrieved June 23, 2015 from http://ec.europa.eu/health/rare_diseases/expert_group/index_en.htm

EuroPlan. (n.d.). Retrieved June 23, 2015 from http://www.europlanproject.eu/

EURORDIS. (n.d.). Retrieved June 23, 2015 from http://www.eurordis.org/

FEDER. (n.d.). *Federación Española de Enfermedades Raras*. Retrieved June 23, 2015 from http://www.enfermedades-raras.org/

Ferguson, T., & The e-Patients Scholars Working Group. (n.d.). *e-Patients: How They Can Help Us Heal Healthcare*. Retrieved October 5, 2014, from e-patients.net: http://e-patients.net/

Findacure. (n.d.). Retrieved June 23, 2015 from http://www.findacure.org.uk/

Fondation Maladies Rares. (n.d.). Retrieved June 23, 2015 from http://fondation-maladiesrares.org/

Forsström, J., Eklund, P., Virtanen, H., Waxlax, J., & Lähdevirta, J. (1991). DIAGAID: A connectionist approach to determine the diagnostic value of clinical data. *Artificial Intelligence in Medicine*, *3*(4), 193–201. doi:10.1016/0933-3657(91)90011-Y

Frawley, W., Piatetsky-Shapiro, G., & Mathews, C. (1992). Knowledge discovery in databases: An overview. *AI Magazine*, 57-70. Retrieved June 23, 2015 from http://www.fundacionmehuer.es/

GARD. (n.d.). Retrieved June 23, 2015 from https://rarediseases.info.nih.gov/gard

Gheware, S. D., Kejkar, A. S., & Tondare, S. M. (2014). Data Mining: Task, Tools, Techniques and Applications. *International Journal of Advanced Research in Computer and Communication Engineering, 3*(10), 8095–8098. doi:10.17148/IJARCCE.2014.31003

Girdea, M., Dumitriu, S., Fiume, M., Bowdin, S., Boycott, K., Chénier, S., & Brudno, M. et al. (2013). PhenoTips: Patient Phenotyping Software for Clinical and Research Use. *Human Mutation, 34*(8), 1057–1065. doi:10.1002/humu.22347 PMID:23636887

Groth, R. (1998). *Data mining. A hands-on approach for business professionals.* Prentice-Hall, Inc.

Groza, T., Hunter, J., & Zankl, A. (2013). Mining Skeletal Phenotype Descriptions from Scientific Literature. *PLoS ONE, 8*(2), 1–8. doi:10.1371/journal.pone.0055656 PMID:23409017

Health Institute Carlos III. (n.d.). Retrieved June 23, 2015 from https://registroraras.isciii.es/Comun/Inicio.aspx

Hilbert, J., Kissel, J., Luebbe, E., Martens, W., McDermott, M., Sanders, D., & Moxley, R. T. III et al.. (2012). If you build a rare disease registry, will they enroll and will they use it? Methods and data from the National Registry of Myotonic Dystrophy (DM) and Facioscapulohumeral Muscular Dystrophy (FSHD). *Contemporary Clinical Trials, 33*(2), 302–311. doi:10.1016/j.cct.2011.11.016 PMID:22155025

IRDiRC. (n.d.). Retrieved June 23, 2015 from http://www.irdirc.org/

ISS. (n.d.). *Instituto Superiore di Sanitá, Italia.* Retrieved June 23, 2015 from http://www.iss.it/

Jacob, S. G., & Ramani, R. (2012). Data Mining in Clinical Data Sets: A Review. *International Journal of Applied Information Systems, 4*(6), 15–26. doi:10.5120/ijais12-450774

Jegga, A., Zhu, C., & Aronow, B. (2012). Orphan diseases, bioinformatics and drug discovery. In J. Hutton (Ed.), Pediatric Biomedical Informatics: Computer Applications in Pediatric Research (pp. 287-307). Dordrecht: Springer Science+Business Media. doi:10.1007/978-94-007-5149-1_16

Johnson, K., Hussain, I., Williams, K., Santens, R., Mueller, N., & Gutmann, D. (2013). Development of an international internet-based neurofibromatosis Type 1 Patient registry. *Contemporary Clinical Trials, 34*(2), 305–311. doi:10.1016/j.cct.2012.12.002 PMID:23246715

Jovic, A., & Bogunovic, N. (2011). Electrocardiogram analysis using a combination of statistical, geometric, and nonlinear heart rate variability features. *Artificial Intelligence in Medicine, 51*(3), 175–186. doi:10.1016/j.artmed.2010.09.005 PMID:20980134

Jovic, A., Brkic, K., & Bogunovic, N. (2014). An overview of free software tools for general data mining. *Information and Communication Technology, Electronics and Microelectronics (MIPRO), 2014 37th International Convention on* (pp. 1112–1117).

JPA. (n.d.). *Japan Patients Association.* Retrieved June 23, 2015 from http://nanbyo.jp/

JRC. (n.d.). *Joint Research Centre.* Retrieved June 23, 2015 from https://ec.europa.eu/jrc/en/research-topic/public-health?searchterm=rare%2520diseases

Koh, H., & Tan, G. (2005). Data mining applications in healthcare. *Journal of Healthcare Information Management, 19*(2), 64–72. PMID:15869215

Kumar, V., & Ahmed, E. (2011). An Empirical Study of the Applications of Web Mining Techniques in Health Care. *International Journal of Advanced Computer Science and Applications, 2*(10), 91–94. doi:10.14569/IJACSA.2011.021015

Martínez, V., Navarro, C., Cano, C., Fajardo, W., & Blanco, A. (2015). DrugNet: Network-based drug–disease prioritization by integrating heterogeneous data. *Artificial Intelligence in Medicine, 63*(1), 41–49. PMID:25704113

Mazzucato, M., Visonà Dalla Pozza, L., Manea, S., Minichiello, C., & Facchin, P. (2014). A population-based registry as a source of health indicators for rare diseases: The ten-year experience of the Veneto Region's rare diseases registry. *Orphanet Journal of Rare Diseases, 9*(37), 1–12. PMID:24646171

Munson, M., Wrobel, J., Holmes, C., & Hanauer, D. (2014). Data Mining for Identifying Novel Associations and Temporal Relationships with Charcot Foot. *Journal of Diabetes Research*, 1-13.

NCATS. (n.d.). *National Center for Advancing Translational Sciences*. Retrieved June 23, 2015 from https://ncats.nih.gov/

NIH. (n.d.). *National Institutes of Health*. Retrieved June 23, 2015 from http://www.nih.gov/

NORD. (n.d.). Retrieved June 23, 2015 from https://www.rarediseases.org/

NZORD. (n.d.). Retrieved June 23, 2015 from http://www.nzord.org.nz/

ORDR. (n.d.). Retrieved June 23, 2015 from http://rarediseases.info.nih.gov/

Orphadata. (n.d.). Retrieved June 23, 2015 from http://www.orphadata.org/

Orphanet. (n.d.). Retrieved June 23, 2015 from http://www.orpha.net/

Patients Like Me. (n.d.). Retrieved June 23, 2015 from http://www.patientslikeme.com/

Patnaik, D., Butler, P., Ramakrishnan, N., Parida, L., Keller, B., & Hanauer, D. (2011). Experiences with Mining Temporal Event Sequences from Electronic Medical Records: Initial Successes and Some Challenges. *Proceedings of the 17th ACM SIGKDD international conference on Knowledge discovery and data mining*. San Diego, CA: ACM.

Paul, R., Groza, T., Hunter, J., & Zankl, A. (2012). Decision Support Methods for Finding Phenotype-Disorder Associations in the Bone Dysplasia Domain. *PLoS ONE, 7*(11), e50614. doi:10.1371/journal.pone.0050614 PMID:23226331

Perner, P. (2006). Intelligent data analysis in medicine-Recent advances. *Artificial Intelligence in Medicine, 37*(1), 1–5. doi:10.1016/j.artmed.2005.10.003 PMID:16338124

PhenomeCentral. (n.d.). Retrieved June 23, 2015 from https://phenomecentral.org/

Polat, K., & Güneş, S. (2007). Detection of ECG Arrhythmia using a differential expert system approach based on principal component analysis and least square support vector machine. *Applied Mathematics and Computation, 186*(1), 898–906. doi:10.1016/j.amc.2006.08.020

Pro Rare Austria. (n.d.). Retrieved June 23, 2015 from http://www.prorare-austria.org/

Rabasco, A. M., León, J. M., González-R, P. L., Calle, M., Cózar-Bernal, M., Ojeda, M., & González-Rodríguez, M. L. (2013a). *Un sistema de información para la gestión del conocimiento en enfermedades raras. ER 2.0. 2° Congreso Nacional de Servicios Farmacéuticos, XIX Jornadas de Farmacia Hospitalaria.* Montevideo, Uruguay: V Jornadas Rioplatenses de Farmacia Hospitalaria.

Rabasco, A. M., Cózar-Bernal, M. J., Ojeda, M., González-Rodríguez, M. L., Calle, M., León, J. M., & González-R., P. L. (2013b). ER 2.0: Gestión del conocimiento vía web. *VI Congreso Internacional de Medicamentos Huérfanos y Enfermedades Raras.* Sevilla. Rare Disease Dot Org. Retrieved June 23, 2015 from http://raredisease.org/

RARECARENET. (n.d.). Retrieved June 23, 2015 from http://www.rarecarenet.eu/

RareConnect. (n.d.). Retrieved June 23, 2015 from http://www.rareconnect.org/

RARELINK. (n.d.). Retrieved June 23, 2015 from http://rarelink.org/

RD Connect. (n.d.). Retrieved June 23, 2015 from http://rd-connect.eu/

RD-NeurOmics. (n.d.). Retrieved June 23, 2015 from http://rd-neuromics.eu/

RDRD. (n.d.). Retrieved June 23, 2015 from http://www.fda.gov/ForIndustry/DevelopingProductsforRareDiseasesConditions/HowtoapplyforOrphanProductDesignation/ucm216147.htm

RE(ACT). (n.d.). Retrieved June 23, 2015 from http://react-community.org/

Robinson, P., & Mundlos, S. (2010). The Human Phenotype Ontology. *Clinical Genetics, 77*(6), 525–534. doi:10.1111/j.1399-0004.2010.01436.x PMID:20412080

Rodwell, C., & Aymé, S. (Eds.). (2014). *Report on the state of the art of rare disease activities in Europe.* RVA, Rare Voices Australia. Retrieved June 23, 2015 from https://www.rarevoices.org.au/

Santoro, M., Coi, A., Lipucci Di Paola, M., Bianucci, A. M., Gainotti, S., Mollo, E., & Bianchi, F. et al. (2015). Rare Disease Registries Classification and Characterization: A Data Mining Approach. *Public Health Genomics, 18*(2), 113–122. doi:10.1159/000369993 PMID:25677717

SKELETOME Project. (n.d.). University of Queensland, Australia. Retrieved June 23, 2015 from http://www.itee.uq.edu.au/eresearch/projects/skeletome

Spain R. D. R. (n.d.). Retrieved June 23, 2015 from https://spainrdr.isciii.es/

Taboada, M., Martínez, D., Pila, B., Jiménez-Escrig, A., Robinson, P., & Sobrido, M. (2012). Querying phenotype-genotype relationships on patient datasets using semantic web technology: The example of cerebrotendinous xanthomatosis. *BMC Medical Informatics and Decision Making,* 1–11. PMID:22849591

Taruscio, D., Vittozzi, L., Choquet, R., Heimdal, K., Iskrov, G., Kodra, Y., & Van Oyen, H. et al. (2015). National registries of rare diseases in europe: An overview of the current situation and experiences. *Public Health Genomics, 18*(1), 20–25. doi:10.1159/000365897 PMID:25228300

Tomar, D., & Agarwal, S. (2013). A survey on Data Mining approaches for Healthcare. *International Journal of Bio-Science and Bio-Technology, 5*(5), 241–266. doi:10.14257/ijbsbt.2013.5.5.25

Weka. (n.d.). Retrieved June 23, 2015 from http://www.cs.waikato.ac.nz/ml/weka/

Witten, I., & Frank, E. (2000). *Data Mining: Practical Machine Learning Tools and Techniques with Java Implementations*. San Francisco, CA: Morgan Kaufmann.

Ye, J., Chen, K., Wu, T., Li, J., Zhao, Z., Patel, R., & Reiman, E. (2008). *Heterogeneus Data Fusion for Alzheimer Disease Study. In Knowledge Discovery in Databases 2008* (pp. 1025–1033). Las Vegas, NV: ACM.

Yoo, I., Alafaireet, P., Marinov, M., Pena-Hernandez, K., Gopidi, R., Chang, J., & Lei, H. (2012). Data mining in healthcare and biomedicine: A survey of the literature. *Journal of Medical Systems*, *36*(4), 2431–2448. doi:10.1007/s10916-011-9710-5 PMID:21537851

Recent Advances in Microprompting Technology

Catherine Best
University of Stirling, UK

Brian O'Neill
Brain Injury Rehabilitation Trust, UK

Alex Gillespie
London School of Economics, UK

INTRODUCTION

Assistive technology for cognition (ATC) is technology to extend mental capacity. The majority of people reading this article will use technology to support their everyday cognitive function; by setting appointment reminders on their phone to support prospective memory, using a SatNav to support navigational skills or an search engine as an alternative to storing information in long term memory. If technology can support the cognition of ordinary individuals, potentially it can have an even greater role in assisting the cognition of people who through illness, injury or developmental disorders live with cognitive impairment. In these cases technology can act as a cognitive prosthetic or orthotic supporting or replacing lost or impaired cognitive function (Cole, Dehdashti, Petti, & Angert, 1994).

Research on Assistive Technology

Research on assistive technology for cognition has been accelerating over the last twenty years and has already been the subject of a number of authoritative reviews (LoPresti, Mihailidis, & Kirsch, 2004). It is common for reviews to restrict their scope to a single clinical group e.g. dementia (Bharucha et al., 2009) or technology type e.g. electronic portable devices (Charters, Gillett, & Simpson, 2014) or type of cognitive impairment e.g. memory disorders (Jamieson, Cullen, McGee-Lennon, Brewster, & Evans, 2013). However there is no reason why the application of ATC devices should be limited by the etiology of the cognitive disorder. A device that supports prospective memory is just as likely to work for someone with traumatic brain injury as it is for someone with intellectual disabilities. Likewise devices such as a smart phone can perform a myriad of functions. Therefore examining the effectiveness of smart phones as an ATC lacks specificity. To counter these difficulties Gillespie, Best & O'Neill (2012) classified ATC by the function of the device and looked across all the ways technology can act as a cognitive prosthesis for the diverse etiologies of cognitive impairment. ATC devices were classified into: reminding, storing and displaying, navigating, distracting, biofeedback and micro prompting technologies (see (Best, O'Neill, & Gillespie, 2013; Gillespie, Best, & O'Neill, 2012). This review focuses on one type of assistive technology 'microprompting technologies'.

DOI: 10.4018/978-1-4666-9978-6.ch060

Microprompting Technologies

Microprompting technologies are a type of assistive technology for cognition that support the planning and execution of complex behavioral sequences. Even mundane tasks such as getting dressed, hand washing or making a cup of tea require complex prioritization of action, goal monitoring, decision making and problem solving for their successful execution. Microprompting devices break down complex tasks into steps and prompt the user through each step of the sequence and continually check that the activity goal is being achieved. Microprompting devices guide the user through an immediately present task step-by-step usually using either verbal and/or visual prompts. In this chapter we aim to review existing studies of microprompting devices and discuss the limitations of these studies. We will then cover how these limitations have been addressed by the most recent work in this area and outline the most pressing research priorities. Section 1 of this chapter describes and evaluates existing research on microprompting devices; section 2 discusses how recent research addresses the limitations of previous work and section 3 outlines future research priorities.

BACKGROUND

Gillespie, Best and O'Neill's 2012 review identified 22 trials of microprompting technologies. These studies are shown in Table 1.

Table 1. Studies of microprompting technologies

Authors	Year	Device	Type of Activity Supported	Clinical Group	Sign Rating	N	
Bergman	2002	Computer	Economic self-sufficiency	Traumatic Brain Injury	3	1	Qualitative
Carmien	2005	Alarm	Social & civic - Leisure	Intellectual disability	3	7	Qualitative
Cihak, Kessler & Alberto,	2008	Computer	Major life area - Employment	Intellectual disability	2-	4	Yes
Davies, Stock & Wehmeyer	2002	Alarm	Major life area - Employment	Intellectual disability	2-	12	Yes
Ferguson, Myles & Hagiwara	2005	Alarm	Major life area - Education	Neurodevelopmental disorders	2-	1	Yes
Ferreras et al.	2010	Alarm	Major life area - Employment	Intellectual disability	3	8	Qualitative
Fish, Manly & Wilson	2008	Alarm	General tasks - Daily routine	ABI-other	2-	1	Yes
Furniss et al.	1999	Computer	Major life area - Employment	Intellectual disability	2-	6	Yes
Gorman, Dayle, Hood & Rummell	2003	Computer	General tasks - Daily routine	ABI-other	3	2	Qualitative
Kirsch, Levine, Fallon-Krueger & Jaros	1987	Computer	Domestic life - Household tasks	ABI-other	2+	1	Yes
Kirsch, Levine, Lajiness-O'Neill & Schnyder	1992	Computer	Major life area - Employment	Traumatic Brain Injury	2+	4	Mixed

continued on following page

Table 1. Continued

Authors	Year	Device	Type of Activity Supported	Clinical Group	Sign Rating	N	
Kirsch, Shenton, Spirl, Rowan Simpson & Lo Presti	2004	Computer	Domestic life - Household tasks	Traumatic Brain Injury	2-	1	Yes
Lancioni et al.	2006	Audio visual	Self-care - Dressing	Intellectual disability	2+	2	Yes
Lancioni, O'Reilly, Seedhouse, Furniss & Cunha	2000	Computer	Major life area - Employment	Intellectual disability	2-	6	Yes
Lancioni, O'Reilly, Van den Hof, Furniss, Seedhouse & Rocha	1999	Computer	Major life area - Employment	Intellectual disability	2-	4	Yes
Lancioni, van den Hof, Boelens, Rocha & Seedhouse	1998	Computer	Major life area - Employment	Intellectual disability	2-	3	Yes
Lancioni, Van den Hof, Furniss, O'Reilly & Cunha	1999	Computer	Domestic life - Household tasks	Intellectual disability	2+	4	Yes
Lemoncello	2009	Other	Self-care - Personal health	Stroke	2-	3	Yes
Mihailidis, Barbenel & Fernie	2004	Computer	Self-care - Washing	Dementia & older people	2+	9	Yes
Mihailidis, Boger, Craig & Hoey.	2008	Computer	Self-care - Washing	Dementia & older people	2+	6	Yes
O'Neill & Gillespie	2008	Computer	Self-care - Personal health	ABI-other	2+	1	Yes
O'Neill, Moran & Gillespie	2010	Computer	Self-care - Personal health	ABI-other	2+	8	Yes

Microprompting technologies have been used to support a range of activities including household (Kirsch, Levine, Fallon-Krueger, & Jaros, 1987) vocational (Lancioni, O'Reilly, Seedhouse, Furniss, & Cunha, 2000) and personal care (Mihailidis, Barbenel, & Fernie, 2004; O'Neill, Moran, & Gillespie, 2010) tasks. Researchers have used purpose-designed (Davies, Stock, & Wehmeyer, 2002; Ferreras et al., 2010) 'off the shelf' software (Cihak, Kessler, & Alberto, 2008) to develop prompting systems.

Limitation of the Reviewed Studies

As can be seen from Table 1 the number of participants in the identified trials was generally very small with only one study recruiting more than ten participants. This is in part a natural consequence of the degree of impairment present in people who require microprompting devices. Recruiting and deploying these devices in such populations is difficult and time consuming so recruiting large samples is unusual.

The methodological quality of the studies was rated using the SIGN (Scottish Intercollegiate Guidelines Network, 2001) ratings of levels of evidence. The eight ratings are:

1++: High quality meta-analyses, systematic reviews of RCTs, or RCTs with a very low risk of bias.
1+: Well-conducted meta-analyses, systematic reviews, or RCTs with a low risk of bias.
1-: Meta-analyses, systematic reviews, or RCTs with a high risk of bias.
2++: High quality systematic reviews of case control or cohort or studies or high quality case control or cohort studies with a very low risk of confounding or bias and a high probability that the relationship is causal.

2+: Well-conducted case control or cohort studies with a low risk of confounding or bias and a moderate probability that the relationship is causal.

2-: Case control or cohort studies with a high risk of confounding or bias and a significant risk that the relationship is not causal.

3: Non-analytic studies, such as case reports or case series.

4: Expert opinion.

All the studies in Table 1 are categorized as 2+ or below. There is a lack of high quality research designs e.g. randomized controlled trials, in this field. The next section addresses how recent advances address these limitations.

RECENT ADVANCES

Use of 'Off the Shelf' Prompting Systems to Increase Sample Size

The widespread availability at relatively low cost of multifunctional devices such as smart phones coupled with access to a large array of applications means that using 'off the shelf' applications to support people with cognitive impairment is becoming more feasible. This enables larger trials with more robust methodologies. For example Gentry and colleagues (Gentry, Kriner, Sima, McDonough, & Wehman, 2015) used an individually selected set of apps on an apple iPod touch to support people with autism in a vocational setting. Through their randomized controlled trial with 50 users they found that people using the ATC required fewer hours of vocational support than people without the ATC. This was over and above the time spent selecting and training users with the ATC. This approach has the potential to increase the methodological quality of studies of microprompting technologies by enabling larger sample sizes and more robust designs

Research with People with High Levels of Impairment

Use of off the shelf applications in unlikely to be feasible for all users of microprompting technologies. People with the highest level of support needs may not be able to provide the required feedback to the device. The micro prompting devices identified by Gillespie, Best and O'Neill (2012) differ in the amount and type of user feedback required during task performance. All the devices mentioned in Table 1, with the exception of Guide (O'Neill, Best, Gillespie,, & O'Neill, 2013) and COACH (Mihailidis, Boger, Craig, & Hoey, 2008), require the user to interrupt the task they are performing and physically interact with the device in order to progress to the next step. For example, someone using the VICAID system (Lancioni, O'Reilly, Seedhouse, Furniss, & Cunha, 2000), given the prompt to 'brush the floor', will have to assess when they have adequately completed that step and then remember to push the button on the device to receive the next prompt. In contrast microprompting devices such as COACH are becoming more advanced in their ability to register user progress through the task automatically. COACH uses movement detection (Hoey et al., 2010). This opens up the use of micro prompting devices to people with high levels of impairment in their ability to self-monitor. It has been commented that having to learn to use any new device is a barrier to ATC adoption for people with cognitive impairments therefore the lower the burden on the user to learn new behaviors, for example, pushing a button after each step for VICAID or restricting their responses to 'yes or no' for Guide the more useable the device will be for people with the greatest degree of cognitive impairment. However this may mean that research into microprompting will bifurcate with less impaired users who are able to self-monitor using 'off the shelf' devices whereas the more impaired will use purpose-designed individually tailored support that takes over the monitoring aspect of task performance. It is unlikely that large scale trials of the more individually-tailored intensive support devices will be feasible but robust evaluation can be undertaken using intensive repeated measures designs.

FUTURE RESEARCH DIRECTIONS

Existing reviews of micro prompting devices have found that there are already effective devices for improving independent of task performance in people with cognitive impairment (Charters et al., 2014; Jamieson et al., 2013). The most important next stage in research is to find out how to improve the implementation of existing microprompting devices. This covers the prescription, adoption and maintenance of such ATC in rehabilitation programs and services to people with cognitive impairment (O'Neill & Gillespie, 2015). This can be achieved through additional research on users' views on barriers to implementation, addressing known barriers, user training and support, and addressing the needs of carers and professionals. These areas will be further discussed below.

User Views

As mentioned in the introduction, use of ATC is ubiquitous among some sections of society. Researchers have investigated the extent of technology use in people with cognitive impairment. These, usually small scale studies, indicate that a small proportion of people with acquired brain injury do use ATC (de Joode, van Boxtel, Verhey, & van Heugten, 2012) but they have many have difficulties with its use (Chu et al., 2014) and do not utilize its full potential with significant unmet needs in this population which could be addressed by ATC (Chu, Brown, Harniss, Kautz, & Johnson, 2014). As would be expected it is the people with the most severe impairments who have the greatest difficulties with use of technology after brain injury (Engström, Lexell, & Lund, 2010). In people with dementia the picture is worse with very low use of electronic ATC to support cognitive function but carers and people with dementia reporting many unmet needs and very low awareness of what ATC is available (Boger, Dunal, Quraishi, & Turcotte, 2014). We need more detailed information on why people with cognitive impairment, who could potentially benefit from using microprompting devices, are not using them. This is particularly urgent when there are 'off the shelf' technologies that could be effective in many cases.

Barriers to Use

One known barrier to technology use in people with cognitive impairment is the burden of individually tailoring the prompts to the users' needs. A difficulty with detailed prompting systems is that someone has to design and program the individually specific recipe of instructions, and this can be a potential burden on carers or clinical staff. The possibility of having a library of prompting templates online that can be easily downloaded might attenuate this barrier to access, by providing high quality generic templates for people with cognitive impairment that can be easily tailored to the individual. The Guide system now has capability of providing a menu of online task instructions for various personal tasks such as laundry and performing the morning routine.

User Training and Support

For devices that require users to interact with the device, research on training of users with cognitive impairment has shown that a structured program better is better than trial and error approach to ATC device familiarization (Svoboda, Richards, Polsinelli, & Guger, 2010). Implementation support is at least, if not more important, as the device itself. People with cognitive impairment may require significant input from researchers/health professionals to:

- Recognize the potential benefits of ATC,
- To develop their confidence in being able to use ATC, and
- Gradual introduction to the device using established rehabilitation techniques such as errorless learning.

There is a strong existing literature on how to select and provide assistive technology (Scherer, Jutai, Fuhrer, Demers, & Deruyter, 2007). There is a need for further research from a psychological perspective to develop optimal methods to support people to recognize the need for, learn to use and to promote generalization and maintenance of ATC in people with cognitive impairment.

Support of Professionals and Carers

People who require micro prompting devices will be people who have considerable on-going support needs therefore the wider support network of carers, clinicians, need to be on side for device adoption to be successful (de Joode et al., 2012). The aim of ATC adoption is frequently reduction in carer burden and increased independence for the user. For users, carers and health professionals ATC have many potential benefits but to achieve these benefits requires change in behavior involving effort and new learning. Research in other areas of health behavior has shown it is very difficult to get people to change established behavior patterns (Michie, van Stralen, & West, 2011). Behaviour change in the form of adoption of ATC (for users, carers and health professionals) may require specific psychosocial interventions. That is to say, developing ATC is only the first (albeit major) hurdle, we also need reliable knowledge about how to embed these potentially beneficial technologies in people's everyday lives.

REFERENCES

Bergman, M. M. (2002). The benefits of a cognitive orthotic in brain injury rehabilitation. *The Journal of Head Trauma Rehabilitation, 17*(5), 45–51. doi:10.1097/00001199-200210000-00005 PMID:12802253

Best, C., O'Neill, B., & Gillespie, A. (2013). Assistive Technology for Cognition: Enabling Activities of Daily Living. In M. M. Cruz-Cunha, I. M. Miranda, & P. Gonçalves (Eds.), *Handbook of Research on ICTs for Human-Centered Healthcare and Social Care Services* (pp. 112–129). IGI Global. doi:10.4018/978-1-4666-3986-7.ch006

Bharucha, A. J., Anand, V., Forlizzi, J., Dew, M. A., Reynolds, C. F., Stevens, S., & Wactlar, H. (2009). Intelligent Assistive Technology Applications to Dementia Care: Current Capabilities, Limitations, and Future Challenges. *The American Journal of Geriatric Psychiatry: Official Journal of the American Association for Geriatric Psychiatry, 17*(2), 88–104. doi:10.1097/JGP.0b013e318187dde5

Boger, J., Quraishi, M., Turcotte, N., & Dunal, L. (2014). The identification of assistive technologies being used to support the daily occupations of community-dwelling older adults with dementia: A cross-sectional pilot study. *Disability and Rehabilitation. Assistive Technology, 9*(1), 17–30. doi:10.3109/17 483107.2013.785035 PMID:23607569

Charters, E., Gillett, L., & Simpson, G. K. (2014). Efficacy of electronic portable assistive devices for people with acquired brain injury: A systematic review. *Neuropsychological Rehabilitation*, 1–40. doi: 10.1080/09602011.2014.942672 PMID:25121394

Chu, Y., Brown, P., Harniss, M., Kautz, H., & Johnson, K. (2014). Cognitive support technologies for people with TBI: Current usage and challenges experienced. *Disability and Rehabilitation. Assistive Technology, 9*(4), 279–285. doi:10.3109/17483107.2013.823631 PMID:23919409

Cihak, D. F., Kessler, K. B., & Alberto, P. A. (2008). Use of a handheld prompting system to transition independently through vocational tasks for students with moderate and severe intellectual disabilities. *Education and Training in Developmental Disabilities, 43*(1), 102–110.

Cole, E., Dehdashti, P., Petti, L., & Angert, M. (1994). Design and outcomes of computer based cognitive prosthetics for brain injury : A field study of three subjects. *NeuroRehabilitation, 4*(3), 174–186. PMID:24525366

Davies, D. K., Stock, S. E., & Wehmeyer, M. L. (2002). Enhancing independent task performance for individuals with mental retardation through use of a handheld self-directed visual and audio prompting system. *Education and Training in Mental Retardation and Developmental Disabilities, 37*(2), 209–218.

De Joode, E. A., van Boxtel, M. P. J., Verhey, F. R., & van Heugten, C. M. (2012). Use of assistive technology in cognitive rehabilitation: Exploratory studies of the opinions and expectations of healthcare professionals and potential users. *Brain Injury, 26*(10), 1257–1266. doi:10.3109/02699052.2012.6675 90 PMID:22571738

Engström, A.-L. L., Lexell, J., & Lund, M. L. (2010). Difficulties in using everyday technology after acquired brain injury: A qualitative analysis. *Scandinavian Journal of Occupational Therapy, 17*(3), 233–243. doi:10.3109/11038120903191806 PMID:19707949

Ferreras, A., Belda, J. M., Barberà, R., Poveda, R., Urra, M., García, N., … Valero, M. (2010). PDA Software Aimed at Improving Workplace Adaptation for People with Cognitive Disabilities. *Computers Helping People with Special Needs*, 13–20.

Gentry, T., Kriner, R., Sima, A., McDonough, J., & Wehman, P. (2015). Reducing the need for personal supports among workers with autism using an iPod Touch as an assistive technology: Delayed randomized control trial. *Journal of Autism and Developmental Disorders, 45*(3), 669–684. doi:10.1007/s10803-014-2221-8 PMID:25212414

Gillespie, A., Best, C., & O'Neill, B. (2012). Cognitive Function and Assistive Technology for Cognition: A Systematic Review. *Journal of the International Neuropsychological Society, 18*(01), 1–19. doi:10.1017/S1355617711001548 PMID:22152338

Hoey, J., Poupart, P., von Bertoldi, A., Craig, T., Boutilier, C., & Mihailidis, A. (2010). Automated handwashing assistance for persons with dementia using video and a partially observable Markov decision process. *Computer Vision and Image Understanding, 114*(5), 503–519. doi:10.1016/j.cviu.2009.06.008

Jamieson, M., Cullen, B., McGee-Lennon, M., Brewster, S., & Evans, J. J. (2013). The efficacy of cognitive prosthetic technology for people with memory impairments: A systematic review and meta-analysis. *Neuropsychological Rehabilitation*. PMID:23957379

Kirsch, N. L., Levine, S. P., Fallon-Krueger, M., & Jaros, L. A. (1987). Focus on clinical research: The microcomputer as an "orthotic" device for patients with cognitive deficits. *The Journal of Head Trauma Rehabilitation*, 2(4), 77–86. doi:10.1097/00001199-198712000-00012

Lancioni, G. E., O'Reilly, M. F., Seedhouse, P., Furniss, F., & Cunha, B. (2000). Promoting Independent Task Performance by Persons with Severe Developmental Disabilities through a New Computer-Aided System. *Behavior Modification*, 24(5), 700–718. doi:10.1177/0145445500245005 PMID:11036735

LoPresti, E. F., Mihailidis, A., & Kirsch, N. (2004). Assistive technology for cognitive rehabilitation: State of the art. *Neuropsychological Rehabilitation*, 14(1/2), 5–39. doi:10.1080/09602010343000101

Michie, S., van Stralen, M. M., & West, R. (2011). The behaviour change wheel: A new method for characterising and designing behaviour change interventions. *Implementation Science; IS*, 6(1), 42. doi:10.1186/1748-5908-6-42 PMID:21513547

Mihailidis, A., Barbenel, J. C., & Fernie, G. (2004). The efficacy of an intelligent cognitive orthosis to facilitate handwashing by persons with moderate to severe dementia. *Neuropsychological Rehabilitation*, 14(1-2), 135–171. doi:10.1080/09602010343000156

Mihailidis, A., Boger, J. N., Craig, T., & Hoey, J. (2008). The COACH prompting system to assist older adults with dementia through handwashing: An efficacy study. *BMC Geriatrics*, 8(1), 28. doi:10.1186/1471-2318-8-28 PMID:18992135

O'Neill, B., Best, C., Gillespie, A., & O'Neill, L. (2013). Automated prompting technologies in rehabilitation and at home. *Social Care and Neurodisability*, 4(1), 17–28. doi:10.1108/20420911311302281

O'Neill, B., Moran, K., & Gillespie, A. (2010). Scaffolding rehabilitation behaviour using a voice-mediated assistive technology for cognition. *Neuropsychological Rehabilitation*, 20(4), 509–527. doi:10.1080/09602010903519652 PMID:20182951

Scherer, M., Jutai, J., Fuhrer, M., Demers, L., & Deruyter, F. (2007). A framework for modelling the selection of assistive technology devices (ATDs). *Disability and Rehabilitation. Assistive Technology*, 2(1), 1–8. doi:10.1080/17483100600845414 PMID:19263548

Scottish Intercollegiate Guidelines Network. (2001). *SIGN 50: A guideline developer's handbook - SIGN grading system 1999–2012*. Retrieved from http://www.sign.ac.uk/guidelines/fulltext/50/annexoldb.html

Svoboda, E., Richards, B., Polsinelli, A., & Guger, S. (2010). A theory-driven training programme in the use of emerging commercial technology: Application to an adolescent with severe memory impairment. *Neuropsychological Rehabilitation: An International Journal*, 20(4), 562–586. doi:10.1080/09602011003669918 PMID:20425664

KEY TERMS AND DEFINITIONS

E

Alerting ATC: These are devices which draw attention to something present in the environment.

Assistive Technology for Cognition: Use of technology to extend human mental capacity.

Biofeedback ATC: Provide the user with information about their own bodies.

Cognition: Thinking, remembering, and knowing.

Distracting ATC: Distracting devices are those which distract users from anxiety provoking stimuli.

Executive Function: Specific mental functions that enable goal directed behavior. This includes the functions of planning, engaging and disengaging attention, postponing reward and sequencing complex behaviors.

Micro Prompting ATC: Micro-prompting devices provide detailed step-by-step prompts, guiding the user through an immediately present task. The supported tasks are usually complex with multiple embedded stages so the devices often require feedback on task progress in order to generate the next prompt in the sequence.

Navigating ATC: These devices help the user to be aware of their location.

Reminding ATC: Those devices providing a one-way, usually one-off, time-dependent reminder about something not in the immediate environment which is intended to be an impetus to action (e.g., reminder about an appointment).

Storing and Displaying ATC: These devices store and present stimuli that are personally relevant. These devices are not time bound i.e. they do not present information in a time dependent fashion but instead are always used in an interpersonal context. These devices are never an impetus to action.

Remote Patient Monitoring Technologies

Marília Dourado
Faculty of Medicine, University of Coimbra, Portugal

Rui Garcia
Faculty of Medicine, University of Coimbra, Portugal

INTRODUCTION

Over the last decades we experienced a paradigm shift from acute to chronic diseases, mainly due to the aging of population. However, the training of doctors, and other health professionals, kept the traditional educational models that focused in diagnosis and treatment of acute pathologies. In the second half of the 20th century, since the 1960's, new information and communication technologies began to develop and they have emerged in the health context, with positive and negative effects. It is therefore important to develop new approaches, technologies, skills and knowledge to address this new reality. (Ruiz et al. (2006); Strandberg et al. (2007); Wholihan et al. (2012)).

Despite the fact that acute conditions require specific medical attention at the current conjuncture we cannot continue to control chronic diseases in the same way we do for acute diseases. It is essential to develop an educational model that turns to the chronicity and long-term care, to the disease prevention and to palliative care (Celler et al. (2003)).

In this context doctor-patient communication develops a new and a highest reputation and, also, has evolved throughout the last decades from paternalism to individualism. The fundamental objective of any doctor-patient communication is to improve the patient's health and medical care. (Bertakis (1977); Nilsson (2010)) Current model of information exchange shared decision making and patient-centered communication is currently considered to be the best model (Cline et al. (2001); Herndon et al. (2002); Sawyer et al. (2003)). The main objective is learning to negotiate therapeutic and care plans, to support patients in self-management, to use information systems and to work as members of multidisciplinary teams. Increasing patient involvement in supervision and documentation process of their own health may lead to a greater involvement and accountability from the patient. This is certainly a new way to look at the doctor-patient relationship (Reis et al. (2013); Albernethy et al. (2010)).

Also, with the same purpose, efficient and reliable measurement technology and sensor technology in physiology will gain a lot of importance for the assessment of human functional state. The registration of physiological signals or biosignals is important not only for timeless classical applications concerning medical diagnosis and subsequent therapy, but also for future applications such as daily monitoring (Kaniusas (2012)).

Bearing in mind the importance and current of this theme, in this chapter, a definition of biosignals will be given as well as possible classifications of commonly used biosignals in order to perceive a nearly unlimited diversity of biosignals, their usefulness for remote monitoring patients, followed by future trends in biosignal monitoring.

DOI: 10.4018/978-1-4666-9978-6.ch061

BIOSIGNALS DEFINITION AND MONITORING

The use of human biosignals, or physiological signals, in medicine had a great evolution over the centuries determined by patient and physician needs as well as by other problems that were encountered, namely those related with changes in disease pattern associated with population aging.

A biosignal can be defined as a description of a physiological phenomenon that can be used in both diagnosis and therapy. The first were historically evaluated by *inspection* (through which patient is carefully observed, with necked eye, for example as regards skin colour, nutritional state), *palpation* (to feel and to determine body size, shape, location of organs, and so on, with hands applying a small of pressure), *percussion* (involves striking the body directly or indirectly with short and sharp knocks of a finger. The produced sounds indicate the presence of a solid mass or an air-containing structures, and are also helpful in determining the size and position of various internal organs) and *auscultation* (in which the physician listens to internal body sounds to detect pathologies). With technological progress these procedures were improved with the support of instruments used by the physician on the patient (e.g. stethoscope, otoscope, ophthalmoscope) spreading to the spectrum of functions to evaluate. However, these acquisition methods of biosignals are not objective, and in this way an objective evaluation essential for a good diagnosis is not possible. Likewise, reproducibility, analysis, comparison and circulating biosignals information is not possible due to the subjective and variability of physicians and it's instantaneous impression, as well as due to the lack of storage for future applications (Kaniusas (2012); Loewe et al. (2013)).

Considering that a biosignal is any signal in living beings that can be continually measured and monitored, problems related with the objectivity of their evaluation were recognized, and efforts to avoid them were made in order to be objective and any assessment can be reproducible, recorded, compared with other assessments and communicated on a large scale for global assessment. (Shalevet et al. (2011)

In a simple way we have in extreme poles verbal and individualized description of a signal, which is inaccurate and subject to interferences by the experience and sensibility of who makes the evaluation. On the other hand we have technology assessment with precise, quantitative measurements where hardly occurs interference of the observer.

The question is how and what to monitor? Nowadays, the surveillance of chronic diseases is a problem for the organization of health systems because of their high costs.

With the progressive aging of the population, associated with errors held in lifestyle (sedentary lifestyle, improper diet, smoking habit, among others), the need to care for patients with chronic and progressively disabling weaknesses increased. In this context hospitalization and costs associated with the recovery, rehabilitation and control of diseases and their complications also increased. Thus the idea of permanently monitoring health status of patients emerged,. With this we intend to identify and detect any change as early as possible and to intervene early and prevent further deterioration in the health status of the patient.

Currently more and more biosignals monitoring tended to depend on the use of new mobile communication technologies that allow continuous transmission of information on the health status of the patient to health professionals, generating responses for individual control of each patient and timely policy planning of global health. The first step of this process depends on the definition of what should be monitored and how such monitoring can be made. (Bull et al. (2010))

It is important to reaffirm that the use of means of monitoring physiological functions to evaluate the state of health is not new. The use of regular analytical controls, the determination of capillary blood glucose, regular measurement of weight or blood pressure is widely known.

Although these measurements are more frequent in the control of chronic conditions and outpatient also acute conditions are subject to monitoring processes, usually in hospital environments using invasive and complex methods as well as excessive acquisition of information. In both cases a desired and opportune response does not always occur either by default or delay in response.

The monitoring processes often depend on the registration by patients as well as their willingness to do it, what can cause data errors and measuring devices use. In order to avoid errors associated with information mismanagement it is necessary to define what kind of data is useful for assessing and monitoring a specific health condition. A biosignal often means bioelectrical signals, but it may refer to both electrical and non-electrical signals. On the other hand, the usual understanding is to refer only to time-varying signals, although spatial parameter variations, e.g. the nucleotide sequence determining the genetic code, are sometimes subsumed as well. (Kaniusas (2012); Cooper et al. (1990); Twork et al. (1990)).

It is concluded that there is an almost endless number of what can be monitored and within each one many possible parameters or signals to measure physiological processes. For this reason it is important to determine what physiological mechanism is intended to monitor and what signs should be used in this assessment to develop the method of acquiring information, being sure that there are several possibilities for this ranging from patient's visual inspection to biosensor application. A widely known example of this is the study of respiratory function. It can be measured by chest auscultation, using radiological methods, plethysmographic functional studies, blood gas determinations, assessment of peripheral oxygen saturation, among others.

In practice there is no interest of using all these processes on continuous assessment of an individual. A judicious choice of what to use and when to use is necessary in order to get useful information to generate practical applications, whether diagnostic or therapeutic.

Nevertheless biosignals having been used since a long time further advancement of their acquisition, interpretation and diagnostic approaches continues to be a subject on the agenda. The reason for that *never ending improvements* in biosignal monitoring results from the fact that biosignals reflect human health and wellbeing. They are essential for point vital physiological phenomena and so mankind and not just for increased comfort. Also, they are relevant for the pre-screening of the human functional state and diagnosis of disease as well as for subsequent therapy, follow-up treatment, and assessment of its efficiency.

When analysing data from a set of individuals one can also consider using applications on health policies.

Biosignals: Classification

For the classification of biosignals, intrasubjective and intersubjective variability in the measurement signals play an important role. Because of them, the classification accuracy of biosignal is not simple and the algorithm used for it needs to be evaluated with large population's studies. In addition, to demonstrate the general applicability of the algorithms, they must be validated with different data than those used for the design of the algorithm.

They can be measured as physical quantities such as temperature or pressure, electrical quantities such as currents and voltages and biochemical quantities such as concentrations..In this way they can contribute to quantify physiological processes. Thus they can be classified as Physical, Electrical and Biochemical biosignals (Table 1).

Table 1. Biosignals classification according their measured characteristics

Biosignals Classification
• Physical, • Electrical, • Biochemical.

Nevertheless, a diversity of biosignals is almost unlimited. For that reason a single classification is not possible. Another possible approach to classify it divides them in three categories according "the existence" of biosignals, the "dynamic nature of biosignals" and the "origin of biosignals" as it is represented in Table 2.

There are many other possibilities to classify biosignals, for instance, the one that divides it into: *continuous signals*, defined by a continuous functions, most biomedical signals are continuous; *discrete signals*, which will show information exactly at a particular time; *deterministic signals*, which can be determined and described exactly using mathematics or graphics and *stochastic signals* that can be expressed only in terms of probabilities. All of them, in one way or another are based on physiological characteristics of these biological variables that can be captured and translated into a value.

A diversity of signal types can be found, including image, audio and other biological sources of information. The analysis and use of these signals is a multidisciplinary area including signal processing, pattern recognition and computational intelligence techniques, amongst others.

BIOSENSORS AND NETWORK MONITORING

The clinical need for monitoring biosignals arises from the fact that dysfunctions in the biological processes cause changes that usually lead to pathological processes. Also nonpathological changes in the status of the body can cause changes in physiological processes, for example, speaking causes, irregularities in the breathing rhythm.

To treat and follow up patients in their own home and provide them medical assistance can partly be accomplished to a defined level, by the use of new bio-medical sensors and wireless communication, in

Table 2. Biosignals classification according their existence, dynamic nature, and origin

Existence of Biosignals	Dynamic Nature of Biosignals	Origin of Biosignals
• **Permanent Biosignals:** Always present and available. The source is inside the body. • **Examples:** Electrocardiographic signal induced by electrical myocardial excitation	• **Static Biosignals:** Transmits information in its steady state level, which may exhibit slow changes over time. • **Example:** Body temperature and it's circadian rhythm	• **Electric:** Electroencephalogram, electromyogram, electrocardiogram • **Magnetic:** Magnetocardiogram • **Mechanic:** Mechanorespirogram • **Optic:** Optoplethysmogram • **Acoustic:** Phonocardiogramphonocardiogram • **Chemical:** Course of cortisolover 24h in humans • **Thermal:** Heat loss/absorption mechanisms in the body • Others.
• **Induced Biosignals:** Artificially induced. Exists roughly for the duration of the excitation. As soon as artificial stimulus is over biosignal it decays with a certain time. • **Example:** Electric plethysmography.	• **Dynamic Biosignals:** Show extensive changes in the time domain, with dynamic processes conveying the physiological information of interest. • **Example:** Heart rate	

this trend to use virtual instrumentation, in a sense of reducing costs, increase flexibility and biological signal processing systems modularization. Designing a medical product that has necessary structures and capabilities to be used by a particular customer is very difficult. (Cibuk et al. (2012)) monitoring physiological functions To overcome this challenge, a new approach that allows increased modularity of design complexity, while allowing the implementation of innovative ideas from non-technical specialists is needed. (Postolache et al. (2007); Jaana et al. (2007); Branzila et al. (2013); Brooks et al. (2011))

According to the nature of biosignal to monitor a proper evaluation strategy must be created. From a technical point of view, the quality assessment is openly connected with the acceptance of the sensor by the patient, with the number of sensors to be used and its sensitivity and ability to simultaneously assess multiple parameters.

Modern biosensors are integrated in electronic medical equipment that converts various forms of *stimuli* into electrical signals for analysis. There are three directions that influence the development of medical instruments that can establish what can be considered to be the ideal biosensor. It should be asafe, high-quality device to generate a signal, whose intensity should be proportional to the intensity of the biosignal/*stimulus* to assess, which should be reproducible, specific, rapid and sensitive and low cost. (Artero-Delgado et al. (2013)

Schematically a sensor includes a contact element for assessing the biological *stimulus* and a "transducer" that transforms the *stimulus* into quantifiable and measurable electrical signal.

The advantages of modern biosensors lies in its low cost, light weight, smallest size (nanometers) and integration in electronic circuits with low energy consumption and the possibility of interaction with intelligent communication networks.

The first developed biosensors allowed evaluating temperature, pressure, vibration, light intensity. The technological development allowed them to be adapted to the continuous monitoring of physiological functions such as blood glucose tests or troponin.

Biosensors can be integrated in daily routine of patients in a little intrusive, unobtrusive manner. They may be applied to the patient, in clothing or in the living environment.

Once the parameters and the method to use it were determined it is important to integrate the gathered information when managing the patient's condition. At this stage the new information and communication technologies allow data to be directly transferred to doctor's office. At the distance, messages could be sent to patient via mobile applications with therapeutic guidelines, recipes, and other. The implementation of wireless biosignals processing and monitoring by Bluetooth technology is a good example. With this technology biosignals are acquired to a sever and transmitted via Bluetooth. The signals will be sent and received in a remote monitoring centre and a specialist can attend to this centre without the inconvenience of leaving the hospital or office. This requires a robust wireless link. Although many wireless standards can be used, there are important considerations such as variety, security, quantity and ease implementation and low cost, that has to be taken into account. (Dehghani et al. (2010))

The experience of Ambient Assisted Living (AAL) program has multiplied, in which new information and communication technologies are used to support chronic patients, enabling them to stay in their homes, promoting their autonomy and independence when managing the information captured by the sensors and generate responses to the detected needs.

It is well known that assessment tools that can be used to monitoring biosignals have been developed for patient and clinician use. It is a true continuous monitoring that will provide information about the health status of the patient (almost) in real time, symptoms recognition and medication related side effects. However, chronic diseases tend to progress and there is a need for another type of monitoring, with regular intervals, assisted by additional data, laboratory and imaging studies, among others, that will support medical team in its regular observation of the patient. It allows redefining stadiums and new needs to be monitored remotely.

This phenomenon is bringing new challenges to physicians and health policy makers, enabling a better patients' orientation based on an accurate and ongoing information, which will approach patient from his/her doctor, but also involving him/her more, pointing him/her the responsibility for his/her state of health. However there are still barriers to implement in these procedures on a large scale. There is ignorance and suspicion about these methodologies, confusing them with intrusion in his/her privacy. There is the concern about data security and the maintenance of confidentiality. Patient monitoring outside conventional clinical settings is undoubtedly a challenge to be overcame. New information and communication technologies will enable to improve the human health condition, resulting on the changes of paradigms of health systems and structures.

CONCLUSION

There is the need to prove that the cost-benefit ratio is useful for implementing health policy measures based on these technologies.

The work to be done in order to overcome these barriers is ongoing and will allow everyone to benefit from the role of new technologies in the continuous monitoring of patients.

REFERENCES

Abernethy, A. P., Wheeler, J. L., & Currow, D. C. (2010). Utility and use of palliative care screening tools in routine oncology practice. *Cancer Journal (Sudbury, Mass.), 165*(5), 444–460. doi:10.1097/PPO.0b013e3181f45df0 PMID:20890140

Artero-Delgado, C., Nogueras-Cervera, M., & Mànuel-Làzaro, A. (2013). pH Sensor Calibration Procedure. *Proceedings of the 19th Symposium IMEKO TC 4 Symposium and 17th IWADC Workshop - Advances in Instrumentation and Sensors Interoperability.*

Bertakis, K. D. (1977). The communication of information from physician to patient: A method for increasing patient retention and satisfaction. *The Journal of Family Practice, 5*(2), 217–222. PMID:894226

Branzila, M., & David, V. (2013) Wireless Intelligent Systems for Biosignals Monitoring Using Low Cost Devices. *Proceedings of the 19th Symposium IMEKO TC 4 Symposium and 17th IWADC Workshop - Advances in Instrumentation and Sensors Interoperability.*

Brooks, D. J., Hunter, P. J., Smaill, B. H., & Titchener, M. R. (2011). BioSignalML – a meta-model for biosignals. *33rd Annual International Conference of the IEEE EMBS.*

Bull, J., Zafar, S. Y., Wheeler, J. L., Harker, M., Gblokpor, A., & Hanson, L. (2010). Establishing a regional, multisite database for quality improvement and service planning in community-based palliative care and hospice. *Journal of Palliative Care, 13*(8), 1013–1020. PMID:20649439

Celler, B. G., Lovell, N. H., & Basilakis, J. (2003). Using information technology to improve the management of chronic disease. *The Medical Journal of Australia, 179*(5), 242–246. PMID:12924970

Cibuk, M., & Balik, H. H. (2012). Implementation of web based biotelemetry applications on WiMax networks. *Advances in Engineering Software*, *49*, 14–20. doi:10.1016/j.advengsoft.2012.02.014

Cline, R. J., & Haynes, K. M. (2001). Consumer health information seeking on the Internet: The state of the art. *Health Education Research*, *16*(6), 671–692. doi:10.1093/her/16.6.671 PMID:11780707

Cooper, J. M., & Cass, A. E. G. (1990). *Biosensors, a practical approach*. Oxford University Press.

Dehghani, M. J., Shahabinia, A. R., & Safavi, A. A. (2010). Implementation of wireless data transmission based on Bluetooth technology for biosignals monitoring. *World Applied Science Journal*, *10*(3), 287–293.

Herndon, J. H., & Pollick, K. J. (2002). Continuing concerns, new challenges, and next steps in physician-patient communication. *The Journal of Bone & Joint Surgery*, *84*(2), 309–315. PMID:11861738

Jaana, M., & Paré, G. (2007). Home telemonitoring of patients with diabetes: A systematic assessment of observed effects. *Journal of Evaluation in Clinical Practice*, *13*(2), 242–253. doi:10.1111/j.1365-2753.2006.00686.x PMID:17378871

Kaniusas, E. (2012) Fundamentals of biosignals. In E. Kaniusas (Ed.), Biomedical and sensors I - Linking Physiological Phenomena and Biosignals, (pp. 1-25). Springer-Verlag, Berlin Heidelberg. doi:10.1007/978-3-642-24843-6_1

Loewe, S. A., Rodríguez-Molinero, A., Glybb, L., Breen, P. P., Baker, P. M., Sanford, J., & Ólaighin, G. et al. (2013). New technology-based functional assessment tools should avoid the weaknesses and proliferation of manual functional assessments. *Journal of Clinical Epidemiology*, *66*(6), 619–632. doi:10.1016/j.jclinepi.2012.12.003 PMID:23415867

Nilsson, C., Skär, L., & Söderberg, S. (2010). Swedish district nurses' experiences on the use of information and communication technology for supporting people with serious chronic illness living at home–a case study. *Scandinavian Journal of Caring Sciences*, *24*(2), 259–265. doi:10.1111/j.1471-6712.2009.00715.x PMID:20030770

Postolache, O., Girão, P. S., & Postolache, G. (2007). New approach on cardiac autonomic control estimation based on BCG processing. *Proceedings of the Canadian Conference on Electrical Computer Engeneering*. doi:10.1109/CCECE.2007.224

Reis, A., Pedrosa, A., Dourado, M., & Reis, R. (2013). Information and Communication Technologies in Long-term and Palliative Care. *Procedia Technology*, *9*, 1303–1312. doi:10.1016/j.protcy.2013.12.146

Ruiz, J. G., Mintzer, M. J., & Leipzig, R. M. (2006). The impact of e-learning in medical education. *Academic Medicine*, *81*(3), 207–212. doi:10.1097/00001888-200603000-00002 PMID:16501260

Sawyer, S., & Aroni, R. (2003). Sticky issue of adherence. *Journal of Paediatrics and Child Health*, *39*(1), 2–5. doi:10.1046/j.1440-1754.2003.00081.x PMID:12542804

Shalevet, V., Chodick, G., Goren, I., Silber, H., Kokia, E., & Heymann, A. D. (2011). The use of an automated patient registry to manage and monitor cardiovascular conditions and related outcomes in a large health organization. *International Journal of Cardiology*, *152*(3), 345–349. doi:10.1016/j.ijcard.2010.08.002 PMID:20826019

Strandberg, E. L., Ovhed, I., Borgquist, L., & Wilhelmsson, S. (2007). The perceived meaning of a holistic view among general practitioners and district nurses in Swedish primary care: A qualitative study. *BMC Family Practice, 8*(1), 8. doi:10.1186/1471-2296-8-8 PMID:17346340

Twork, J., & Yacynych, A. M. (1990). *Sensors in bioprocess control.* New York: Marcel Dekker, Inc.

Wholihan, D. J., & Pace, D. J. (2012). Community discussions: a vision for cutting the costs of end-of-life care. *Nurse Economics, 30*(3), 170-5, 178.

A Review of Existing Applications and Techniques for Narrative Text Analysis in Electronic Medical Records

Alexandra Pomares-Quimbaya
Pontificia Universidad Javeriana, Colombia

Rafael A. Gonzalez
Pontificia Universidad Javeriana, Colombia

Santiago Quintero
Pontificia Universidad Javeriana, Colombia

Oscar Mauricio Muñoz
Pontificia Universidad Javeriana, Colombia

Wilson Ricardo Bohórquez
Pontificia Universidad Javeriana, Colombia

Olga Milena García
Pontificia Universidad Javeriana, Colombia

Dario Londoño
Pontificia Universidad Javeriana, Colombia

INTRODUCTION

Electronic Medical Records (EMR) contain information that is typically stored in structured (coded) attributes as well as unstructured narrative data. These narrative data or free text includes: discharge notes, progress notes, radiology reports, pathology reports, nursing notes, and general clinical notes. These texts contain valuable patient information, but are often underused and only looked at for a particular patient, remaining hidden for population studies, clinical studies or administrative analysis. As a consequence, finding and using evidence contained in medical records remains fragmented due to the fact that narrative text is cumbersome to analyze.

To face this challenge, different research projects have applied natural language processing techniques and/or text mining techniques to improve the quantity and quality of the information extracted from EMR aimed at supporting clinical research and administration. From the content point of view, many such projects are focused on the analysis of a specific disease, while others try to improve the pharmacovigilance process. From the technical point of view, most of them deal with the extraction of patterns from narrative texts, while others propose methods for de-identification (anonymization). Another group emphasizes on solving co-reference and redundancy aspects. Lastly, others work on the generation of summaries from original texts.

DOI: 10.4018/978-1-4666-9978-6.ch062

The objective of this chapter is to present a thorough exploration of these projects and synthesizes this diversity into a coherent classification. To achieve this, the chapter is organized as follows: in Section 2 we present the background of the work and the method used to obtain the projects that were included in the study. Then, Section 3 presents different applications of natural language processing to improve the analysis of specific diseases or process, and Section 4 explores generic tools and methods that have been propose for the analysis of narrative medical information or narrative information in general. Finally, Section 5 explores future challenges and research perspectives, and Section 6 concludes the chapter proposing a classification of recent works around natural language processing and text mining applied on the analysis of narrative text contained in medical records.

BACKGROUND

The obstacles for using the extensive narrative data found within EMR in research projects, mainly due to their lack of structure and standardization, have motivated different types of works. This chapter presents projects that have demonstrated successful use of Natural Language Processing (NLP) and/or data mining techniques for the exploitation of EMR narrative data. These works can be classified into two broad groups: the first group uses NLP or data mining techniques in the context of a disease or a process; for instance, the analysis of a specific disease or within a pharmacovigilance process; this group is called *NLP applications for medical analysis*. The second group, called *Generic NLP Methods and Tools*, comprises works that propose methods or techniques to improve the analysis of texts regardless of the context, including, generating summaries, de-identifying narrative texts and solving redundancy aspects.

This chapter surveys recent work in NLP and text mining over medical records. The period of the analysis ranges from 2008 to the beginning of 2014. Even though there are previous works on this subject, we decided to restrict the dates considering the recent advances on NLP and text mining the last years.

Papers were identified using Web of Science database[1], and specifically the results obtained from the following query: TS=(EHR or Electronic Health Record or Medical Health Record) and TS=(text mining or natural language processing or information retrieval) and TS= (text-free or free-text or free text or narrative text or text or medical notes or nursery notes)) <i> AND </i>LANGUAGE: (English). From the obtained list of paper we selected interesting publications by analyzing the titles and their abstracts.

Besides the works identified though this query, we identified other previous works that recognizes the importance of applying text mining techniques to biomedical literature in order to recognize entities, their relationships, create summaries and enhance question-answer systems from scientific publications, like the work presented by (Zweigenbaum, Demner-Fushman, Yu & Cohen, 2007), and using ontologies to facilitate associations between genomic data and information from biomedical texts, as is the case of the paper presented by (Tiffin, 2005). However, we decided not to include them in this study because they were more focused on the analysis of literature and not the analysis of medical records, which is the focus of this chapter.

NLP APPLICATIONS FOR MEDICAL ANALYSIS

In health domain NLP applications have been used for the analysis of a specific disease with successful results. The first group of solutions is focused on the application and/or evaluation of NLP processes or data mining techniques to improve the knowledge of a disease or healthcare process.

Overview of Related Projects

These projects analyze a specific disease or condition using NLP tools and NLP techniques. They take advantage of the opportunities that the increasing availability of EMRs gives, and develop solutions to improve a specific treatment.

One of these projects developed an NLP - based system to process electronic clinical notes for women in early-stage breast cancer to identify whether and when recurrences were diagnosed. In this case, narrative information has been used to improve epidemiological studies. The NLP system replaced the manual method, which was expensive and infringe the patient's privacy. It was developed with the open source Apache clinical Text Analysis and Knowledge Extraction System (cTAKES), Python and SQL. The complete system was applied at the Group Health in the Pacific Northwest, from 2007 to 2012. The results showed that NLP could identify cases of recurrent breast cancer at a rate comparable to traditional abstraction with up to 90% reduction in the number of charts requiring manual review (Carrell, Halgrim, Tran, Buist, & Chubak, 2014). Similarly, another work proposes the use of NLP to automate the process of identifying trauma patients using as input the information from injured patients (Day, Christensen, Dalto & Haug P, 2007).

An interesting project identified patients who need colorectal cancer (CRC) tests by applying four methods: Setting, Patient eligibility, Manual EMR abstraction and NLP System to detect CRC testing. NLP was applied to detect four kinds of CRC testing using a system that identifies Unified Medical Language System (UMLS) concepts from biomedical text documents and produces XML-tagged output containing lists of UMLS concepts found in each sentence with relevant context called KMCI. Using KMCI to detect CRC testing is more efficient than other methods used before (Denny, Choma, Peterson, Miller, Bastarache, & Peterson, 2012).

Similarly, NLP was applied to assess the performance on colonoscopy quality measures and how to enhance the procedure that is currently being applied. This study used a previously validated NLP program, called C-QUAL, to analyze this kind of reports. The program was tested showing excellent accuracy on nine different quality measures advocated by specialty societies (Ateev Mehrotra, Evan S. Dellon, Robert E. Schoen, Melissa Saul, Faraz Bishehsari, & Carrie Farmer, 2012).

Besides these projects, NLP and artificial intelligence has been used to evaluate the prevalence of comorbid conditions among patients with alopecia areata (AA) using a novel algorithm to collate data on disease associations in a large retrospective patient cohort. The algorithm is based on an artificial intelligence program, the Automated Retrieval Console (ARC), which performed natural language processing and machine learning technology to review free-text medical records and select for the diagnosis of AA. After applying this model in the 3568-patient set, ARC identified 2115 patients with AA (Kathie P. Huang, Samyukta Mullangi, Ye Guo, & Abrar A. Qureshi, 2013).

In addition, a support vector machine (SVM)-based system for identifying EMR progress notes pertaining to diabetes is an additional project related to a specific disease. This classifier is based on a SVM for searching and classifying EMR progress notes applying this method to the task of identifying notes about diabetes (Wright, McCoy, Henkin, Kale, & Sittig, 2013).

Another project describes the construction and validation of an EMR-based algorithm to identify subjects with age-related cataracts. Cataract cases were selected if the subject had either a cataract surgery, or two or more cataract diagnoses, or one cataract diagnosis with either an indication found using NLP or optical character recognition (OCR). The results of the EMR-based cataract phenotyping algorithm was successfully developed and validated, resulting in positive predictive values (PPVs) >95% (Peissig, et al., 2011).

A set of projects is focused in ADEs (Adverse Events Detection) using Name Entity Recognition (NER) – tagger and data mining techniques. The objective of the first one was to identify situations at risk of ADE using data mining of routinely collected data of previous hospitalizations (Chazard, Ficheur, Bernonville, Luyckx, & Beuscart, 2011); the second one identified possible adverse events (AEs) and, specifically, possible adverse drug events (ADEs), improving and simplifying the steps involved as they occur in the clinical setting using a NER tagger to identify dictionary matches in the text and post-coordination rules to construct ADE compound terms (Eriksson, Jensen, Frankild, Jensen, & Brunak, 2013).

For post–operative complications we mention here two related projects. The goal of the first study was to build electronic algorithms using a combination of structured data and NLP of text notes for potential safety surveillance of nine post-operative complications and to develop a Post-Operative Event Monitor (called POEM) to detect surgical complications using the full electronic health record across six hospitals (Fern, et al., 2014). The second study objective is to evaluate a NLP search–approach to identify postoperative surgical complications within a comprehensive EMR using MedLEE to identify 45 adverse events tracked as part of the New York Patient Occurrence Reporting and Tracking System (Murff, et al., 2011).

Other projects analyze the use of certain drugs, like is the case of a study of warfarin. This study uses DNA biobanks linked to comprehensive EMRs systems; these are potentially powerful resources for pharmacogenetic studies. The authors developed two algorithms to extract weekly warfarin doses from both data sets: a regular expression-based program for semi structured Coumadin Clinic notes; and an advanced weekly dose calculator based on an existing medication information extraction system (MedEx) for narrative providers' notes. The results show that the MedEx-based system could determine patients' warfarin weekly doses with 99.7% recall, 90.8% precision, and 93.8% accuracy (Xu, et al., 2011).

A recent work aims at identifying drug and food allergies automatically. To achieve this goal they developed a high-performance, easily maintained algorithm to identify medication and food allergies and sensitivities from unstructured allergy entries in EMR systems. This algorithm used RxNorm and NLP techniques (Epstein, Jacques, Stockin, Rothman, Ehrenfeld, & Denny, 2013).

In addition, another project characterized the environment and phenotypic associations using information theory and EMR. This project developed methods that were generated based on use of NLP to encode clinical information in narrative patient records followed by statistical methods. They developed methods using mutual information (MI) and its property, the data processing inequality (DPI), to help characterize associations that were generated based on the use of NLP to encode clinical information in narrative patient records followed by statistical methods. MedLEE was used to parse and transform discharge summaries into structured representations consisting of UMLS codes with modifiers. Evaluation based on a random sample consisting of two drugs and two diseases indicates an overall precision of 81% (Wang, Hripcsak, & Friedman, 2009).

Finally, there is a project whose objective was to undertake a proof of concept that demonstrated the use of primary care data, NLP and term extraction to assess emergency room use. Free text notes were extracted from a primary care clinic in Guelph, Ontario and analyzed with a software toolkit that incorporated General Architecture for Text Engineering (GATE), and MetaMap components for NLP and term extraction (St-Maurice, Kuo2, & Gooch, 2013).

Table 1 summarizes the main aspects of each project including its objectives, NLP tools used, Data source, trainings, other tools used in the project and the reference associated. The field called Disease/ Objective stores the particularly disease, the algorithm used or the state of the art objectives. The NLP tool field stores the software used in each project. The data source field stores the initial data required to start the project. The training/dataset field stores the type of datasets required, in the case the NLP

Table 1. NLP tools for specific disease

Reference	Disease/Objective	NLP Tool	Data Source	Trainings/Data Sets	Other Tools/Techniques
(Carrell, Halgrim, Tran, Buist, & Chubak, 2014)	Breast Cancer Recurrence	cTAKES	Electronic clinical notes, clinical notes, pathology reports, progress notes, and radiology reports.	Its initial entries were gathered from a review of the training corpus and the National Cancer Institute's online vocabulary services	Python and SQL
(Denny, Choma, Peterson, Miller, Bastarache, & Peterson, 2012)	Colorectal Cancer	KMCI	EHR: medical notes, radiology and pathology reports, laboratory outcomes, medical history, procedure background, family medical history and social history.	NAI	NONE
(Ateev Mehrotra, Evan S. Dellon, Robert E. Schoen, Melissa Saul, Faraz Bishehsari, & Carrie Farmer, 2012)	Colonoscopy	C - QUAL	Colonoscopy and pathology reports in the electronic health record (EHR)	Relevant information from randomly selected colonoscopy reports, and these samples of manually abstracted data	NONE
(Kathie P. Huang, Samyukta Mullangi, Ye Guo, & Abrar A. Qureshi, 2013)	Alopecia Areata	ARC	Information included demographics, diagnoses, medications, pathology reports, and the complete longitudinal medical record notes.	To validate this model they randomly selected 40 patients	NONE
(Wright, McCoy, Henkin, Kale, & Sittig, 2013)	Diabetes	SVM	EHR progress notes	They trained SVM using a bag of words approach	ROCR, LIBSVM 3.126
(Epstein, Jacques, Stockin, Rothman, Ehrenfeld, & Denny, 2013)	Drug and food allergies	Algorithm based on NLP to compare strings and substrings of a free - text note	Allergy and sensitivity EHR	The training dataset consisted of 9445 cases performed from 1 January to 31 March	RxNorm, SQL, Transact -SQL, Soundex and Double Metaphone
(Fern, et al., 2014)	Post-operative complications	POEM	EHR	VASQIP outcomes	VASQIP, SQL

continued on following page

Table 1. Continued

Reference	Disease/ Objective	NLP Tool	Data Source	Trainings/Data Sets	Other Tools/ Techniques
(St-Maurice, Kuo2, & Gooch, 2013)	Assess emergency room use	MetaMap, GATE	Patient Records, text notes, patient surveys, interviews or questionnaires	Metamap do not need any training model	MySQL database
(Wang, Hripcsak, & Friedman, 2009)	Phenotypic and environmental associations	MedLEE	Process EHR	NAI	MI (Mutual Information), DPI (Data Processing Inequality)
(Chazard, Ficheur, Bernonville, Luyckx, & Beuscart, 2011)	ADEs (Adverse Events Detection)	NONE	EHR	Set of drugs in combination with a clinical background, in the form of ADE detection rules	Data Mining, XML
(Eriksson, Jensen, Frankild, Jensen, & Brunak, 2013)	ADEs (Adverse Events Detection)	NER - Tagger	summary of product characteristics (SPC)	NAI	NONE
(Xu, et al., 2011)	Warfarin	MedEx	Drug-dose information	Randomly selected 200 warfarin sentences from Coumadin Clinic notes and 500 sentences from providers' notes.	NONE
(Peissig, et al., 2011)	Cataract	eMERGE, MedLEE	EHR	100 documents.	OCR (Optical Character Recognition), XML, Cypress tool version 1.0
(Hahn, Cohen, & Shah, 2012)	Pharmacogenomics	TM (text mining)	UMLS, EMR	NAI	Several NLP tools review
(Lua, et al., 2009)	Syndromic surveillance	NONE	470 Chinese key phrases	NAI	NONE
(Murff, y otros, 2011)	Postoperative surgical complications	NLP General	EHR	VASQIP outcomes	VASQIP, SQL

tool or the project needed an initial training, and the Other Tools/Techniques field stores the software or algorithms to complete the study of the project.

As it can be seen in Table 1, most of the projects use a different NLP tool to improve the evaluation of EMRs and to do it automatically for a specifically disease. Therefore, most of the projects need to train their applications so they can evaluate the accuracy after testing the results of the training. NLP is a common technology to analyze EMRs and it demonstrates the feasibility, performance and variety of tools by using it.

NLP Tool Categorization

As Table 1 presented, current projects use different NLP tools. Some of these tools are generic; others are specialized on the processing of narrative texts containing health domain information. Both are explained below.

Health Specialized NLP Tools

- **cTAKES (Open-Source Apache Clinical Text Analysis and Knowledge Extraction System):** An NLP platform with components specifically trained on clinical text. Each one has unique qualities and capabilities and includes at least one analysis engine (annotator).
- **KMCI System:** A general-purpose medical NLP system developed by several authors. The system identifies Unified Medical Language System (UMLS) concepts from biomedical text documents and produces XML-tagged output containing lists of UMLS concepts found in each sentence with relevant context.
- **C-QUAL:** An NLP-based computer software application for measuring performance on colonoscopy quality indicators. It automatically analyzes both colonoscopy and pathology reports in the EMR and abstract the necessary information.
- **ARC (Automated Retrieval Console):** An algorithm based on an artificial intelligence program, which performed NLP and machine learning technology to review free-text medical records and select for the diagnosis of alopecia areata.
- **POEM (Post-Operative Event Monitor):** It detects surgical complications using the EMR for post-operative care.
- **MetaMap:** A NLP and term extraction tool. Its strength is its ability to map text to the Unified Medical Language Syntax (UMLS) database, forming a standard terminology.
- **MedLEE (The Medical Language Extraction and Encoding System):** The goal of MedLEE is to extract, structure, and encode clinical information in textual patient reports so that subsequent automated processes can use the data (Friedman, et al., 1995). It has been used in different projects that aim to extract knowledge from medical narrative cases (Friedman, Knirsch, Shagina & Hripcsak, 1999).
- **MedEx:** A process free-text clinical records to recognize medication names and signature information, such as drug dose, frequency, route, and duration. It uses a context-free grammar and regular expression parsing to process free text clinical notes.
- **REX:** A rule-based NLP system written in Java for extracting and coding clinical data from free text reports such as admission notes, radiology and pathology reports, and discharge summaries. It has been used successfully used to extract and code clinical concepts related to congestive heart failure (Friedlin, Grannis & Overhage 2008) and methicillin-resistant Staphylococcus Aureus (MRSA) (Friedlin, & McDonald, 2006), among others.

Generic Tools

- **GATE (General Architecture for Text Engineering):** The GATE tool is part of a collaborative project that is broadly used for text processing in several domains and is freely available. It supports a full-featured Application Programming Interface (API) and has been used in different decision support systems as the ones presented in (Rijo, Silva, Pereira, Gonçalves & Agostinho, 2014) and (Pomares Quimbaya, 2014), among others.
- **SVM (Support Vector Machine)-Based System:** An algorithm based on the statistical learning theory to analyze data and recognize patterns, used for classification and regression analysis.
- **NER (Named Entity Recognizer)-TAGGER:** A java implementation that comes with well-engineered feature extractors for Named Entity Recognition, and different options for defining feature extractors.

GENERIC NLP METHODS AND TOOLS

This section presents the proposals of methods and/or tools that aim to improve the NLP of medical narrative texts. As in the review of the projects in the NLP applications for medical analysis, this section classifies the proposals into four groups: the first one includes proposals for the summarization of medical narratives texts. The second one emphasizes works that ensure the anonymisation of medical texts. The third one describes proposals that aim to improve the quality of texts. The last group illustrates briefly proposals that intend to extract or to store the medical narrative texts.

Summarization

A proposal of summarization described a framework that aggregates and extracts findings and attributes from free-text clinical reports. This framework maps findings to concepts in available knowledge sources, and generates a tailored presentation of the record based on the information needs. The framework is a system called Adaptive EHR and it was implemented to demonstrate its capabilities to present and synthesize information from neuro-oncology patients (Hsu et al., 2012).

Similarly, a system was developed which automatically generates partial neonatal intensive care unit (NICU) summaries using data-to-text technology. The results in an on-ward evaluation have showed that a substantial majority of the summaries was found by outgoing and incoming nurses to be understandable (90%), and a majority was found to be accurate (70%), and helpful (59%) (Hunteret al., 2012).

Anonymisation

A variety of works investigated anonymisation in narrative text with different mechanisms to ensure that patient's data to be analyzed remain confidential. One of the methods proposes is an automated method for de-identifying medical notes, which don't require a lot of private information. They developed a model to recognize Protected Health Information (PHI) on private notes, recognize no-PHI words and recognize phrases that appear in the public medical texts. In this work they analyzed the public and private medical texts sources to distinguish common medical words and phrases from PHI. The main identifiers from patients are names and numbers that appear frequently in the medical literature and to quantify its relation, they compared the magazine publications and the physician notes, and examined standard medical concepts and phrases in ten medical dictionaries. Finally, 28 characteristics were used to train decision tree classifiers. The evaluation of the tool shows that the model recognized successfully 98% of the PHI cards from 220 reports (Mc-Murry et al., 2013).

Another related project that investigates methods for de-identifying medical texts describes an experiment to create a system for de-identifying medical reports using the open source MITRE Identification Scrubber Toolkit (MIST) with two medical registry types: history and physical notes and social work notes. The result shows that the accuracy of the history and physical notes outperformed the social work notes. That result suggested that the major variety and contexts for the PHI in the social work notes is more difficult to model, so they can say that it is possible to build a functioning de-identification system using MIST (Hanauer et al., 2013).

In addition to the de-identification techniques, there are two methods for different purposes talking about languages: FASDIM, a fast and simple de-identification method for French medical free text records that consists in the elimination of the entire words that do not exist in the list of authorized words and all the numbers except those that match with a pattern list of protection The corresponding lists increase in the course of the iteration of the method. The authorized words list building is progressive: 12 hours for the first 7000 letters, 16 additional hours for 20.000 additional letters. The recall of this method is 98.1%, the accuracy 79.6% and the F-Measure is 87.9%. On average 30.6 terminology codes were codified by each letter and 99.02% of these codes are preserved despite de-identification. FASDIM shows good results in French, and doesn't require any dictionary (Chazard et al., 2014). The second method is a manual and automatic PHI-annotation trial for EMR written in Swedish that consists in two parts. The first part is the creation of a manually PHI-annotated gold standard and the second one is the evaluation of existing software. As a result, the study shows fairly results in the Inter-Annotator Agreement (IAA) manually created on the gold standard. Conversely, the portable existing software yielded poor results and demonstrated that new de-identification software needs to be developed (Velupillaiet al., 2009).

De-identification can be applied in other fields like for Veterans Health Administration (VHA). An automatic text de-identification system for (VHA) is based on a previous study about best documents-VHA de-identification methods whose aim was to evaluate existing de-identification of automated texts methods and tools applied to medical notes of VHA to determine performance in which methods are better than others over each PHI category, and when new methods are needed to improve performance (Ferrandez et al., 2012). In this study, they evaluate "out-of-the-box" De-Identification system using medical VHA documents. Systems were based on automated learning methods and were trained with the 2006 i2b2. These methods were also evaluated with a cross-validation experiment using their own VHA corpus (Ferrandez et al., 2012).

The De-Identification medical text automated system treats the problem as two different and independent tasks: the first one, maximizes confidentiality of patients writing PHI as possible as they can, and the second one, leaves documents identified in a usable state and preserve as much medical information as possible. The system was evaluated manually writing a variety of VHA medical notes and as a result they showed detailed system main components. On the other hand, another De-Identification system was also included in the evaluation. The VHA system was successfully completed and its hybrid design demonstrates its ruggedness and efficiency, giving priority to the patient's confidentiality leaving more safe medical information (Ferrandez et al., 2013).

Another research project did a cross-sectional study that included 3503 stratified medical notes random selected of the five million documents produced in one of the biggest hospitals of the United States. They calculated the sensibility, accuracy and the F-Measure of two automated De-Identification systems for PHI removing and evaluated performance against a manually generated one and the statistical significance was proved. The PNL-based De-Identification shows an excellent performance (Deleger et al., 2013).

Personal information is a concern especially if it is personal health information. Many times this kind of information are published or treated without any caution or just without intention. In (Sokolova et al., 2012) a system that prevents leaks of PHI in heterogeneous text data is presented. From an empirical testing they applied string matching and character-based N-gram modeling methods. After a few steps of texts stages analysis like titles and body, they found that the system helps to prevent leaks of PHI and is able to work within the complex environment of previously unseen data types.

In (Morrison et al., 2009) uses NLP and MedLEE tool to evaluate its utility on the removal of PHI by comparing 100 medical notes with the corresponding XML- tagged output. The results of this study shows that from 100 medical notes analyzed, 26 pieces of PHI slipped through and appear in MedLEE's output and demonstrated that an existing NLP system can be used to remove PHI from medical notes.

Quality Improvement

Quality improvement can be accomplished by a deep analysis over historical texts. There are two proposals that focus on the identification of regular expressions: the first one worked in identifying clinical events as problems, test or treatments for example and associated temporal expressions as dates and time. These are relevant tasks to extract and manage data from EMR. This project developed a system that automatically extracts temporal expressions and events from clinical narratives. As a result, the system achieved micro F scores of 90% for the extraction of temporal expressions and 87% for clinical event extraction (Kovacevic et al., 2013). The second one extended an open source software for the temporal ordering of events within narrative text documents, TTK, to support medical notes using veteran's affairs clinical notes and compared it to TTK. TTK is The Temporal Awareness and Reasoning System for Question Interpretation (TARSQI) Toolkit. They create Med-TTK using a development set consisting of 200 veteran's affairs clinical notes. After Med-TTK was created, they compared both tools performance using the reference standard consisting of 3146 temporal expressions and TTK identified 1595 expression and Med-TTK identified 3174 expressions. These results show that Med-TTK improved performance compared to TTK (Reeves et al., 2013).

There is also a project that worked to correct misspellings of queries using an efficient method. The method includes the combination of two approximate string comparators, Stoilos and Levenshtein. The objective of this method is to increase the number of matched medical terms in French and the results of this work shows that the combination of the normalized edit distance of Levenshtein and the Stoilos algorithm improved the results for misspelling corrections of user queries (Soualmia et al., 2012).

Likewise, solving existing coreference is another important component to improve the quality of clinical free text. Coreference objective is to link related data from the texts and to explain this relationship. The analysis presented in (Zheng et al., 2011) reviewed coreference resolution approaches in the English domain and contrasted them with those in the clinical domain and the related biomedical domain. They conclude that undoubtedly this technique will advance the methodologies for information extraction.

Furthermore, there is an investigation that works to take out redundant text to improve the quality of the analysis of clinical notes. A novel of variant Latent Dirichlet Allocation (LDA) topic modeling, called Red-LDA, is proposed. Red-LDA takes the inherent redundancy of patient records when modeling content of clinical notes. The investigation seeks to solve the problem when clinicians copy information in the same clinical note, duplicating relevant data creating a negative impact on the quality of the text mining. They experimented on different topic modeling techniques and the inherent redundancy of clinical notes indicate that while redundancy is harmful to traditional topic modeling technique, it is possibly to solve the problem (Cohen et al., 2014).

Text Storage and Extraction

New proposals to improve the data storage for effective clinical data management evaluated three databases: NoSQL, XML-enabled and native XML and found that the NoSQL was best for query speed (Lee et al., 2013).

Finally, there is a proposal to improve the text extraction of medical information using mobile applications with SMS. The proposed system extracts medical information from patient's SMS. As a result they verified and found that the overall medication name F – Measure was 79.8% and the medication action term F – Measure was 90%. They also found that other studies that extract medical information using semantic tagging, regular expression-based approaches or a combination of both approaches were successfully demonstrated (Stenner et al., 2012).

RESEARCH OPPORTUNITIES

As previous sections presented, healthcare analysis has been improved enormously through the use of NLP and text mining. While there has been significant innovation and progress, challenges and opportunities remain. This section summarizes the challenges and research opportunities, from the point of view of the authors, in the field of text mining and NLP applied to the analysis of EMR.

Incorporating domain knowledge is a must in this kind of systems; however, we believe that one important challenge is to enrich this knowledge taking into account the informal vocabulary, terms and jargon used in this domain. The recognition of events and patterns in medical narrative texts depends vastly on the inclusion of this terminology, which it is not well documented. Currently, the projects that recognize events or specific characteristics from narrative texts, beyond the coded concepts, consume an important period of time configuring the expressions necessary to detect what they are looking for. The challenge here is how to build these enriched knowledge bases or ontologies automatically or semi-automatically for each language in such a way that any NLP or text mining project can use it.

Data quality is an important barrier to NLP and text mining. Unfortunately, medical narrative texts disregarded grammatical rules; they frequently contained incomplete words, incomplete sentences, spelling errors, duplicate information, and sometimes they lacked proper punctuation. One interesting research opportunity is to create integrated strategies able to recognize and correct this quality issues typical in the medical domain. Even though there are some works around the improvement of quality, they are not well integrated or do not produce good results.

The analysis of natural language is one of the most time consuming tasks in terms of computation. Some algorithms for text pre-processing and for semantic entity recognition are well known for being complex and very time consuming. There is then a tremendous potential in using Big Data technologies to improve NLP and text mining time response. The challenge is how to integrate these two worlds without increasing the complexity of the assembly solutions.

Finally, and related to the previous challenges, it is important to improve the analysis of narrative text using the structured information that is related to them. Although medical records contain an important portion of text, they usually contain structured information. The challenge is to contextualize the analysis of medical texts using as input the well-structured information contained in the record. Contextualizing the analysis may improve time responses and allow adapting the kind of algorithm that should be applied to the texts.

Figure 1. Classification of projects related to narrative text analysis in EMR

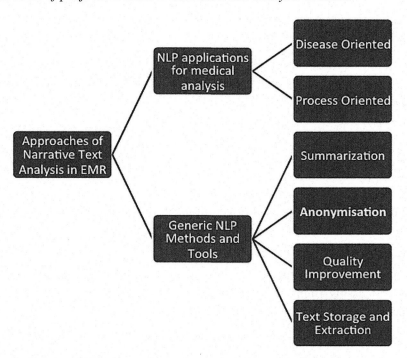

CONCLUSION

This chapter presents a review of existing applications and techniques for narrative text analysis in EMR. Figure 1 synthesizes the classification of current initiatives in this area, considering the publications and tools available. As it can be seen, there are two big groups of projects. The first one applies NLP and text mining tools to explore and analyze a specific disease (or diagnosis group) or an important clinical process using an existing software tool (see Section NLP Applications for Medical Analysis); the second group includes proposals of new tools and methods that enhance the analysis of narrative texts in the health domain (see Section Generic NLP Methods and Tools).

The area of NLP over medical narrative information has been evolving extremely rapidly. However, the analysis of current works led us to conclude that is important to produce user-oriented applications that can be employed to analyze any diagnosis or process using narrative text as the main source of information. Current tools are limited to a specific disease or are very difficult to configure by a final user. These facts hinder the use of these tools in research or medical institutions.

REFERENCES

Carrell, D. S., Halgrim, S., Tran, D.-T., Buist, D. S., & Chubak, J. (2014). Using Natural Language Processing to Improve Efficiency of Manual Chart. *American Journal of Epidemiology*, 10. PMID:24488511

Chazard, E., Ficheur, G., Bernonville, S., Luyckx, M., & Beuscart, R. (2011). Data Mining to Generate Adverse Drug Events Detection Rules. IEEE, 8.

Chazard, E., Mouret, C., Ficheur, G., Schaffar, A., Beuscart, J.-B., & Beuscart, R. (2014). Proposal and evaluation of FASDIM, a Fast And Simple De-Identification Method for unstructured free-text clinical records. *International Journal of Medical Informatics*, *83*(4), 303–312. doi:10.1016/j.ijmedinf.2013.11.005 PMID:24370391

Cohen, R., Aviram, I., Elhadad, M., & Elhadad, N. (2014). Redundancy-Aware Topic Modeling for Patient Record Notes. *PLoS ONE*, *9*(2), e87555. doi:10.1371/journal.pone.0087555 PMID:24551060

Day, S., Christensen, L. M., Dalto, J., & Haug, P. (2007). Identification of trauma patients at a level 1 trauma center utilizing natural language processing. *Journal of Trauma Nursing*, *14*(2), 79–83. doi:10.1097/01. JTN.0000278792.20913.82 PMID:17579326

Deleger, L., Molnar, K., Savova, G., Xia, F., Lingren, T., Li, Q., & Solti, I. et al. (2013). Large-scale evaluation of automated clinical note de-identification and its impact on information extraction. *JOURNAL OF THE American Medical Informatics Association*, *20*(1), 84–94. doi:10.1136/amiajnl-2012-001012 PMID:22859645

Denny, J. C., Choma, N. N., Peterson, J. F., Miller, R. A., Bastarache, L., & Peterson, M. L. (2012). Natural Language Processing Improves Identification of Colorectal Cancer Testing in the Electronic Medical Record. *Medical Decision Making*, 10. PMID:21393557

Epstein, R. H., Jacques, P. S., Stockin, M., Rothman, B., Ehrenfeld, J. M., & Denny, J. C. (2013). Automated identification of drug and food allergies entered using non-standard terminology. *American Medical Informatics Association*, 8.

Eriksson, R., Jensen, P. B., Frankild, S., Jensen, L. J., & Brunak, S. (2013). Dictionary construction and identification of possible adverse drug events in Danish clinical narrative text. American Medical Informatics Association, 8.

Fern, F., Fielstein, N. G., Steven, B., Ruth, R.,... Speroff, T. (2014). Exploring the Frontier of Electronic Health Record Surveillance: The Case of Post-Operative Complications. *Medical Care*, 15.

Ferrandez, O., South, B. R., Shen, S., Friedlin, F. J., Samore, M. H., & Meystre, S. M. (2012). Evaluating current automatic de-identification methods with Veteran's health administration clinical documents. *BMC Medical Research Methodology*, 12. PMID:22839356

Ferrandez, O., South, B. R., Shen, S., Friedlin, F. J., Samore, M. H., & Meystre, S. M. (2013). BoB, a best-of-breed automated text de-identification system for VHA clinical documents. *Journal of the American Medical Informatics Association*, *20*(1), 77–83. doi:10.1136/amiajnl-2012-001020 PMID:22947391

Friedlin, J., Grannis, S., & Overhage, J. M. (2008). Using Natural Language Processing to Improve Accuracy of Automated Notifiable Disease Reporting. *AMIA... Annual Symposium Proceedings / AMIA Symposium. AMIA Symposium*, *2008*, 207–211. PMID:18999177

Friedlin, J., & McDonald, C. J. (2006). A Natural Language Processing System to Extract and Code Concepts Relating to Congestive Heart Failure from Chest Radiology Reports. *AMIA... Annual Symposium Proceedings / AMIA Symposium. AMIA Symposium*, *2006*, 269–273. PMID:17238345

Friedman, C., Hripcsak, G., DuMouchel, W., Johnson, S. B., & Clayton, P. D. (1995). Natural language processing in an operational clinical information system. *J Natural Language Engineering*, *1*(1), 83–108. doi:10.1017/S1351324900000061

Friedman, C., Knirsch, C., Shagina, L., & Hripcsak, G. (1999). Automating a severity score guideline for community-acquired pneumonia employing medical language processing of discharge summaries. *Proceedings of the AMIA Symposium*, (pp. 256–260).

Hahn, U., Cohen, K. B., & Shah, Y. G. (2012). Mining the pharmacogenomics literatureça survey of the state of the art. Oxford University Press, 35.

Hanauer, D., Aberdeen, J., Bayer, S., Wellner, B., Clark, C., Zheng, K., & Hirschman, L. (2013). Bootstrapping a de-identification system for narrative patient records: Cost-performance tradeoffs. *International Journal of Medical Informatics, 82*(9), 821–831. doi:10.1016/j.ijmedinf.2013.03.005 PMID:23643147

Hsu, W., Taira, R. K., El-Saden, S., Kangarloo, H., & Bui, A. A. T. (2012). Context-Based Electronic Health Record: Toward Patient Specific Healthcare. *IEEE Transactions on Information Technology in Biomedicine, 16*(2), 228–234.

Hunter, J., Freer, Y., Gatt, A., Reiter, E., Sripada, S., & Sykes, C. (2012). Automatic generation of natural language nursing shift summaries in neonatal intensive care: BT-Nurse. *Artificial Intelligence in Medicine, 56*(3), 157–172. doi:10.1016/j.artmed.2012.09.002 PMID:23068882

Kathie, P., Huang, M., Samyukta Mullangi, B., Ye Guo, M., & Abrar A. Qureshi, M. M. (2013). Autoimmune, Atopic, and Mental Health Comorbid Conditions Associated With Alopecia Areata in the United States. *JAMA Dermatology*, 6.

Kovacevic, A., Dehghan, A., Filannino, M., Keane, J. A., & Nenadic, G. (2013). Combining rules and machine learning for extraction of temporal expressions and events from clinical narratives. *Journal of the American Medical Informatics Association, 20*(5), 859–866. doi:10.1136/amiajnl-2013-001625 PMID:23605114

Lee, K. K.-Y., Tang, W.-C., & Choi, K.-S. (2013). Alternatives to relational database: Comparison of NoSQL and XML approaches for clinical data storage. *Computer Methods and Programs in Biomedicine, 110*(1), 99–109. doi:10.1016/j.cmpb.2012.10.018 PMID:23177219

Lua, H.-M., Hsinchun Chena, D. Z., King, C.-C., Shih, F.-Y., Tsung-Shu Wub, & Hsiao, J.-Y. (2009). Multilingual chief complaint classification for syndromic surveillance: An experiment with Chinese chief complaints. *International Journal of Medical Informatics*, 13.

McMurry, A. J., Fitch, B., Savova, G., Kohane, I. S., & Reis, B. Y. (2013). Improved de-identification of physician notes through integrative modeling of both public and private medical text. *BMC Medical Informatics and Decision Making*, 13. PMID:24083569

Mehrotra, , Dellon, Schoen, Saul, Bishehsari, & Farmera. (2012). Applying a Natural Language Processing Tool to Electronic Health Records to Assess Performance on Colonoscopy Quality Measures. *Gastrointestinal Endoscopy*, 12.

Morrison, F. P., Lai, A. M., & Hripcsak, G. (2009). Repurposing the Clinical Record: Can an Existing Natural Language Processing System De-identify Clinical Notes? *Journal of the American Medical Informatics Association, 16*(1), 37–39. doi:10.1197/jamia.M2862 PMID:18952938

Murff, H. J., FitzHenry, F., Matheny, M. E., Gentry, N., Kotter, K. L., Crimin, K.,... Speroff, T. (2011). Automated Identification of Postoperative Complications Within an Electronic Medical Record Using Natural Language Processing. American Medical Association, 8.

Peissig, P. L., Rasmussen, L. V., Berg, R. L., Linneman, J. G., McCarty, C. A., Waudby, C.,... Starren, J. B. (2011). Importance of multi-modal approaches to effectively identify cataract cases from electronic health records. *Am Med Inform Assoc*, 10.

Pomares Quimbaya, A., Gonzalez, R.A., Bohórquez, W.R., Muñoz, O.M., García, O.M., & Londoño, D. (2014). *Engineering and Management of IT-based Service Systems*. Academic Press.

Reeves, R. M., Ong, F. R., Matheny, M. E., Denny, J. C., Aronsky, D., Gobbel, G. T., & Brown, S. H. et al. (2013). Detecting temporal expressions in medical narratives. *International Journal of Medical Informatics*, *82*(2), 118–127. PMID:22595284

Rijo, R., Silva, C., Pereira, L., Gonçalves, D., & Agostinho, M. (2014). Decision Support System to Diagnosis and Classification of Epilepsy in Children. *Journal of Universal Computer Science*, *20*(6), 907–923.

Sokolova, M., El Emam, K., Arbuckle, L., Neri, E., Rose, S., & Jonker, E. (2012). P2P Watch: Personal Health Information Detection in Peer-to-Peer File-Sharing Networks. *Journal of Medical Internet Research*, *14*(4), 225–237. doi:10.2196/jmir.1898 PMID:22776692

Soualmia, L. F., Prieur-Gaston, E., Moalla, Z., Lecroq, T., & Darmoni, S. J. (2012). Matching health information seekers' queries to medical terms. *BMC Bioinformatics*, *13*(14). PMID:23095521

St-Maurice, J., Kuo, M.-H., & Gooch, P. (2013). A Proof of Concept for Assessing Emergency Room Use with Primary Care Data and Natural Language Processing. *Methods of Information in Medicine*, 10. PMID:23223678

Stenner, S. P., Johnson, K. B., & Denny, J. C. (2012). PASTE: Patient-centered SMS text tagging in a medication management system. *Journal of the American Medical Informatics Association*, *19*(3), 368–374. doi:10.1136/amiajnl-2011-000484 PMID:21984605

Tiffin, N., Kelso, J. F., Powell, A. R., Pan, H., Bajic, V. B., & Hide, W. A. (2005). Integration of text- and data-mining using ontologies successfully selects disease gene candidates. *Nucleic Acids Research*, *33*(5), 1544–1552. doi:10.1093/nar/gki296 PMID:15767279

Velupillai, S., Dalianis, H., Hassel, M., & Nilsson, G. H. (2009). Developing a standard for de-identifying electronic patient records written in Swedish: Precision, recall and F-measure in a manual and computerized annotation trial. *International Journal of Medical Informatics*, *78*(12), E19–E26. doi:10.1016/j.ijmedinf.2009.04.005 PMID:19482543

Wang, X., Hripcsak, G., & Friedman, C. (2009). Characterizing environmental and phenotypic associations using information theory and electronic health records. *BioMed Central*, 7.

Wright, A., McCoy, A. B., Henkin, S., Kale, A., & Sittig, D. F. (2013). Use of a support vector machine for categorizing free-text notes: assessment of accuracy across two institutions. American Medical Informatics Association, 5.

Xu, H., Jiang, M., Oetjens, M., Bowton, E. A., Ramirez, A. H., Jeff, J. M.,... Denny, J. C. (2011). Facilitating pharmacogenetic studies using electronic health records and natural-language processing:a case study of warfarin. *Am Med Inform Assoc*, 6.

Zheng, J., Chapman, W. W., Crowley, R. S., & Savova, G. K. (2011). Coreference resolution: A review of general methodologies and applications in the clinical domain. *Journal of Biomedical Informatics*, *44*(6), 1113–1122. doi:10.1016/j.jbi.2011.08.006 PMID:21856441

Zweigenbaum, P., Demner-Fushman, D., Yu, H., & Cohen, K. B. (2007). Frontiers of biomedical text mining: Current progress. *Briefings in Bioinformatics*, *8*(5), 358–375. doi:10.1093/bib/bbm045 PMID:17977867

ENDNOTE

[1]   http://wokinfo.com/

The Role of Audio in Two Accessible Vision-Rehabilitation Games for Blind Teenage Users

Sofia Cavaco
NOVA LINCS, Department de Informática, Faculdade de Ciências e Tecnologia, Universidade Nova de Lisboa, Portugal

Frederico Ferreira
NOVA LINCS, Department de Informática, Faculdade de Ciências e Tecnologia, Universidade Nova de Lisboa, Portugal

Diogo Simões
NOVA LINCS, Department de Informática, Faculdade de Ciências e Tecnologia, Universidade Nova de Lisboa, Portugal

Tiago Silva
NOVA LINCS, Department de Informática, Faculdade de Ciências e Tecnologia, Universidade Nova de Lisboa, Portugal

INTRODUCTION

Often computer (and other electronic) games are considered as an addictive way of entertainment for youngsters, with many disadvantageous effects. Yet, well designed computer games can have very positive effect on the players. In particular, computer games can be used for vision rehabilitation purposes. By definition, vision rehabilitation is concerned about giving blind and low vision people the ability to live independently and improve their quality of life. This includes training orientation and mobility skills and educational related issues, among others.

The advantages of training orientation and mobility skills with a game include the motivation that a fun environment can bring to the patient, and the possibility of training the skills in a safe environment. Also, the fact that a game can help the patient forget (or not think about) the real purpose of the game, can help surpass inhibition of these patients.

Computer games can also be used for educational purposes. In fact, well designed educational games can lead to an improvement on school performance. Educational games contribute to making students feel more motivated and engaged in the learning process. This promotes studying and influences the effort students put on learning the school curriculum.

Unfortunately, since most educational computer games are designed for sighted students and have a very strong visual component, blind students are not always able to take full advantage of these games and benefit from them. However it would be desirable that these students could have access to the games not only to guarantee that all students have equal opportunities but also because nowadays blind students attend inclusive schools. Ultimately, access to well designed educational computer games for blind students can contribute to the improvement on the quality of life of this special needs group, as good school performance is the key for more and better opportunities in the student's future.

DOI: 10.4018/978-1-4666-9978-6.ch063

In this paper we focus on the role of audio in computer games accessible to visually impaired users. In particular we focus on two vision rehabilitation games we have designed for blind and low vision middle school users. One of these games was designed to help blind and low vision students on learning mathematics and the other for developing and training orientation and mobility skills.

In order to guarantee accessibility to blind users, we have designed games that can be played without the need to see the graphics. These games use speech and non-speech audio to convey information, and use 3D spatialized audio for orientation purposes. All the features, like questions and feedback, instructions, etc. are complemented with audio, and the games use audio localization cues for orientation. In particular, the game designed for developing mobility skills uses 3D spatialized audio obtained with head related transfer functions.

BACKGROUND

Most computer games have a strong visual component. While the majority of these games also use audio, most (relevant) information is provided through images. This way, it is very difficult for low vision users, and impossible for blind users, to play the games independently. This is also true for serious computer games for education and health, which are usually designed for sighted users. Nonetheless, it would be desirable that these games would be accessible to visually impaired users, allowing these users to take advantage of these applications in the same way that sighted users do.

In order to allow visually impaired users to enjoy and take advantage of computer games, these must use non-visual modalities as means of interaction with the user. Some possibilities include using sound, touch screens, haptic equipment, and specially designed hardware. For example, the TIM project used a specially designed keyboard and a scripting language to adapt existing educational games for visually impaired children (Archambault & Burger, 2000).

The clock reference system is another possibility, which combined with voice, can be used to let the blind users know about the location of items in the screen and for orientation purposes. This technique has been used successfully to indicate the position of atoms in molecular structures in a molecular editor that helps chemistry students with molecules interpretation (Fartaria, et al., 2013). Another example that uses this system is the MOVA3D game, which was designed to help visually impaired children with their mobility skills (Sánchez, Sáenz, & Garrido, 2010). This game uses 3D spatialized audio and a special haptic controller (a digital clock carpet) that uses the clock reference system for orientation purposes. This game was tested by blind and low vision school children in over three-hour eight sessions during a period of three months. It was observed that children who played the game could better estimate their location and orientation in the navigated space.

Haptic screens can be used as input devices for applications to the visually impaired. Provided that the users understand what regions of the screen they have to touch and how to touch them, users can interact with the application in this way. AudioPuzzle is game for the visually impaired that uses the Android's haptic screen as an input device (Carvalho, Guerreiro, Duarte, & Carriço, 2012). It consists of an audio puzzle, more specifically, it is a musical puzzle, in which the pieces are music segments. The players have to place the music pieces in the correct order by touching the screen with sliding movements.

Sound can be used in many ways to convey information to the blind. That includes speech and non-speech sounds. Non-speech sounds can be used to give information about location of a destination, a target to catch, of something approaching, the presence of an object or character, etc. One interesting possibility is to use spatialized audio, in particular 3D audio. When listening to these sounds, the user perceives that sounds are coming from different locations around him/her. In other words, the listener is able to indicate the approximate location of the sound sources.

AudioDoom is an example of a game accessible to the visually impaired that uses spatialized audio and has a very rich acoustic environment (Lumbreras & Sánchez, 1988). The goal of this game was to verify if some abilities of blind children, like spatial representation, can improve when the children have access to a highly interactive acoustic environment. During the game, the children have to save planet Earth from an alien invasion. For that the users have to locate the position of sound sources and coordinate haptic equipment (a joystick).

Terraformers is another game accessible to the visually impaired that uses very rich audio (Westin, 2004). It uses voice and spatialized audio, and demonstrates that audio can be used in several ways to convey information to the blind. Voice is used to give users access to objects, obtained through a system of voiced hierarchical menus. 3D spatialized audio is used to simulate an acoustic compass and a sonar. The sonar can be used to localize objects as it gives the perception of their direction and distance. The exact position (coordinates) of the objects and the main character's position can also be found with a simulated GPS.

The sound-based games AudioVida and AudioChile aim at helping children developing problem-solving capabilities and orientation and mobility skills (Sanchéz, 2008). These games use sound to help the user understand his location. AudioVida associates sounds to walls. When the user learns this association, he recognizes when he is close to an intersection. AudioChile uses variations on the intensity of the spatialized sounds to help the user understand his location. It was observed that blind children who use either of these games can show improvements on their problem-solving capabilities.

BlindFarm is another game developed for orientation and mobility training (Magnusson, et al., 2010). In this game, children have to localize the sounds of (virtual) animals that are placed in specific locations to help the children learn paths. Since the tests were done with only a couple of children, not many conclusions about the use of the game can be made.

Sound can also be used to code the color and light information in the images. The color information, or other properties in the images, can be converted into sound attributes, such that the sound reflects the properties of the images. This possibility has been explored by a few researchers. Though in order to learn how to associate colors to sounds requires training, and this possibility has been explored mainly in tools that are not games, we feel that this is a topic that it is worth discussing here because it can be used to convey visual information to the blind through sound.

Payling and his colleagues created HueMusic, a tool that associates hue values to timbres (Payling, Mills, & Howle, 2007). Their goal was to create sounds that reflected the color composition of the images. SeeColor is another tool that uses hue. It was created by Bologna and his colleagues, who have mapped the hue, saturation and lightness (HSL) attribute values into the pitches of known musical instruments (Bologna, Deville, & Pun, 2010). They argue that with familiar pitches it is easier to learn an association between colors and pitches. In addition to sonifying color, they also take into account depth, which is coded into rhythm.

An alternative is to map colors into sound location, as explored by Capalbo and Glenney in the Kromophone tool (Capalbo & Glenney, 2009). This tool detects color blobs and converts the red, green and blue (RGB) values of the detected colors, into pitch and pan. For each color, the tool plays three sounds simultaneously, one for each of the RGB values. Each sound has a different pitch and is played as if it were located in a different position of the auditory space (left, front and right).

Another possibility is to map the hue, saturation and value (HSV) attributes into sound parameters related to pitch, timbre and volume (Cavaco, Henriques, Mengucci, Correia, & Medeiros, 2013) (Cavaco,

Mengucci, Henriques, Correia, & Medeiros, 2013). The authors also used a fourth parameter in the tool, the pixel's abscissa, which was mapped into azimuth and was added to indicate the location the sound within the horizontal plane. This tool was able to deal with more hue values than HueMusic and SeeColor, which allows synthesizing richer sounds. Also, unlike the Kromophone, this tool can play more than one color at a time.

Finally, there is also the possibility of mapping the shapes in the images into sounds (Auvray, Hanneton, & O'Regan, 2007; Bach-y-Rita & Kercel, 2003; Meijer, 1992). The tool proposed by Auvrey et al. also considers the colors of the shapes. The tool converts color images and video frames into gray scale (with 16 gray tones) and then maps the position and brightness of the pixels into frequency and amplitude of the sound, respectively. Black is mapped into silence and white is mapped into the loudest sound.

ACCESSIBILITY THROUGH SOUND

In order to be effective, educational and rehabilitation games for the visually impaired must be accessible and fun. There are several options to make software accessible to blind and low vision users, and one of the most popular options is to use sound. This is one of the easier options to implement since it does not require special hardware.

Sound can be used in many ways to make software accessible to blind users. As seen above, the use of voice, spatialized audio and color sonification can give the user many different types of information usually available through text and images.

In particular, voice can be used to give the user information about everything that is happening in the game, instructions, and other relevant information. Below (section 4.1) we discuss the accessibility characteristics of the game "Código Pitágoras", a 9th grade math game that uses voice.

Spatialized audio is also a very powerful tool which can give the games an immersive feeling. The Audio Space Station game is a vision rehabilitation game that uses 3D audio to motivate blind and low vision users to train their orientation and mobility skills. This game is discussed in section 4.2.

Voice

The "Código Pitágoras" illustrates well how to use voice for transmitting different types of information. This is a mathematics game designed for 9th grade students and it is accessible to blind and low vision students. Though it uses some 2D sounds to guide the users through the scenes where they have to walk from a certain point to a specific destination, the most important accessibility feature of this game is the use of voice.

This game consists of a treasure hunt in the streets of Lisbon and nearby locations. The users have to discover a series of clues in order to solve the mystery and find a treasure. In order to discover the clues, they have to answer math questions. The game alternates between three distinct modes: story, adventure and learning mode. The objective of having these three modes is to keep the user motivated and interested while at the same time assuring that he/she has several learning moments.

In order to lead the blind and low vision user through the game's distinct modes, to explain what is happening and what the user's options are, the game uses mainly voiced audio. In particular, the game uses (recorded) speech to complement all its features: the menus, the dialogs between the game's characters, the questions, the results (correct/incorrect), feedback on the questions explaining the correct solution, etc. Figure 1 to Figure 3 show examples of the game's different screens[1].

Figure 1. Main menu

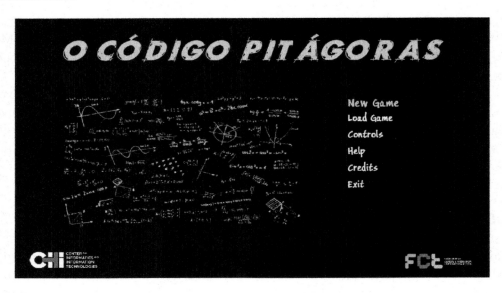

Figure 2. Learning mode: screen with a math question

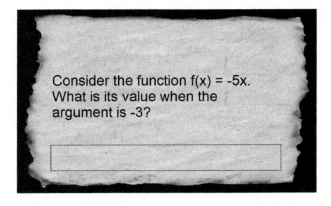

Figure 3. Story mode: an indoor conversation scene

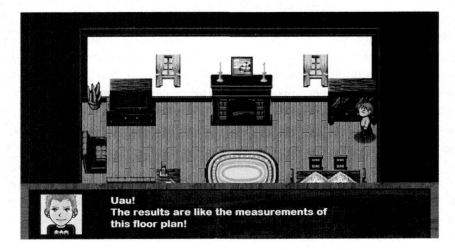

All written information is complemented with voice, such as the information in dialog boxes, menus, etc. Figure 1 shows the main menu, where the options appear written in the right hand side of the screen and are read with recorded voice. During learning mode, several math questions are presented to the user. All the math questions that the player has to answer throughout the game are written in the screen and complemented with voice (Figure 2). The user can introduce his/her answer with the keyboard. The answer will show up in the box that appears below the questions and all introduced characters are indicated with voice to allow blind users to double check what they are writing.

Once the user finishes writing the answer, the game indicates whether the answer is correct or wrong. If the answer is not correct, the game will explain (with written text and voice) what is the correct way of solving the problem. This feedback on wrong answers is an important feature of the game, the goal is that the student understands why he/she failed and learns how to solve the problems properly.

Story mode and adventure mode are also complemented with voice to allow the blind user to understand what is happening. After the user answers a set of questions in learning mode, the game jumps to story mode, in which a new clue is revealed along with instruction on where to go to find the next clue. Figure 3 shows an indoor scene in story mode, where the characters have a conversation about the math questions they have just solved.

Afterwards the user has to lead the main character in a map towards the location where the next clue is hidden (adventure mode). The next clue will only be revealed after the user answers a new set of math questions (learning mode). Due to difficulties found during the testing period in leading the main character in a map (in the adventure mode), we have included a new feature in the game: whenever the character bumps into a wall, there is a voiced indication of what happens.

As the reader may have noticed, all the screens include graphics and written text (for the menu, math questions, dialogs, etc.) The game was designed not only for blind users but also for low vision users. Therefore it has very simple, non-cluttered graphics with no overlapping objects and with big characters (when compared to the size of other objects in the scene). The characters have bright color clothes and hair. The choice of graphics was discussed with the teachers of blind and low vision students from two inclusive schools in the Lisbon area.

A second reason to include graphics is that we wanted the game to be sufficiently interesting for sighted students because we wanted to promote interaction between blind and sighted students. The written text was included because, though this game was especially designed for blind and low vision students, we also wanted to make it accessible to deaf students.

Results

The game was tested by students of two inclusive schools[2] following Virvou et al. and Ketamo's testing methodology (Virvou, Katsionis, & Manos, 2005) (Ketamo, 2003). Before the students had access to the game, they answered a nine-questions math quiz. After the testing period, in which the students had access to the game, they answered another nine-questions math quiz with the same level of difficulty as the first quiz. The game was installed in the student's laptops and during the testing period they could play as much as they wished and with no restrictions.

In addition, we divided the students in three groups, in which some students had access to the game's full version, some students had no access to the game and others had access to a test version which did not include feedback on wrong answers. Unfortunately, we could not use the results of all participants in the test, because, due to a very busy schedule and several school tests, some participants did not perform the complete test, i.e., they did not perform at least one of the quizzes or did not use the game during the testing period. So, even though initially each group had a few students, we only used the results of five students. The final groups were organized as follows: there was one group of two visually impaired students (one was totally blind and the other had low vision) who had access the complete version of the game; one group of two students (one sighted and one visually impaired) who did not play the game, and one sighted student with access to the game's no-feedback version.

Comparing the results from the two quizzes from the different groups (Figure 4) we can observe that the group of visually impaired students with access to the game's full version (that is, with feedback on wrong answers) was the group that improved the most. This group had an average of 3.5 correct answers in the first quiz and 6 correct answers in the second quiz. The student who played the game with no feedback, showed no improvement. The group of students who did not play the game also showed some improvements, yet the average improvement (0.6 questions) was lower than for the group with access to feedback on wrong answers (which improved on average 2.5 questions).

These results suggest that providing feedback on wrong answers is an important feature of the game. This helps the students understand where they are failing and helps them to consolidate the learned material. Moreover, the results also suggest that using voice is appropriate to provide information on what is happening in the game, on the options the user has, on the math questions and feedback. The visually impaired students who had access to the game's full version could understand all stages of the game and could take full advantage of the game which led to an improvement of their quizzes results. In addition, the students reported that they were able to play without the help of sighted colleagues or their parents and teachers, which seemed to be an important factor. Also, they enjoyed the game and the fact that this was specifically designed for them.

3D Spatialized Audio

Spatialized audio is a very powerful tool that can be used to give games an immersive feeling. On the other hand, it can also be used with rehabilitation purposes, such as for training orientation and mobility

Figure 4. Results from the two nine-questions quizzes

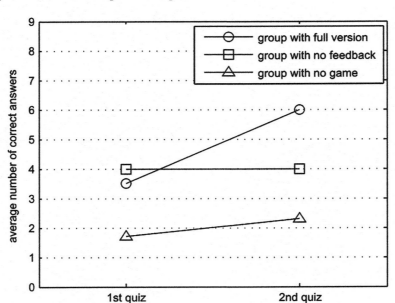

skills. The Audio Space Station game is a good example on how 3D sound can be used for this purpose. While other orientation and mobility training games have been developed, such as those proposed by Magnusson et al. (Magnusson, et al., 2010) and Sánchez et al. (Sánchez, Sáenz, & Garrido, 2010), (Sanchéz, 2008), these do not use 3D audio. As a consequence they lack the immersion needed to train certain orientation and mobility skills.

The Audio Space Station game is about a scientist working in a space station. This game, which was developed for the Android operating system, has three scored challenges in which the scientist has to capture or photograph live alien insects for latter analysis, or perform other tasks in the space station. The game was especially designed for blind and low vision users (Figure 5a). Therefore, the game can (and should) be played without seeing the graphics. Nonetheless, for the convenience of teachers and parents, the game has very simple graphics (Figure 5b).

The game uses 3D spatialized sound and requires the player to do accurate sound localization to catch insects or follow a robot in a virtual environment. The users should wear headphones and hold the smartphone in front of them. They do not need to walk (in the real world) but they have to turn around in order to face the sounds they hear. The main goal of the game is to train to perform accurate sound localization, while orienting oneself towards the sound. The game also aims at having the users do a simple rotation movement when turning to face the sounds.

The game uses the smartphone's gyroscope to determine the direction the user is facing, and the users interact with the game by turning and touching the phone's screen. Apart from 3D spatialized audio, the game also uses speech for the menus and vibrations of the device to indicate when an insect has escaped.

In the two first challenges, the player has to catch the insects by turning himself/herself and the phone towards the location of the insects and touching the screen to catch them. The sounds are either static (challenge 1) or move up and down around the player with a sinusoidal motion (challenge 2).

As an illustration, Figure 5b shows a scene of the first challenge. Note that the graphics are not used to play the game, these can be used by the teachers or parents just to have an idea of what is going on in the game and be able to help the child. The image shows the player in the middle of the room with an insect between 0° and 90° (where 0° is defined by the player's nose, 90° by the right ear and -90° by the left ear). Here the player should turn a bit towards the right (clockwise) in order to face and catch the insect.

Figure 5. Audio space station challenge 1: (a) a blind student playing the game; (b) a scene from challenge 1. The cylinder in the middle of the room represents the player, and the ball represents the insect.

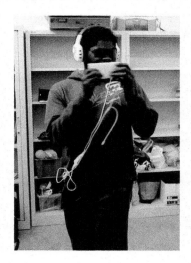
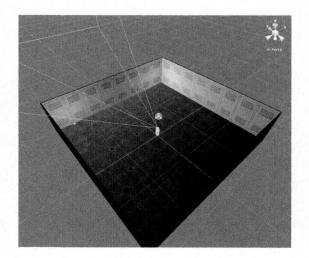

In the first two challenges the azimuth (challenge 1 and 2) and elevation (challenge 2) of the insects can vary. In the third challenge, in which the player has to follow a robot in a laboratory, the distance of the sound sources can also change. While the players do not have to walk in the real world, they have to simulate that they are walking in the virtual environment. Here the players can turn themselves and the phone to face the sound source and they can touch the screen to walk in the virtual environment. The sound of footsteps is heard when the players are walking in the virtual environment so that players know that they are moving.

Figure 6a shows a scene from the third challenge. Here the player (the thin cylinder) has to follow a robot (the fat cylinder) while avoiding the obstacles in the room (the two parallelepipeds). All objects in the room (robot and obstacles) produce sound so that they can be identified and localized. Also note that there are three types of floor in this room. The user can identify in which part of the room he/she is by the sound of the footsteps, which varies according to the flooring. Figure 6b shows the user's perspective for the same scene.

Audio Localization Cues

The signals that reach our right and left ears are not exactly the same and the brain uses their differences to determine the location of the sound source. In order to produce spatialized audio we can change the right and left channel signals to simulate what happens in the real world.

The differences processed by the brain include some simple cues like interaural differences, which measure the differences between the signal arriving at the left ear and the signal arriving at the right ear. These can be for instance time differences (interaural time differences) and intensity differences (interaural intensity differences). While these simple cues can be used to determine the azimuth of the sound source, they do not provide enough information to determine the exact location of the sound source in 3D space, namely its elevation and distance. In addition, there can also be ambiguity to determine if a sound is ahead or behind the listener. For instance, sounds at the front of the listener and back of the listener at angles x and $180°-x$ (Figure 7a), produce the same differences (when we do not consider the effects of the pinnae). In fact, there is a ear-centered cone of confusion in each side of the head (Figure 7b), such that the location of sounds coming from any point on the surface of the cone cannot be unambiguously determined based solely on interaural differences (Woodworth, 1938).

Figure 6. Audio space station challenge 3: (a) the tall cylinder represents the player, the large cylinder represents the robot and the other shapes represent obstacles; (b) the same scene from the player's perspective. The cylinder represents the robot.

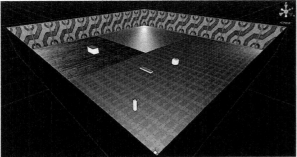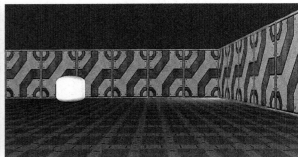

Figure 7. Representation of the head (facing 0°) and the direction of sound: (a) the location of sounds coming from ahead (from x degrees) and behind the head (from 180° - x) cannot be distinguished based solely on interaural differences; (b) Cone of confusion

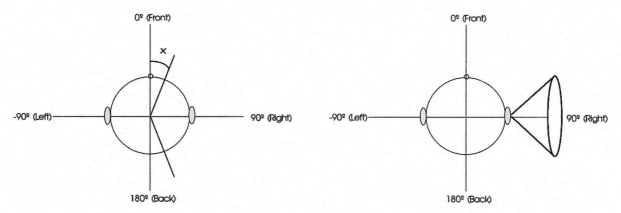

The signals that reach our ears are modified by the head, torso and pinnae. These changes are another cue that our brain uses to localize sound. In fact, we are able to distinguish whether a sound source is behind or ahead of us, as well as determining its elevation, due to the changes that the sound waves suffer when they transverse the pinnae. The pinnae act like filters that change the intensity of the high frequency components of the sound (Handel, 1989). The strange shape of the pinnae generates a series of reflected waves and the phase differences between the direct and reflected waves depend on the sound source's location. The final sound wave that results from the mixture of the direct and reflected waves is a new waveform whose frequency components have different amplitudes (when compared to the direct waveform). When a sound is known, these slight differences in its spectrum, along with the delays of the reflected waves, are used by the brain to determine if the sound source is ahead or behind of us and also to determine its elevation.

Experience is also important to judge distance. Though we are not very accurate at judging it, we can have a rough idea of the sound source's distance based on sound pressure, the spectrum and reverberation (Handel, 1989).

The Head Related Transfer Functions (HRTFs) characterize the spectral changes that the head, torso and pinnae cause to the sound. These functions are used to reproduce the direction-dependent acoustic filtering of the sound waves caused by the head, torso, and pinnae. More specifically, the HRTFs are acoustic frequency filters that depend on the source's azimuth, elevation and distance relative to the listener (Blauert, 1983). An individual HRTF characterizes the left or right ear frequency response to the audio signals coming from a specific location relative to that ear.

By changing the left and right channel signal with HRTFs, we obtain a pair of signals that when heard simultaneously (at the left and right ear) produce the perception of 3D spatialized sound. The Audio Space Station game uses HRTFs to produce 3D spatialized audio. In order to process the sounds with HRTFs we used OpenAL[3].

Results

We performed two tests to validate the Audio Space Station. The first was a preliminary test that aimed at determining if the students enjoyed the game and could understand and play it easily. The second was a usability test to determine if the players showed improvements in localization and mobility. Both tests were performed in an inclusive school. The tests were run indoors. In both tests, the participants played the game on a smartphone while wearing headphones (Figure 5a).

Preliminary Test

Five students, two girls and three boys between 8 and 19 years old, participated in the preliminary test. Two of the participants were totally blind, while the other three had very low vision. Some of the students needed a little help on the first trials (that is, to catch the first few insects), but after that they could play the game with little or no difficulties.

The results from this test showed that the students' estimation of the insects' locations improved. In the first challenge, the insects escape if the user does not catch them within a few seconds. We observed that while the first insect is hard to capture (4 subjects failed this insect), the subjects quickly adapted to the game and did not fail many insects from the first challenge. In this test, the insects in the second challenge did not escape and the players could take as long as necessary to catch them. It was observed that in average the users took 8.3 seconds to catch these insects and that the time needed to catch the insects improved as the users got accustomed to the game.

The test showed that the students understood how to play easily and enjoyed the theme of the game, except for the younger 8 year girl, which suggests that another more girly theme would be more adequate for younger girls. This test was also important to detect some features that needed improvement. Namely, we introduced a scoring system (already used in the usability test described below) that did not favor students who continuously pressed the screen in the hope of quickly catching the insects but without trying to perform accurate localization.

Usability Test

The second test had six participants, one girl and five boys between 11 and 14 years old. None of these students had participated in the preliminary test. Four of the participants were blind and two had low vision. The two students with low vision played the game without seeing the graphics. Other identified problems of the students were: Bardet-Biedl syndrome (one student), cerebral palsy (one student) and hyperactivity (one student). Four of the students had independent mobility, that is, they walked independently, while two of them were dependent on the help of a friend or teacher, that is, they held someone's arm while walking. A special education teacher was present in all trials of the test. She observed the reactions of the students and gave us very valuable feedback.

Each student played the game four times, that is, there were four trials at different times during two or three weeks. Only the first and second challenges were used in this test. Each trial consisted of playing the two challenges once, each with 15 insects (15 static insects in challenge 1 and 15 flying insects in challenge 2).

While some students had very good results (high number of caught insects) in all four trials, others showed an improvement on the number of caught insects from the first to subsequent trials. Also, it was observed that, in average, the number of missed attempts to catch the insects decreased from the first to subsequent trials. This later observation does not mean that the students were faster to catch the insects, just that when they decided to press the screen to catch the insect they chose incorrect directions less often. These observations show a learning pattern on the students characterized by an improvement on their localization estimation and/or their confidence on their estimations.

Along with these observations the students showed an improvement of freedom of movements and decrease in the inhibition to move independently both in rotation movements as well as in walking independently. While low vision users had no difficulty on turning themselves to face the sounds, blind users tended to fix their feet on the floor and only turned the upper body. This behavior was observed in the preliminary test and in the first trial of the usability test, but disappeared in subsequent trials. As noted by the special education school teacher who accompanied the testing, the game can have a positive impact in such motor coordination details.

It is interesting to note that the students who showed an improvement pattern on the number of caught insects, were the two students with dependent mobility. These students were not used to move independently, that is they were used to holding someone's arm or hand when walking. This led us to conclude that either at the beginning of the test they were apprehensive on turning around by themselves to catch the insects or they were also used to rely on a friend or adult to do the localization for them. Either way, the results from these two students, together with the observations from the special education teacher who watched the tests, suggest that the game can help children and teenagers with dependent mobility to gain more confidence on moving by themselves without the need to hold a friend's arm.

Above we referred that we noticed a decrease in the inhibition of walking independently. While the users did not have to walk in the real world, some students, including that with dependent mobility and cerebral palsy, got so enthusiastic with the game and so eager to catch the insects that they actually walked (a few steps) in the real world to try to get closer to the insects. The game made the students forget about their limitations and compelled them to move freely in the room.

CONCLUSION

Here we discussed the ways in which sound can be used in vision rehabilitation games for blind children and teenagers. These include the use of voice, spatialized audio and color sonification. In particular, we presented two computer games that use these techniques: one is a mathematics educational computer game, while the other is an orientation and mobility game.

The first game consists of an educational 9th grade math game that uses speech. This game uses voice signals to inform the user about everything that is happening in the game, instructions, information in the dialog boxes and menus, the dialogs between the game's characters, the math questions, the results (correct/incorrect), feedback on the questions explaining the correct solution, help to navigate in the adventure maps, and other relevant information.

The game was tested in two inclusive schools. The results showed that using voice to provide all the information mentioned above is appropriate. The visually impaired students who played the game's full version could understand all stages of the game and could take full advantage of the game, which, together with the feedback provided on wrong answers, led to an improvement of their results in a test quiz. The feedback the game gives on wrong answers is another important characteristic of the game. The aim of these explanations is to help the student understand the math material and learn how to solve the questions properly. In addition, the students reported that they were able to play by themselves with no help of sighted people. They also reported that they had fun while playing the games and wanted to reach the treasures. This together with the results from the two quizzes shows that this type of accessible games can help blind and low vision students spend time on practicing mathematics while enjoying the process.

The second game consists of an orientation and mobility game. The aim of this game is to train and develop orientation skills and a simple mobility skill (rotation towards sound sources). This game uses

3D spatialized audio obtained with HRTFs to motivate blind and low vision users to train their orientation and mobility skills. The 3D sounds give the game an immersive feeling.

The results from two tests with blind and low vision subjects in an inclusive school showed that the localization estimations improved with the game. We noticed an improvement on the number of correct location estimations and orientation towards the sounds.

This game is also especially useful to train motor coordination details related to rotating the body and to lose inhibition on moving independently. We, together with the special education teacher who accompanied the tests, observed improvements on the mobility of the players while they were playing. However when they returned to their normal routines, the mobility inhibition returned. This suggests that playing the game just four times is not enough but playing it further may have benefits on the students' independent mobility.

The results from the tests of both games show that this type of well designed fun applications can be important to the rehabilitation process of blind and low vision young people, also improving their self confidence and helping on their integration in the classroom, and ultimately in society. Well designed educational games can help the students spend more time practicing the school subjects and help them on learning the school curriculum, have higher grades and better opportunities in their future lives, which contribute to improve their quality of life. On the other hand, while orientation and mobility games can help blind students in general to train motor coordination details, these games can be especially useful to children and teenagers with dependent mobility.

Finally, we noticed that the blind and low vision students who participated in the tests described here were happy to have these games especially designed for them, and to be chosen to participate in the tests. The attention they were given helps the vision rehabilitation process. The fact that the students can play both games without the help of a sighted friend or teacher is also an important aspect of the games, which contributes to help the students on improving their self confidence and on learning to be independent.

REFERENCES

Archambault, D., & Burger, D. (2000). TIM (tactile interactive multimedia): Development and adaptation of computer games for young blind children. *Proceedings of the Workshop on Interactive Learning Environments for Children*, (pp. 1-3).

Auvray, M., Hanneton, S., & O'Regan, J. K. (2007). Learning to perceive with a visuo-auditory substitution system: Localization and object recognition with the vOICe. *Perception*, *36*(3), 416–430. doi:10.1068/p5631 PMID:17455756

Bach-y-Rita, P., & Kercel, S. W. (2003). Sensory substitution and the human-machine interface. *Trends in Cognitive Neuroscience*, *7*(12), 541–546. doi:10.1016/j.tics.2003.10.013 PMID:14643370

Blauert, J. (1983). *Spatial Hearing*. The MIT Press.

Bologna, G., Deville, B., & Pun, T. (2010). Sonification of Color and Depth in a Mobility Aid for Blind People. *Proceedings of the International Conference on Auditory Displays (ICAD)*.

Capalbo, Z., & Glenney, B. (2009). Hearing color: Radical pluralistic realism and SSDs. *Proceedings of AP-CAP*, (pp. 135–140).

Carvalho, J., Guerreiro, T., Duarte, L., & Carriço, L. (2012). Audio-Based Puzzle Gaming for Blind People.*Proceedings of the Mobile Accessibility Workshop at MobileHCI (MOBACC).*

Cavaco, S., Henriques, J., Mengucci, M., Correia, N., & Medeiros, F. (2013). Color sonification for the visually impaired. In M. Cruz-Cunha, J. Varajão, H. Krcmar, & R. Martinho (Eds.), *Procedia Technology. 9* (pp. 1048–1057). Elsevier.

Cavaco, S., Mengucci, M., Henriques, J. T., Correia, N., & Medeiros, F. (2013). From Pixels to Pitches: Unveiling the World of Color for the Blind.*Proceedings of the IEEE International Conference on Serious Games and Applications for Health (SeGAH).* doi:10.1109/SeGAH.2013.6665305

Fartaria, R., Pereira, F., Bonifácio, V., Mata, P., Aires-de-Sousa, J., & Lobo, A. (2013). NavMol 2.0 – A Molecular Structure Navigator/Editor for Blind and Visually Impaired Users. *European Journal of Organic Chemistry, 2013*(8), 1415–1419. doi:10.1002/ejoc.201201458

Handel, S. (1989). *Listening, An Introduction to the Perception of Auditory Events.* MIT Press.

Ketamo, H. (2003). An adaptive geometry game for handheld devices. *Journal of Educational Technology & Society, 6*(1), 83–95.

Lumbreras, M., & Sánchez, J. (1988). 3D aural interactive hyperstories for blind children. *International Journal of Virtual Reality,* 119-128.

Magnusson, C., Waern, A., Grohn, K., Bjernryd, A., Bernhardsson, H., Jakobsson, A., & Hedvall, P.-O. et al. (2010). Navigating the world and learning to like it: mobility training through a pervasive game. *Proceedings of the 13th International Conference on Human Computer Interaction with Mobile Devices and Services* (pp. 285–294). ACM.

Meijer, P. (1992). An Experimental System for Auditory Image Representations. *IEEE Transactions on Bio-Medical Engineering, 39*(2), 112–121. doi:10.1109/10.121642 PMID:1612614

Payling, D., Mills, S., & Howle, T. (2007). HueMusic – creating timbral soundscapes from colored pictures.*Proceedings the of International Conference on Auditory Displays (ICAD).*

Sanchéz, J. (2008). User-centered technologies for blind children. *Human Techn. J., 45*(2), 96–122. doi:10.17011/ht/urn.200810245832

Sánchez, J., Sáenz, M., & Garrido, J. (2010). Usability of a multimodal video game to improve navigation skills for blind children. *ACM Transactions on Accessible Computing, 3*(2), 1–29. doi:10.1145/1857920.1857924

Virvou, M., Katsionis, G., & Manos, K. (2005). Combining software games with education: Evaluation of its educational effectiveness. *Journal of Educational Technology & Society, 8*(2), 54–65.

Westin, T. (2004). Game accessibility case study: Terraformers – a real-time 3D graphic game.*Proc. of the The Fifth International Conference on Disability, Virtual Reality and Associated Technologies,* (pp. 95-100).

Woodworth, R. (1938). *Experimental Psychology.* New York: Henry Holt & Co, Inc.

ENDNOTES

[1] Since the game was tested in Portuguese schools, the original game is written and spoken in Portuguese. Yet, for convenience of the reader, here the figures were adapted to English.

[2] Inclusive schools are schools where special needs children are integrated in the same classrooms as regular children.

[3] http://openal.org/

Simulation for Medical Training

Cecilia Dias Flores
Federal University Health Science of Porto Alegre, Brazil

Ana Respício
Universidade de Lisboa, Portugal

Helder Coelho
Universidade de Lisboa, Portugal

Marta Rosecler Bez
Feevale University, Brazil

João Marcelo Fonseca
Federal University Health Science of Porto Alegre, Brazil

INTRODUCTION

General Perspective

In a recent meeting held in London in April, Wired Health 2014, it was discussed the future of medicine, along the fusion of healthcare with technology and under the motto "What gets measured gets done". Three elements are key now for envisaging artifacts, namely data, technology and design. Sensors, algorithms, big data, machine learning, nanotechnology, neurosciences, behavioral psychology and economics, are now adequate triggers for changing radically health and putting it under new tracks. All these topics are within the so-called Social Computation area where several disciplines come together to support aggressive applications for education, entertainment, business or healthcare. The goal is to build social systems, kind of artificial structures, designed and transformed by human action. In what concerns health, these systems may be very complex covering behaviors (predictions and explanations) and artifacts (e.g. for policies, methodologies for organization change, or transition management projects).

The aim is to boost efficiency in the services (monitoring vital signs remotely to detect impending problems) and, at the same time, to transform patient experiences with innovative tools capable to predict dis-functions before they happen (the data uploaded to distance servers where it is run through preprogrammed rules that flag up early signs of trouble). The idea is taking earlier decisions before things have actually gone wrong, and builds interventions we have never had the opportunity to consider before, tailored to a person´s profile. The vision of a connected and intelligent approach covers the ability to deal with illness, aging and fitness, by articulating detect with intervene and prevent.

Objectives

Part of the illness around us may be mitigated by education and changes of our own behaviours. But it is also necessary help patients to move from physical to digital (and connected) healthcare, by getting them to take their medicine when alarms are activated on account of simple symptoms. A policy of

DOI: 10.4018/978-1-4666-9978-6.ch064

early indicators (disrupted patterns) with tacking technology insures the follow-up of new diagnostic and therapeutic approaches. The innovation drive consists of moving from conservative and traditional social information processes toward emphasizing social intelligence, and by inventing new roles for information, Internet and mobile technology. Social intelligence and technology improves also our understanding about human behave and social interactions in human society at the individual, interpersonal and community levels.

This chapter focus on simulation for medical training. The literature review examines simulators in the area of healthcare and medical simulation. The chapter describes SimDeCS, the Intelligent Simulator for Decision Making in Health Care Services (in Portuguese, Simulador Inteligente para a Tomada de Decisão em Cuidados de Saúde) which is an end result of a large project for medical learning (Flores, Fonseca, Bez, Respício, & Coelho, 2014). Special focus is given to its architecture and the methodology employed in building clinical cases. SimDeCS plays the role of a virtual patient (Orton & Mulhausen, 2008; McLaughlin et al., 2008) and has been extensively evaluated (Barros, Cazella, & Flores, 2015; Flores et al., 2014; Maroni, Flores, Cazella, Bez, & Dahmer, 2013). Examples of clinical cases are presented. In addition, the chapter proposes future research directions in simulation for medical training and draws final conclusions.

BACKGROUND

Many studies have confirmed the effectiveness of simulation in the teaching of medicine and clinical knowledge as well as in the assessment at the undergraduate and graduate medical education levels (Okuda et. al., 2009). Several currently existing simulators propose to offer students safe virtual environments, where they can test and consolidate recently acquired theoretical knowledge in simulated clinical situations (Brookfield, 2005; Botezatu et al., 2010; Holzinger et al., 2009).

Table 1 presents examples of several types of simulators for healthcare from the literature.

Simulators provide learning environments for the playful application of acquired knowledge and eventually the evaluation of that process. The simulator can also be an open space where students exercise the decision making process in a more realistic framework; not only achieving a goal – such as making a diagnosis or choosing a therapy – but also understanding that different decisions will imply different financial costs, risks to the virtual patient and time expenditures. A simulation can, therefore, also show the student that although excessive research can lead to the correct final result, shorter and cheaper strategies may also lead to adequate results.

The development of simulators for healthcare is to a large extent on the use and refinement of Artificial Intelligence (AI). Simulators integrate AI in the form of algorithms that can handle concepts, heuristics use, knowledge representation, support for computation with inaccurate data, multiple solutions, and integrate machine learning mechanisms. According to Bourg and Seemann (2004), AI techniques can be divided into two groups: deterministic and non-deterministic. The first are predictable, easy and quick to implement, however, predictability restricts the simulation, after a few iterations the users realizes what the next states and events. Non-deterministic techniques facilitate learning by providing an unpredictable end to the simulation. Their difficulty lies in the implementation, computational tests, and validation of specific events. The types of simulators using AI are divided by Machado et al. (2009) according to their performance on two levels: the upper level control, referring to the decisions related to the course

Table 1. Examples of simulators for healthcare

Focus/Type	Software/Subject	Language/Environment	Validation
Motivational serious game	• Happy Farm (Gamberini, Marchetti, Martino, & Spagnolli, 2009) • Intensive glycemic control (Thompson et al., 2010)	Two-dimensional, side-scrolling, "platform" games and 3D environment	
Skills/Artifacts	• Videolaparoscopic simulator (Seymour et al., 2002) • The Emory Neuro Anatomy Carotid Training (ENACT)(Nicholson et al., 2006) • Personal patient simulation (Gibson, Grimson, Kanade, & Kikinis, 2000) – Simulator patented • Pressure Ulcer Simulator and Related Methods (Sparks, Sanger, & Conner-Kerr, 2012) • Patient Specific Planning and Simulation of Ablative Procedures (Mansi et al., 2014)	Virtual Reality	Best performance/ Error minimizations; Quantification of the learning curve
Strategies	• Cognitive forcing strategies in Emergency Room (Bond et al., 2004) • Training triage of incidents (Huizinga, 1971)		Assessment exercise based on tagging accuracy
3D Simulators	• JDoc (Sliney & Murphy, 2008) • *HAEMOdynamics SIMulator* (Holzinger et al., 2009)	• C++ • Several light-weighted JAVA2-Applets	Usability Questionnaire
Training	Cardiopulmonary resuscitation (Creutzfeldt, Hedman, Medin, Heinrichs, & Felländer-Tsai, 2010)	Massively multiplayer virtual world	A test-retest (6-month interval between sessions)
Educational Software	• Online virtual patients (Dewhurst, Borgstein, Grant, & Begg, 2009) • Web-based Simulation of Patients application (Web-SP) (Botezatu, Hult, Tessma, & Fors, 2010) • The Clinical Health Economics System Simulation (CHESS) (Voss, Nadkarni, & Schectman, 2005)	• Computerized team-based quasi-competitive simulator • Explorative linear-interactive virtual patient simulation	Usability Questionnaire

of action of the simulation, and the lower level of control, referring to the decentralized decisions in the course of the internal simulator decision making process. These systems, also known as knowledge-based systems have rules that replicate the knowledge of human experts, and are used to solve problems in specific domains. The main characteristics of simulators using AI are listed by (Plemenos & Miaoulis, 2009) and include: manipulation of concepts far beyond numerical data; use of heuristic methods to solve problems for which there are no known exact solutions; ability to representing knowledge explicitly; capability to manipulate inaccurate or incomplete data; possibility to obtain multiple solutions; ability to learn, including machine learning mechanisms that imitate human reasoning

Bayesian networks (BN), an approach in AI to emulate clinical reasoning, are an option to provide the structure of a medical simulator (Vicari et al., 2003). Achieving the most adequate diagnosis (and treatment) for a given scenario and changing choices, based on new evidence, make BN be similar to several features of medical cognition (Flores et al., 2005; Simel, 2007; Schwartz and Elstein, 2008; Niedermayer, 2008; Pearl, 2009). This advantage has been explored with other clinical decision support tools. A widely known experiment is the Quick Medical Reference – Decision Theoretic, which consists of a model wherein 600 diseases are related with approximately 4000 symptoms (Jaakkola & Jordan, 1999). Over the last two decades, the use of BN, as a basis for algorithms applied in medicine, was reinvigorated, including the addition of learning resources and automatic calibration based on existing clinical records (Ananthaswamy, 2011). The certification examination in family practice of the American Board of Family Practice was enlarged to consider computer-based case simulations (Hagen et. al., 2003).

INTELLIGENT SIMULATOR FOR DECISION MAKING IN HEALTH CARE SERVICES: SIMDECS

SimDeCS is a multi-agent computational environment that simulates patient care in a Basic Health Unit or during a house call, where the patient is a virtual character and the player is a medical student. During the process, the player receives interventions from an instructor whose goal is to drive the performance. Clinical cases are modeled based on clinical protocols and therapeutic guidelines that are formulated with rigorous quality parameters and represent the technical-scientific consensus.

The development of this virtual environment supports the medical teaching and learning processes, both at the graduate and specialization level. Trainee doctors in groups led by more experienced doctors discuss patient information, obtained by anamnesis and physical and subsidiary exams. Scientific literature is also used as a support source. This volume of data is analyzed, mainly by a teacher (or a group of teachers) who indicates which information should receive greatest weight in the decision process and which subsequent research and treatment stages are necessary.

Medical doctors, based on the information collected from the above described sources, attempt to establish a differential diagnosis from among the pathologies that may have led to the clinical findings found in the patient. Often new exams are necessary to supply supplementary information in order to narrow the scope of the diagnostic alternatives.

SimDeCS Architecture

The SimDeCS architecture (see Figure 1) consists of three layers. The lowest level is the content layer, which includes the techniques applied for knowledge representation and that supply the knowledge data base. Above the content layer is the communication layer that manages the interaction between the different system agents. The upper layer is the presentation one, developed in Flash, able to exchange information with the user and the communication layer through a Java Servlet. This servlet is a component, like a server, that manages HTML and XML data for the presentation layer of a Web application, a class in the programming language Java that dynamically processes requisitions and responses, thereby affording new resources to the multi-agent environment.

The *Domain Agent* represents the domain of the specialist's knowledge, represented by the clinical cases in the Presentation layer, while the *Learner Agent* represents the knowledge of the student. If the decisions taken by the student are different from the case information, the *Mediator Agent* – representing the tutor/instructor – attempts to motivate the learner to review their decision or obtain additional information on the case. The *Mediator Agent* guides the student using pedagogical strategies selected by an Influence Diagram (ID), explained below.

The content layer represents the storage of information about the clinical cases, the logs (records) of student navigation in the simulation as well as the dialog records of the characters and the processing of the ID (Bez et al., 2012) and BN (Flores et al., 2012).

The exchange of information among agents is essential for the simulator performance. The SimDeCS agents communicate on a Foundation for Intelligent Physical Agents (FIPA) platform.

BN and ID are representations, for communication purposes, in an XML (XBN) based format. In order to establish communication among agents a common structure of references and shared ontologies is necessary. This will determine how a specific message should be interpreted. From an implementation point of view, the format to encode probabilistic knowledge like BN and ID was the HUGIN[1] 's BN representation format.

Figure 1. SimDeCS architecture

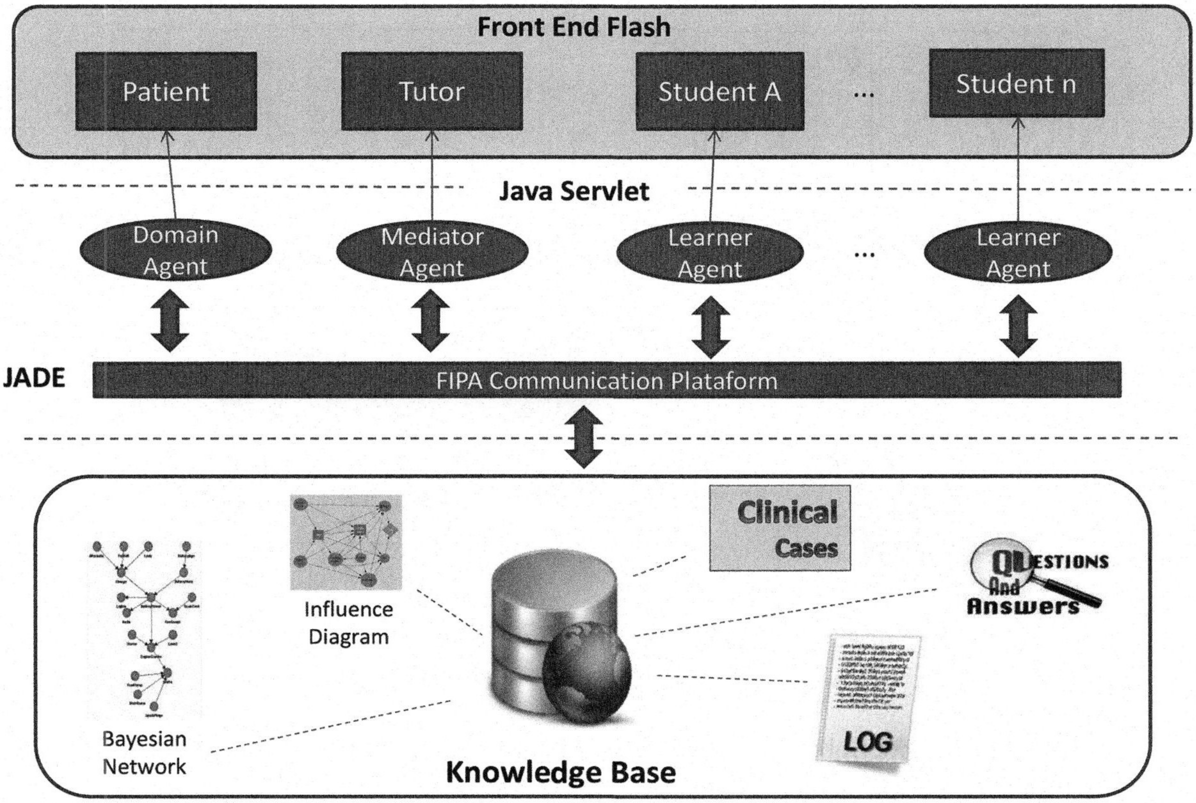

Communication along SimDeCS is established using a JADE[2] (JAVA Agent Development) framework that supplies alternatives for the development of agent-based technologies, accelerating the development process.

The Method for Building Simulations in SimDeCS

SimDeCS relies on three steps to build a simulation, as presented in Figure 2 and detailed in the following.

Step 1: Modeling the Knowledge Specialist.

In Step 1, the specialist practitioner structures the medical knowledge into a BN, using the Clinical Practice Guidelines as a basic resource. Some of the Brazilian Society of Family and Community Medicine guidelines were adopted for modeling by BN within the framework of the SimDeCS project. The clinical guideline for Headache, used as a testbed in the project, was written by Family Medicine doctors and offers the perspective of the specialty for the diverse ambulatory issues of the Headache problem (Pinto et al., 2012).

The elaboration of the BN is summarized as having three main moments (Pearl, 1988):

1.   Identification of the pertinent and relevant variables;

Figure 2. Steps of building a simulation in SimDeCS
Bez et al., 2012.

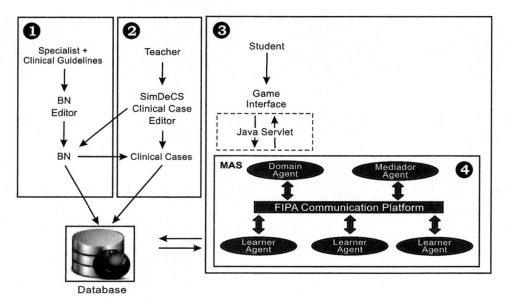

Database

2. Organization of these variables into the structure of a directed acyclic graph that represents their relationships; and

3. For each variable (node), obtaining the possible conditional probability values and prior probabilities for model propagation.

Guided by the presented semantic issues and with the three tasks in mind, one can define a method for building BN.

The database, the literature and the knowledge of the domain specialists are the usually accepted sources for the attribution of numeric values for the probabilities of each network node (Druzdzer & Van Der Gaag, 2000).

The method used to generate the BN begins by reading the text and isolating the clinical information that can influence the medical diagnosis or is related with the steps to be adopted. This bibliography search and choice of variables is performed by a domain specialist, using their knowledge as a reference for the choice of variables and the future connection among them. For the clinical guidelines about Headache, 30 variables were used to compose the nodes of the BN – some of which are described in Table 2.

The BN built according to this clinical guideline is presented in Figure 3. After separating important variables, nodes corresponding to clinical evidence reinforcing a diagnosis are connected to the corresponding diagnosis node (such the ones presented in Table 2). The calibration of probabilities is also done by the domain specialist doctor, using a specific tool for building the BN.

As a diagnosis emerges as predominant over others, a node also emerges as the most adequate. Note that analgesics ("Analgesia" in Figure 3), for instance, are the pertinent treatment for several diagnoses in the headache domain. On the other side, the frequency of crises can, within the diagnosis of migraine, determines the pertinence of a prophylactic treatment.

Once the network is built, the domain specialist simulates several typical and non-typical presentations of the diagnoses in questions. That allows for the adjustment of node probabilities so that the most probable diagnosis emerges, according to specialist clinical experience.

Table 2. Examples of nodes of the BN

Node	Description
Aneurysmal history	Family history of central nervous system aneurysm in more than one first degree relative
Facial pain	Pain in face not related with mastication
Fever	Presence of the symptom in patient anamnesis
Prophylaxy *	Prescription of prophylactic medication to decrease recurrence
Specialist *	Decision by the family doctor to solicit consultation by a specialist
Temporomandibular #	Dysfunction of the temporomandibular articulation
Tension-type Headache #	Tension headache

Represents a diagnosis node.
* Represents a clinical procedure node.
Remaining nodes represent anamnesis findings.

Figure 3. Bayesian Network built based upon the headache clinical guideline

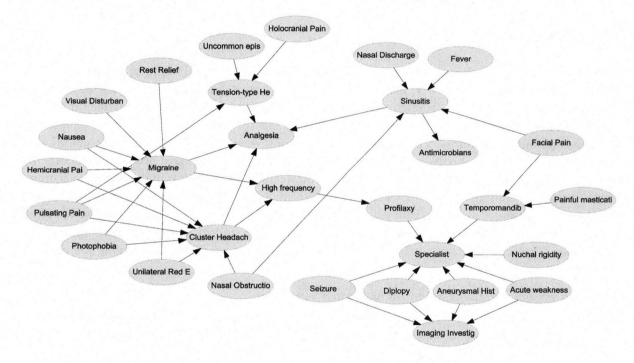

Each node of the BN has a colloquial phrase associated. Table 3 includes some examples of these sentences. The interface in which the player interacts is composed of characters in a medical office or a home environment. As the player inquires the virtual patient about their symptoms, using structured phrases, the player receives a response, in the form of a colloquial term, as modeled in the clinical case. The BN is inferred by the system and the probability of each node is converted, using a mapping of the answers into probabilities, as follows "always" and "almost always" are mapped into [90%-100%], "most times" and "part of the time" into [50% - 90%]; "few times" and "sometimes" into [10-50%]; and "never", "almost never", and "rarely" into [0-10%].

When the clinical interview is concluded, the player can formulate their diagnostic hypothesis given the options present in the game – these are highlighted as the most prevalent in the clinical guideline.

Subsequently, the player is led to take decisions about supplementary research, leading to a specialist or prescription of medication.

Step 2: Modeling clinical cases.

In Step 2, clinical cases are created by the teacher based on BN previously built by the domain specialist. By freely including symptoms and signs available on the network, the teacher propagates the probabilities and causes one or more diagnoses and their respective treatments to emerge, thus modeling the case that will be simulated by the students. The clinical cases are stored in the Knowledge Base. They are composed of the nodes selected by the teacher, and make up all the phases of the game (simulation): research, diagnosis and treatment. Additional information about the clinical case like exam images, auscultations and biological signs can be stored at Knowledge Base.

Some examples of clinical cases:

Case 1: Maria José

This case was to create a female character with complaints suggestive of a migraine. By adding Hemicranial Pain, as present in the BN, the default value of Migraine increases. By adding the Pulsating Pain symptom, Migraine will increase to a probability of 89%, becoming the predominant diagnosis, in contrast with others. The expected treatment is prophylaxis (given the frequency of crisis), followed by analgesics and, secondarily, a follow-up with a specialist (neurologist) given the magnitude of the symptoms. If the student directs his diagnostic hypothesis to the second most probable diagnosis, the decision system of the ID will consider the distance between the probabilities in the network according to the symptoms and signs modeled by the teacher. If the diagnoses have close probabilities (alternative diagnoses or differential diagnoses), the pedagogical strategies will take that similarity into consideration. If they are very discrepant, the strategies chosen to redirect the student will tend to be more incisive. The Figure 4 presents four screens from the SimDeCS simulator interface, representing the interface

Table 3. Some of the colloquial phrases associated with nodes

Node	Questions and Associated Answers
High frequency	Do you have more than four headache crises per month? _____I have more than four headache crises per month.
Tension-type Headache	"I think your headache is a type called tension headache."
Analgesia	"I'm going to prescribe analgesics. This is a medication that will relieve pain when it arises."
Uncommon episodes	Do your headaches occur approximately four times per month or less? _____ I have headaches four time per month or more.
Holocranial Pain	Does your whole hear hurt? Is the pain spread throughout the head? Does it hurt on both sides of your head? _____ all my head hurts. I feel pain _____ throughout my head.
Painful mastication	When you eat, do you feel pain or discomfort in your masticating articulation? _____ it hurts to chew. _____ feel discomfort or pain when I chew.
Specialist	"Considering your symptoms, I think it is necessary to refer you to a specialist for examination and treatment."
Nuchal rigidity	Is your nape hard, such that you can't touch your chest with your chin? _____ I feel my nape hard.

module of simulation construction, the research process, which is separated into groups: medical history (anamnesis), physical, and requesting (or not) complementary exams; the viewing of medical records of the patient; and the intervention of the simulator (*Mediator Agent*).

Case 2: Dirceu Cruz

When modeling, in the BN editor, a virtual patient called Dirceu Cruz, the intent was to create a young male patient with complaint of a Tension-type cephalalgia. The Holocranial pain and Nasal obstruction nodes were selected as present. When these two symptoms are propagated in the network, Tension-type cephalalgia arises as the most probable diagnosis (98%), followed at a distance (15%) by Sinusitis.

Step 3: Use of SimDeCS by students.

Step 3 corresponds to the execution of clinical cases by the final user (medical student). In this stage the *Learner Agent* interacts with the student through a kind of game with two players (student and simulator).

The student selects the clinical case to be solved and the simulator presents a summary of the case, the patient file and the interaction possibilities in the three phases of the simulation (Research, Diagnosis and Treatment). In the diagnosis phase, when the student asks the virtual patient a question, the simula-

Figure 4. Interface of the SimDeCS

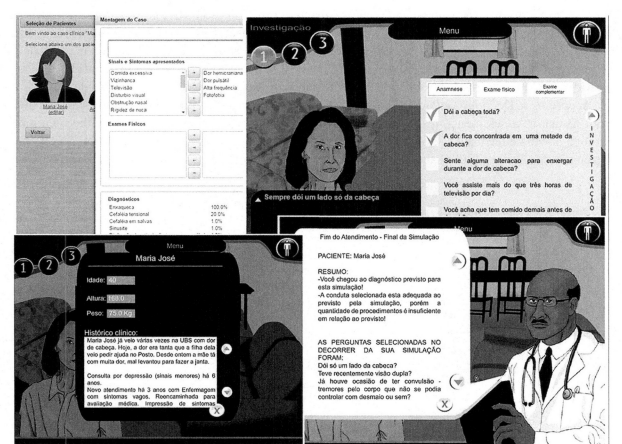

tor checks the network propagated by the teacher and obtains an answer that expresses colloquially the node probability referred to by the question.

Under the dialog form, the student has the possibility of formulating his diagnostic hypotheses by selecting the questions asked of the virtual patient, thus reinforcing or refuting them. The *Learner Agent* collects all the concrete evidence about the status of its learning process. Based on this evidence, the *Learner Agent* elaborates and updates the student mode, inferring the credibility (expectation) the system may have about the student, and also records the level of self-confidence declared by the student. A question concerning student self-confidence is asked at the beginning of the clinical case and at the end of the research, diagnosis and treatment phases. Credibility is obtained throughout the whole simulation process.

The *Domain* and *Mediator Agent* also interact reinforcing the role of the teacher in SimDeCS. The *Domain Agent* evaluates the student decisions. The result is sent to the *Mediator Agent*, in order to coordinate the whole interaction process. The interactions between the student and SimDeCS are viewed as a process of pedagogical negotiation (PN), wherein the *Mediator Agent* resolves differences using several pedagogical strategies. The role of the *Mediator Agent* is to measure the interactions between the student (*Learner Agent*) and the teacher (*Domain Agent*) in each phase. This agent uses an ID to choose the strategy that will demonstrate the best usefulness in each moment. The parameters used are the level of confidence declared by the student and the credibility (inferred by the *Learner Agent* given the actions of the student during a Simulation). The ID, pedagogical strategies and messages sent to the student are presented in Bez et al. (2012) as shown in Figure 5.

The ID is a variation on the BN (Flores et al., 2012; Pearl 1988; An et al., 2007). Its objective is to monitor the actions of the student and what is expected. From this comparison, pedagogical strategies emerge (Bez et al., 2012; Flores et al., 2005) that are sent to the student to positively reinforce him during the research phase, suggest corrections and manage the performance report. Between each phase of research, diagnosis and treatment the student is asked to declare his degree of self-confidence. This confidence modulates the interventions of the ID, through the pedagogical strategies (Table 4).

According to DePaola (DePaola, 2008), a way of improving metacognitive skills is to provide students with formative assessments, resources and opportunities that allow them to reflect on their learning through adequate feedback. Several authors of Virtual Patient simulators as Botezatu et al. (2010) and Orton and Mulhausen (2008) show the importance of feedback in the evolution of the clinical case. In

Figure 5. Influence diagram for pedagogical strategy selection

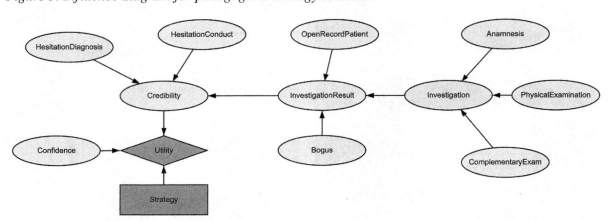

Table 4. Available strategies in the influence diagram

		Credibility		
		High	**Medium**	**Low**
Confidence	**High**	Extension	Contestation	Proof
	Medium	Proof	Contestation	Orientation
	Low	Support	Support	Orientation

Bez et al., 2012.

SimDeCS, feedback is provided by an intelligent agent, which monitors the progress during the simulation and adopts pedagogical strategies. The simulator provides interventions of the *Mediator Agent* between in each phase of the medical interview, physical exams, diagnostic hypothesis, conduct (comprised of prescription medication, new exams or forwarding to specialist).

Pilot Experiment

In a preliminary analysis of SimDeCS, we used an ongoing distance education environment directed towards health professionals in the field of Family and Community Medicine.

A pilot analysis of the simulator compared with the traditional testing method. Nineteen family physicians received individual usernames and passwords to access the virtual learning environment. They were invited to make a formal evaluation or to play with the simulator. The formal evaluation was composed of 15 multiple-choice questions based exclusively on the content of the clinical guideline. The simulation was composed of several clinical cases of headache in the context of community medicine. Of the 19 invited practicing family doctors only 12 completed both stages of the procedure.

The scores of the formal test and the simulator were compared. We did not obtain sufficient participation to allow for a Gaussian statistical evaluation of results. The small number of participants was insufficient for a comparison of performance using the simulator and in the formal test. In spite of this, the experiment could evaluate the pedagogical agent that selects and issue pedagogical strategies for students to undergo simulations of complex clinical cases in the SimDeCS. This evaluation got some interesting results published by Maroni (Maroni et al., 2013). Another evaluation done from this pilot experiment was the evaluating software based on the ISO / IEC 9126 standards and the ten golden rules for software in medical education published in (Barros et al., 2015).

FUTURE RESEARCH DIRECTIONS

The importance of (educational) technology in a digital world is greater than a decade ago. For example in education, MOOC´s (Massive Online Open Courses) increased their relevance, from 2012 on, and they present now advantages in what concerns traditional courses because they may be watched every time the students desire, playing an entirely different game at each time (see YouTube for a variety of these courses). MOOC´s expect that their participants will be motivated and will have learned how to learn. It is reasonable to assume they will learn to take responsibility when they are given responsibilities.

Also simulation tools seem suitable for medical education by creating virtual worlds easily switched on in several situations to face a young doctor and push him to think about the best options. BN´s, and other tools with intelligent agents, one of the powerful technologies around, may create environments where students can practice their skills by interacting with each other. In such virtual environments, students can learn by watching and joining in, and so to learn to be better reasoners, motivators and arguers.

Each individual is unique. Yet, we are cared as we were all identical. Today, any illness requires fast and acute diagnostics, in order to keep patients in a safer environment. A new look of healthcare requires new kinds of personalized medicines, towards precision and anticipation. For example, more tests are needed to reveal cancer presence (biological signature), drug resistance or bacteria transmission. Also, a new generation of tools will be capable to support sharp ways (earlier prescriptions, prognostic evaluation, therapeutic targeting, controllable and dynamic devices to detect malfunctions and infections in the body) to foresee what comes next.

A different line of research for medical diagnosis is to follow inspiration, and no longer causality. A doctor is always looking for ideas (ideation and action) when he is facing a complex case. Therefore, a different tool able to foster creativity is needed to draw ideas from a stream by generating opportunities to connect him to inspiration anytime and anywhere. The app Pinterest (2014) is very suggestive to help build another sort of tools, where discovery is articulated with guided search. The aim is to facilitate a kind of fluid creativity, and a short path is the curating ability of handling personalized streams of images. Collecting is a part of the creative process because collectors often recognize patterns, and this tool may spot patterns and make connections.

CONCLUSION

This chapter presents our perspective on simulation for medical training based on our experience on the development of SimDeCS, an educational tool that simulates providing medical care to a patient using a virtual character. This experience promoted the study whether the use of BNs as a pedagogical resource would be feasible. In addition, we investigated whether BNs would enable the student to model properly his knowledge, follow the student's actions during the learning process, make inferences through a probabilistic agent, and, also, select pedagogical actions that have the maximum utility for each student at each moment of his knowledge construction process. All these processes involve all the complexity and dynamics of a human agent learning process, but with the possibility of being followed by artificial agents and, therefore, are assumed to be probabilistic.

In addition, our research has been supported by our own vision on how to analyse, interpret and model the complex phenomena that occurs in the whole teaching-learning process, through modelling the student and even the process of pedagogical negotiation (Flores et al., 2005).

The temporality of the relationships among the nodes in BN generates problems in assembling the networks, on account of the false causal nexuses (Pearl, 2009). This problem is especially relevant for networks that express this type of causal relationship among variables (nodes) through time. Time dimension can be explored along two directions, one toward the past (to check the spectrum of alternatives), and another for the future (to advance predictions). Nevertheless, multiple causality can arise from contexts where each one and several different nodes have influence over a child node. The structural contingencies that can modify these influences, if modified through time, make it difficult to adequately represent this knowledge in the form of a BN (Pearl, 2009). Many of the correct medical practices have an ideal moment to be applied, behaving as if there were an adequacy time gradient that can be increasing, decreasing or vary irregularly. A procedure may benefit a patient admitted to the emergency room if done in good time, yet not benefit the patient (or potentially even be harmful) if performed later.

The current SimDeCS architecture does not integrate the time factor in the analysis of student performances. We envisage an improvement by relying on the Fuzzy Logic concept association. Many clinical decisions have a temporal relation, because adequate measures in the beginning stages of pathology can be inadequate at later stages, or vice-versa. In addition, often used concepts are context dependent and may have imprecise and variable meanings in different scenarios. To sum up, in our perspective there still are challenges and opportunities to increase the trustworthiness of the simulator as a learning environment, namely, by widening it for clinical situations even closer to real ones which encompass complex decision-making processes.

ACKNOWLEDGMENT

During 2010, the Brazilian educational agency CAPES through an open Call (Edital 024/2010) invited all the universities to propose projects in the area of healthcare education. This research around a simulator with probabilistic networks (SimDeCS) was accomplished in the following where a methodology to build up clinical cases with this simulator was further developed. We would like to acknowledge CAPES for all the supplied aid. We acknowledge FCT funding under project UID/MAT/04561/2013. We also acknowledge the anonymous reviewers of a previous version of the chapter.

REFERENCES

An, N., Liu, J., & Bai, Y. (2007, August). Fuzzy Influence Diagrams: An Approach to Customer Satisfaction Measurement. In *Fuzzy Systems and Knowledge Discovery, 2007. FSKD 2007. Fourth International Conference on* (Vol. 4, pp. 493-497). IEEE.

Ananthaswamy, A. (2011). I, algorithm: A new dawn for AI. *New Scientist, 209*(2797), 28–31. doi:10.1016/S0262-4079(11)60216-9

Barros, P. R. M., Cazella, S. C., & Flores, C. D. (2015). *Analyzing Softwares in Medical Education Focusing on Quality Standards*. Academic Press.

Bez, M. R., Flores, C. D., Fonseca, J. M., Maroni, V., Barros, P. R., & Vicari, R. M. (2012). Influence Diagram for selection of pedagogical strategies in a multi-agent system learning. In. Lecture Notes in Computer Science: Vol. 7637. *Advances in Artificial Intelligence–IBERAMIA 2012* (pp. 621–630). Springer Berlin Heidelberg. doi:10.1007/978-3-642-34654-5_63

Bond, W. F., Deitrick, L. M., Arnold, D. C., Kostenbader, M., Barr, G. C., Kimmel, S. R., & Worrilow, C. C. (2004). Using simulation to instruct emergency medicine residents in cognitive forcing strategies. *Academic Medicine, 79*(5), 438–446. doi:10.1097/00001888-200405000-00014 PMID:15107283

Botezatu, M., Hult, H., Tessma, M. K., & Fors, U. (2010). Virtual patient simulation: Knowledge gain or knowledge loss? *Medical Teacher, 32*(7), 562–568. doi:10.3109/01421590903514630 PMID:20653378

Brookfield, S. (2005). *The Power of Critical Theory: Liberating Adult Learning and Teaching* (1st ed.). San Francisco, CA: Jossey-Bass.

Ceccim, R. B., & Feuerwerker, L. (2004). A four-way approach to training in the health field: Teaching, management, care, and social control. *Physis (Rio de Janeiro, Brazil), 14*(1), 41–65.

Creutzfeldt, J., Hedman, L., Medin, C., Heinrichs, W. L., & Felländer-Tsai, L. (2010). Exploring virtual worlds for scenario-based repeated team training of cardiopulmonary resuscitation in medical students. *Journal of Medical Internet Research, 12*(3), e38. doi:10.2196/jmir.1426 PMID:20813717

DePaola, D. P. (2008). The revitalization of U.S. dental education. *Journal of Dental Education, 72*(2Suppl), 28–42. PMID:18250375

Dewhurst, D., Borgstein, E., Grant, M. E., & Begg, M. (2009). Online virtual patients - A driver for change in medical and healthcare professional education in developing countries? *Medical Teacher, 31*(8), 721–724. doi:10.1080/01421590903124732 PMID:19811208

Druzdel, M. J., & Van Der Gaag, L. C. (2000). Building probabilistic networks:" Where do the numbers come from? *IEEE Transactions on Knowledge and Data Engineering, 12*(4), 481–486. doi:10.1109/TKDE.2000.868901

Flores, C. D., Bez, M. R., Respício, A., & Fonseca, J. M. (2012). Training Clinical Decision-Making through Simulation. In Hernandez, J et al., Decision Support Systems–Collaborative Models and Approaches in Real Environments, Lecture Notes in Business Information Processing (vol. 121, pp. 59-73). Springer Berlin Heidelberg. doi:10.1007/978-3-642-32191-7_5

Flores, C. D., Fonseca, J. M., Bez, M. R., Respício, A., & Coelho, H. (2014). Method for Building a Medical Training Simulator with Bayesian Networks: SimDeCS. *Studies in Health Technology and Informatics, 207*, 102–114. PMID:25488216

Flores, C. D., Seixas, L. J., Gluz, J. C., & Vicari, R. M. (2005). A model of pedagogical negotiation. In. Lecture Notes in Computer Science: Vol. 3808. *Progress in Artificial Intelligence* (pp. 488–499). Springer Berlin Heidelberg. doi:10.1007/11595014_49

Frenk, J., Chen, L., Butta, Z., & Cohen, J. et al.. (2010). Health professionals for a new century: Transforming education to strengthen health systems in an interdependent world. *Lancet, 376*(9756), 1923–1958. doi:10.1016/S0140-6736(10)61854-5 PMID:21112623

Gamberini, L., Marchetti, F., Martino, F., & Spagnolli, A. (2009). Designing a serious game for young users: The case of happy farm. *Studies in Health Technology and Informatics, 144*, 77–81. PMID:19592735

Gibson, S. F. F., Grimson, W. E. L., Kanade, T., & Kikinis, R. (2000). *Personal patient simulation.* Google Patents.

Hagen, M. D., Sumner, W., Roussel, G., Rovinelli, R., & Xu, J. (2003). Computer-based testing in family practice certification and recertification. *The Journal of the American Board of Family Practice, 16*(3), 227–232. doi:10.3122/jabfm.16.3.227 PMID:12755250

Holzinger, A., Kickmeier-Rust, M. D., Wassertheurer, S., & Hessinger, M. (2009). Learning performance with interactive simulations in medical education: Lessons learned from results of learning complex physiological models with the HAEMOdynamics SIMulator. *Computers & Education, 52*(2), 292–301. doi:10.1016/j.compedu.2008.08.008

Huizinga, J. (1971). *Homo ludens: o jôgo como elemento da cultura.* Editora da Universidade de S. Paulo, Editora Perspectiva.

Jaakkola, T. S., & Jordan, M. I. (1999). Variational Probabilistic Inference and the QMR-DT Network. *Journal of Artificial Intelligence Research, 10*, 291–322.

Machado, L. S., Moraes, R. M., & Nunes, F. (2009). Serious Games para Saúde e Treinamento Imersivo. In Abordagens Práticas de Realidade Virtual e Aumentada. Porto Alegre: SBC.

Mansi, T., Sharma, P., Mihalef, V., Kamen, A., Rapaka, S., & Comaniciu, D. (2014). *Patient Specific Planning and Simulation of Ablative Procedures*. Google Patents.

Maroni, V., Flores, C. D., Cazella, S. C., Bez, M. R., & Dahmer, A. (2013). Development and Evaluation of an Intelligent Pedagogical Agent for the SimDeCS Software. *Procedia Technology, 9*, 1217–1226. doi:10.1016/j.protcy.2013.12.136

McLaughlin, S., Fitch, M. T., Goyal, D. G., Hayden, E., Kauh, C. Y., Laack, T. A., & Gordon, J. A. (2008). Simulation in graduate medical education 2008: A review for emergency medicine. *Academic Emergency Medicine, 15*(11), 1117–1129. doi:10.1111/j.1553-2712.2008.00188.x PMID:18638028

Nicholson, W. J., Cates, C. U., Patel, A. D., Niazi, K., Palmer, S., Helmy, T., & Gallagher, A. G. (2006). Face and content validation of virtual reality simulation for carotid angiography: Results from the first 100 physicians attending the Emory NeuroAnatomy Carotid Training (ENACT) program. *Simulation in Healthcare, 1*(3), 147–150. doi:10.1097/01.SIH.0000244457.30080.fc PMID:19088583

Niedermayer, D. (2008). An Introduction to Bayesian Networks and Their Contemporary Applications. In D. E. Holmes & L. C. Jain (Eds.), *Innovations in Bayesian Networks* (Vol. 156, pp. 117–130). Springer Berlin Heidelberg. doi:10.1007/978-3-540-85066-3_5

Okuda, Y., Bryson, E. O., DeMaria, S., Jacobson, L., Quinones, J., Shen, B., & Levine, A. I. (2009). The utility of simulation in medical education: what is the evidence?. *Mount Sinai Journal of Medicine: A Journal of Translational and Personalized Medicine, 76*(4), 330-343.

Orton, E., & Mulhausen, P. (2008). E-learning virtual patients for geriatric education. *Gerontology & Geriatrics Education, 28*(3), 73–88. doi:10.1300/J021v28n03_06 PMID:18215989

Pearl, J. (1988). *Probabilistic Reasoning in Intelligent Systems*. San Mateo, CA: Morgan Kaufmann.

Pearl, J. (2009). *Causality: Models, Reasoning and Inference* (Vol. 29). Cambridge University Press. doi:10.1017/CBO9780511803161

Pinterest. (2014). Retrieved September 9, 2014 from https://www.pinterest.com/

Pinto, M. E. B., Wagner, H. L., Klafke, A., Ramos, A., Stein, A. T., & de Castro Filho, E. D. (2007). Diagnóstico e tratamento das cefaléias em adultos na Atenção Primária à Saúde. *Sociedade Brasileira de Medicina de Família e Comunidade, 17*.

Schwartz, A., & Elstein, A. S. (2008). Clinical reasoning in medicine. In J. Higgs, M. A. Jones, S. Loftus, & N. Christensen (Eds.), *Clinical reasoning in the health professions* (3rd ed.; pp. 223–234). Edinburgh, UK: Elsevier.

Seymour, N. E., Gallagher, A. G., Roman, S. A., O'Brien, M. K., Bansal, V. K., Andersen, D. K., & Satava, R. M. (2002). Virtual reality training improves operating room performance: results of a randomized, double-blinded study. *Ann Surg, 236*(4), 458-463; discussion 463-454.

Simel, D. L. (2011). Approach to the patient: history and physical examination. In L. Goldman & A. I. Schafer (Eds.), *Goldman's Cecil Medicine* (24th ed.). Philadelphia, PA: Elsevier Saunders.

Sliney, A., & Murphy, D. (2008). *JDoc: A Serious Game for Medical Learning.* Paper presented at the Advances in Computer-Human Interaction, 2008 First International Conference on.

Thompson, D., Baranowski, T., Buday, R., Baranowski, J., Thompson, V., Jago, R., & Griffith, M. J. (2010). Serious Video Games for Health How Behavioral Science Guided the Development of a Serious Video Game. *Simulation & Gaming, 41*(4), 587–606. doi:10.1177/1046878108328087 PMID:20711522

Vicari, R. M., Flores, C. D., Silvestre, A. M., Seixas, L. J., Ladeira, M., & Coelho, H. (2003). A multiagent intelligent environment for medical knowledge. *Artificial Intelligence in Medicine, 27*(3), 335–366. doi:10.1016/S0933-3657(03)00009-5 PMID:12667742

Voss, J. D., Nadkarni, M. M., & Schectman, J. M. (2005). The Clinical Health Economics System Simulation (CHESS): A teaching tool for systems- and practice-based learning. *Academic Medicine, 80*(2), 129–134. doi:10.1097/00001888-200502000-00004 PMID:15671315

ENDNOTES

[1]   HuginR, avaliable at http://www.hugin.com
[2]   JAVA Agent Development available at http://jade.tilab.com/

Towards a Framework for Measuring E–Health Status across the World

Marina Jovanovic-Milenkovic
University of Belgrade, Faculty of Organizational Sciences, Serbia

Veljko Jeremic
University of Belgrade, Faculty of Organizational Sciences, Serbia

INTRODUCTION

The evaluation and development of health systems of countries and provinces is frequently elaborated in various articles (Sang, Wang & Yu, 2014). All of them share a general thought of health sector as the concept of immense importance for well-being of nations (Arber, Fenn & Meadows, 2014). With the exponential growth in information-communication technologies (ICTs), which created a wealth of opportunities for societies around the world (Ayanso, Cho & Lertwachara, 2014), ICTs introduction in the health care system has led to many changes and has consequently provided a powerful platform for changing the way people deal with health issues (Kuehn, 2011). Accordingly, more than 60% of Americans have used the platform to acquire health information (Mackart, Champlin, Holton, Munoz & Damasio, 2014). Today's medical field is very different from what it was just a decade ago as exemplified by the use of medical informatics, novel surgical equipment and modern testing techniques (Yadav & Poel-labauer, 2012). The technological advances, medical development, better, and more efficient services have improved the human quality of life and life expectancy, leading to a new paradigm for health care service providers (Gomes, Sperandio, Peles, Borges, Brito, & Almada-Lobo, 2013).

Our chapter is firstly oriented towards emphasizing the importance of health-care system evaluation. Due to the importance and impact the status of health has for its population, a state implements a large number of measures in health-care system planning and management in order to ensure steady financing and a rational, high-quality health-care system, and to provide basic health protection to its citizens within available resources (Jovanovic-Milenkovic, 2011; Frenk, 2010; Vujin & Jovanovic-Milenkovic, 2012). Consequently, the introduction of information system increases the efficiency, productivity and work quality of a health organisation; it also evaluates the work done, eliminates data duplication, and provides a more comprehensive use of data (Jovanovic Milenkovic, Milenkovic & Dobrota, 2012; Jeremic & Jovanovic-Milenkovic, 2014). Nowadays there are many attempts to enhance the quality of e-Health concept even more by implementing cloud computing (Sultan, 2014; Zapater, Arroba, Ayala, Moya & Olcoz, 2014; Vilaplana, Solsona, Abella, Filgueira & Rius, 2013; Milenkovic, Jovanovic Milenkovic, Vujin, Aleksic & Radojicic, 2012; Jeremic, Jovanovic-Milenkovic, Radojicic & Martic, 2013).

Secondly, we will point out to a continuous need for a comparison as an imperative for validating the progress over time (Kell & Kell, 2014). Hence, an appropriate methodology for evaluation and ranking of countries e-Health progress is a necessity.

DOI: 10.4018/978-1-4666-9978-6.ch065

BACKGROUND

The rapid usage of the Internet is also altering the traditional relationship between doctors and their patients. More and more people use the Internet to address their health and wellness needs and concerns, and the Internet enables patients to assume much greater responsibility for their health care (Ballas, 2001).

Application of information-communication technologies (ICT) in health care tends to expand the focus of resource management to knowledge management and process management. Integration of information-communication technologies in health care was performed to provide better health services for patients, by achieving mobility of people. ICT in health care providing the opportunity to control and analyse the total healthcare system in terms of quality and economy, and thus to the possibility of managing total health systems. Depending on its socio-economic opportunities, each country makes efforts to find out the best way to solve problems of management and control of its health system (Milenkovic, Jovanovic Milenkovic, Vujin, Aleksic & Radojicic, 2012).

The electronic health system called e-Health. It was created by the application of ICT, which fundamentally changed medical practice, enabling a significant increase in efficiency and quality of health service through a more logical and effective use of available resources. The term "e-Health" encompasses a wide purview of medical services used with the help of information technologies.

Today there are many definitions of e-Health. Eysenbach (2001) defined e-Health as "an emerging field in the intersection of medical informatics, public health and business, referring to health services and information delivered or enhanced through the Internet and related technologies. The term characterizes not only a technical development, but also a state-of-mind, an attitude, a way of thinking, and a commitment for networking, global thinking, improving health care locally, regionally, and worldwide by using information-communication technology" (Eysenbach, 2001).

E-Health is a term used to describe the use of information-communication technologies over a wide spectrum of health-care system functions. Innovative and well-thought-out applications of this new technology are able to increase the consistency, reliability, and quality of information delivered (Robertson, Ann et al. 2010; Milenkovic, Jovanovic Milenkovic, Vujin, Aleksic & Radojicic, 2012). The features and solutions of e-Health include products, systems, and support services that go by and simple Internet-based applications: in addition to those designed for medical experts and professionals, there are also ones designated to include the active participation of patients in their own healthcare (Jovanovic-Milenkovic, Jeremic & Martic, 2014).

The e-Health system encompasses the following essential services (Milenkovic, Jovanovic Milenkovic, Vujin, Aleksic & Radojicic, 2012):

- An electronic medical record is the first step towards more efficient and higher quality healthcare system. It contains useful information for all actors in the system.
- Electronic medical records are typically computerized regular medical records created in an organization that delivers care, such as hospitals or doctor's surgeries. An electronic medical record tends to be part of a local stand-alone health information system that allows storage, retrieval and manipulation of records.
- Telemedicine is a service that includes all types of physical and psychological measurements that do not require a patient' visit to a specialist. Owing to this service, a patient doesn't have to travel often, and a specialist can cover a wider geographical area.

- Evidence-based medicine is a service which includes a system that contains information about the current state of a patient. A specialist can check whether the diagnosis coincides with the current scientific research achievement. The advantage of this service is that data is always up-to-date.
- Citizen-oriented information provision is a service that potentiates physicians and patients to be informed about the latest medical knowledge.
- Specialist-oriented information provision is a service that permits physicians to follow the best experience in practice, the most recent editions of medical journals and epidemiological monitoring.
- A virtual healthcare team is a virtual service representing a team of physicians who collaborate with each other and ensure necessary information to patients via e-mail (e-mail, web portals, forums).
- The main benefits derived from the use of e-Health system are the following: efficiency in giving health care – the initiation of electronic communication model between patients and physicians; health care costs reduction; employees' productivity growth; maintenance of medical service quality by the use of electronic knowledge management; providing the right information in real time by the use of the internet.

E-Health has been under development for four decades. In the European Union, the first foundations of e-Health were determined in the late 1980s. Pilot studies were co-financed as early as the second stage of the European Union. From an initial funding of €20 million in 1988, the investment in this domain of research and development later outspreaded tenfold during its Sixth Framework Programme (2002 to 2006). The Commission co-financed the Seventh Framework Programme that run from 2007 to 2013. (Eucarinet, 2012; Whitehouse & Duquenoy, 2011). Large amounts of co-financed funds are now being invested in the deployment of e-Health. The research and development commitment of the Commission has been paralleled by the work on the practical aspects of e-Health in the Competitiveness and Innovation Framework Programme (CIP) Information and Communication Technologies Policy Support Programme (PSP) (Whitehouse & Duquenoy, 2011).

The European Union formulated the program of action for the electronic health system, both to the benefits of employees in healthcare as well as to patients. It included a survey of best practices for e-Health (2005), setting up pilot projects and common standards for exchanging electronic patient records (2006). It also made a request for "better provision of information to patients on how to obtain treatment in other Member States" (Van Dijkum & Vegter, 2010). Later on (2007, 2008) a number of targets were formulated such as: providing implementation of clinical tools such as tele-consultation; creating a European electronic health card; the fulfillment of Health Information Networks to expedite the flow of health information through a healthcare system. The European Union took care of the patient's side. It is crucial that health information can be transferred with patients' agreement and securely. In the case of the provision of healthcare through electronic means, it is considered that a citizen is someone who has a legitimate desire to access health information in general and/or his or her own health information specifically" (Angaran, 2006; Van Dijkum & Vegter, 2010).

In recent years, the actors - patients, health providers, government health departments, pharmaceutical industry and others – have become aware of opportunities to use the Internet and related technologies with several levels of benefits to different users. Many pilot projects throughout the world showed the clinical and organisational benefits that can be achieved through the application of e-Health technologies (Carrasqueiro & Monteiro, 2010).

FRAMEWORKS FOR MEASURING E-HEALTH STATUS

Composite Index

Measuring the area of e-Health status, as many researchers argue, is dominated by economic and organizational aspects, without a standard framework for evaluating the effects and outputs of implementation and use, and the area, in general, is both under-developed and under-managed in theory and practice (Hamid & Sarmad, 2011). Most of the existing frameworks for measuring that have been proposed or used in e-Health context are suffering from several limitations. In particular, the aspect of integrating variables/indicators with different measurement units proved to be an issue of a great concern. In order to provide more impartial rankings and adequate policy implications, the use of the composite index (Arndt et al., 2013; Guttorp & Kim, 2013; Saisana et al., 2011) emerged as a viable solution. Composite indicators as tools to compare countries' performances are increasingly common (Saisana & Tarantola, 2002; Saisana & D'Hombres, 2008). Oversimplified, a composite indicator synthesizes the information included in a selected set of indicators and variables (Paruolo et al., 2013).

The output of a composite indicator is a set of scores indicating the relative performance of a country within a set of countries (Brügermann & Patil, 2011). A composite is thus a measure of similarity (Saltelli, 2007; Paruolo et al., 2013). The primary virtue of composite indicators is their usefulness for policy analysis in that they can summarise complex and sometimes inaccessible issues in wide ranging fields, e.g., environment, society, technological or economy development. Composites often appear easier to interpret than finding a common trend in many separate indicators and have proven useful in benchmarking country performance (Maricic & Kostic-Stankovic, 2014).

Each multi-criteria performance measurement is formed as a certain composite indicator, and its stability ensures the amount of safety of the observed system. The selection of an appropriate methodology is crucial to any attempt to capture and summarize the interactions among the individual indicators included in a composite indicator or a ranking system (Saisana & Tarantola, 2002; Saisana & D'Hombres, 2008; Dobrota, Bulajic, Bornmann & Jeremic, 2015c). The e-Health evaluation framework emerges as one of the potential application of composite index. Although Europe's countries have made substantial progress towards modern e-Health infrastructures and implementations, the need to formalize a framework for evaluating the progress in the area of e-Health is not fully met. Even though there have been attempts to provide e-Health ranking models (Moghad-Dasi & Rabiei, 2013), the issues with composite indicators remain. Among others, the choice of variables and weights has been frequently elaborated in various publications (Soh, 2013a, 2013b). In this chapter we will emphasize the significance of selecting appropriate indicators, which can provide an in-depth picture of the e-Health status of a country. However, the main focus of our work will be on how to provide a statistically sound rationale for weight choice in producing a composite index score, thus providing more impartial results.

An important area of research is measuring e-Health status. It could contribute to significant knowledge that can be used to support the value of available e-Health projects, and to enhance the quality and efficiency of future e-Health initiatives (Hamid & Sarmad, 2011). Measuring e-Health services bring to the main objective. It includes, among others (Codagnone & Lupiañez-Villanueva, 2011):

- Reduce medical errors, associated costs and drug adverse events (i.e. through computerised reporting systems for adverse events, electronic health records, ePrescription of diagnostic procedures, etc);

- Minimize in-patient costs while improving health outcomes (telemonitoring);
- Improve adherence to prescriptions (through telemonitoring and reminders);
- Support and improve the work of professionals in different ways (PACS systems, tele-radiology, computerised physician order entry, online transmission of clinical tests results);
- Streamline and make hospital administration more efficient (Integrated computerised systems for order entry, billing, discharging, etc);
- Enhance access and convenience for users (access to their electronic health records, eBooking, portability of their information across the system, etc).

Naturally, the European Commission is not the only stakeholder focusing on or prioritizing e-Health and a lot of studies (Stroetmann, Artmann & Stroetmann, 2011) have shown how an increasing number of Member States have developed their own e-Health strategies and supporting instruments. Industry is also very present with several initiatives and nine European Technology Platforms (ETPs) (Codagnone & Lupiañez-Villanueva, 2011).

Composite Indexes represent a way of providing more compact information from large quantity of data. Composite Indexes have their advantages such as the following:

- Summarize complex or multi-dimensional issues for decision-makers
- Provide the big picture and are easier to interpret than trying to find a trend in many separate indicators, facilitating so the task of ranking countries on complex issues.
- Help attracting public interest by providing a summary figure with which to compare the performance across countries and their progress over time.
- Help reduce the size of a list of indicators or to include more information within the existing size limit.

I-Distance Method

As a possible remedy to the subject of subjectively given weights, here we used the I-distance method. Ivanovic originally devised this method to rank countries according to their level of development on the basis of several indicators (Ivanovic, 1977, Al-Lagilli, Jeremic, Seke, Jeremic & Radojicic, 2011). Many socio-economic development indicators had first been taken into consideration, whereupon the problem of how to utilize all of them in order to calculate a single synthetic indicator that would thereafter represent the rank was addressed.

For a selected set of variables $X^T = \left(X_1, X_2, \ldots X_k \right)$ is chosen to characterize the entities, the I-distance between the two entities $e_r = \left(X_{1r}, X_{2r}, \ldots X_{kr} \right)$ and $e_s = \left(X_{1s}, X_{2s}, \ldots X_{ks} \right)$ is defined as

$$D(r,s) = \sum_{i=1}^{k} \frac{\left| d_i(r,s) \right|}{\sigma_i} \prod_{j=1}^{i-1} \left(1 - r_{ji.12\ldots j-1} \right)$$

where $d_i(r,s)$ is the distance between the values of variable X_i for e_r and e_s, e.g. the discriminate effect,

$$d_i(r,s) = x_{ir} - x_{is}, i \in \left\{ 1, \ldots k \right\}$$

σ_i the standard deviation of X_i, and $r_{ji.12...j-1}$ is a partial coefficient of the correlation between X_i and X_j, $(j < i)$ (Dobrota, Jeremic, & Markovic, 2012).

The construction of the I-distance is iterative and is calculated through the following steps (Jovanovic, Jeremic, Savic, Bulajic & Martic, 2012):

- Calculate the value of the discriminate effect of the variable X_1 (the most significant variable that provides the largest amount of information on the phenomena which is to be ranked).
- Add the value of the discriminate effect of X_2 which is not covered by X_1.
- Add the value of the discriminate effect of X_3 which is not covered by X_1 and X_2.
- Repeat the procedure for all variables.

In some instances it proves impossible to achieve the same sign mark for all variables in all sets, and, as a result, a negative correlation coefficient and a negative coefficient of partial correlation may occur (Radojicic & Jeremic, 2012). This makes the use of the square I-distance even more desirable. Therein, the square I-distance is given as:

$$D^2\left(r,s\right) = \sum_{i=1}^{k} \frac{\left|d_i^2\left(r,s\right)\right|}{\sigma_i^2} \prod_{j=1}^{i-1} \left(1 - r_{ji.12...j-1}^2\right)$$

In order to rank the selected entities, it is essential to have one entity fixed as a referent in the perceiving set using the I-distance methodology (Dobrota et al., 2015b). The entity with the minimal value for each indicator or a fictive minimal entity should be then utilized as the referent entity, as the ranking of the entities in the set is based on the calculated distance from the referent entity (Seke, Petrovic, Jeremic, Vukmirovic, Kilibarda, & Martic, 2013).

RESULTS AND DISCUSSION

As the basis of measuring e-Health status across the world, we analyzed the data on European countries. There are several reasons for this approach. It was done comparing the data obtained in the paper of the authors Codagnone and Lupiañez-Villanueva (2011). The data were collected in hospitals in 30 countries in Europe in 2010, more precisely, in each of the 27 EU member states, plus Croatia, Iceland and Norway.

The survey measured values grouped into four dimensions:

- **A:** Infrastructure:
  - **A1:** Physical oriented (Sub-dimension).
  - **A2:** Services oriented (Sub-dimension).
- **B:** Applications and integration:
  - **B1:** Clinical & Image (Sub-dimension).
  - **B2:** EPR & patient management Intramural (Sub-dimension).
  - **B3:** Patient access and safety (Sub-dimension).
  - **B4:** PHR & tele-monitoring Extramural.
- **C:** Information flow:
  - **C1:** Country (Sub-dimension).

- ◦ **C2:** Health professionals (Sub-dimension).
- ◦ **C3:** Medication list (Sub-dimension).
- ◦ **C4:** Hospital (Sub-dimension).
- **D:** Security and privacy:
  - ◦ **D1:** Encryption.
  - ◦ **D2:** Regulation.
  - ◦ **D3:** Workstation.

Intelligent technology infrastructure contibutes each patient's journey through the healthcare process. In many areas of the world patients now have more choices as to where they obtain their healthcare. Neverethless, the experience a patient has while in hospital will likely impact their decision to comeback when they next need care (Robertson, 2013). The different parts of an infrastructure are often acquired by individual actors and independently. To make the overall infrastructure work they must fit together. Consequently, standardized interfaces (protocols) between components are crucial for making infrastructures (Hanseth & Lundberg, 2001). When we say the infrastructure, we mean the Physical oriented and Services oriented infrastructure. The term physical infrastructure is used to refer to a very wide array of systems and infrastructure that makes it possible for goods, services and people to be transferred from one geographical place to another. The physical infrastructure can have a major impact on the performance, efficiency and reliability of data center. Service oriented infrastructure is a systematic means for reporting Information Technology infrastructures in terms of services. Where Service Oriented Infrastructure manages to distinguish itself is the way in which it ensures a framework for making Business benefits measurable. Physical infrastructure represents Computer system connected and Broadband above 50MBps. Service oriented infrastructure represents two factors: wireless communication and videoconference facilities (Zhang, Yu & Chin, 2005).

The use of IT applications is thus rapidly evolving beyond what in the past was considered a clinical information system. Healthcare IT now covers new tools and healthcare services that are delivered or enhanced through the Internet and other advanced networking technologies. These applications have been deployed to support particular functions in healthcare organizations (Khoumbati & Themistocleous, 2006). Applications and integration have four sub-dimensions: Clinical & Image, EPR & patient management Intramural, Patient access and safety, Personal Health Record (PHR) & tele-monitoring Extramural. Clinical & Image includes applications more directed to the professional side of core clinical activities such as: clinical tests; diagnostics results; Picture archiving and communication systems (PACS) and tele-radiology. Electronic Patient Record (EPR) & patient management Intramural captures an orientation to the patient for what concerns his/her intramural management. Patient access and safety means that the information is protected. Finally, Personal Health Record (PHR) & tele-monitoring Extramural include access to health data that is monitored and used in an emergency situation. By this we mean the use of the following applications: Electronic Patient Record (EPR), Integrated system for billing management, Electronic appointment booking system, Electronic Clinical Tests, Picture archiving and communication systems (PACS), Electronic service order placing (e.g. diagnostic results/test), Integrated system to send electronic discharge letters, Adverse health events report system, Integrated system for tele-radiology, Integrated system to send or receive electronic referral letter, Computerized system for ePrescribing, Tele-homecare/tele-monitoring services to outpatients (at home), Personal Health Record (PHR). Consumer health IT applications that permit gathering and integrating data from different health care sources. Consumer health IT applications can also be important in emergency situations to provide critical health information to medical staff (AHRQ National Resource Center, 2014).

Hospitals exchange different types of information electronically (clinical information; laboratory results; medical list information and/or radiology reports) with different types of external actors (another hospital, general practitioners, specialists, healthcare providers in other EU or non EU countries). Information flow has four sub-dimensions: Country, Health professionals, Medication list and Hospital. Factor 'Country' relates to electronic exchange of information across countries within and outside EU boundaries. It is essential that information can be accessed from anywhere in the health system, even in remote locations, to facilitate seamless communications between care providers (Suter, Oelke, Adair & Armitage, 2009). 'Health professionals' is about information flow among doctors. Physicians need to be effectively integrated at all levels of the system and play leadership roles in the implementation and operation of an integrated health system (Suter, Oelke, Adair & Armitage, 2009). 'Medication list' identifies a drug oriented focus of electronic exchange, and finally Factor 'Hospital' captures information flows between hospitals. Electronic exchange health information facilitates the electronic sharing of patient level information among different providers in a community. Therefore, access to a Health Information system could potentially avert unnecessary admissions by providing relevant clinical data. This information could also potentially prevent unnecessary admissions by providing access to the medical opinions of previous physicians as well as access to lists of medications and problems (Vest, Kern, Campion, Silver, & Kaushal, 2014).

The issue of information security and privacy in the healthcare sector is of growing importance. The adoption of digital patient records, increased regulation, provider consolidation, and the increasing need for information between patients, providers, and payers, all strives for better information security. Privacy is an underlying governing principle of the patient – physician relationship for effective delivery of healthcare (Appari & Johnson, 2008; Jin, Ahn, Hu, Covington & Zhang, 2011). This section provides a description of the dimensions Security and Privacy, which has three sub-dimensions: Encryption, Regulation and Workstation. Security and privacy dimension represents:

- Protect the patient data Workstations with access only through a password.
- Security and privacy of electronic patient data at national level.
- Protect the patient data Encryption of all transmitted data.
- Protect the patient data Encryption of all stored data.
- Security and privacy of electronic patient data at regional level.
- Protect the patient data Data entry certified with digital signature.
- Protect the patient data Workstations with access only through health professional cards.
- Protect the patient data Workstations with access only through fingerprint information.

This paper uses multivariate statistical methods to analyze e-Health services. The objectives are three-fold:

- To elaborate upon the results of a composite index (Codagnone & Lupiañez-Villanueva, 2011);
- To compare the official results with the ones obtained using the I-distance method; and
- To extract key policy messages and new directions for future research.

First step, we analyze the results of a composite index that gave authors Codagnone & Lupiañez-Villanueva. Figure 1 shows the three best and worst ranked countries in relation to the four dimensions (Codagnone & Lupiañez-Villanueva, 2011). As it can be seen, Infrastructure has a direct impact on personal and economic health, and the infrastructure crisis is endangering nation's future prosperity. As a

Figure 1. Overview of the three best-and-worst ranked states and their dimensions scores

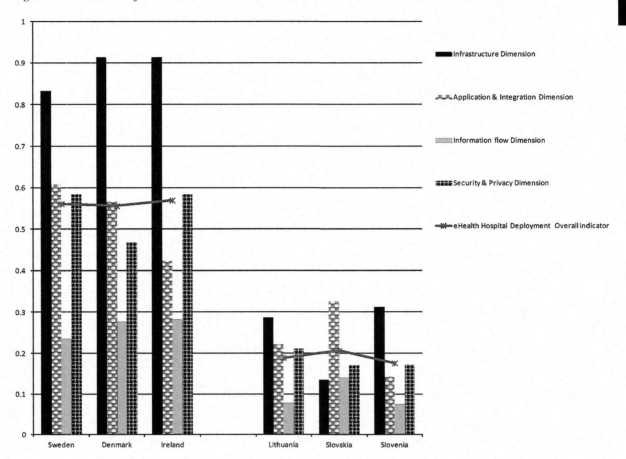

society, we must become better stewards of the environment through the use of sustainable infrastructure practices. The quality of life for future generations depends on willingness to rise to the challenge. A healthy infrastructure will enable us to stay a strong and prosperous nation, but only if we move forward with vision and community involvement and support. The investing in infrastructure is essential to support healthy communities. Infrastructure is also analytical for long-term economic growth, employment, household income, increasing GDP and exports. The reverse is also true – without prioritizing nation's infrastructure needs, deteriorating conditions can transfer on the economy (Report Card for America's Infrastructure, 2013). Quality of life is a central focus of infrastructure policy. The National Council on Public Works Improvement during the 1980s emphasized the importance of infrastructure to the economy (Aschaue, 1990).

Looking at the different summary indexes of the four dimensions it is clear that infrastructure is the domain where more progress has been achieved, whereas electronic information flows and exchange lag behind. Application and Integration tend to be relatively well developed and come second after infrastructure, although in some countries security and privacy issues seem to be prioritized over integrated applications (Codagnone & Lupiañez-Villanueva, 2011).

In the second step, we apply I-distance method and compare the official results with the ones obtained using the I-distance method. In order to aggregate the framework indicators, the aggregation method was applied in several steps. First, we applied the I-distance method to the indicators of dimensions. Secondly, the I-distance method was again applied, but now on the previously obtained dimension results in order to calculate the Total I-distance values (Table 1).

The multilevel analysis allows ranking of countries on two criteria: by dimensios and in Total. In addition, we examined the underlying dynamics of multilevel I-distance framework by calculating the Pearson correlations between the I-distance values and input variables. By using the Pearson correlations, we emphasized a particular feature of the I-distance method, i.e. presenting the relevance of input

Table 1. Results of the total I-distance rank, I-distance ranks for each dimension, and Composite Index (CI) rank

Country	Total I-Dist Rank	CI Rank	I-Dist Rank Dimension A	I-Dist Rank Dimension B	I-Dist Rank Dimension C	I-Dist Rank Dimension D
Denmark	1	2	1	1	6	9
Norway	2	4	4	8	1	6
Sweden	3	1	7	2	8	4
Ireland	4	3	5	7	2	3
UK	5	5	8	12	5	1
Finland	6	7	2	3	9	16
Estonia	7	12	25	6	12	2
Netherlands	8	8	11	4	7	11
Belgium	9	11	13	5	4	17
Austria	10	9	3	15	10	10
Island	11	6	9	13	13	5
Spain	12	10	12	10	11	7
Portugal	13	13	15	11	25	8
Luxembourg	14	14	10	9	15	19
Latvia	15	23	21	25	3	29
Croatia	16	22	6	19	27	27
Italy	17	15	19	18	20	12
Hungary	18	19	22	14	19	18
Germany	19	17	18	22	24	14
Cyprus	20	20	23	17	14	26
Malta	21	21	24	16	17	22
France	22	16	16	23	23	15
Romania	23	24	28	30	26	13
Czech Republic	24	18	20	20	18	20
Greece	25	26	26	21	29	23
Bulgaria	26	25	14	28	30	30
Lithuania	27	28	17	27	21	25
Slovakia	28	29	30	24	16	28
Poland	29	27	29	26	28	21
Slovenia	30	30	27	29	22	24

variables. Instead of assigning subjective weights to input indicators, the I-distance method determines which of the input indicators are most important for the ranking process (Jovanovic Milenkovic et al., 2015, Dobrota et al., 2015a).

Table 1 shows the results giving the Total I-distance rank and Composite Index rank. The differences in the ranks can also be noted. After applying I-distance method, the results pointed out that Denmark, Norway, Sweden are the most successful countries. According to the I-distance methodology Denmark is in the first place and in the second according to the rank of composite indicators. Norway is the second, or the fourth. On the other hand, Slovakia, Poland and Slovenia are listed at the bottom of the rank list. Generally, the top five countries remain the same according to both ranking methods, with slight changes in positions.

Besides providing ranks, our methodology provides a correlation coefficient of each indicator with its I-distance value (Jovanovic Milenkovic et al., 2015), thus making it clear to the general public which e-Health indicators are the most important ones (Table 2).

When we look at a graphical presentation of the multilevel I-distance framework of measuring e-health status (Figure 2), we can observe crucial indicators for each sub-dimension and dimension score. In addition, correlation coefficients are also presented.

As the model shows, sub-dimension *Infrastructure physical oriented* is the most significant variable, with $r=0.925$. This is understandable, considering that e-Health brings together the technologies of unique identification, authentication and encryption to ensure the foundations and solutions for the safe and secure replacement of healthcare information. The infrastructure set-up consists of connected virtual networks, special centralized infrastructure services, modernised hard-/software in doctors' offices, hospitals, pharmacies and other locations, special secure connectors to the network. To allow for the ubiquitous, but secure access to health data across jurisdictional boundaries, an all-embracing e-Health infrastructure is indispensible. The second most significant variable is the sub-dimension *Emphasis on clinical and image*, with $r = 0.847$. Insight into the clinical image is important for establishing the correct diagnosis of patients. This service provides authorised clinicians immediate access to full-

Table 2. Correlation coefficient of each dimension with the total I-distance value and correlation coefficient of each indicator (sub-dimension) with its dimension I-distance value

Dimensions	r	Sub-Dimension	r
A. Infrastructure	0.812	A1. Infrastructure physical oriented	0.925
		A2. Infrastructure service oriented	0.774
B. Application and Integration	0.875	B1. Emphasis on clinical and image	0.847
		B2. Emphasis on EPR and patient management (intramural)	0.807
		B3. Emphasis on patient demand and safety	0.646
		B4. Emphasis on PHR and tele-monitoring (extramural)	0.680
C. Information flow	0.770	C1. Country	0.646
		C2. Health professionals	0.850
		C3. Medication list	0.730
		C4. Hospital	0.706
D. Security and Privacy	0.706	D1. Encryption	0.784
		D2. Regulation	0.906
		D3. Workstation	0.756

Figure 2. Two-phase I-distance framework for evaluating e-health development index

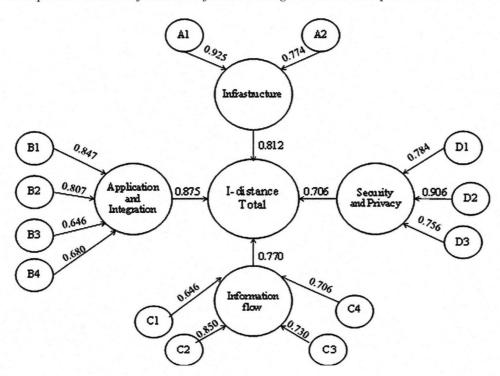

resolution diagnostic-quality images at any time, from anywhere they are needed. Medical images are collected and integrated into the Exchange, allowing authorised clinicians access to a comprehensive patient medical history remotely (Stonehenge Growth Capital, 2011). The least significant variables are two sub-dimensions *Emphasis on patient demand and safety* and *Country*, with r=0.646. Managing in patient demand implies reducing nursing stress and improving patient safety (Litvak, Buerhaus, Davidoff, Long, McManus & Berwick, 2005). It addresses the need in the healthcare system for an emphasis on patient quality and safety.

As the model shows, sub-dimension *Infrastructure physical oriented* is the most significant variable, with *r*=0.925. This is understandable, considering that e-Health brings together the technologies of unique identification, authentication and encryption to ensure the foundations and solutions for the safe and secure replacement of healthcare information. The infrastructure set-up consists of connected virtual networks, special centralized infrastructure services, modernised hard-/software in doctors' offices, hospitals, pharmacies and other locations, special secure connectors to the network. To allow for the ubiquitous, but secure access to health data across jurisdictional boundaries, an all-embracing e-Health infrastructure is indispensable. The second most significant variable is the sub-dimension *Emphasis on clinical and image*, with r = 0.847. Insight into the clinical image is important for establishing the correct diagnosis of patients. This service provides authorised clinicians immediate access to full-resolution diagnostic-quality images at any time, from anywhere they are needed. Medical images are collected and integrated into the Exchange, allowing authorised clinicians access to a comprehensive patient medical history remotely (Stonehenge Growth Capital, 2011). The least significant variables are two sub-dimensions *Emphasis on patient demand and safety* and *Country*, with r=0.646. Managing in patient demand implies reducing nursing stress and improving patient safety (Litvak, Buerhaus, Davidoff, Long, McManus & Berwick, 2005). It addresses the need in the healthcare system for an emphasis on patient quality and safety.

When we look at the dimensions, we see that the most important dimension to determine e-Health status of a country is *Application & Integration*, with r =0.875. Dimension *Application & Integration* is to connect electronic health data from different sources (patient's electronic records from healthcare hospitals and pharmacies), to form a complete „image" of the patient's health condition. It enable such interconnected data to be available to physicians in order to provide quick insight into data crucial for the medical treatment – health problems, allergies, reactions to certain drugs etc. Subsequently, the *Application & Integration* enables different ways of data availability – insights into general health condition for physicians, aggregated for statistics, analytically processed for decision makers (managers), multidimensional correlated for researchers etc. Dimension *Application & Integration* is an integral factor of the e-Health system because it connects various systems of electronic records in healthcare centres into an information-organized image of the patient's treatment (Jovanovic-Milenkovic, Radojicic, Milenkovic, & Vukmirovic, 2009).

In conclusion, the synthetic information that can be extracted from the Composite Index and from the I-distance methodology represents a unique contribution to the field of e-Health. If e-Health is to have its maximum positive impact on a country's entire health system, the institutions need to work closely together so that the e-Health profession in the country is adequately supported, well organized and efficient (Kwankam, 2012).

FUTURE RESEARCH DIRECTIONS

E-Health system ensures a foundation for a new approach to organising and carrying out business processes in healthcare systems supported by information and communication technologies. The primary characteristics of the new approach are orientation to a patient, exchange of information about the health of a patient in order to make better health services, health care based on evidence and reduce costs.

Economic (growing health costs), structural (move towards less acute to more preventative models of care) and technological (improvements in health technology) trends are converging in the health sector to continue the growth and further transformation of health settings through technological developments (Gapenski et al., 2003).

The results of our study present a new perspective on the measuring e-health status. By applying the multilevel I-distance approach we were able to present a more in-depth approach to measuring the e-health status of countries. In the proposed multilevel I-distance framework, we can see the most important indicators, i.e. correlations, for dimensions and sub-dimensions. This paper describes a model that considers which of the variables is the most important. Calculating the correlation coefficient, the most important variable is certainly Infrastructure. Adequate infrastructure contributes to better electronic exchange of data between physicians, hospitals, patients. Certainly, for a complete development of e-Health across the world there need to be cooperation and exchange of information among other states.

There are several directions for future research. I-distance post-hoc analysis (Markovic et al., 2015) could be done to revise the number of indicators. Also, uncertainty and sensitivity analysis (Dobrota et al., 2015a; Dobrota & Dobrota, 2015) with weights proposed by our methodology could be a step in the right direction.

CONCLUSION

The results of our chapter could be of significance for e-Health policy makers as well, since they can provide an in-depth analysis of e-Health performance and potentials of each evaluated country. Understanding the multi-disciplinary nature of measuring e-Health status and the challenges that it faces is the prerequisite towards dealing effectively with the complexities and overcoming the barriers of e-Health services evaluation.

The paper provides a set of clear and useful e-Health evaluation criteria that can be used as part of e-Health evaluation framework. It also addresses areas that require further attention in the development of future e-Health initiatives.

Everything about health care is complex. There are complex care processes, complex organizations, complex health care technologies, complex patient needs and responses to therapeutic interventions. There are vast opportunities and challenges in improving the quality and safety of health care, but the majority require crucial redesign of health care organizations and processes (Hughes, 2008).

REFERENCES

AHRQ National Resource Center. (2014). Consumer Health IT Applications. *Health Information Technology: Best practices transforming quality, safety and efficienty.* Available at: http://healthit.ahrq.gov/key-topics/consumer-health-it-applications

Al-Lagilli, S., Jeremic, V., Seke, K., Jeremic, D., & Radojicic, Z. (2011). Evaluating the Health of Nations: A Libyan Perspective. *Libyan Journal of Medicine, 6,* 6021. doi:10.3402/ljm.v6i0.6021 PMID:21526042

Angaran, D. (2006). Electronic Communication in Health Care. In R. S. Beardsley, C. L. Kimberlin, & W. N. Tindall (Eds.), Communication Skills in Pharmacy Practice (pp. 196–211). Baltimore, MD: Lippincott Williams & Wilkins. Available at http://downloads.lww.com/wolterskluwer_vitalstream_com/sample-content/9780781765985_beardsley/samples/samplechapter2.pdf

Appari, A., & Johnson, E. (2008). *Information Security and Privacy in Healthcare: Current State of Research.* Available at http://www.ists.dartmouth.edu/library/416.pdf

Arber, S., Fenn, K., & Meadows, R. (2014). Subjective financial well-being, income and health inequalities in mid and later life in Britain. *Social Science & Medicine, 100,* 12–20. doi:10.1016/j.socscimed.2013.10.016 PMID:24444834

Arndt, S., Acion, L., Caspers, K., & Blood, P. (2013). How reliable are county and regional health rankings? *Prevention Science, 14*(5), 497–502. doi:10.1007/s11121-012-0320-3 PMID:23400846

Aschaue, D. A. (1990). Why is infrastructure important? *Federal Reserve Bank of Boston, 34,* 21-68. Available at http://www.bostonfed.org/economic/conf/conf34/conf34b.pdf

Ayanso, A., Cho, D., & Lertwachara, K. (2014). Information and Communications Technology Development and the Digital Divide: A Global and Regional Assessment. *Information Technology for Development, 20*(1), 60–77. doi:10.1080/02681102.2013.797378

Ballas, M. S. (2001). The impact of the Internet on the healthcare industry: A close look at the doctor-patient relationship, the electronic medical record, and the medical billing process. *The Einstein Journal of Biology and Medicine; EJBM, 48*(2), 79–83.

Brügermann, R., & Patil, G. P. (2011). *Ranking and Prioritization for Multi-indicator Systems*. Dordrecht: Springer. doi:10.1007/978-1-4419-8477-7

Carrasqueiro, S., & Monteiro, M. H. (2010). E-Health Strategic Planning: Defining the E-Health Services' Portfolio. In M. M. Cruz-Cunha, A. J. Tavares, & R. J. Simoes (Eds.), *Handbook of Research on Developments in E-health and Telemedicine: Technological and Social Perspectives* (pp. 451–474)., doi:10.4018/978-1-61520-670-4.ch021

Codagnone, C., & Lupianez-Villanueva, F. (2011). *A Composite Index for the Benchmarking of e-Health Deployment in European Acute Hospitals*. Luxembourg: JRC Scientific and Technical Reports; doi:10.2791/5846

Dobrota, M., Bulajic, M., Bornmann, L., & Jeremic, V., (2015c). A New Approach to QS University Ranking Using Composite I-distance Indicator: Uncertainty and Sensitivity Analyses. *Journal of the Association for Information Science and Technology*. doi: 10.1002/asi.23355

Dobrota, M. & Dobrota, M. (2015). ARWU ranking uncertainty and sensitivity: What if the award factor was Excluded?. *Journal of the Association for Information Science and Technology*. doi: 10.1002/asi.23527

Dobrota, M., Jeremić, V., Bulajić, M., & Radojičić, Z. (2015b). Uncertainty and Sensitivity Analyses of PISA Efficiency: Distance Based Analysis Approach. *Acta Polytechnica Hungarica, 12*(3), 41–58. doi:10.12700/APH.12.3.2015.3.3

Dobrota, M., Jeremic, V., & Markovic, A. (2012). A New Perspective on the ICT Development Index. *Information Development, 28*(4), 271–280. doi:10.1177/0266666912446497

Dobrota, M., Martic, M., Bulajic, M., & Jeremic, V. (2015a). Two-phased composite I-distance indicator approach for evaluation of countries' information development. *Telecommunications Policy, 39*(5), 406–420. doi:10.1016/j.telpol.2015.03.003

Eucarinet. (2012). *Handbook on European Funding for research and innovation*. EL&I, APRE, UNIBE. Available at http://www.eucarinet.eu

Eysenbach, G. (2001). What is e-health? *Journal of Medical Internet Research, 3*(2), e20. doi:10.2196/jmir.3.2.e20 PMID:11720962

Frenk, J. (2010). The Global Health System: Strengthening National Health Systems as the Next Step for Global Progress. *PLoS Medicine, 7*(1), e1000089. doi:10.1371/journal.pmed.1000089 PMID:20069038

Gapenski, L. C. (2003). *Technology, health care, and management in the hospital of the future*. Santa Barbara, CA: Greenwood Publishing Group.

Gomes, C., Sperandio, F., Peles, A., Borges, J., Brito, A. C., & Almada-Lobo, B. (2013). An Operating Theater Planning Decision Support System. In R. Martinho, R. Rijo, M. Cruz-Cunha, & J. Varajão (Eds.), *Information Systems and Technologies for Enhancing Health and Social Care* (pp. 69–86). Hershey, PA: Medical Information Science Reference; doi:10.4018/978-1-4666-3667-5.ch005

Guttorp, P., & Kim, T. Y. (2013). Uncertainty in ranking the hottest years of US surface temperatures. *Journal of Climate, 26*(17), 6323–6328. doi:10.1175/JCLI-D-12-00760.1

Hamid, A., & Sarmad, A. (2011). Multi-Dimensional Criteria for the Evaluation of E-Health Services. In M. Guah (Ed.), *Healthcare Delivery Reform and New Technologies: Organizational Initiatives* (pp. 172–189). Hershey, PA: Information Science Reference; doi:10.4018/978-1-60960-183-6.ch010

Hanseth, O., & Lundberg, N. (2001). Designing Work Oriented Infrastructures. *Computer Supported Cooperative Work, 10*(3-4), 347–372. doi:10.1023/A:1012727708439

Hughes, G. R. (2008). Nurses at the "Sharp End" of Patient Care. In Patient Safety and Quality: An Evidence-Based Handbook for Nurses. AHRQ Publication No. 08-0043. Rockville, MD: Agency for Healthcare Research and Quality.

Ivanovic, B. (1977). *Classification Theory*. Belgrade: Institute for Industrial Economics.

Jeremic, V., & Jovanovic-Milenkovic, M. (2014). Evaluation of Asian university rankings: Position and perspective of leading Indian higher education institutions. *Current Science, 106*(12), 1647–1653.

Jeremic, V., Jovanovic-Milenkovic, M., Radojicic, Z. & Martic, M. (2013). Excellence with Leadership: the crown indicator of SCImago Institutions RankingsIber report. *El profesional de la información, 22*(5), 474-480.,10.3145/epi.2013.sep.13

Jin, J., Ahn, G. J., Hu, H., Covington, J. M., & Zhang, X. (2011). Patient-centric authorization framework for electronic healthcare services. *Computers & Security, 30*(2–3), 116–127. doi:10.1016/j.cose.2010.09.001

Jovanovic, M., Jeremic, V., Savic, G., Bulajic, M., & Martic, M. (2012). How does the normalization of data affects the ARWU ranking? *Scientometrics, 93*(2), 319–327. doi:10.1007/s11192-012-0674-0

Jovanovic-Milenkovic, M. (2011). Interest of the Population in Electronic Communication in the Health Services Provision – Research Results. *Management, 16*(59), 79.

Jovanovic Milenkovic, M., Brajovic, B., Milenkovic, D., Vukmirovic, D., Jeremic, V. (2015). Beyond equal-weight framework of the Networked Readiness Index: a multilevel I-distance methodology. *Information Development*. doi: 10.1177/0266666915593136

Jovanovic-Milenkovic, M., Jeremic, V., & Martic, M. (2014). Sustainable Development in the e-Health Sector of the European Union. *Journal of Environmental Protection and Ecology, 15*(1), 248-256.

Jovanovic Milenkovic, M., Milenkovic, D., & Dobrota, M. (2012). Communication via the Web and SMS Services in the Health Care System in the Republic of Serbia. *Actual Problems* of *Economics, 138*(12), 364-369.

Jovanovic-Milenkovic, M., Radojicic, Z., Milenkovic, D., & Vukmirovic, D. (2009). Applying electronic Documents in Development of the Healthcare Information System in the Republic of Serbia. *Computer Science and Information System., 6*(2), 111–126. doi:10.2298/CSIS0902111J

Kell, M., & Kell, P. (2014). League Tables and the Politics of Ranking. *Literacy and Language in East Asia – Education in the Asia-Pacific Region: Issues, Concerns and Prospects, 24*, 25–32.

Khoumbati, K., & Themistocleous, M. (2006). Integrating the IT Infrastructures in Healthcare Organisations: A Proposition of Influential Factors. *The Electronic Journal of E-Government, 4*(1), 27–36.

Kuehn, B. M. (2011). Patiens go online seeking support, practical advice on health conditions. *Journal of the American Medical Association, 205*(16), 1644–1645. doi:10.1001/jama.2011.509 PMID:21521841

Kwankam, S. Y. (2012). Successful partnerships for international collaboration in e-health: The need for organized national infrastructures. *Bulletin of the World Health Organization, 90*(5), 395–397. doi:10.2471/BLT.12.103770 PMID:22589576

Litvak, E., Buerhaus, P. I., Davidoff, F., Long, M. C., McManus, M. L., & Berwick, D. M. (2005). Managing unnecessary variability in patient demand to reduce nursing stress and improve patient safety. *Joint Commission Journal on Quality and Patient Safety, 31*(6), 330–338. PMID:15999963

Mackart, M., Champlin, S. E., Holton, A., Muñoz, I. I., & Damásio, M. J. (2014). eHealth and Health Literacy: A Research Methodology Review. *Journal of Computer-Mediated Communication, 19*(3), 516–528. doi:10.1111/jcc4.12044

Maricic, M., & Kostic-Stankovic, M. (2014). Towards an impartial Responsible Competitiveness Index: A twofold multivariate I-distance approach. *Quality & Quantity*. doi:10.1007/s11135-014-0139-z

Markovic, M., Zdravkovic, S., Mitrovic, M., & Radojicic, A. (2015). An iterative multivariate post hoc I-distance approach in evaluating OECD Better Life Index. *Social Indicators Research*. Epub ahead of print 18 January 2015. doi:10.1007/s11205-015-0879-8

Milenkovic, D., Jovanovic Milenkovic, M., Vujin, V., Aleksic, A., & Radojicic, Z. (2012). Electronic Health System: Development and Implementation into the Health System of the Republic of Serbia, *Vojnosanitetski Pregled. Military Medical and Pharmaceutical Journal of Serbia, 69*(10), 880–890. PMID:23155610

Moghad-Dasi, H., & Rabiei, R. (2013). A model for measuring e-health status across the world. *Telemedicine Journal and e-Health, 19*(4), 322–327. doi:10.1089/tmj.2012.0147 PMID:23506327

Paruolo, P., Saisanam, M., & Saltellim, A. (2013). Ratings and rankings: Voodoo or science? *Journal of the Royal Statistical Society. Series A, (Statistics in Society), 176*(3), 609–634. doi:10.1111/j.1467-985X.2012.01059.x

Radojicic, Z., & Jeremic, V. (2012). Quantity or Quality: What Matters More in Ranking Higher Education Institutions? *Current Science, 103*(2), 158–162.

Report Card for America's Infrastructure. (2013). *Executive summary*. Available at http://www.infrastructurereportcard.org/a/#p/overview/executive-summary

Robertson, A., Cresswell, K., Takian, A., Petrakaki, D., Crowe, S., Cornford, T., & Sheikh, A. et al. (2010). Implementation and adoption of nationwide electronic health records in secondary care in England: Qualitative analysis of interim results from a prospective national evaluation. *British Medical Journal, 341*(sep01 3), c4564. doi:10.1136/bmj.c4564 PMID:20813822

Robertsonm, G. (2013). *Effect of Intelligent Technology Infrastructure on Hospital Operating Costs and Patient Care*. Available at: http://www2.schneider-electric.com/documents/support/white-papers/healthcare/Healthcare-intelligent-architecture-high-level.pdf

Saisana, M. & D'Hombres, B. (2008). *Higher education rankings: robustness issues and critical assessment. How much confidence can we have in higher education rankings?* EUR23487, Joint Research Centre, Publications Office of the European Union, Italy. doi:10.2788/92295

Saisana, M., D'Hombres, B., & Saltelli, A. (2011). Rickety numbers: Volatility of university rankings and policy implications. *Research Policy, 40*(1), 165–177. doi:10.1016/j.respol.2010.09.003

Saisana, M., & Tarantola, S. (2002). State-of-the-art report on current methodologies and practices for composite indicator development. EUR Report 20408 EN. European Commission, JRC-IPSC, Italy.

Saltelli, A. (2007). Composite indicators between analysis and advocacy. *Social Indicators Research, 81*(1), 65–77. doi:10.1007/s11205-006-0024-9

Sang, S., Wang, Z., & Yu, C. (2014). Evluation of Heath Care System Reform in Hubei Province, China. *International Journal of Environmental Research and Public Health, 11*(2), 2262–2277. doi:10.3390/ijerph110202262 PMID:24566052

Seke, K., Petrovic, N., Jeremic, V., Vukmirovic, J., Kilibarda, B., & Martic, M. (2013). Sustainable Development and Public Health: Rating European Countries. *BMC Public Health, 13*(1), 77. doi:10.1186/1471-2458-13-77 PMID:23356822

Soh, K. (2013a). Rectifying an honest error in world university rankings: A solution to the problem of indicator weight discrepancies. *Journal of Higher Education Policy and Management, 35*(6), 574–585. doi:10.1080/1360080X.2013.844670

Soh, K. (2013b). Nominal versus attained weights in Universitas 21 Ranking. *Studies in Higher Education.* doi:10.1080/03075079.2012.754866

Stonehenge Growth Capital. (2011). *Impressive Growth in 2011 for eHealth Global Technologies, Stonehenge Growth Capital.* Available at http://www.stonehengegrowthcapital.com/stonehenge_new_detail.cfm?id=109

Stroetmann, K.A., Artmann, J., & Stroetmann, V.N. (2011). European countries on their journey towards national eHealth infrastructures - evidence on progress and recommendations for cooperative actions. *eHealth Strategies Report.*

Sultan, N. (2014). Making use of cloud computing for healthcare provision: Opportunities and challenges. *International Journal of Information Management, 34*(2), 177–184. doi:10.1016/j.ijinfomgt.2013.12.011

Suter, E., Oelke, D. N., Adair, E. C., & Armitage, D. G. (2009). Ten Key Principles for Successful Health Systems Integration. *Healthcare Quarterly, 13*(sp), 16–23. doi:10.12927/hcq.2009.21092 PMID:20057244

Van Dijkum, C., & Vegter, L. (2010). A Client Perspective on E-Health: Illustrated with an Example from The Netherlands. In M. M. Cruz-Cunha, A. J. Tavares, & R. J. Simoes (Eds.), *Handbook of Research on Developments in E-health and Telemedicine: Technological and Social Perspectives* (pp. 357–377). Hershey, PA: IGI Global; doi:10.4018/978-1-61520-670-4

Vest, J. R., Kern, L. M., Campion, T. R. Jr, Silver, M. D., & Kaushal, R. (2014). Association between use of a health information exchange system and hospital admissions. *Appled Clinical Informatics., 5*(1), 219–231. doi:10.4338/ACI-2013-10-RA-0083 PMID:24734135

Vilaplana, J., Solsona, F., Abella, F., Filgueira, R., & Rius, J. (2013). The cloud paradigm applied to e-Health. *BMC Medical Informatics and Decision Making, 13*(35). doi:10.1186/1472-6947-13-35 PMID:23496912

Vujin, V., & Jovanovic-Milenkovic, M. (2012). Implementation of Cloud Computing in the Health Care System. *Metalurgia International, 17*(9), 161–165.

Whitehouse, D., & Duquenoy, P. (2011). EHealth and Ethics: Theory, Teaching, and Practice. In D. M. Haftor & A. Mirijamdotter (Eds.), *Information and Communication Technologies, Society and Human Beings: Theory and Framework* (pp. 454–465)., doi:10.4018/978-1-60960-057-0.ch037

Yadav, N., & Poellabauer, C. (2012). Challenges of Mobile Health Applications in Developing Countries. In K. M. Watfa (Ed.), *E-Healthcare Systems and Wireless Communications: Current and Future Challenges* (pp. 1–22)., doi:10.4018/978-1-61350-123-8.ch001

Zapater, M., Arroba, P., Ayala, J. L., Moya, J. M., & Olcoz, K. (2014). A novel energy-driven computing paradigm for e-health scenarios. *Future Generation Computer Systems-The International Journal of Grid Computing and Escience, 34*, 138–154. doi:10.1016/j.future.2013.12.012

Zhang, D., Yu, Z., & Chin, C. (2005). Context-Aware Infrastructure for Personalized Healthcare. In Personalised Health Management Systems: The Integration of Innovative Sensing, Textile, Information and Communication Technologies, (pp. 154-163). IOS Press.

KEY TERMS AND DEFINITIONS

Composite Index: Synthesizes the information included in a selected set of indicators/variables.

Correlation Coefficient: Provides a closer look at indicators that are the most important for determining the e-Health status of the country.

E-Health: The delivery of health services and information across the Internet and related technologies.

E-Health Services: Applications using Internet technologies with the aim to provide health care services to patients.

I-Distance Method: Method to rank countries according to their level of development on the basis of several indicators.

Measuring E-Health Status: Involves measuring the progress in the use of electronic services for health purposes.

Towards Interoperable and Extendable Clinical Pedigrees in Healthcare Information Systems

João Miguel Santos
University of Aveiro, Portugal

Leonor Teixeira
University of Aveiro, Portugal

Beatriz Sousa Santos
University of Aveiro, Portugal

INTRODUCTION

Since ancient times, it has been evident that several diseases are more prevalent in some families. It is now know that genetic traits are passed from generation to generation and that many common diseases and clinical conditions are linked to genetic factors. This allows some degree of predictability when dealing with such diseases, provided that clinical family history data is available. Recording patients' clinical family histories is therefore recognized as an important step in the diagnosis and risk assessment of many diseases. In some cases, clinical family histories also allow the identification of at-risk individuals before diseases manifest, potentially minimizing or completely avoiding diseases or symptoms. Though there are several ways to record clinical family histories, such as checklists, forms, descriptive test, etc., clinical pedigrees are a particularly well-accepted tool, standing out for their balance of expressivity and ease of use. These graphical representations illustrate both family structure and clinical conditions of family members, allowing important information to be quickly assessed by observers, such as disease heredity patterns, penetrability, mortality and at-risk individuals.

Given the usefulness of clinical family histories, one would expect this tool to be widely used by practitioners, yet recent studies attest otherwise. Existing literature suggests that one of the main reasons for this underutilization is the fact that most Healthcare Information Systems (HIS) do not yet include adequate tools to record this information. Though clinical pedigrees can easily be drawn by hand or in external drawing software packages – and indeed some practitioners do resort to these alternatives – this results in representations that are disconnected from current health records and consequently difficult to integrate with existing HIS and keep up-to-date.

Some proprietary solutions do exist that allow the creation of clinical pedigrees within certain HIS, but their closed-source nature makes the integration with other HIS a difficult and potentially expensive task.

This chapter presents an alternative solution: the usage of open, interoperable and extendable clinical pedigree information systems that can be easily and freely integrated with existing HIS.

DOI: 10.4018/978-1-4666-9978-6.ch066

BACKGROUND

It has long been observed that a number of diseases and clinical conditions are more prevalent in some families than in others. In colloquial terms, it is said that such conditions "run in families". It is now known that genetic are being passed from generation to generation. In fact, developments in Genetics have unveiled links between genetic factors and hundreds of common diseases, such as diabetes, Alzheimer, deafness, schizophrenia and many others (Kmiecik & Sanders, 2009; Rich et al., 2004). It is likely that efforts in human DNA sequencing and gene mutation identification, collection and interpretation, such as those carried out by Human Variome Project (2014) and Human Genome Project (U.S. Department of Energy Human Genome Project, 2014), will expose more and more links between genetic factors and medical conditions.

The significance of combining family history information with patients' clinical data has also been recognized for a long time, before specific links between genetics and diseased were even established. Based solely on the observation of increased occurrence of certain medical conditions within families, Hippocrates (460 B.C. – 370 B.C.) reportedly included family history information in "case studies", complementing the clinical evaluation of disease manifestations and providing an early form of risk stratification, (Hinton, 2008).

Naturally, a better understanding of the genetic nature of some conditions has increased the importance of family history information in modern healthcare. On the one hand, this information provides additional insight to patients' clinical conditions, which may ease prognostics and promote optimal choice of treatment (Morales, Cowan, Dagua, & Hershberger, 2008; Rich et al., 2004). On the other hand, family history information allows the identification of at-risk individuals within the patient's family, when genetic links exist, serving as a cost-effective risk assessment tool (R.L. Bennett, 2010). This discoverability of at-risk individuals fosters the application of predictive medicine, namely monitoring, counseling, genetic testing, suggestion of behavior changes or a combination of these, which can delay, diminish or completely avoid diseases or their symptoms (Frezzo, Rubinstein, Dunham, & Ormond, 2003).

CLINICAL FAMILY HISTORY REPRESENTATIONS

Clinical family history information can be recorded in several formats with varying degrees of detail. Text formats, such as forms, checklists or free text are common (American College of Obstetricians and Gynecologists, 2011) and relatively easy to register but lack the immediate expressivity that visual representations may provide. Free text in particular lacks structure, and important clues about conditions or family structure may be overlooked. Forms and checklists may also be limiting in the presence of uncommon symptoms or family structures. Graphical formats are also used to record family history information, such as genograms, ecomaps and pedigrees. Genograms and ecomaps include not only family structure and clinical conditions but also social relations with external individuals, as well and data regarding emotional symptoms, educational achievements, occupational history, ethnicity, religion, race, migration, class, and sexual orientation (Butler, 2008; Rempel, Neufeld, & Kushner, 2007). Not surprisingly, these tools are commonly used by therapists and clinical practice with families but, as Bennet (2010) puts it, they are not as multifunctional as pedigrees, particularly for disease risk assessment, since non-clinical information frequently clutters the representation, making relevant health information difficult to discern.

The clinical pedigree (from here onwards referred as pedigree) appears to be the most understood and accepted graphic representation for recording, analyzing and communicating family history information (R. L. Bennett, French, Resta, & Doyle, 2008; Hinton, 2008). Pedigrees are visual representations of family histories denoting individuals and their family relations, clinical conditions, genetic characteristics, external factors and other pertinent information relating to the health condition of represented individuals (R.L. Bennett, 2010). Based on existing work reviews and expert opinions, the Pedigree Standardization Work Group (PSWG) has proposed standard symbols for the representation of affected, non-affected, asymptomatic, carrier and deceased individuals and their biological and non-biological family relations, as well as notation for representing age, birth and death dates, causes of death, results of genetic tests and other relevant information (R. L. Bennett et al., 2008; R.L. Bennett et al., 1995). Figure 1 presents an example pedigree in standard PSWG notation where a family tendency for sickle cell disease (a hereditary blood disorder, also known as sickle cell anemia) can be observed on the leftmost branch.

As a key to understanding the example pedigree, a brief introduction to PSWG notation follows. Squares and circles are used to represent males and females, respectively, while diamonds represent individuals of unknown gender. Filled or semi-filled shapes indicate the presence of a certain condition or trait (according to visual codes indicated in the pedigree's legend) and diagonal strikes indicate deceased individuals. The proband is identified by the letter P and a diagonal arrow pointing towards the respective individual. As for the layout of individuals, it is closely tied to the family relations amongst them. Marriage or union is represented by a horizontal line connecting the participating individuals at their sides. A line descending from the union line represents offspring. When there is more than one offspring, this line is branched so that a horizontal line connects all siblings from the same union. Individuals within a generation are identified (or distinguished, as pedigree representation are usually anonymous) using arabic numerals, while generations themselves are identified with roman numerals. This makes it easy to refer to individuals in the pedigree, for instance, individual 4 on generation II is a 57 year-old female with sickle cell disease diagnosed at age 37. Optionally, as is the case in the example

Figure 1. Example pedigree demonstrating a family tendency for sickle cell disease

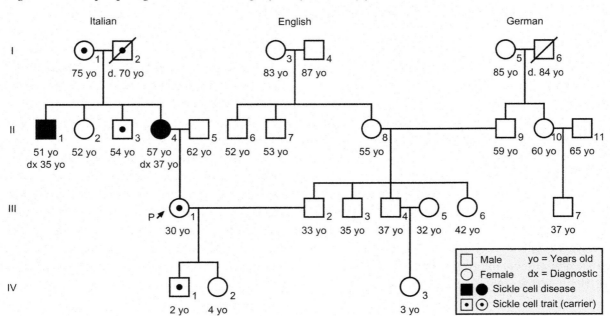

pedigree, ethnicity of ancestor branches can be indicated at the top of those branches. This is relevant since the prevalence of some conditions is related to the ethnical background. For example, sickle cell disease is particularly present in sub-Saharan Africa, India, Saudi Arabia and Mediterranean populations (World Health Organization, 2006).

Being a visual representation, pedigrees allow observers to quickly recognize important information regarding heredity patterns, as well as penetrability and mortality rates of clinical conditions affecting family members (Wattendorf & Hadley, 2005). A pedigree also helps in the diagnosis, risk estimation, identification of at-risk individuals and choice of treatment and medical vigilance options (R.L. Bennett, 2010).

Given the benefits of using pedigrees to assist medical care, coupled with the relatively low cost of producing them, it would be expectable to find near-universal usage of this tool in healthcare and medical practice organizations and, consequently, in Healthcare Information Systems (HIS). Yet several studies and authors' personal experience attest that pedigrees remain underused (Feero, Bigley, & Brinner, 2008; Hinton, 2008). The reasons and possible solutions for this contradiction will be detailed in the coming sections.

UNDERUSAGE OF FAMILY HISTORY AND PEDIGREES IN HEALTHCARE

The relevance of recording and using patients' family history information in healthcare has been increasingly recognized. Nevertheless, this tool is not as widely used as would be desirable. Several studies have focused on identifying the causes of this discrepancy. One of the prime reasons appears to be the lack of time by physicians to record family histories – a task that may take between 15-30 minutes on average for new patients (Frezzo et al., 2003; Rich et al., 2004). Unless these times are reduced or offloaded, it is understandable how they may pose a barrier towards the collection of family history information. To this extent, the Cancer Genetics Service for Wales proposes an interesting alternative: the use of non-clinical staff to record most of the pedigree data (Tempest et al., 2005). This study has found that pedigrees constructed by "data administrators" (non-clinical staff responsible for recording pedigree data) mostly mirrored those created by genetic counselors, in terms of disease confirmation. In fact, data administrators' information collection was often more detailed, in terms of names, dates of birth and the like, possibly due to time constraints on the part of genetic counselors. These are promising results, hinting that usage of non-clinical staff to record pedigrees eases, or may even solve, the problem of the time required to gather and record family history information. Another possibility is to have patients record some or most of the family history themselves, using tools such as My Family Health Portait (Owens, Marvin, Gelehrter, Ruffin, & Uhlmann, 2011; U.S. Department of Health & Human Services, 2009) or MeeTree (Orlando et al., 2013). My Family Health Portait is a publically available website that guides users (assumed to be non-practitioners) though a series of forms that allow the construction of pedigrees containing users' family histories. The resulting pedigrees and their data can be exported for integration with Healthcare Information Systems (HIS) and Electronic Health Record (EHR) systems. MeeTree uses Web-based surveys to establish family structure and allows users to identify affected relatives, out of 48 potential conditions. The quality of resulting pedigrees is sufficient to allow risk assessments for most patients (Wu et al., 2014).

Another frequently reported problem is that many EHR and HIS are not able to record pedigrees or family history data in a structured manner (Feero et al., 2008; Kmiecik & Sanders, 2009; Rich et al., 2004). Practitioners that want to record patients' family histories in a structured manner must resort to external tools, such as hand-drawn pedigrees or standalone drawing software. This is problematic, as it causes data duplication and makes it difficult to keep family histories up-to-date. A recent study reports that the lack of pedigree drawing capabilities or integration with existing pedigree drawing software is one of the main barriers towards the adoption of family history tools in EHR, along with time constraints, privacy concerns and a lack of knowledge, on the part of some clinicians, on how to use family history information (Scheuner et al., 2009). The same study reports that pedigree drawing capabilities and decision support/risk assessment tools are amongst the most useful genetic-related features that clinicians currently miss in their EHR systems. The lack of adequate family history tools helps explain why most practitioners end up using unstructured formats, such as plain text fields, to digitally record family history information. Though easy to implement, unstructured formats do not offer a complete solution because they neither offer the expressivity of visual representations nor allow automatic decision support or risk assessment processes.

While time constraints can be potentially solved resorting to the aforementioned practice of having non-clinical staff record most of the family history information, and the lack of knowledge on how to use family history information tends to be surpassed as awareness on the utility of this tools continues to increase, the lack of adequate family history or pedigree drawing tools in HIS and EHR systems is a complex problem yet to be fully resolved.

Practitioners' desire for better family history tools in HIS is well justified. The presence of this information, alongside other patient information, allows for better and more personalized treatment options for affected patients, as well as preventive measures for unaffected at-risk individuals (Bonacina, Marceglia, Bertoldi, & Pinciroli, 2010; Glaser, Henley, Downing, & Brinner, 2008). Currently, practitioners resort to external pedigree-drawing tools or unstructured formats to overcome the lack of adequate family history tools. Some pedigree drawing tools, such as Progeny Clinical, allow some form of integration with existing HIS/EHR systems, but integration is link-based, allowing a pedigree to be displayed within the HIS/EHR system through a hyperlink (Progeny Software, 2014). My Family Health Portrait offers interesting integration capabilities, exporting data using HL7 (Health Level Seven International, 2014) and other standards which can be integrated in existing HIS/EHR systems, but the tool itself is limiting for practitioner's use, which is understandable given its current intended audience (the general public). These workarounds are therefore not completely satisfactory, and mode adequate solutions are needed to fully address the problem.

INTEGRATION OF FAMILY HISTORY INFORMATION WITH EXISTING HIS

Ideally, HIS would include family history/pedigree capabilities "out of the box", so that integration would not be a concern. But, as aforementioned, most HIS do not yet include such tools. In this context, family history tools that integrate with existing HIS provide a solution, at least a temporary one. Should integration reach a degree where users are not aware or disturbed by the presence of external tools, the use of such tools could provide a definitive solution for many HIS, in the same manner that productivity tools, like word processors and spreadsheets, are not re-implemented by every system that needs that functionality.

Existing pedigree drawing tools with integration capabilities export, and sometimes import, family history information in XML-based formats that adhere to a particular schema, such as HL7 standards. In other words, the interchange document contains a specific set of information formatted in a pre-specified manner. Extensions are possible (tools can include their own data that is not part of the standard), but understanding the content present in extensions depends on the existence of documentation, as the expressivity of a XML document is somewhat limited.

Though there is nothing wrong with XML – quite the contrary, as it helped achieve unparalleled levels on interoperability between heterogeneous systems – its expressivity is limited. XML is, after all, a structured document format which can be verified against a schema, but conferring meaning to the actual data depends on human interpretation of the schema. As Berners-Lee and colleagues put it, in the article presenting the Semantic Web vision, *"XML allows users to add arbitrary structure to their documents but says nothing about what the structures mean."* (Berners-Lee, Hendler, & Lassila, 2001). Briefly put, the Semantic Web vision points towards a better, more interoperable Web, filled with information that can be understood by computers and humans alike. One of its key points is defining formats that allow machines to understand information, such as Resource Description Format (RDF) and Ontologies. These formats build on XML, extending it to offer additional expressivity and capabilities to structured and semi-structured information.

Though initially conceived with the Semantic Web in mind, RDF and ontologies can be – and frequently are – used in information systems not directly related to the Web. In the Biomedical area in particular, ontologies have been playing an important role in knowledge management, interoperability and data integration, computer reasoning and decision support (Bodenreider, 2008). Given their greater expressivity, using ontologies to represent and reason with family history data can help achieve higher degrees of integration between pedigree drawing systems and existing HIS. The potential benefits of using ontologies in this fashion include higher expressivity and interoperability of family history information, greater extensibility, powerful and flexible queriability and the possibility of automatic inference and computer reasoning (Santos, Santos, & Teixeira, 2014).

SOLUTIONS AND RECOMMENDATIONS

This section presents the architecture for an ontology-based, interoperable clinical pedigree information system, which addresses the issues raised in the previous sections. The high-level view of the proposed system architecture is represented in Figure 2. This design follows a typical n-tier architecture, albeit resorting to ontologies and Semantic Web technology for storing and reasoning with data.

Figure 2. High-level view of system architecture

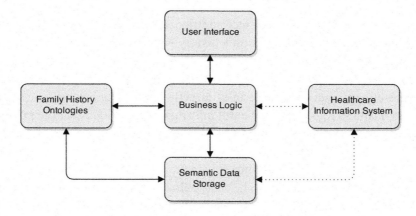

The role of the user interface layer is to display pedigrees and patient data to the user, as well as allowing pedigrees to be constructed and patient data to be entered. The business logic layer mediates the user interface and data storage layers. It gathers, translates and transfers data between these layers as needed. It uses ontologies to reason with family history information, validate new data and infer information whenever possible. Optionally, it also interfaces with existing HIS to retrieve patient data or send family history information. The interface is plugin based, allowing it to be tailored to specific systems, if necessary. A few preset plugins should be included in the system, allowing data do be transferred in RDF and HL7 formats, as well as a generic database plugin that can be configured to match systems' particular schemas. The data layer plays the standard role of storing and retrieving data, using Semantic Web storage tools such as Triple Stores (databases optimized for storing and querying triple-based data like RDF). This layer also interfaces with family history ontologies to allow automatic inference from existing triples and contextualize semantic queries. The HIS interface can be performed at the business logic layer, as previously mentioned, but it may also connect directly to the data layer to access the family history information.

Integration with existing HIS can therefore be achieved in several ways, with varying degrees of interoperability:

- **Using a Plug-In to Directly Access the HIS Data:** This allows the pedigree information system to access patient data without changing the HIS codebase. A generic database plug-in coupled with configuration files to map patient information to the database layout should suffice for most database-oriented HIS. As an alternative, specific plug-ins can be designed to gather data using available HIS outputs or Application Programming Interfaces (APIs).
- **Invoking the Pedigree Information System to Display a Patient's Pedigree:** Assuming the HIS code can be changed, an option can be provided to invoke the pedigree information system and display the clinical pedigree of a patient. If the pedigree information system is implemented as a Web application, this would be as easy as opening a web page with a link containing the patient ID.
- **Directly Accessing the Pedigree Data:** To achieve a higher degree of interoperability, the HIS can be enhanced to access the pedigree information system APIs to directly access, interpret and complement pedigree data.
- **Using the Pedigree Information System as Standalone:** If direct interoperability between the systems is not possible or desired, the pedigree information system can be used in standalone mode and its data can be exported in RDF or HL7 formats for future manual integration.

Because ontologies can be extended, and since additional ontologies can be mixed with existing information, the HIS is also able to complement family history with additional, context-specific information. For example, if a particular HIS needs to record results of genetic tests for which the pedigree information system was not originally conceived, that HIS can define a new ontology (or reuse an existing one that fits the purpose) and either inject the extra triples directly in the data layer or use the ontology-based interface to send the business logic layer the extra information. Provided that the pedigree information system is allowed access to the respective ontology, it may even continue to reason and validate this extra information.

A Web-based implementation of this architecture is presently underway in the University of Aveiro, in the form of a project dubbed OntoFam. The materialization of the proposed system architecture is represented in Figure 3. To test its validity, the system is being integrated with Hemo@Care, a previ-

Figure 3. OntoFam's implementation of the proposed system architecture

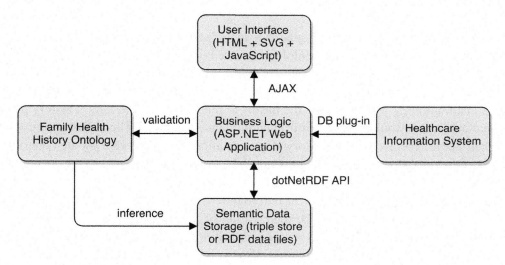

ously existing HIS specific for Hemophilia care (Teixeira, Ferreira, & Santos, 2012). For the sake of easing future implementations of the proposed architecture, a brief description of the most relevant implementation aspects of OntoFam follows.

Given the choice of building a new or reusing an existing ontology, the latter is generally favorable, as it promotes knowledge reuse and refinement of existing ontologies. Accordingly, the Family Health History Ontology (FHHO) was selected, as it closely matched the requirements for the project and had previously been submitted to instance testing, with favorable results (Peace & Brennan, 2008, 2009). The ontology was then extended to incorporate specificities related to Hemophilia patients, required by the Hemo@Care integration. The open-source Madeline engine was chosen as the base component of the user interface layer (Trager et al., 2007). This engine uses text-based input to gather family history data and outputs Standard Vector Graphics (SVG) pedigrees adhering to the PSWG proposed notation. Since browsers can operate with SVG graphics on the individual shape level, client-side scripts allow users to interact with the represented individuals and add new individuals and family relations to the pedigree. The pedigree representation is therefore interactive, allowing both input and output of family history information. Additional patient information, such as personal data and health state, is entered in popup forms activated when creating or editing individuals. The business logic layer makes intensive use of dotNetRDF, an open-source library that handles the actual processing of semantic data (Vesse, Zettlemoyer, Ahmed, Moore, & Pluskiewicz, 2014). This library also abstracts semantic data storage by providing a single interface to many triple stores, such as AllegroGraph, 4store, Fuseki, Virtuoso, Stardog and Sesame-based stores. A plug-in allows patient data to be gathered from Hemo@Care's database, ensuring that patient information on the pedigree is correct and up-to-date.

OntoFam implementation and integration with Hemo@Care are currently in a functional prototype stage. Internal testing suggests that the aforementioned technological choices are valid and allow a successful concretization of the proposed architecture. Preliminary expert reviews have been favorable, hinting that a finalized system will indeed be welcomed by practitioners that wish to integrate family history/pedigree drawing capabilities in their HIS/EHR systems.

FUTURE RESEARCH DIRECTIONS

At present, no publically available ontology appears to include all the aspects that a clinical pedigree should cover. Combining and extending existing ontologies solve this problem – and that was the route chosen in the current OntoFam implementation – but to truly achieve a high degree of interoperability between HIS/EHR systems a single more complete ontology (or a small set of ontologies) would be preferable.

Ideally, a main ontology would include the means to represent the core family history information, and additional ontologies would describe information relative to specific clinical areas or use scenarios. The Core Data Set for Family Health History Representation, recommended by the American Health Information Community Personalized Health Care Workgroup (Feero et al., 2008), is a good starting point for the sort of information that the main ontology should define.

Once a common ontology (or small set of ontologies) is established for describing clinical family histories, an interesting extension would be the creation of logic and probabilistic rules according to known hereditary patterns and probabilities of specific conditions. Combined with existing Semantic Web inference and reasoning tools, this addition would allow the clinical pedigree information system to infer and estimate at-risk individuals, aiding practitioners in risk estimation and treatment choice processes.

CONCLUSION

At present, a contradiction exists between the utility and usage levels of clinical family history tools, such as pedigrees. Practitioners recognize the importance of these tools in the diagnosis, risk estimation and choice of treatment processes, yet studies attest that pedigrees remain underused by most health professionals. The most important reasons for this contradiction appear to be the time taken to collect and record family history information and the lack of adequate tools in most HIS/EHR systems. While potential solutions for the former problem have already been considered – such as using non-clinical staff to record family history information – the latter problem remains mostly unsolved.

This chapter points at a possible solution: the creation of interoperable and extendable clinical pedigrees. By resorting to Semantic Web technology, ontology-based clinical pedigrees can be managed in specific information systems that integrate with existing HIS/EHR systems with relative ease. An implementation of these principles has been materialized in the OntoFam project and its integration with Hemo@Care, an existing HIS for Hemophilia care. Preliminary testing suggests that this integration is successful in bringing the necessary family history tools onto the HIS with little adaptation to the latter. Therefore, it is expectable that implementations of the proposed system architecture will alleviate or solve the lack of adequate family history tools in HIS/EHR systems and, in so doing, remove one of the major barriers towards efficient family history usage in healthcare.

REFERENCES

American College of Obstetricians and Gynecologists. (2011). Committee Opinion No. 478: Family History as a Risk Assessment Tool. *Obstetrics and Gynecology, 117*(3), 747–750. doi:10.1097/AOG.0b013e318214780e PMID:21343792

Bennett, R. L. (2010). The Practical Guide to the Genetic Family History (2nd ed.). Wiley-Blackwell. doi:10.1002/9780470568248

Bennett, R. L., French, K. S., Resta, R. G., & Doyle, D. L. (2008). Standardized Human Pedigree Nomenclature: Update and Assessment of the Recommendations of the National Society of Genetic Counselors. *Journal of Genetic Counseling, 17*(5), 424–433. doi:10.1007/s10897-008-9169-9 PMID:18792771

Bennett, R. L., Steinhaus, K. A., Uhrich, S. B., O'Sullivan, C. K., Resta, R. G., Lochner-Doyle, D., & Hamanishi, J. (1995). Recommendations for Standardized Human Pedigree Nomenclature. *Journal of Genetic Counseling, 4*(4), 267–279. doi:10.1007/BF01408073 PMID:24234481

Berners-Lee, T., Hendler, J., & Lassila, O. (2001). The Semantic Web. A new form of Web content that is meaningful to computers will unleash a revolution of new possibilities. *Scientific American, 284*(5), 1–5.

Bodenreider, O. (2008). Biomedical ontologies in action: Role in knowledge management, data integration and decision support. *Yearbook of Medical Informatics, 47*(Suppl 1), 67–79. PMID:18660879

Bonacina, S., Marceglia, S., Bertoldi, M., & Pinciroli, F. (2010). Modelling, Designing, and Implementing a Family-Based Health Record Prototype. *Computers in Biology and Medicine, 40*(6), 580–590. doi:10.1016/j.compbiomed.2010.04.002 PMID:20444443

Butler, J. F. (2008). The Family Diagram and Genogram: Comparisons and Contrasts. *The American Journal of Family Therapy, 36*(3), 169–180. doi:10.1080/01926180701291055

Feero, W. G., Bigley, M. B., & Brinner, K. M. (2008). New Standards and Enhanced Utility for Family Health History Information in the Electronic Health Record: An Update from the American Health Information Community's Family Health History Multi-Stakeholder Workgroup. *Journal of the American Medical Informatics Association, 15*(6), 723–728. doi:10.1197/jamia.M2793 PMID:18755994

Frezzo, T. M., Rubinstein, W. S., Dunham, D., & Ormond, K. E. (2003). The Genetic Family History as a Risk Assessment Tool in Internal Medicine. *Genetics in Medicine, 5*(2), 84–91. doi:10.1097/01.GIM.0000055197.23822.5E PMID:12644777

Glaser, J., Henley, D. E., Downing, G., Brinner, K. M., & Brinner,. (2008). Advancing Personalized Health Care through Health Information Technology: An Update from the American Health Information Community's Personalized Health Care Workgroup. *Journal of the American Medical Informatics Association, 15*(4), 391–396. doi:10.1197/jamia.M2718 PMID:18436899

Health Level Seven International. (2014). *Introduction to HL7 Standards.* Retrieved 2014-09-04, from http://www.hl7.org/implement/standards/index.cfm?ref=nav

Hinton, R. B. Jr. (2008). The Family History: Reemergence of an Established Tool. *Critical Care Nursing Clinics of North America, 20*(2), 149–158. doi:10.1016/j.ccell.2008.01.004 PMID:18424345

Human Variome Project. (2014). *Human Variome Project International Limited.* Retrieved 2014-09-18, from http://www.humanvariomeproject.org/about/

Kmiecik, T., & Sanders, D. (2009). *Integration of Genetic and Familial Data into Electronic Medical Records and Healthcare Processes.* Northwestern Medical Faculty Foundation, Northwestern University. Retrieved from www.surgery.northwestern.edu/docs/KmiecikSandersArticle.pdf

Morales, A., Cowan, J., Dagua, J., & Hershberger, R. E. (2008). Family History: An Essential Tool for Cardiovascular Genetic Medicine. *Congestive Heart Failure (Greenwich, Conn.), 14*(1), 37–45. doi:10.1111/j.1751-7133.2008.08201.x PMID:18256568

Orlando, L. A., Buchanan, A. H., Hahn, S. E., Christianson, C. A., Powell, K. P., Skinner, C. S., & Henrich, V. C. et al. (2013). Development and validation of a primary care-based family health history and decision support program (MeTree). *North Carolina Medical Journal, 74*(4), 287–296. PMID:24044145

Owens, K., Marvin, M., Gelehrter, T., Ruffin, M., & Uhlmann, W. (2011). Clinical Use of the Surgeon General's "My Family Health Portrait" (MFHP) Tool: Opinions of Future Health Care Providers. *Journal of Genetic Counseling, 20*(5), 510–525. doi:10.1007/s10897-011-9381-x PMID:21701956

Peace, J., & Brennan, P. F. (2008). Instance testing of the family history ontology. *AMIA... Annual Symposium Proceedings/AMIA Symposium. AMIA Symposium*, 1088. PMID:18999123

Peace, J., & Brennan, P. F. (2009). Formalizing nursing knowledge: From theories and models to ontologies. *Studies in Health Technology and Informatics, 146*, 347–351. PMID:19592863

Progeny Software. (2014). *Progeny Clinical: Data Integration*. Retrieved 2014-09-04, from http://www.progenygenetics.com/clinical/integration.html

Rempel, G. R., Neufeld, A., & Kushner, K. E. (2007). Interactive use of genograms and ecomaps in family caregiving research. *Journal of Family Nursing, 13*(4), 403–419. doi:10.1177/1074840707307917 PMID:18180467

Rich, E. C., Burke, W., Heaton, C. J., Haga, S., Pinsky, L., Short, M. P., & Acheson, L. (2004). Reconsidering the Family History in Primary Care. *Journal of General Internal Medicine, 19*(3), 273–280. doi:10.1111/j.1525-1497.2004.30401.x PMID:15009784

Santos, J. M., Santos, B. S., & Teixeira, L. (2014). Using Ontologies and Semantic Web Technology on a Clinical Pedigree Information System. In V. Duffy (Ed.), *Digital Human Modeling. Applications in Health, Safety, Ergonomics and Risk Management* (Vol. 8529, pp. 448–459). Springer International Publishing. doi:10.1007/978-3-319-07725-3_45

Scheuner, M. T., de Vries, H., Kim, B., Meili, R. C., Olmstead, S. H., & Teleki, S. (2009). Are Electronic Health Records Ready for Genomic Medicine? *Genetics in Medicine, 11*(7), 510–517. doi:10.1097/GIM.0b013e3181a53331 PMID:19478682

Teixeira, L., Ferreira, C., & Santos, B. S. (2012). User-centered requirements engineering in health information systems: A study in the hemophilia field. *Computer Methods and Programs in Biomedicine, 106*(3), 160–174. doi:10.1016/j.cmpb.2010.10.007 PMID:21075471

Tempest, V., Iredale, R., Gray, J., France, L., Anstey, S., & Steward, J. (2005). Pedigree Construction and Disease Confirmation: A Pilot Study in Wales Exploring the Role of Nonclinical Personnel. *European Journal Of Human Genetics: EJHG, 13*(9), 1063–1070. doi:10.1038/sj.ejhg.5201454 PMID:15956999

Trager, E. H., Khanna, R., Marrs, A., Siden, L., Branham, K. E. H., Swaroop, A., & Richards, J. E. (2007). Madeline 2.0 PDE: A new program for local and web-based pedigree drawing. *Bioinformatics (Oxford, England), 23*(14), 1854–1856. doi:10.1093/bioinformatics/btm242 PMID:17488757

U.S. Department of Energy Human Genome Project. (2014). *Human Genome Project Information Archive: About the Human Genome Project*. Retrieved 2014-09-18, from http://www.ornl.gov/hgmis

U.S. Department of Health & Human Services. (2009). *My Family Health Portrait*. Retrieved 2014-09-12, from http://familyhistory.hhs.gov/

Vesse, R., Zettlemoyer, R. M., Ahmed, K., Moore, G., & Pluskiewicz, T. (2014). *dotNetRDF - Semantic Web, RDF and SPARQL Library for C#/.Net* (Version 1.0.3). Retrieved from http://www.dotnetrdf.org/

Wattendorf, D. J., & Hadley, D. W. (2005). Family History: The Three-Generation Pedigree. *American Family Physician*, *72*(3), 441–448. PMID:16100858

World Health Organization. (2006). Sickle-cell anaemia: Report by the Secretariat. 59th World Health Assembly.

Wu, R. R., Himmel, T. L., Buchanan, A. H., Powell, K. P., Hauser, E. R., Ginsburg, G. S., & Orlando, L. A. et al. (2014). Quality of family history collection with use of a patient facing family history assessment tool. *BMC Family Practice*, *15*(1), 31. doi:10.1186/1471-2296-15-31 PMID:24520818

KEY TERMS AND DEFINITIONS

Clinical Pedigree: A graphical representation of a clinical family history capable of representing the individuals belonging to a certain family and the family relations between them, as well as the relevant clinical and environmental information.

DNA: Deoxyribonucleic acid, a molecule containing the genetic code of living organisms.

Hemo@Care: A Healthcare Information System (HIS) built specifically for hemophilia care which has been integrated with OntoFam to provide clinical pedigree building tools.

HL7: Health Level Seven International, a non-profit organization that develops standards for exchange, integration, sharing, and retrieval of electronic health information. The organization has created a number of standards suited for different health-related purposes, which are collectively known as HL7.

OntoFam: An ontology-based clinical pedigree information system built using the principles described in this chapter. It allows the interactive creation and visualization of standards-based clinical pedigrees and uses Semantic Web technology to store, index, retrieve and reason with family history data.

Ontology: A description of a knowledge domain in a machine-understandable format, using classes, attributes, relations, restrictions and logic rules.

RDF: Resource Definition Framework, an XML-based representation of semantic data.

Triple: The fundamental unit of semantic data representation. A triple is a statement asserting that an entity (*subject*) has a certain relation (*predicate*) with another entity (*object*).

XML: Extensible Markup Language, a standard text-based format used to represent structured data.

Understanding Customer Behavior through Collaboration RFM Analysis and Data Mining Using Health Life Center Data

Numan Çelebi
Sakarya University, Turkey

Musa Efe Erten
Istanbul Technical University, Turkey

Hayrettin Evirgen
Istanbul University, Turkey

INTRODUCTION

Sports provides an outlet for athleticism and competitions, such as the Olympics and World Cup, as well as personal activities done for health reasons. In turn, sports activities generate a nearly infinite amount of data, such as individual player performance, managerial decisions, and the income sports organizations derive. For that, the most important question remains, "How can we use this data efficiently?" Sport center managers can turn this data into meaningful and useful knowledge using several techniques, and they can use it against their competitors to create a competitive advantage. Data mining tray to extract previously unknown and potentially useful information from data (Fayyad, et al., 1996) and tray to find relations, patterns and predictive rules hidden in databases. In the past, sports data-mining did not attract considerable attention (Solieman, 2006) because of a resistance and lack of faith by sports clubs and organizational managers who focussed primarily on the results of athletes and team scores. The enormous variety of sources providing data made anecdotal opinions based on the data insufficient, however, for most sports organizations; they needed more powerful methods to extract significant information from the collected data. This lead to a need to measure athletes' performance more precisely and to establish better decision-making by using statistical analysis. More recently, however, data-mining techniques have emerged as an important technology for revolutionizing a wide range of applications, including sports. These techniques are preferred instead of statistical methods because of their superior properties as a generalization of present condition and for making predictions -allowing sports managers to create better strategies for their teams or facilities.

Most of the work regarding sports data-mining has occurred in regard to professional sports, while life centers or amateur sports organizations, the centers of individual sports involvement, have not been analyzed as much. Nowadays, sports, fitness and health life centers have become a big and growing sector. People, especially in metropolitan areas try to stay healthy, using fitness, sauna and massage areas in these centers. To survive, these businesses, having gained strength economically and increased in numbers, need tools to maintain their customers and to predict their future needs.

As competition for sales grows tense, companies and organizations have started to appreciate their customers as their most valuable assets (Poel and Bart, 2004). The difficulty and expense of acquiring new customers exceeds that for retaining old ones (Krivobokova, 2009). Because of increasing the number

DOI: 10.4018/978-1-4666-9978-6.ch067

of customers and rising competition, the health life sport centers have begun to take into consideration customers' needs as a priority. Customers may each prefer different services or products. Therefore, companies should first classify customers according to their prior transactions involving services and products. Firms can identify their customers' profiles using Customer Relations Management's (CRM) concept and data-mining techniques. CRM aims to reveal customers' needs, choices and behaviours and to provide a basis for making long-lasting relationships with customers (Tsiptsis and Chorianopoulos, 2009). For that reason, with segmentation being based on customers' values and grading different relationships among different segments is important. For segmentation, customer loyalty is a suitable property, and customers' past buying behaviour shows their customer loyalty (Chang, et al., 2011). A customer who has a positive attitude towards a firm or organization and makes frequent transactions is a loyal customer. Positive attitude alone is not enough for customer loyalty - there must be an inclination for future transactions. Some experts evaluate customer loyalty with Recency, Frequency and Monetary (Seyed, et al., 2010). Customer Lifetime Value is defined as the net profit gained from a customer by an organization in the customer's total lifetime (Gupta and Lehmann, 2003). Also, RFM has recently become one of the most popular CLV model in order to extend the relationship with customers (Khajvand, et al. 2011).

There are usually two variables for evaluating customer loyalty. The first one is demographic variables such as age, gender, etc. The second one is RFM variables which express the customers' behaviours. In the RFM, Recency is a certain time from the last service transaction. Frequency is the number of transactions in a certain time. And, Monetary is fiscal benefit from the customer to the company in a certain time. Customers' behaviour can be analysed by using RFM variables. It is well known that customer past behaviour's score gives tips to predict the customer's behaviour for future (Birant, 2011). According to RFM variable scores, a company can segment customer groups and identify their most profitable customers. In this chapter, RFM scors first are used as an input for clustering algorithm to specify customer loyalty groups. Then, these groups are analyzed based on the customers' demographic variables to extract classification rules. After that, an association rule mining algorithm applied to these rules to express the relationship between customers' transactions and theirs demographic variables.

The remainder of this paper is organized as follows: A literature review about data-mining techniques and RFM applications is presented in Section 2. A description of the research methodology is given in Section 3. In Section 4, all the steps of the proposed model are expressed in detail using a real case study. The proposed model's results appear in section 5. The last section is the conclusion of the paper.

LITERATURE REVIEW

Data-mining techniques have been used for solving problems related to customers in areas such as engineering, finance and business (Written and Frank, 2005). In recent years, data-mining applications based on RFM concepts have been proposed for different areas. Liu and Shih (2005) developed a novel product recommendation methodology combining group decision making and data-mining techniques by using AHP, clustering and association rule mining techniques. Lo et al. (2008) adopted an RFM model to analyze members of a sports store. The results showed that higher transaction customers are male and aged between 26 and 35. Sohrabi and Khanlari (2007) used k-means clustering techniques to develop a customer live-value model and segmented the customers by taking into account their RFM values. Cheng and Chen (2009) combined quantitative values of RFM attributes and k-means algorithm with rough set theory to extract classification rules. They applied RFM to understand customer consuming behavior so they could segment groups of customers. Ha and Park (1998) applied data-mining techniques to increase the amount of sales of a shop based on RFM data extracted from customer transaction data. Hsieh (2004) proposed an integrated data-mining and behavioral scoring model to manage existing credit card customers in a bank by a self-organizing maps neural network to predict profitable groups of customers based on repayment information and RFM behavioral scoring predictors. The result showed the values of RFM affected customer segmentation.

Integration of RFM analysis and data-mining techniques provides useful knowledge about customers. Clustering based on RFM values provides more behavioral knowledge of customers` actual marketing levels than other cluster analysis. Classification rules discovered from customer demographic variables and RFM variables provides useful knowledge for managers to predict future customer behavior, such as how soon the customer will probably purchase, how often the customer will purchase, and what will be the values of the customer's purchases. Association rule mining based on RFM values analyzes the relationships of product properties and customers`contributions/loyalties to provide better recommendations to satisfy customers`needs.

RESEARCH METHODOLOGY

The proposed approach is based on data-mining and customer value analysis techniques to improve customer relationship management based on RFM variables and with Two-step, C5.0 and association rules mining algorithms. It has five stages: (1) Selecting the dataset and preprocessing, (2) Calculating the RFM values to give numeric values to clustering analysis, (3) Using a Two-step algorithm to cluster the customers by RFM values to specify the customer loyalty degree, (4) Using the C5.0 algorithm to create classes which shows the relationships between customers' demographic attributes and RFM values, (5) Applying association rule mining to extract useful rules for service recommendations. Finally, interpreting the results and comparing the rules from different classes. With the help of this model, old data can be analysed and thus detailed knowledge about customers can be obtained. Fitness and life center managers can use this knowledge when they promote new marketing strategies. Figure 1 shows the required steps for the proposed model as we will discuss further.

1. Data Preprocessing

First, a dataset is chosen for empirical case work. To extract knowledge from the data, it must be prepared. Data preprocessing involves data cleaning, data integration and data reduction as its three main activities. In the data cleaning phase, wrongs and blanks in the dataset are changed to suitable forms or removed. In the data integration phase, all data is made compatible with each other. Finally, in the data reduction phase, data having the same meaning is removed to arrive at a more meaningful and less complicated dataset.

2. Calculating RFM Values

RFM analysis consists of dividing, sorting and grading a dataset by RFM parameters into five groups. Sorting methods include basic, nested and weighted sorting (Sellers and Hughes, 2013); in this study, a basic sorting method is used. For this method, in every parameter from top to bottom, let slices of 20%

Figure 1. Proposed combined model

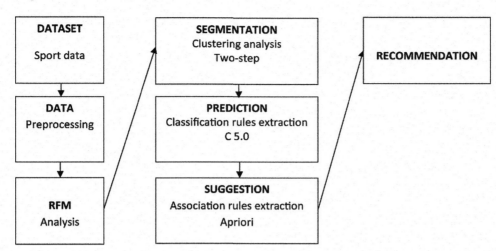

have points decreasing from 5 to 1. The point '5' corresponds to the customer point with maximum benefit, whereas the point '1' corresponds to minimum benefit. Thus, records could divide into 125 (5x5x5) different RFM labels. A label having the maximum scores is '555', whereas a label having the minimum score is '111'.

3. Clustering Customers Based on RFM Values

In this stage, to determine high-valued customers, the dataset is fragmented into segments of customers having the same or close to the same RFM scores. This approach allows the manager to recognize market segments in a more comprehensive manner so they can apply different marketing strategies to their different customer clusters. Most of the clustering algorithms have limitations and weaknesses. For example, in a k-means algorithm results are often related to clusters selected as start points (Shih et al., 2010). In this study, because of its advantages, a two-step algorithm has been used instead of a k-means clustering algorithm. This algorithm has several desirable features differentiating it from traditional clustering techniques (Li and Sun, 2011). It is an exploratory tool designed to reveal natural groupings (or clusters) within a dataset. The two-step cluster analysis developed by Chiu, et al., (2001) has been specifically designed to handle very large datasets. The name "two-step clustering" already indicates the algorithm relies on two-phases: (1) preclustering and (2) agglomerative clustering.

4. Extracting Classification Rules Considering Customers' Demographic Attributes

In this stage, classification rules are discovered by classifying customers into segments according to theirs demographic variables. When choosing a classification algorithm, the total number of variables, the compability of variables and algorithms are taken into account. Decision Tree (Kotsiantis, 2007) is an important model to carry out the classification. The first concept of Decision Tree comes from Concept Learning System (CLS) as proposed by Hunt et al., (1966) when they researched human concept modeling early in the 1960s. Based on it, numerous improved algorithms have emerged. Among these, the most famous algorithm is ID3 with a choosing policy according to entropy based information gain as put forward by Quinlan (1986). In 1993, Quinlan developed C4.5 algorithm on the basis of the ID3 algorithm (Quinlan, 1994). C4.5 takes information gain ratio as the selecting criterion to overcome the defect of ID3, which is apt to use attributes having more values. C5.0 is another new Decision Tree algorithm developed by Quinlan as an improved version of the well-known and widely used C4.5 classifier (Chiang, 2012). It has several important advantages over C4.5 based on efficiency and memory (Bujlow et al. 2012); the generated rules are more accurate, and the time used to generate them is lower (even around 360 times on some data sets). For these reasons, in this study, using demographic variables and RFM parameters, classification rules are extracted by a C5.0 Decision Tree algorithm. The realization process of the algorithm can be described as follows: "C5.0 model works by splitting the sample, based on the field providing the maximum information gain. The C5.0 model can split samples on the basis of the biggest information gain field. The sample subset obtained from the former split will be split afterward. The process will continue until the sample subset cannot be split more or according to another field. Finally, examining the lowest level split, those sample subsets without remarkable contribution to the model will be rejected" (Patil, et al. 2012).

5. Extracting Association Rules

This step aims to determine association rules between customer segments, customer profiles and products or services customers have bought. Association rule mining is one of the most popular data-mining approaches to find frequent item sets from a transaction dataset. Apriori algorithm is used to extract interesting correlations, frequent item sets, and association rules in the transaction databases. The apriori algorithm was first introduced by Agrawal, et al. (1993) and has become an important data-mining algorithm studied extensively by database and data-mining researchers. The most often cited application of association rules is market basket analysis using transaction databases from supermarkets (Nandagopal, et al. 2010). Association rules are also used in other areas, such as telecommunication networks, health, risk management and inventory control, etc. After these phases, clusters, demographic classification rules and association rules are interpreted together. For meaningless and unrealistic results, data and phases should be reviewed. If the method is not efficient enough, other methods and data-mining models should be created.

AN ILLUSTRATIVE EXAMPLE

This section presents a case study demonstrating how our proposed model was applied to real world data collected by a fitness and sport center. All steps of the proposed model are expressed in detail.

Step 1: Data Preprocessing

Data used in this case study was provided from a health life center in Istanbul, Turkey. The data consists of customer records covering the nine year period between January 1, 2003 and January 1, 2012. In the dataset for every record identified with an ID number, there are three different demographic variables covering age, gender and educational length and three different RFM data scores covering the length of time from the date of the last extension of the membership, the duration of the membership itself and the payment of the customer to the company within the membership period. Moreover, there is a "purchased product-service" dataset showing the consumption of customers as well as products or services and their dates. Age range runs between seven and ninety and, for the Recency calculation starting point of January 1, 2012, the records of every customer between seven and ninety years old on January 1, 2012, are taken into account. Gender is divided between "Male" and "Female" and, the educational length ranges between six and nineteen years. Data preprocessing simply has three main activities, namely, data cleaning, data integration and data reduction. At the data cleaning phase, wrong or missing records are changed into suitable ones or removed. At the data integration phase, data types are changed into compatible ones. Finally, at the data reduction phase, data types are reduced to simplify the dataset. Table 1 shows data types and records at the beginning of our proposed process.

Step 2: Calculating RFM Value

RFM analysis is adapted according to models established due to data types and extracted from the data set. In this chapter, the logic behind the RFM analysis is based on the renewal of memberships in a health sport center. According to this idea, Recency means that from the length of time the last renewal of membership to recent time. Frequency means that the length of the membership in years between 2003 and 2012. Monetary means that the purchasing of services which are taken by customers of a health life center having standard membership revenues. The longer the membership time length, the more benefit to the company from the customer. Therefore, frequency is selected as "the duration of the membership". For every attribute (R-F-M), records are split and sorted into five equal pieces. All customers were ranked by considering their RFM labels, and they were represented by RFM codes. According to the first row in Table 2, the customer with ID number 1 has an RFM label of 225. This customer renewed his or her membership 1555 days ago, this membership lasted 605 days, and the customer's contribution to the health center is 957.50. The customers separated into five equal groups, each one account for 20% of all data. Based on his separation, the RFM labels of customers are determined by RFM analysis as shown in Table 2.

Table 1. Initial table

ID	Age	Gender	The length of Education	The Length of Membership Renewal	The Length of MembeWrship	Monetary Contribution
1	34	Male	8	1555	605	957.5
2	42	Male	15	2019	373	45
3	54	Male	15	2346	1837	1498
4	45	Male	17	288	879	65
5	47	Female	11	536	792	115
6	50	Male	15	468	791	425
7	46	Male	19	1934	737	5
8	39	Female	17	397	1186	15
9	44	Male	17	48	791	15
10	53	Male	17	554	880	795
.	.	.	.	.	.	.
3412	49	Female	15	621	833	75

Table 2. RFM labels of customers after RFM analysis

ID	R (Day)	F (Day)	M (Income)	R (Score)	F (Score)	M (Score)	RFM Label
1	1555	605	957.5	2	2	5	225
2	2019	373	45	1	1	4	114
3	2346	1837	1498	1	5	5	155
4	288	879	65	4	3	4	434
5	536	792	115	4	3	4	434
6	468	791	425	4	2	5	425
7	1934	737	5	1	2	2	122
8	397	1186	15	4	4	3	443
9	2142	1836	65	1	5	4	154
10	139	1187	2201	5	4	5	545
.	.	.	.	.	.	.	.
3412	295	750	75	4	3	4	434

Step 3: Clustering Customers with Similar RFM Values by Two-Step Algorithm

Two-step clustering, a hierarchical clustering method, was employed to group customers with similar RFM labels. In this method, the number of clusters is not applied to the algorithm before the clustering process. The two-step algorithm first starts partitioning the data into separate clusters, then merges customers having similar RFM labels in the same cluster or vice versa. Finally, the algorithm finds automatically the optimal number of clusters where clusters are meaningful and different from each other. The two-step algorithm found five clusters (C1, C2, C3, C4 and C5) automatically based on RFM labels of the customer data. Table 3 shows the average of the cluster center according to RFM labels.

According to Table 3, the RFM characteristic (center) of Cluster1 is 213 since the average number in R row is 2 (at 31.62%), in F row is 1 (at 77.65%) and in M row is 3 (at 42.65%). By the same method, the RFM labels of the other cluster centers are 324, 445, 531 and 111, respectively. After finding the cluster centers, we can add customers into clusters according to their RFM label. To determine the cluster of the customers, we consider minimizing the distance measure between the customer RFM label and the cluster center RFM point. The minimization of distance measure has the following form:

$$\min dis\tan ce = \sum_{i=1}^{n}\sum_{j=1}^{m}\left|x_i - c_j\right|$$

where x represents customers and c represents cluster centers. i is the index of the customers $(i = 1, 2, \ldots\ldots, n)$, j is the index of the cluster center $(j = 1, 2, \ldots\ldots, m)$. In this study, we developed an algorithm for assigning customers to the appropriate cluster. The algorithm works as follows: first, it finds the minimum distance between each customer and all cluster centers, and then it assigns the customer to the cluster having the minimum distance based on RFM labels between customer and cluster centers as shown in Table 4.

Table 4 presents the result of the clustering analysis with the corresponding RFM label of each customer. Each cluster has different size; the clusters have 680 (C1), 754 (C2), 975 (C3), 666(C4) and

E

Table 3. Average of cluster centers based on RFM labels

Clusters No	RFM Labels (%)					Total
Cluster 1	**1**	**2**	**3**	**4**	**5**	
Recency	12.79	31.62	23.97	17.94	13.68	100
Frequency	77.65	0.00	22.35	0.00	0.00	100
Monetary	32.20	1.91	42.65	5.74	17.50	100
Cluster 2	**1**	**2**	**3**	**4**	**5**	
Recency	7.56	15.52	39.52	37.40	0.00	100
Frequency	17.24	32.63	27.45	3.45	19.23	100
Monetary	25.99	35.68	0.00	38.33	0.00	100
Cluster 3	**1**	**2**	**3**	**4**	**5**	
Recency	15.28	26.56	22.46	28.62	7.08	100
Frequency	0.00	13.75	0.00	51.79	34.46	100
Monetary	13.44	2.15	32.82	14.87	36.72	100
Cluster 4	**1**	**2**	**3**	**4**	**5**	
Recency	8.26	13.81	0.00	0.00	77.93	100
Frequency	0.00	33.93	41.59	9.16	15.32	100
Monetary	36.64	8.26	12.61	11.71	30.78	100
Cluster 5	**1**	**2**	**3**	**4**	**5**	
Recency	100.00	0.00	0.00	0.00	0.00	100
Frequency	44.81	0.00	0.00	26.11	29.08	100
Monetary	65.88	0.00	0.00	34.12	0.00	100

Table 4. Cluster determination with RFM label

ID	R (Day)	F (Day)	M (Income)	R (Score)	F (Score)	M (Score)	RFM Label	Cluster
1	1555	605	957.50	2	2	5	225	C1
2	2019	373	45	1	1	4	114	C5
3	2346	1837	1498	1	5	5	155	C5
4	288	879	65	4	3	4	434	C3
5	536	792	115	4	3	4	434	C3
6	468	791	425	4	2	5	425	C3
7	1934	737	5	1	2	2	122	C4
8	397	1186	15	4	4	3	443	C3
9	2142	1836	65	1	5	4	154	C5
10	139	1187	2201	5	4	5	545	C4
.	.	.	.	.	.	.	.	.
3412	295	750	75.00	4	3	4	434	C3

337(C5) customers, respectively. While cluster C3 contains the maximum number of customers (28%), C5 includes the minimum, only 337 cutomers (9%).

Step 4: Extracting Classification Rules Considering Customers' Demographic Attributes

After clustering analysis, every record has been gathered into clusters as much as "k" with a unique RFM label. The k parameter was set to five, the optimal cluster number obtained by the two-step algorithm. Then, to predict future customer behavior from customer segments, the model wants to extract classification rules using RFM labels and demographic attributes. At this phase, every record is subject to "classification" with its demographic attributes. So, if some of the customers have the same demographic attributes, then very likely they have the same RFM labels. At this phase, we understand the relation between RFM labels and demographic attributes of records. Finding classification rules helps managers to determine target customer profiles effectively. Besides, if they analyze these results, they can improve health life center's service strategies. In this chapter, we used cluster number, age, gender and education length variables to extract classification rules. We get the classification rules for each cluster as shown between in Table 5 and Table 8.

Seven extracted classification rules exist for cluster 1. The first rule tells us that if a customer's age is 30 or 31, the gender is male and the educational length is greater than 15 years, then this record belongs to cluster 1 whose RFM label we know from RFM analysis. As shown in Table 8, some rows's columns representing attributes are blank; the algorithm did not find a sufficiently significant pattern. For example, in Table 5 rule 3 shows there is no meaningful relationship between gender and educational length in cluster 1 for the 19 - 21 age interval. Other rules in that table and the following tables (Table6, Table7 and Table8) should be interpreted as we just did.

The algorithm could not extract classification rules for cluster5.

Table 5. Classification rules for cluster1

Rule No.	Age	Gender	Educational Length
1	=30 || =31	Male	>15
2	>35 &&<=38	Male	>17
3	>19 &&<=21		
4	>32 &&<=35	Female	>11
5	>33 &&<=35	Male	<=11
6	<=32	Male	<=12
7	<=28	Female	

Table 6. Classification rules for cluster2

Rule No.	Age	Gender	Educational Length
1	>28 &&<=30		>12
2	>30 &&<=32	Male	<=11
3	>22 &&<=29	Male	<=8
4	>37 &&<=38		>=15
5	>24 &&<=32	Female	<7

Table 7. Classification rules for cluster3

Rule No.	Age	Gender	Educational Length
1	>24		

Step 5: Extracting of Association Rules

After identifying the best clustering results and their characteristics, the next step is to extract association rules from these five clusters. That is, the extracted rules can be used to predict customers who are going to purchase services or products and have high profitability. Thus, for every cluster we can see which product or service relations are dense. Therefore, the association rules algorithm is used for this purpose. In our study, after the experimental analysis, we determined the most convenient confidence ratio as 10% and support ratio as 2%, respectively. Table 9 lists the extracted rules of the five clusters for helath life sport center to identify the more profitable cluster customers.

The prediction results indicate that the extracted association rules from the identified five clusters are highly dependent on educational length and age variables. The gender variables have no effect on the rules.

SOLUTIONS AND RECOMMENDATIONS

This paper focuses on examining customers at one sport and health life center in Istanbul, Turkey, by taking advantage of data-mining combined with RFM analysis. In this section, the experimental results and the contribution of this paper are explained. Except from the whole function of the proposed model, knowledge can be understood and extracted from any phase of our study. For example, some knowledge can be interpreted after the RFM analysis and Two-Step algorithm as below:

Cluster 1: With a 2-1-3 RFM label, second most contributive customers;
Cluster 2: With a 3-2-4 RFM label, customers who have balanced consumption habits;
Cluster 3: With a 4-4-5 RFM label, most uncontributive customers;
Cluster 4: With a 5-3-1 RFM label, customers who have not made transactions recently; and
Cluster 5: With a 1-1-1 RFM label, most contributive customers.

Customers who are in clusters 1 or 5 are very important for the company because of their transactions. The company should be extremely sensitive to these customers' needs or wants. Otherwise, the company will face the greater cost of finding new customers. Clusters 3 and 4, contain the potential customers of the company, thus they should be drawn in by marketing. Cluster 3 consists of customers who have not made lots of transactions, so to get these customers is relatively less expensive. Cluster 4 consists of

Table 8. Classification rules for cluster4

Rule No.	Age	Gender	Educational Length
1	<=26	Female	>15
2	<=26	Male	>8 &&<=12
3	>26 &&<=28		>12 &&<=15
4	>29 &&<=30		<=8
5	>21 &&<=24	Female	
6	<36 &&>=37		<=11
7	<=32	Male	>12

Table 9. Results of association rule mining

Dependent Variable	Independent Variable	Support (%)	Confidence (%)
Fee of Pilates	age_53.0 = 1	2.107	49.781
Fee of Pilates	educational length_19.0 = 1 and clusters_3 = 1	3.487	30.606
Fee of Bonnet	clusters_1 = 1 and educational length_11.0 = 1	3.459	19.680
Fee of Bonnet	clusters_2 = 1 and educational length_15.0 = 1	3.146	17.543
Fee of Turkish Bath	clusters_5 = 1	5.253	16.637
Fee of Bonnet	age_30.0 = 1	2.116	16.086
Fee of Bonnet	clusters_2 = 1 and educational length_11.0 = 1	3.726	15.802
Fee of Bonnet	age_32.0 = 1	3.146	15.497
Fee of Pilates	educational length_19.0 = 1	7.103	15.025
Fee of Bonnet	clusters_1 = 1	15.891	14.244
Fee of Bonnet	educational length_6.0 = 1 and clusters_2 = 1	2.493	14.022
Fee of Private Sports Assistant	age_45.0 = 1	3.579	13.624
Fee of Bonnet	clusters_1 = 1 and educational length_17.0 = 1	3.229	13.390
Fee of Bonnet	clusters_2 = 1	16.148	13.162
Fee of Bonnet	age_31.0 = 1	2.337	12.992
Fee of Bonnet	age_41.0 = 1 and clusters_3 = 1	2.153	12.820
Fee of Bonnet	educational length_6.0 = 1 and clusters_1 = 1	3.110	12.721
Fee of Private Fitness Lesson	educational length_8.0 = 1 and clusters_4 = 1	3.993	12.442
Fee of Bonnet	educational length_17.0 = 1 and clusters_4 = 1	3.257	12.429
Fee of Private Fitness Lesson	educational length_6.0 = 1 and clusters_4 = 1	2.530	12.363
Fee of Bonnet	educational length_11.0 = 1	21.991	12.133
Fee of Private Fitness Lesson	educational length_12.0 = 1 and clusters_3 = 1	2.603	12.014
Fee of Bonnet	age_35.0 = 1	3.395	11.653
Fee of Bonnet	educational length_12.0 = 1	6.505	11.598
Fee of Bonnet	age_37.0 = 1	3.441	11.497
Fee of Bonnet	age_52.0 = 1	2.097	11.403
Fee of Bonnet	age_46.0 = 1	2.603	11.307
Fee of Pilates	educational length_12.0 = 1 and clusters_3 = 1	2.603	11.307
Fee of Private Fitness Lesson	age_43.0 = 1 and clusters_3 = 1	2.705	11.224
Fee of Slippers	clusters_1 = 1 and educational length_17.0 = 1	3.229	11.111
Fee of Bonnet	age_33.0 = 1	4.085	11.036
Fee of Slippers	age_31.0 = 1	2.337	11.023
Fee of Bonnet	clusters_5 = 1	5.253	10.858
Fee of Slippers	age_35.0 = 1	3.395	10.840
Fee of Private Fitness Lesson	educational length_11.0 = 1 and clusters_3 = 1	8.483	10.629
Fee of Bonnet	clusters_1 = 1 and educational length_15.0 = 1	2.723	10.472
Fee of Private Fitness Lesson	age_39.0 = 1 and clusters_3 = 1	2.548	10.469
Fee of Bonnet	age_42.0 = 1	3.606	10.459
Fee of Slippers	clusters_2 = 1 and educational length_17.0 = 1	3.091	10.416

continued on following page

Table 9. Continued

Dependent Variable	Independent Variable	Support (%)	Confidence (%)
Fee of Bonnet	educational length_15.0 = 1	19.617	10.272
Fee of Bonnet	educational length_12.0 = 1 and clusters_3 = 1	2.603	10.247
Fee of Bonnet	educational length_15.0 = 1 and clusters_3 = 1	7.554	10.231
Fee of Bonnet	educational length_17.0 = 1	19.001	10.169
Fee of Pilates (10 package)	educational length_8.0 = 1 and clusters_4 = 1	3.993	10.138
Fee of Private Sports Assistant	age_52.0 = 1	2.097	10.087
Fee of Slippers	clusters_2 = 1	16.148	10.085

customers who have made dense transactions earlier, however, but for some reason have stopped. If the company is not very careful about this cluster, the customers will stop making transactions.

After extracted classification rules, knowledge has become more sophisticated, more precise and more understandable. Cluster 1 consists of relatively young (28-38 years) and intellectual people (their educational length is more than 11 years); these people are very likely in the labor market. If we think this cluster is important to the company, there should be a suitable sport schedule and activities for their work life. After long work hours, they want to relax, so the company could create sport and exercise activities which relax them. This would increase service quality.

Demographic attributes of cluster 2 are parallel to cluster 1, but cluster 2 has a different RFM label; consumption habits create this difference. These habits can be related to the customers' social or cultural background. For that reason, the propositions given for cluster 1 are also appropriate for cluster 2. Cluster 3 is the cluster which the company should work on. On the other hand, from classification rule analysis, we cannot extract detailed rules. The reasons for this can be either narrow demographic attributes data or lack of patterns. To make this work better, the number of demographic variables should be increased. Cluster 4 consists of unsatisfied customers as shown from the low RFM label. This cluster is the same as cluster 1 according to age, but the customers in this cluster have limited educational length (8-15 years). The company should end the churn situation in this cluster.

If we blend our knowledge of demographic attributes and RFM labeled clusters with products and services, we reach more detailed information covering customer profiles and consumption habits. Pilates service is popular among the customers who are near 50 or who belong to cluster 3. For them, the company should arrange different sport activities or pilates sessions for the different age groups. As pointed out before, for cluster 3 there should be a new approach.

Another popular pattern is the consumption of slippers and bonnets regardless of clusters or demographic attributes. For this reason, purchasing of these materials could be reviewed. Knowing these materials are often sold, their quality is very important. And, among the low educational length group, there is routine purchasing of fitness lessons. In this situation, for children there can be special sessions or club activities scheduled on the weekends.

Because of the elasticity of our model, there can be different syntheses. There are given some suggestions for different situations for future studies as follows:

- If we increase the number of data variables, more sensitive results can be reached (for example, there could be variables such as health problems, purchasing sport programs, diets, jobs, etc.).

- The company could give weight to any RFM label (for example, R can be more important compared to F and M, so Recency scores could be multiplied with any ratio).
- Besides our model, "Churn Analysis" can be done regarding RFM scores.

In some sectors needing one-to-one analysis (like sport centers), with proper methods and synthesis, customers can be evaluated better. After this evaluation, our knowledge based on a numeric basis gives managers the opportunity to make better strategies.

CONCLUSION

This study aimed at analyzing customer behavior in a sport and life center. We introduced a well-designed data-mining approach using RFM analysis and three data-mining techniques - clustering, classification and association rule mining. Determination of the customer behavior is of great importance, especially in issues such as retail marketing and the tourism sector. Using RFM along with three data-mining techniques gives our model the advantage of identifying customers and profiles more subjectively. To the best of our knowledge, there has been no previous study investigating customer behavior in a sports and life fitness center using this approach. In order to evaluate the proposed model, a case study was carried out using a sport and life center database of stored customer transactions. The experimental results indicated the proposed approach works well to determine customer behavior for sport marketing use, and it helps the decision makers to improve the service quality. The proposed model is effective, yet certain modifications are needed to make it more suitable for different cases; this will be discussed in detail in future work ongoing in this regard.

REFERENCES

Agrawal, R., Imielinski, T., & Swami, A. N. (1993). Mining association rules between sets of items in large databases. In *Proceedings of the 1993 ACM SIGMOD International Conference on Management of Data* (pp. 207-216). doi:10.1145/170035.170072

Birant, D. (2011). *Data Mining using RFM Analysis. Knowledge-Oriented Applications in Data Mining* (pp. 91–108). Crotia, InTech.

Bujlow, T., Riaz, T., & Pedersen, J. M. (2012). A method for classification of network traffic based on C5.0 Machine Learning Algorithm.*Workshop on Computing, Networking and Communications*. IEEE. doi:10.1109/ICCNC.2012.6167418

Chang, H. C., & Tsai, H. P. (2011). Group RFM analysis as a novel framework to discover better customer consumption behavior. *Expert Systems with Applications*, 38(12), 14499–14513. doi:10.1016/j. eswa.2011.05.034

Cheng, C. H., & Chen, Y. S. (2009). Classifying the segmentation of customer value via RFM model and RS Theory. *Expert Systems with Applications*, 36(3), 4176–4184. doi:10.1016/j.eswa.2008.04.003

Chiang, W. Y. (2012). Applying a New Model of Customer Value on International Air Passengers' Market in Taiwan. *International Journal of Tourism Research*, 14(2), 116–123. doi:10.1002/jtr.840

Chiu, T., Fang, D., Chen, J., Wang, Y., & Jeris, C. (2001). A Robust and Scalable Clustering Algorithm for Mixed Type Attributes in Large Database Environment.*Proceedings of the seventh ACMSIGKDD International conference on knowledge discovery and data-mining* (pp. 263–268). San Francisco, CA: ACM. doi:10.1145/502512.502549

Fayyad, U., Piatetsky-Shapiro, G., & Smyth, P. (1996). *From Data-Mining to Knowledge Discovery, An Overview: Advances in Knowledge Discovery and Data-Mining*. AAAI Press.

Gupta, S., & Lehmann, D. R. (2003). Customers as assets. *Journal of Interactive Marketing*, *17*(1), 9–24. doi:10.1002/dir.10045

Ha, S. H., & Park, S. C. (1998). Application of data-mining tools to hotel data mart on the Intranet for database marketing. *Expert Systems with Applications*, *15*(1), 1–31. doi:10.1016/S0957-4174(98)00008-6

Han, J., Kamber, M., & Pei, J. (2012). *Data-Mining Concepts and Techniques*. MA, USA: Morgan Kaufman Publisher.

Han, J., Pei, J., & Yin, Y. (2000). Mining Frequent Patterns without Candidate Generation.*SIGMOD Conference* (pp. 1-12). ACM.

Hsieh, N. C. (2004). An integrated data-mining and behavioral acoring model for analyzing bank customers. *Expert Systems with Applications*, *27*(4), 623–633. doi:10.1016/j.eswa.2004.06.007

Hunt, E. B., Marin, J., & Stone, P.J. (1966). Experiments in induction. New York: Academic Press.

Khajvand, M., Zolfaghar, K., Ashoori, S., & Alizadeh, S. (2011). Estimating customer lifetime value based on RFM analysis of customer purchase behavior: Case study. *Procedia Computer Science.*, *3*, 57–63. doi:10.1016/j.procs.2010.12.011

Kotsiantis, S. B. (2007). Supervised Machine Learning: A Review of Classification Techniques. *Informatica*, *31*, 249–256.

Krivobokova, O. V. (2009). Evaluating Customer Satisfaction as an Aspect of Quality Management. *International Journa of Network Security Application*, *2*, 9–20.

Li, H., & Sun, J. (2011). Mining business failure predictive knowledge using two-step clustering. *African Journal of Business Management*, *5*(11), 4107–4120.

Liu, D. R., & Shih, Y. Y. (2005). Integrating AHP and data-mining for product recommendation based on customer lifetime value. *Information & Management*, *42*(3), 387–400. doi:10.1016/j.im.2004.01.008

Lo, C. F., Wu, H. H., Chang, E. C., & Cheng, Y. Y. (2008). Applying data-mining to an outfitter's customer loyalty and value analysis. *Journal of Quality*, *15*(4), 293–300.

Nandagopal, S., Karthik, S., & Arunachalam, V. P. (2010). Mining of Meteorological Data Using Modified Apriori Algorithm. *European Journal of Scientific Research*, *47*(2), 295–308.

Patil, N., Lathi, R., & Chitre, V. (2012). Customer Card Classification Based on C5.0 & CART Algorithms. *International Journal of Engineering Research and Applications*, *2*(4), 164–167.

Quinlan, J. R. (1986). Induction of decision trees. *Machine Learning*, *4*(1), 81–106. doi:10.1007/BF00116251

Quinlan, J. R. (1994). C4.5: Programs for machine learning. *Machine Learning*, *3*, 235–240.

Sellers, J., & Hughes, A. M. (2013). *RFM Migration Analysis - A New Approach to a Proven Technique*. Retrieved April 25, 2013, from http://www.dbmarketing.com/articles/Art123.htm

Seyed Hosseini, S. M., Maleki, A., & Gholamian, M. R. (2010). Cluster analysis using data-mining approach to develop CRM methodology to assess the customer loyalty. *Expert Systems with Applications*, *37*(7), 5259–5264. doi:10.1016/j.eswa.2009.12.070

Shih, M. Y., Jheng, J. W., & Lai, L. F. (2010). A Two-Step Method for Clustering Mixed Categorical and Numeric Data. *Tamkang Journal of Science and Engineering*, *13*(1), 11–19.

Sohrabi, B., & Khanlari, A. (2007). Customer lifetime value (CLV) measurement based on RFM model. *Iranian Accounting & Auditing Review*, *14*(47), 7–20.

Solieman, O. K. (2006). *Data-Mining in Sports: A Research Overview*. Retrieved April 25, 2013, from http://ai.arizona.edu/mis480/syllabus/6_Osama-DM_in_Sports.pdf

Tsiptsis, K., & Chorianopoulos, A. (2009). *Data-Mining Techniques in CRM: Inside Customer Segmentation*. John Wiley & Sons Ltd.

Van den Poel, D., & Bart, L. (2004). Customer attrition analysis for financial services using proportional hazard models. *European Journal of Operational Research*, *157*(1), 196–217. doi:10.1016/S0377-2217(03)00069-9

Witten, I. H., & Frank, E. (2005). *Data-Mining, Practical Machine Learning Tools and Techniques*. Morgan Kaufmann Publishers.

KEY TERMS AND DEFINITIONS

Association Rule: Association rule analysis is a data mining technique to find frequent item sets from customers' transaction database.

Clustering: Clustering is a techniques to segment the items which they have similiar values or attributes.

Customer Life Time Value (CLV): CLV is a measure value to find the organization's gain are taken from the customer based on his/her expenses.

Customer Relationship Management (CRM): CRM is an approach to reveal cutomers' needs and making beter relationship along time with them.

Data Manipulation: It is a step in datamining process with the aim of data cleaning, data transformation and finding missing values etc. in database.

Datamining: Datamining is a knowledge extraction method from the databases. It uses the machine learning techniques and algorithms such as apriori algorithm, decision tree and clustering techniques etc.

RFM (Recency, Frequency, Monetary): RFM is a popular segmentation variable in marketing management that measures the loyalty of customers.

Using Big Data in Healthcare

Georgios Lamprinakos
National Technical University of Athens, Greece

Ioanna A. Aristeidopoulou
Intracom Telecom, Greece

Stefan Asanin
Anticimex, Greece

Andreas P. Kapsalis
National Technical University of Athens, Greece

Angelos-Christos G. Anadiotis
National Technical University of Athens, Greece

Dimitra I. Kaklamani
National Technical University of Athens, Greece

Iakovos S. Venieris
National Technical University of Athens, Greece

INTRODUCTION

The healthcare sector is undergoing fundamental changes recently. The vision of transforming the healthcare system from a treatment-oriented system to a patient-centered system based on prevention, ubiquitous monitoring and continuous multi-level support is considered to be a key point towards the improvement of the provided services and the reduction of healthcare costs, mainly attributed to the expected reduction in the number of hospitalizations. Throughout the new pathways, data volume and complexity are increasingly augmenting and require the use of the emerging big data analytics technologies in order to be significantly exploited. Health and social care services integration, continuity of care to the home, behavioral analysis and remote monitoring based on sensing devices are just a few elements of the new generation healthcare domain that all lead to the management of large, complex and frequently heterogeneous data.

In this chapter, the authors will summarize the trends of the modern healthcare ecosystem and present the current application categories, as well as challenges posed, concerning the high volume, variety and velocity healthcare data manipulation.

BACKGROUND

The term 'big data' refers to high volume and complexity data, which have become extremely difficult to process using traditional techniques. One of the earliest definitions of big data was provided by Laney

DOI: 10.4018/978-1-4666-9978-6.ch068

(2001), describing the new data growth challenges as three-dimensional (*Volume, Velocity, Variety*). The three-dimensional model, which stands as the most adopted definition up to date, regards big data as data that are massive in size (*Volume*), need to be quickly acquired and processed (*Velocity*), and are unstructured, loosely coupled and cannot be handled by traditional RDBMS (*Variety*). Another 'V' term that frequently accompanies the definition of big data is *Veracity*, indicating the need of processing clean and quality data, in order to achieve meaningful results from the big data use (cf. e.g., Buhl et al., 2013).

Nowadays, various sectors have transformed their way of functioning and they are collecting and exploiting large amounts of data, that may offer groundbreaking insights. Traditional services, such as weather forecasting, now require the manipulation of large amounts of data in order to provide better models, more accurate predictions, profiling and decision support. Many other paradigms exist where big data analytics can reshape well established operations. Power grids, for example, are beginning to evolve into smart grids, which are able to analyze data acquired from smart home appliances and smart sensors in order to sustain resources and energy and prevent service downtime during peak hours (Balac et al., 2013).

The aforementioned achievements, would not be made possible using legacy software methods and database systems. During the last years, extensive research has been conducted in order to invent new programming paradigms and software that would improve the manipulation, processing and analyzing of large scale data. MapReduce is a prevailing programming model for processing large datasets (Dean & Ghemawat, 2008), which usually runs on a cluster by using a parallel/distributed algorithm. Several MapReduce implementations exist, with Apache Hadoop (ASF, 2014a) being the most popular. The Hadoop framework is composed by several modules that include file-system for distributed storage, resource-management services and data processing module which is of course an implementation of the MapReduce algorithm. Among other MapReduce implementations are the CouchDB open source database system (ASF, 2014b), Infinispan (Red Hat, 2014) and MongoDB (MongoDB, 2014). Another fundamental big data technical component is Bigtable (Chang et al., 2006), which proposes a distributed file storage system for managing data that can scale to a very large size. Bigtable uses the distributed Google File System to store logs and data files. Some well-known open-source implementations of Bigtable, are Accumulo (ASF, 2014c), Cassandra (ASF, 2014d) and HBase (ASF, 2014e), all offered by the Apache Software Foundation. The successors of Bigtable are designed to meet the requirements of today's interactive online services. Google's Megastore provides fully serializable ACID semantics within fine-grained partitions of data (Baker et al., 2011), while Spanner is Google's scalable, multi-version, globally-distributed and synchronously-replicated database (Corbett et al., 2013). Other related software projects include Dremel, which is a query system for data analysis, presented by Melnik et al. (2010), Pregel, which is a scalable and fault tolerant graph processing system developed by Malewicz et al. (2010) and Tenzing, which offers an SQL implementation built on top of MapReduce for querying large datasets (Chattopadhyay et al., 2011).

The operations that are required for processing large datasets, as the ones present in the big data era, are computationally intensive and could take an unacceptable amount of time to yield the desired results. Facing this challenge, cloud computing has emerged as an optimal solution for executing jobs and tasks of that magnitude (Armbrust et al., 2010). The cloud computing model offers a collection of heterogeneous computing, storage and network resources as a service. Three basic types of cloud services are offered: IaaS (Infrastructure-as-a-Service), PaaS (Platform-as-a-Service) and SaaS (Software-as-a-Service). Computationally intensive tasks, such as MapReduce jobs, can benefit from the elasticity, high availability, fault-tolerance and transparency features of the Cloud. In fact, many MapReduce implementations are supported and offered out-of-the-box by many Cloud software providers, such as Apache CloudStack

(ASF, 2014f), OpenStack (OpenStack Foundation, 2014) and Microsoft Azure (Microsoft Corporation, 2014). Nowadays, cloud computing solutions are used widely by many organizations that need a reliable and scalable platform for processing, storing and analyzing their ever-growing data.

In parallel to the widespread adoption of the big data culture and the rapid development of the underlying technologies, the healthcare sector is under fundamental restructuring, towards a more efficient and cost-effective technology-assisted care model (Fasano, 2013). Admittedly, one of the main characteristics of the healthcare refactoring is the large augmentation of the collected data, either from the patients or from interconnected healthcare systems, which are expected to revolutionize the established procedures in healthcare (Groves et al, 2013). That data may come from numerous heterogeneous sources. New technological advancements offer new solutions to users as healthcare and environmental measurements can be gathered through smart and intelligent personal devices. As the field of Internet of Things moves forward, modern healthcare platforms in turn need to be able to collect data from these smart devices and process them as effectively and quickly as possible to generate new meaningful data and knowledge (cf. e.g., Bui & Zorzi, 2011). As those personal data derives rapidly from these different sources, what was once regarded as a prohibiting difficulty is now achievable thanks to the techniques that allow for massive and efficient processing of large amounts of heterogeneous and unstructured data. The use of big data is, thus, an emerging and well promising aspect of the modern healthcare sector.

One important initiative in the field is NIH Big Data to Knowledge (BD2K) whose mission is to enable biomedical scientists to capitalize more fully on the big data being generated by those research communities. With advances in technologies, these investigators are increasingly generating and using large, complex and diverse data sets. Consequently, the biomedical research enterprise is increasingly becoming data-intensive and data-driven. However, the ability of researchers to locate, analyze, and use big data (and more generally all biomedical and behavioral data) is often limited for reasons related to access to relevant software and tools, expertise and other factors. BD2K aims to develop the new approaches, standards, methods, tools, software and competencies that will enhance the use of biomedical big data by supporting research, implementation and training in data science and other relevant fields (Ohno-Machado, 2014).

BIG DATA IN HEALTHCARE

Big Data Applications in the Healthcare Domain

The idea of transforming healthcare from a sick care system to a prevention based system, is emerging during the last years (cf. e.g., Fani Marvasti & Stafford, 2012). To that end, there is an increasing need for insights and evidence that could support the decision mechanisms and improve their accuracy. This ongoing shift is expected to offer both greater healthcare outcomes and costs reduction.

The stakeholders rely on the power of the collected data, which become increasingly massive and heterogeneous in the case of healthcare. Firstly, the wider adoption of Electronic Health Record (EHR) systems stands as an important factor in health digital data augmentation (Charles et al., 2013). Significant efforts have been put in the development of mining techniques in order to extract valuable information from the EHR stored data which may include coded data, such as ICD data, laboratory tests results, medication data and clinical notes. Notable mining approaches have been proposed by Jensen, Jensen, & Brunak (2012), Pakhomov, Buntrock, & Chute (2006) and Chapman, Chu, & Dowling (2007). However, it is important to recognize the essential differences between the aforementioned EHR categories. This reinforces the need for the application of novel analytics methods, towards the integrated exploitation of all kinds of EHR data. For instance, clinical notes are mostly unstructured data, often characterized by high level of details, while coded health data are well structured but frequently face information loss (e.g., not all diseases are appropriately coded in all coding schemes).

Apart from the novel techniques in the analysis of the traditional EHR data, the new healthcare era introduces additional data sources, which were never thoroughly examined in the past. To start with, big data analytics can process the large amount of epidemiology data available and correlate them with patient demographic information, such as gender, age and nationality, in order to raise worldwide awareness and, thus, promote targeted campaigns. Moreover, on an infectious disease outbreak, massive information available on the social networks can prove useful for the estimation of the disease's epidemiological patterns (e.g., Chunara, Andrews, & Brownstein, 2012). Going a step beyond, information on the social networks can be processed with new analytics techniques and produce a wide variety of results, such as patients' sentiment analysis (e.g., Greaves et al., 2013), which can lead to more effective healthcare services.

Another novel e-health data source emerges from the behavioral monitoring of patients, aiming at discovering correlations with their health status and recognize early indicators of a possible medical situation worsening. Such recent approaches are described by e.g., Lamprinakos et al. (2015) and Brownsell et al. (2011). Big data technologies are also needed in this domain, since behavioral elements are retrieved from heterogeneous sources, including patient's activity monitoring sensors or mobile applications, which produce a considerably big amount of data. Moreover, big data analytics are a prerequisite in order to group patients' behavioral patterns and correlate them with various diseases. Innovative applications have been recently released in the domain of combined health and behavioral monitoring, which is expected to grow significantly in the near future. For example, Ginger.io (Ginger.io, Inc., 2014) offers a mobile application which enables practitioners to keep track of their patients' habits, such as movement or sleeping patterns.

Last but not least, big data applications are well targeted for two fields of medicine, both handling a huge amount of data: medical imaging and genetic data. To start with, big data technologies can offer a breakthrough in the handling of medical images by analyzing large medical imaging data sets which can provide unprecedented insights, in contrast to the legacy practices in which clinical images tend to be used by a single clinician for a single patient, without any reusability (Moody, 2013). Modern medical imaging analysis is supported by advanced content-based image retrieval features, including semantic representation of images and vector affinity measuring algorithms (Müller, 2004). However, medical image files processing is still challenging; for instance, the wide use of non-splitable compressed image files, such as DICOM (Digital Imaging and Communications in Medicine) files, reduces the effectiveness of big data technologies, since it does not allow the application of parallel computing techniques (Liu & Park, 2014). As far as genetic data are concerned, there is an increasing amount of collected data that could also provide medicine with revolutionary insights, especially when the collection process facilitates the data analysis by duly annotating them (Howe et al., 2008). The identification of genetic factors that are related to human's health and diseases is a computationally intensive task, requiring the application of novel methods (cf. e.g., Shang et al., 2011). Till now, a number of notable platforms have been implemented towards the exploitation of genomic data with regard to the improvement of individual and public health, such as Bina (Bina Technologies, 2014) and NextBio (NextBio, 2014). Another well promising example leveraging the growth of big data is the "precision medicine" initiative, which is strongly supported by President Obama. The program is expected to collect a large amount of anonymized genetic data by U.S. volunteers and accelerate biomedical discoveries at a personalized level (TWH, 2015).

Issues and Challenges

Many sectors have already embraced the big data technology, as it allows them to improve their existing operations, by e.g., optimizing the provided services and costs, improving customer experience, predicting problems or trends. Moreover, modern big data technology is an enabler for the implementation of innovative ideas, which can significantly transform the current state of various domains, including healthcare.

However, the big-data driven healthcare reconstruction has to face some remarkable issues and challenges. To start with, the healthcare industry does not seem ready yet to fully capitalize the available big data technology; according to a report by Oracle (Oracle, 2012), the vast majority of healthcare executives judge their organizations as not yet prepared for large-scale data management, while executives from other domains, such as telecommunications, are far more confident regarding the fruitful big data adoption. Every organization, that is still based on traditional information technology, may not be able to adapt to the emerging needs of modern healthcare. For instance, large-scale data acquisition, data cleansing, data integrity, data analysis and predictive modeling, are indicative elements which require the adoption of the big data technology and tools. What is equally challenging for a healthcare organization aiming at the adoption of the big data technology and practices is that, apart from the necessary investment in the new tools, the new technology also requires migration to a new set of data-driven business processes that extend from data acquisition to knowledge sharing.

Another challenge of the big data technology is the need for a new set of skills and expertise for the professionals who are responsible for the data management. A new discipline has appeared, namely the data science. Data scientists should combine knowledge of data governance, statistics, machine learning, natural language processing and expertise on the applicable domain. The endeavor to find skilled professionals by healthcare companies becomes even harder. Besides the need for the ability to work with the new technology and interpret the data, the candidate healthcare data scientist should also be familiar with medical practices and medical knowledge, in order to gain valuable insights from the available data and be able to contribute to the required refactoring of healthcare processes. Admittedly, such inter-disciplinary skills are hard to find in today's market.

Furthermore, mind-set shift towards data-driven healthcare applications, knowledge sharing and more trust in the technology is needed in order to transform healthcare in a way that all stakeholders can benefit from it. However, regulation is also needed in order to control somehow that no stakeholder will try to benefit only for themselves. Another major change in healthcare, also common to all other disciplines, that requires mind-set shift and openness is the fact that data do not belong to IT anymore, but directly to the end users. This type of "data democratization" unlocks the power of big data and gives the business stakeholders the potential to innovate their business domain or even to create new business. Data has turned into a new type of asset with huge potential of economic and scientific benefits ("data equity"). The data equity is only released when the data is analyzed to reveal these insights, allowing for a business to capitalize upon the resulting opportunities (cf. e.g., Cebr, 2012). Data assets get higher value when they are shared and when they are combined with external data sources. To further support this view, the key to innovation, as expressed by WWW inventor Tim Berners-Lee in his talk "The next web", is "unlock our data and reframe the way we use it together".

The end point challenge in healthcare lies in the security concerns about data protection and patient's privacy (cf. e.g., Rodriguez et al., 2013). Generally, a new set of tools has become available to reassure data protection, like anonymization or de-identification tools (cf. e.g., El Emam & Arbuckle, 2013), but this requirement has made processes more difficult to implement, has created some impacts on performance, but has not yet eliminated the legal concerns.

In sum, modern healthcare processes, like remote health monitoring, preventive medicine and behavioral monitoring, that are enabled by heterogeneous data sources, such as wearable devices, genomic data and social networks, guarantee the availability of large-scale data sets. What is still challenging in the data-driven healthcare process is to guarantee data quality and integrity (cf. e.g., Adler-Milstein et. al, 2013), as well as to avoid any possible misuse of patient's data with respect to their personal privacy.

FUTURE RESEARCH DIRECTIONS

Big data is in fact a new term for a challenge that has existed for many years; that is, how to exploit all this information, which has been made available through heterogeneous sources. Of course, the rapid growth of data size, either because the sources are increasing (e.g., Internet of Things) or because technology has progressed in such a way that new data can now be generated out of existing ones (e.g., signal processing for video/images), has brought the big data challenges into the spotlight. In this context, the research community shows remarkable interest in areas like deep learning, which extends neural networks and allows, for instance, image pattern recognition in an unsupervised manner. The healthcare sector is one of the most characteristic examples where such technologies can have a major impact, both technological and societal. However, in order to leverage all these emerging benefits, novel approaches should be followed in several aspects.

Starting from the representation and the storage of information, there is a need, not only for common schemas that can integrate data coming from heterogeneous sources in order to perform analytics, but also for realizing the appropriate technologies (graph-based/key-based/document-based/etc.) for big data databases, with respect to security and privacy. Especially regarding the latter two, fast cryptographical algorithms have to be devised, which can combine high reliability with computational efficiency. Moreover, the healthcare domain could take advantage of messaging platforms, like Apache Kafka (ASF, 2014g), which enable the accommodation and migration in real-time of all the streamed traffic into the dedicated databases.

Then, after information has been properly stored and represented, it must be leveraged to perform decision making. Artificial intelligence has very strong and long bonds with healthcare; however, the big data era gives it the chance to render itself more efficient with practical applications. Machine learning algorithms need to be devised, which can use information coming from video analysis (e.g. monitoring a patient's house), image analysis (e.g., X-rays), natural language processing and other sensors. These algorithms must be scalable and flexible enough to perform both real-time and offline analysis. IBM Watson supercomputer is a characteristic example in this context, since it is expected to analyze patients' symptoms and, by browsing the international literature, diagnose rare forms of brain cancer (IBM Research, 2014).

Given the large amounts of both raw and processed data, there is a need for classification, compression and aggregation. Existing technologies such as data aggregation and compressed sensing can be exploited and extended here in order to reduce the communication traffic and relax the, anyway much stressed, scalability requirements in the analytics algorithms as well as in the underlying infrastructures.

Finally, new algorithms must be developed that can incorporate all these new pieces and kinds of information, including bioinformatics and spatio-temporal data. Furthermore, these new models have to be aligned with the emerging software development paradigms, such as MapReduce, in order to be scale-out-ready and better exploit the hardware availability, which nowadays has become a de-facto provision due to the growth of cloud computing.

CONCLUSION

The healthcare sector is being transformed by prioritizing prevention, evidence-based medicine, personalized treatment and costs reduction. In this context, the modern healthcare industry is characterized by large and heterogeneous amounts of data, which is currently common to a number of other industries, such as retail, insurance and telecommunications.

As presented in this chapter, state of the art big data technologies can offer unprecedented insights, as well as innovative applications, in the healthcare domain. In parallel to the increasing adoption of big data in healthcare, cross-domain challenges, such as technical, organizational and ethical, have risen, which have been partially or completely tackled. Still, new approaches and, thus, challenges are yet to come. Advances in big data technologies give a boost to various disciplines, like machine learning, natural language processing, bioinformatics algorithms, graph mining and game theory, that are expected to further revolutionize healthcare.

REFERENCES

Adler-Milstein, J., Jha, A. K., Caballero, A. E., Davidson, J., Elmi, A., Gavin, J., & Found, N. R. et al. (2013). Healthcare's "big data" challenge. *The American Journal of Managed Care*, *19*(7), 537–538. PMID:23919417

Apache Software Foundation (ASF). (2014a). *Apache Hadoop*. Retrieved September 15, 2014, from http://hadoop.apache.org/

Apache Software Foundation (ASF). (2014b). *Apache CouchDB*. Retrieved September 15, 2014, from http://couchdb.apache.org/

Apache Software Foundation (ASF). (2014c). *Apache Accumulo*. Retrieved September 15, 2014, from https://accumulo.apache.org/

Apache Software Foundation (ASF). (2014d). *Apache Cassandra*. Retrieved September 15, 2014, from http://cassandra.apache.org/

Apache Software Foundation (ASF). (2014e). *Apache HBase*. Retrieved September 15, 2014, from http://hbase.apache.org/

Apache Software Foundation (ASF). (2014f). *Apache CloudStack*. Retrieved September 15, 2014, from http://cloudstack.apache.org/

Apache Software Foundation (ASF). (2014g). *Apache Kafka*. Retrieved September 15, 2014, from http://kafka.apache.org/

Armbrust, M., Fox, A., Griffith, R., Joseph, A. D., Katz, R., Konwinski, A., & Zaharia, M. et al. (2010). A view of cloud computing. *Communications of the ACM*, *53*(4), 50–58. doi:10.1145/1721654.1721672

Baker, J., Bond, C., Corbett, J. C., Furman, J. J., Khorlin, A., Larson, J., & Yushprakh, V. et al. (2011). Megastore: Providing Scalable, Highly Available Storage for Interactive Services. In *Proceedings of the Conference on Innovative Data system Research (CIDR)* (Vol. 11, pp. 223-234).

Balac, N., Sipes, T., Wolter, N., Nunes, K., Sinkovits, B., & Karimabadi, H. (2013). Large Scale predictive analytics for real-time energy management. In *Proceedings of the IEEE International Conference on Big Data* (pp. 657-664). IEEE. doi:10.1109/BigData.2013.6691635

Bina Technologies. (2014). *Bina Platform.* Retrieved September 15, 2014, from http://www.bina.com/

Brownsell, S., Bradley, D., Cardinaux, F., & Hawley, M. (2011). Developing a systems and informatics based approach to lifestyle monitoring within eHealth: part I-technology and data management. In *Proceeding of the First IEEE International Conference on Healthcare Informatics, Imaging and Systems Biology (HISB 2011)* (pp. 264-271). IEEE. doi:10.1109/HISB.2011.63

Buhl, H. U., Röglinger, M., Moser, D. K. F., & Heidemann, J. (2013). Big Data. *Wirtschaftsinformatik*, *55*(2), 63–68. doi:10.1007/s11576-013-0350-x

Bui, N., & Zorzi, M. (2011). Health care applications: a solution based on the internet of things. In *Proceedings of the 4th International Symposium on Applied Sciences in Biomedical and Communication Technologies* (pp. 1-5). ACM. doi:10.1145/2093698.2093829

Centre for Economics and Business Research (Cebr). (2012). *Data equity: Unlocking the value of big data.* Retrieved September 15, 2014, from http://www.sas.com/offices/europe/uk/downloads/data-equity-cebr.pdf

Chang, F., Dean, J., Ghemawat, S., Hsieh, W. C., Wallach, D. A., Burrows, M., & Gruber, R. E. et al. (2008). Bigtable: A distributed storage system for structured data. *ACM Transactions on Computer Systems*, *26*(2), 1–26. doi:10.1145/1365815.1365816

Chapman, W. W., Chu, D., & Dowling, J. N. (2007). ConText: An algorithm for identifying contextual features from clinical text. In *Proceedings of the Workshop on BioNLP 2007: Biological, Translational, and Clinical Language Processing* (pp. 81-88). Association for Computational Linguistics.

Charles, D., King, J., Patel, V., & Furukawa, M. F. (2013). Adoption of electronic health record systems among US non-federal acute care hospitals: 2008-2012. *ONC Data Brief*, *1*(9), 1–9.

Chattopadhyay, B., Lin, L., Liu, W., Mittal, S., Aragonda, P., Lychagina, V., & Wong, M. et al. (2011). Tenzing A SQL Implementation On The MapReduce Framework. In *Proceedings of the VLDB Endowment* (pp. 1318-1327).

Chunara, R., Andrews, J. R., & Brownstein, J. S. (2012). Social and news media enable estimation of epidemiological patterns early in the 2010 Haitian cholera outbreak. *The American Journal of Tropical Medicine and Hygiene*, *86*(1), 39–45. doi:10.4269/ajtmh.2012.11-0597 PMID:22232449

Corbett, J. C., Dean, J., Epstein, M., Fikes, A., Frost, C., Furman, J. J., & Woodford, D. et al. (2013). Spanner: Google's globally distributed database. *ACM Transactions on Computer Systems*, *31*(3), 8. doi:10.1145/2518037.2491245

Dean, J., & Ghemawat, S. (2008). MapReduce: Simplified data processing on large clusters. *Communications of the ACM*, *51*(1), 107–113. doi:10.1145/1327452.1327492

El Emam, K., & Arbuckle, L. (2013). *Anonymizing Health Data.* O'Reilly Media.

Fani Marvasti, F., & Stafford, R. S. (2012). From sick care to health care—reengineering prevention into the US system. *The New England Journal of Medicine, 367*(10), 889–891. doi:10.1056/NEJMp1206230 PMID:22931257

Fasano, P. (2013). *Transforming Health Care: The Financial Impact of Technology, Electronic Tools and Data Mining.* John Wiley & Sons.

Ginger.io.Inc. (2014), *Ginger.io.* Retrieved September 15, 2014, from https://ginger.io/

Greaves, F., Ramirez-Cano, D., Millett, C., Darzi, A., & Donaldson, L. (2013). Use of sentiment analysis for capturing patient experience from free-text comments posted online. *Journal of Medical Internet Research, 15*(11), e239. doi:10.2196/jmir.2721 PMID:24184993

Groves, P., Kayyali, B., Knott, D., & Van Kuiken, S. (2013). The 'big data' revolution in healthcare. *The McKinsey Quarterly.*

Howe, D., Costanzo, M., Fey, P., Gojobori, T., Hannick, L., Hide, W., & Rhee, S. Y. et al. (2008). Big data: The future of biocuration. *Nature, 455*(7209), 47–50. doi:10.1038/455047a PMID:18769432

Jensen, P. B., Jensen, L. J., & Brunak, S. (2012). Mining electronic health records: Towards better research applications and clinical care. *Nature Reviews. Genetics, 13*(6), 395–405. doi:10.1038/nrg3208 PMID:22549152

Lamprinakos, G. C., Asanin, S., Broden, T., Prestileo, A., Fursse, J., Papadopoulos, K. A., & Venieris, I. S. et al. (2015). An integrated remote monitoring platform towards Telehealth and Telecare services interoperability. *Information Sciences, 308*, 23–37. doi:10.1016/j.ins.2015.02.032

Liu, W., & Park, E. K. (2014). Big Data as an e-Health Service. In *Proceedings of the International Conference on Computing, Networking and Communications (ICNC)* (pp. 982-988). IEEE. doi:10.1109/ICCNC.2014.6785471

Malewicz, G., Austern, M. H., Bik, A. J., Dehnert, J. C., Horn, I., Leiser, N., & Czajkowski, G. (2010, June). Pregel: a system for large-scale graph processing. In *Proceedings of the 2010 ACM SIGMOD International Conference on Management of data (pp. 135-146).* ACM. doi:10.1145/1807167.1807184

Melnik, S., Gubarev, A., Long, J. J., Romer, G., Shivakumar, S., Tolton, M., & Vassilakis, T. (2010). Dremel: interactive analysis of web-scale datasets. In *Proceedings of the VLDB Endowment* (pp. 330-339).

Microsoft Corporation. (2014). *Microsoft Azure.* Retrieved September 15, 2014, from https://azure.microsoft.com/

Mongo, D. B. (2014). *MongoDB.* Retrieved September 15, 2014, from http://www.mongodb.org/

Moody, A. (2013). Perspective: The big picture. *Nature, 502*(7473), S95–S95. doi:10.1038/502S95a PMID:24187705

Müller, H., Michoux, N., Bandon, D., & Geissbuhler, A. (2004). A review of content-based image retrieval systems in medical applications—clinical benefits and future directions. *International Journal of Medical Informatics, 73*(1), 1–23. doi:10.1016/j.ijmedinf.2003.11.024 PMID:15036075

NextBio. (2014). *NextBio Platform.* Retrieved September 15, 2014, from http://www.nextbio.com/

Ohno-Machado, L. (2014). NIH's Big Data to Knowledge initiative and the advancement of biomedical informatics. *Journal of the American Medical Informatics Association, 21*(2), 193–193. doi:10.1136/amiajnl-2014-002666 PMID:24509598

OpenStack Foundation. (2014). *OpenStack.* Retrieved September 15, 2014, from http://www.openstack.org/

Oracle. (2012). *From Overload to Impact: An Industry Scorecard on Big Data Business Challenges.* Retrieved September 15, 2014, from http://www.oracle.com/us/industries/industry-scorecard-1683398.html

Pakhomov, S. V., Buntrock, J. D., & Chute, C. G. (2006). Automating the assignment of diagnosis codes to patient encounters using example-based and machine learning techniques. *Journal of the American Medical Informatics Association, 13*(5), 516–525. doi:10.1197/jamia.M2077 PMID:16799125

Red Hat. (2014). *Infinispan.* Retrieved September 15, 2014, from http://infinispan.org/

Research, I. B. M. (2014). *IBM's Watson takes on brain cancer.* Retrieved September 15, 2014, from http://www.research.ibm.com/articles/genomics.shtml

Rodrigues, J. J., de la Torre, I., Fernández, G., & López-Coronado, M. (2013). Analysis of the security and privacy requirements of cloud-based Electronic Health Records Systems. *Journal of Medical Internet Research, 15*(8). PMID:23965254

Schultz, T. (2013). Turning healthcare challenges into big data opportunities: A use-case review across the pharmaceutical development lifecycle. *Bulletin of the American Society for Information Science and Technology, 39*(5), 34–40. doi:10.1002/bult.2013.1720390508

Shang, J., Zhang, J., Sun, Y., Liu, D., Ye, D., & Yin, Y. (2011). Performance analysis of novel methods for detecting epistasis. *BMC Bioinformatics, 12*(1), 475. doi:10.1186/1471-2105-12-475 PMID:22172045

The White House (TWH). (2015). *FACT SHEET: President Obama's Precision Medicine Initiative.* Retrieved June 28, 2015, from https://www.whitehouse.gov/the-press-office/2015/01/30/fact-sheet-president-obama-s-precision-medicine-initiative

ADDITIONAL READING

Davis, K. (2012). *Ethics of Big Data: Balancing Risk and Innovation.* O'Reilly Media.

Graf, T., Erskine, A., & Steele, G. D. Jr. (2014). Leveraging Data to Systematically Improve Care: Coronary Artery Disease Management at Geisinger. *The Journal of Ambulatory Care Management, 37*(3), 199–205. doi:10.1097/JAC.0000000000000038 PMID:24887520

Kamal, N., Barnard, D. K., Christenson, J. M., Innes, G. D., Aikman, P., Grafstein, E., & Marsden, J. (2014). Addressing Emergency Department Overcrowding Through a Systems Approach Using Big Data Research. *Journal of Health & Medical Informatics.*

Lamprinakos, G., Asanin, S., Rosengren, P., Kaklamani, D. I., & Venieris, I. S. (2012). Using SOA for a Combined Telecare and Telehealth Platform for Monitoring of Elderly People. *In Proceedings of the 2nd International Conference on Wireless Mobile Communication and Healthcare* (pp. 233-239). Springer Berlin Heidelberg. doi:10.1007/978-3-642-29734-2_32

Lupton, D. (2014). The commodification of patient opinion: The digital patient experience economy in the age of big data. *Sociology of Health & Illness*, *36*(6), 856–869. doi:10.1111/1467-9566.12109 PMID:24443847

Meyer, A. M., Olshan, A. F., Green, L., Meyer, A., Wheeler, S. B., Basch, E., & Carpenter, W. R. (2014). Big Data for Population-Based Cancer Research. *North Carolina Medical Journal*, *75*(4), 265–269. doi:10.18043/ncm.75.4.265 PMID:25046092

Peters, S. G., & Buntrock, J. D. (2014). Big Data and the Electronic Health Record. *The Journal of Ambulatory Care Management*, *37*(3), 206–210. doi:10.1097/JAC.0000000000000037 PMID:24887521

Sun, J., & Reddy, C. K. (2013). Big data analytics for healthcare. *In Proceedings of the 19th ACM SIGKDD international conference on Knowledge discovery and data mining* (pp. 1525-1525). ACM. doi:10.1145/2487575.2506178

KEY TERMS AND DEFINITIONS

Anonymization: The severing of links between people in a database and their records, in order to prevent the discovery of the human source of the records.

Big Data: Any kind of data characterized by high volume, variety and/or velocity, which are difficult to process using traditional database management tools or data processing applications.

Big Data Analytics: The application of methods and algorithms in sets of big data in order to gain insights.

Cloud Computing: Internet-based computing, in which large groups of remote servers are networked to allow sharing of data-processing tasks, centralized data storage, and online access to computer services or resources.

De-Identification: The act of removing all data that links a person to a particular piece of information.

E-Health: The provision of healthcare supported by information and communication technologies.

Electronic Health Record (EHR): A systematic collection of digitalized personal or massive health information.

Healthcare: The domain that is associated with the entire life cycle of humans' physical and mental problems, including prevention, diagnosis and treatment.

Unstructured Data: Data that has no identifiable structure, such as the text of an e-mail message.

Category N
New Challenges and Issues

The Decision–Making Processes of Pregnant Women at High Risk

Marta Ferraz
Entidade Reguladora da Saúde, Portugal

Ana Margarida Pisco Almeida
Universidade de Aveiro, Portugal

Alexandra Matias
Universidade do Porto, Portugal

INTRODUCTION

Under the context of the new health communication paradigms, this chapter explores the implications and challenges that the current online search and open publication practices may have on the decision-making process of pregnant women with an associated maternal pathology.

Acknowledging the importance of the concepts of autonomy and mediation in understanding the strategies and mechanisms of e-health information searching, this chapter presents the results of a study which main purpose was understanding how the decision-making process of pregnant women is influenced by the search for information provided by institutional and/or commercial website; moreover we intended to understand whether the nature, quantity and quality of information is taken into account when choosing a source of information and whether the participation of pregnant women in social networks increases the ability of decision-making and if the views and stories shared by other pregnant women influence their decisions; finally our study aimed at comprehend if the decision-making process is supported by the opinions expressed by health professionals or by self-guided web search.

Background

A survey conducted in the United States revealed that over 75% of pregnant women stated they had searched information on pregnancy and labour in digital networks (Declercq, Sakala, Corry, & Applebaum, 2007). Nevertheless, the literature revision points out the lack of reliability and up-to-date of some of the available medical information (Eysenbach & Kohler, 2002; Kunst, Groot, Latthe, Latthe, & Khan, 2002; Weiss & Moore, 2003), as well as the lack of quality (Eysenbach & Kohler, 2002). Indeed, the information available online fails by the absence of regulation, which makes it difficult for the average citizen to distinguish reliable sources from not credible ones (Bernhardt & Felter, 2004; Dhillon, Albersheim, Alsaad, Pargass, & Zupancic, 2003). Some authors even mention the potentially hazardous and damaging nature of the information acquired by the citizen, without the necessary monitoring (Skinner et al., 2003). Many pregnant women have declared to have felt more anxious and confused after reading specific information on the internet (De Santis et al., 2010).

In Japan the decision-making process of pregnant women with a risk pregnancy was analysed. As a result, Usui et al. (Usui, Kamiyama, Tani, Kanagawa, & Fukuzawa, 2011) clarified the main problems

DOI: 10.4018/978-1-4666-9978-6.ch069

of using online medical information during pregnancy in patients of a single Japanese health institution who had been diagnosed with foetal malformation. The authors drew on a survey, via anonymous questionnaire, directed at 155 pregnant women in the aforementioned conditions, during the period between 2005 and 2009. Participants were asked about the diagnosis regarding their foetal complication, the gestational age at which it had been detected, whether they had searched it on the Internet and what type of information they had found, as well as their impression regarding their level of reliability and if they had established a comparison between the online information and that provided by their physician. They were also asked whether they would use the searched information and which particular information they would like to obtain if they lived the situation once again..In terms of results, 57.3% of the respondents resorted to online information during pregnancy. In 60% of the cases, the impression was different concerning the information gathered from the web and the one provided by the health professional. In the first case, 60% of those inquired considered online information more frightening and negative than the one provided by the physician. The authors concluded that the number of pregnant patients who search the Internet has increased significantly in recent years, being these the ones who have experienced feelings of greater anxiety and pessimism, regarding the seriousness of the illness suffered by their babies.

The internet produced a shift in pregnancy policies and it is in this context that the study of Cohen & Raymond emerges (Cohen & Raymond, 2011), analysing the culture of three public online forums in which pregnant women share experiences. According to these authors, pregnancy is a borderline state between health and illness, since the woman can suffer from some pathology derived by her state of pregnancy. In addition, the burden of uncertainty regarding the possibility of spontaneous miscarriages, foetal harm or their own death is carried by the majority of pregnant women. It is in this context that online forums for pregnant women emerge, contributing for their empowerment.

A study conducted in 2012 in China, aiming to understand how Chinese pregnant women use the internet as a tool of information (Gao, Larsson, & Luo, 2012) analysed dimensions such as: the frequency in which health information was searched by pregnant women; the type of searched information; the way it was assessed; the degree of reliability of that information; and whether it was shared with the health professional. Regarding the reliability's level assessment of the information, the interviewed pregnant women elected the matching between the reported facts on other sources as the first reliability factor (64%). The supply of references (42%) and the expert revision (34%) were the second and third factors. It is relevant that 80% of the participants held a university degree and mainly all belonged to the middle class, which might have somehow contributed to the abovementioned findings. Taking into account the interaction with their health professional, 75.1% of the respondents revealed they had not talked to their ob regarding their web search. 32% mentioned to have sought additional information regarding issues which were debated with the childbirth educator.

In "Internet Use in Pregnancy Informs Women's Decision Making: A *Web*-Based Survey", Lagan *et al.* (Lagan, Sinclair, & Kernohan, 2010), present the results of an online questionnaire filled in by 613 women among 24 countries during 12 weeks. Search engines (mainly Google) were used by 97% of the interviewed to identify web pages with pregnancy related information (1), to find support groups (2) and to do online shopping (3). Moreover, about 94% of the sample stated to have resorted to the web to complement the information that had been previously given by their health physician, while 83% declared that the research was carried out with the intention to aid in the decision-making process, especially since about half the interviewed mentioned the lack of time and the little information provided by the health professional as reasons to encourage the online search.

Methods

Aiming to better understand the decision-making process of Portuguese pregnant women, we have conducted an exploratory survey applied to 178 Portuguese pregnant and post-partum women in 2013. Of the 178 overall respondents, 49 answered the section devoted to gestational problems, 32 to maternal pathology and 17 to the foetal pathology. From the 136 respondents who were identified as being frequent users of the web, 37 answered the gestational problems section: 27 regarding maternal problems and 10 regarding foetal problems. From the 34 respondents identified as medium frequency users, 7 answered to that section: 3 regarding maternal problems and 4 regarding foetal problems. From the three respondents who were considered non users: 1 answered to the maternal pathologies and 2 to the foetal ones.

Our paper-based questionnaire was divided in five sections: 1. background demographic and socio-economic information on the individuals; 2. pregnancy separated in two groups, one to be responded by pregnant women and another by post-partum women; 3. the influence of the web on the decision-making processes, includes 11 questions; 4. the relation established with the health professional; 4. pathologies related to gestation.

Survey Results

Web Search

Considering the respondents with associated maternal pathology (AR - 32), 23 stated they had conducted an online search in the context of their condition, 7 claimed the contrary and 2 didn't answer. From the Frequent web users group (FWU - 27), 21 searched in the same context, 4 didn't and 2 didn't answer. In what concerns Medium frequency users (MFU - 3), 2 searched in this context, one did not.

To perform that search, 8 of the 32 AR chose the search engines "often" and 10 "always". 4 selected "sometimes" and 1 "never". FWU: 8 selected "often" to search engines and 9 "always"; 3 selected "sometimes" and 0 "never"; 6 didn't answer. In the MFU group, 1 used search engines "always" using the and one other "sometimes"; The third did not answer (See Table 1).

It is clear that the distinction between institutional/governmental and commercial websites is relevant in any dimension related to health, moreover if an illness is diagnosed. Indeed, 4 of AR "always" used governmental websites. The "often" was chosen by 6, relating to the governmental websites and by 3 relating to the commercial ones. On the FWU group, 4 chose "always" for governmental and 0 for the commercial. The MFU respondents had the following results: 1 selected "hardly ever" for both types of websites and 2 did not answer. Concerning "never", 4 of AR marked it for the governmental websites, however 8 did it for the commercial ones. The same scale was observed for the FWU: 3 for the governmental and 7 for the commercial ones. Hence, the majority of respondents with a maternal pathology diagnosis preferred to search their doubts in governmental websites, over commercial (See Table 2).

Table 1. AR' search engine use

		Always	Often	Sometimes	Hardly Ever	Never
Yes	**22**	10	8	4		
No	2	-	-	-	1	1
N/A	8	-	-	-		-

Table 2. AR's governmental and commercial websites use

	Always	Often	Sometimes	Hardly Ever	Never	N/A
Governmental	4	6	4	4	4	10
Commercial	0	3	6	4	8	11

One of the main goals of this investigation is to evaluate if the peer social support stemming from online communities influences the decision-making process of the pregnant woman. In the context of pathology, this assessment becomes even more relevant, given the understandable state of vulnerability and anxiety. Considering the main AR group, 1 respondent selected "always" for the discussion forums, but not for the online support communities. As for "often", 8 respondents selected it for both spaces. These values match with those of the FWU. "Sometimes" was marked by 6 AR, regarding communities and for 9 regarding the forums. FWU: 5 selected "sometimes" for communities and 7 for forums. MFU: 1 selected "sometimes" for communities and 2 for forums. As for "never", 5 AR selected it for communities and 4 for forums. FWU: 4 selected "never" for communities and 3 for forums.

In what concerns social networks and blogs, our results show that participants did not so frequently use them. 3 of AR selected "often" for social networks and 5 for blogs. "Sometimes" was selected by 3 AR for social networks and by 4 for blogs. In the FWU group 3 respondents selected "often" in both options. 1 MFU also selected it for blogs. "Never" was the most chosen option: 11 AR selected it for social networks and 8 for blogs. 9 of the FWU did the same for social networks and 7 for blogs. One MFU also chose "never" for social networks (See Table 3).

Purpose of the Search

The following question of our questionnaire intended to assess the purpose of the performed search. The result was clear: 18 from AR agreed with the option "to gather additional information" and 7 "fully agreed". In the FWU group, 16 agreed with this statement and 7 fully agreed. Concerning MFU, 2 agreed and the NU did not answer. Likewise, 16 of AR agreed with the options "check the existence of similar cases" and "have access to similar case reports". 3 of these "fully agreed" with both hypotheses. With the FWU the same results were obtained, as 15 agreed with both the checking of identical cases as theirs existence as with the access to the reports and 3 "fully agreed". In the MFU group, 1 agreed with both hypotheses. The NU didn't answer.

It is curious that, despite willing to know or recognise identical cases, AR seem not to be not interested in contacting those individuals: 11 of them wished "to contact other individuals with the same situation", while 7 disagreed and 3 "fully disagreed". Yet 6 of these didn't answer. Peculiarly, the FWU group demonstrated more interest in this contact with peers in an identical situation, possibly due to that same

Table 3. AR's forums, online communities, social networks and blogs use

	Always	Often	Sometimes	Hardly Ever	Never	N/A
Forums	1	8	9	1	4	9
Online communities	0	8	6	3	5	10
Social networks	0	3	3	5	11	10
Blogs	0	5	4	5	8	10

condition. Thus, 11 of them agreed with the statement while only 5 disagreed and 3 "fully disagreed". The 1 MFU who opted to answer this question, disagreed. The NU did not answer.

The option "confirm the information provided by the health professional" was selected by 13 of AR, who agreed, and by 3, who "fully agreed". Nevertheless, 6 disagreed and 5 "fully disagreed". Similar were the figures associated to the FWU: 11 agreed and 2 "fully agreed". However, 6 disagreed and 4 "fully disagreed". One of the MFU agreed with this option, while the other 2 did not answer. The NU "fully agreed" with "confirm the information provided by the health professional".

There is a diffuse attitude concerning the hypothesis of searching the web to validate the information provided by the physician. Combining the "agree" and "fully agree" and contrasting them with "disagree" and "disagree fully", the result is that agreement is superior; nonetheless, the difference is not striking. The answer to this question deals greatly with each of the respondents' sensibility, as well as their previously established correlation with their health professional. Most likely, those who had had a greater proximity with the doctor won't admit the search for validation. Concerning the option "finding contacts of other health professionals", although 7 of AR agreed, 6 disagreed and 7 "fully disagreed". Similarly, 6 of FWU agreed with this search for alternative contacts, but 4 disagreed and 10 "fully disagreed". In the MFU group, 1 "fully agreed", 1 disagreed and the last did not answer, as well as the NU. This last hypothesis was not popular, even because it could be perceived as the will to change doctors and not simply to have a second opinion. The majority of pregnant women with associated maternal pathology wish to have all the available information regarding their case, confirming what had been said by their health professional. Moreover, they also wish to be able to access similar cases, which may provide a greater feeling of comfort and lessen the anxiety. (See Table 4).

Level of Confidence

When questioned about the level of confidence provided by the information found in the internet, 11 of the AR claimed to have felt "reasonably more confident"; 12 felt "slightly more confident"; only 2 felt "much more confident" after having read web information concerning their pathology; 5 considered it "indifferent". In the FWU group, 11 respondents felt "reasonably more confident" after reading digital information and 10 "slightly more confident"; just 1 felt "much more confident". The level of indifference reached 4 of these users. Considering MFU, 1 felt "slightly more confident" and another "much more confident". The searched digital information increased the level of confidence of pregnant women with associated maternal pathology (See Table 5).

Table 4. AR 'purpose of the maternal pathology searches

	Fully Agree	**Agree**	**Disagree**	**Indifferent**	**Fully Disagree**	**N/A**
Gather additional info	7	18	1	1	1	4
Check similar cases	3	16	3	3	2	5
Access similar cases reports	3	16	3	3	2	5
Contact others with same situation	0	11	7	5	3	6
Confirm info provided by HP	3	13	6	1	5	5
Find contacts of other HP	0	7	6	4	10	5

Table 5. AR' level of confidence in the context of a maternal pathology

Much More	Reasonably	Slightly	Indifferent	N/A
2	11	12	5	2

Influence of Web Search and Online Contact

17 of AR felt influenced by the Internet search and 3 were "fully influenced"; 16 of the FWU felt influenced by this search and 3 "fully influenced". Considering the MFU opinions differed: 1 felt "influenced", other "little influenced" and the last "nothing". The NU didn't answer. The FWU had the most expansive mood regarding the digital search influence in the context of their maternal pathology diagnosis.

Online contact was not very influencing. Communication with the physician: 14 AR, the selected "nothing" and 7 selected "little influence"; the remaining 4 selected "indifferent" and only 1 selected "influence". FWU: 11 selected "nothing"; 7 selected "little influence"; 4 selected "indifferent" and just 1 felt "influenced". Two thirds of the MFU selected "nothing". The NU did not answer.

As for the role of the nurse, only the MFU were influenced by this health professional, which cannot be seen as noteworthy. AR: 3 selected "indifferent"; 11 selected "little influence" and 12 selected "nothing". 10 of the WF selected "little influence" and "nothing", whereas 3 selected "indifferent". As mentioned, 1 MFU felt influenced and one other "fully influenced". The NU did not answer.

Other pregnant women were also not very influencing. AR: 2 felt influenced and 1 even felt "fully influenced", however 3 selected "indifferent" and 4 selected "little influence". On the other hand, 17 selected "nothing". The same was observed with the FWU: 1 was "fully influenced" and 2 were influenced. Nevertheless, besides 2 others who selected "indifferent", 4 selected "little influence" and 15 "nothing". Two thirds of the MFU equally selected "nothing" and the NU did not to answer.

It is noteworthy that family and friends were slightly more relevant for the expectant mothers than their peers. Therefore, 2 of AR were even "fully influenced" and 4 were influenced. However, 5 felt "little influence" and 10 selected "nothing". MFU and NU weren't influenced. In fact, pregnant women with a maternal pathology not only intended to find identical cases on the web, as they also seemed to feel better by communicating online with their most inner circle.

Concerning the chemist and doula, the outlook remained steady throughout the whole result presentation. The diagnosis of a maternal pathology did not alter its lack of influence regarding the pregnant and postpartum women. Generally, there was no influence of the chemist in any of the analysis groups. 18 of AR selected "nothing"; 7 selected "little influence"; one selected "indifferent" and 6 did not answer. 15 of the FWU selected "nothing"; 7 selected "little influence", 1 selected "indifferent" and 4 did not answer. 2 MFU selected "nothing" and 1 did not answer as the NU. Regarding the doula, 22 AR selected "nothing" and 4 selected "little influence", but 1 felt "influenced" and 5 did not answer. Also 20 FWU selected "nothing"; 3 felt "little influenced" and 3 did not answer. Still, 1 felt influenced by this labour coach. 3 MFU selected "never" and 1 did not answer (See Table 6).

Influence of Face-to-Face Contact

This kind of contact has different results. The doctor is fully influential for 18 AR and influential of 9; only 2 selected "never". The FWU were substantially influenced by the presence of their doctor: 15 were "fully influenced" and 8 were influenced. These findings are extremely relevant since they show that even skilled web users appreciate face-to-face contact, especially with the health professional and

Table 6. Influence of web search and online contact in AR in the event of a maternal pathology diagnosis

	Fully Influenced	Influenced	Little Influenced	Nothing Influenced	Indifferent	N/A
Internet search	3	17	5	2	3	2
Contact with physician	0	1	7	14	4	6
Contact with nurse	0	1	11	12	3	6
Contact with other pregnant women	1	2	4	17	3	5
Contact with family/ friends	2	4	5	13	2	6
Contact with chemist	0	0	7	18	1	6
Contact with doula	0	1	4	22	0	5

in the context of a maternal pathology. MFU were also influenced and 2 were "fully influenced". The NU was also "fully" influenced.

In second place is the face-to-face contact with a nurse. 13 AR felt "fully influenced" and 6 were influenced, only 2 selected "nothing". 12 FWU were also "fully influenced" and 5 were influenced; having just 2 selected "nothing at all". MFU: 1 was "fully influenced" by the nurse, one other was influenced and the last did not to answer, like the NU. The expectant mother feels closer to the health professional following their advice and clearing her doubts. In the event of a maternal problem, the pregnant women, even searching information on the internet, do not do without the face-to-face contact with the doctor and the nurse.

As far as peers and family/friends are concerned, 1 AR felt "fully influenced" by peers and 9 were influenced, whereas 11 selected "nothing". Similarly, 1 WFU felt "fully influenced, 8 influenced and 9 "nothing". Only 1 MFU was influenced by their counterparts, having the other 2 selected "nothing". The NU did not answer.

Family and friends results' were similar, with exception to the MFU who were not influenced by these agents. Thus, 1 AR was "fully influenced" and 9 were influenced, while 8 selected "never". The NU didn't answer.

The chemist and the doula are left to the end again, due to their complete lack of influence. 21 AR selected "nothing" and "little influence" for the doula. The same is true for 19 FWU who selected "nothing" and 5 selected "little influence" for this professional. 2 MFU selected "nothing" and 1 did not answer, like the NU. This also happened with the chemist, even if with less enthusiastic figures: 15 AR selected "never" and 8 selected "little influence"; 14 FWU also selected "nothing" and 7 selected "little influence". 1 MFU selected "nothing", other "little influence" and the last did not answer, like the NU (See Table 7).

Influence of Media and Scientific Literature

Regarding the last two agents, it can be stated that the media only influenced 2 and 14 AR selected "nothing", 6 selected "little influence" and 5 selected "indifferent". In the FWU group, only 2 felt influenced by the media, whereas 12 were not influenced; 6 were "little influenced" and 4 selected "indifferent". However, 2 MFU were influenced, the other didn't answer, like the NU.

Table 7. Influence of the face-to-face contact in AR in the case of a maternal pathology diagnosis

	Fully Influenced	Influenced	Little Influenced	Nothing Influenced	Indifferent	N/A
Contact with physician	18	9	0	2	1	2
Contact with nurse	13	6	4	2	3	4
Contact with other pregnant women	1	9	6	11	1	4
Contact with family/ friends	1	9	5	10	2	5
Contact with chemist	0	0	8	15	3	6
Contact with doula	0	0	5	21	1	5

Scientific literature, not having influenced 7 AR, influenced 10 and "fully influenced" 6. Concerning FWU, 8 and 6 felt, both, influenced and "fully influenced", having 6 others selected "nothing". It is worth reminding that 46.6% of the respondents to the survey had a university degree, which surely had an impact on these results.

FUTURE RESEARCH DIRECTIONS

Since the questionnaire was distributed throughout the year of 2013, it is important to conduct follow-up analysis, addressing the issue of the influence of online communities and social networks in the pregnant woman decision-making process, since these platforms are, currently, extremely used. Indeed, the results of the survey identify several interesting future research directions, and allowed an already conducted case study of an online community "Rede Mãe". The results of this analysis as well as in-depth interviews conducted will help to build upon the results obtained in the survey and hence characterize more deeply the studied scenario.

CONCLUSION

Pregnant women with associated pathology are influenced by online searches considering their status. However, it is the doctor that still is the most influent agent.

The web search influences pregnant women with associated pathology decisions in several dimensions, but mainly concerning the differences between institutional/governmental and commercial websites as the former seems to be more influential than the latter. Despite some influence, online communities and social networks are promptly overtaken by the contact with relatives and friends and mainly through the face-to-face communication with the physician, whose influence still prevails. Mediation and patients' autonomy are core-concepts when analysing new media influence on health decisions.

REFERENCES

Bernhardt, J. M., & Felter, E. M. (2004). Online pediatric information seeking among mothers of young children: Results from a qualitative study using focus groups. [Evaluation Studies]. *Journal of Medical Internet Research*, 6(1), e7. doi:10.2196/jmir.6.1.e7 PMID:15111273

Cohen, J. H., & Raymond, J. M. (2011). How the internet is giving birth (to) a new social order. *Information Communication and Society*, 14(6), 937–957. doi:10.1080/1369118X.2011.582132

De Santis, M., De Luca, C., Quattrocchi, T., Visconti, D., Cesari, E., Mappa, I., & Caruso, A. et al. (2010). Use of the Internet by women seeking information about potentially teratogenic agents. *European Journal of Obstetrics, Gynecology, and Reproductive Biology*, 151(2), 154–157. doi:10.1016/j.ejogrb.2010.04.018 PMID:20478650

Declercq, E. R., Sakala, C., Corry, M. P., & Applebaum, S. (2007). Listening to Mothers II: Report of the Second National U.S. Survey of Women's Childbearing Experiences: Conducted January-February 2006 for Childbirth Connection by Harris Interactive(R) in partnership with Lamaze International. *Journal of Perinatal Education*, 16(4), 9–14. doi:10.1624/105812407X244769 PMID:18769512

Dhillon, A. S., Albersheim, S. G., Alsaad, S., Pargass, N. S., & Zupancic, J. A. (2003). Internet use and perceptions of information reliability by parents in a neonatal intensive care unit. [Comparative Study]. *Journal of Perinatology*, 23(5), 420–424. doi:10.1038/sj.jp.7210945 PMID:12847540

Eysenbach, G., & Kohler, C. (2002). How do consumers search for and appraise health information on the world wide web? Qualitative study using focus groups, usability tests, and in-depth interviews. *British Medical Journal*, 324(7337), 573–577. doi:10.1136/bmj.324.7337.573 PMID:11884321

Gao, L. L., Larsson, M., & Luo, S. Y. (2012). Internet use by Chinese women seeking pregnancy-related information. *Midwifery*. doi:10.1016/j.midw.2012.07.003 PMID:22958935

Kunst, H., Groot, D., Latthe, P. M., Latthe, M., & Khan, K. S. (2002). Accuracy of information on apparently credible websites: Survey of five common health topics. *BMJ (Clinical Research Ed.)*, 324(7337), 581–582. doi:10.1136/bmj.324.7337.581 PMID:11884323

Lagan, B. M., Sinclair, M., & Kernohan, W. G. (2010). Internet Use in Pregnancy Informs Women's Decision Making: A Web-Based Survey. *Birth-Issues in Perinatal Care*, 37(2), 106–115. doi:10.1111/j.1523-536X.2010.00390.x PMID:20557533

Skinner, T. C., Howells, L., Greene, S., Edgar, K., McEvilly, A., & Johansson, A. (2003). Development, reliability and validity of the Diabetes Illness Representations Questionnaire: Four studies with adolescents. *Diabetic Medicine*, 20(4), 283–289. doi:10.1046/j.1464-5491.2003.00923.x PMID:12675641

Usui, N., Kamiyama, M., Tani, G., Kanagawa, T., & Fukuzawa, M. (2011). Use of the medical information on the internet by pregnant patients with a prenatal diagnosis of neonatal disease requiring surgery. *Pediatric Surgery International*, 27(12), 1289–1293. doi:10.1007/s00383-011-2965-6 PMID:21833721

Weiss, E., & Moore, K. (2003). An assessment of the quality of information available on the Internet about the IUD and the potential impact on contraceptive choices. *Contraception*, 68(5), 359–364. doi:10.1016/j.contraception.2003.07.001 PMID:14636940

Digital Auscultation:
Challenges and Perspectives

Daniel Pereira
Instituto de Telecomunicações CINTESIS, University of Porto, Portugal

Ana Castro
University of Porto, Portugal

Pedro Gomes
Instituto de Telecomunicações, University of Porto, Portugal

José Carlos Neves Cunha Areias
Faculty of Medicine, University of Porto, Portugal

Zilma Silveira Nogueira Reis
Federal University of Minas Gerais, Brazil

Miguel Tavares Coimbra
Instituto de Telecomunicações, University of Porto, Portugal

Ricardo Cruz-Correia
CINTESIS, University of Porto, Portugal

1. INTRODUCTION

Ever since Laënnec invented the stethoscope in 1816 (Laennec, 1819) that auscultation is an essential component of clinical examination. It is both a powerful screening tool, providing a cheap and quick initial assessment of a patient's clinical condition, and a hard skill to master. A number of factors contribute to the difficulty of, for example, cardiac auscultation. Relevant pathological activity is often soft, short-lived and occurs in proximity to loud, normal activity: a typical murmur is 1000 times softer than normal heart sounds and can last for as little as thirty milliseconds (Luisada, 1955). The acoustic information is also inconsistent across the course of an examination, owing to natural variation and noise. These factors make it difficult to precisely pinpoint a sound in the audio signal, and to identify markers indicative of heart disease.

What if we have the ability to digitally record auscultation sounds? Could we create richer electronic health records for future reference? Would we make better diagnostics if we could ask an expert opinion from a remote specialist or from a local clinical decision support system? Could we radically improve the way we train our clinicians in the art of auscultation?

In this article, we will discuss the potential of digital auscultation for answering all these questions, showing how modern interactive technologies can help us improve both current healthcare practice and medical training, transforming an ephemeral sound into something that can be stored, transmitted, analyzed and studied. Reinforced by real case studies in a variety of scenarios, we will discuss how auscultation signals can be systematically recorded for adequate integration into electronic health records

DOI: 10.4018/978-1-4666-9978-6.ch070

(obstetrics cardiac auscultation, Belo Horizonte, Brazil), how digital auscultation can be used in both hospital and field telemedicine scenarios (pediatric cardiac auscultation, Pernambuco - Paraíba, Brazil), how real annotated datasets are boosting research on algorithms for clinical decision support systems (Pascal challenge, Porto-London, Portugal-UK), and how real heart sounds coupled with new interactive technologies are improving the way we teach auscultation to medical students (Sports Cardiology b-learning course, Porto, Portugal).

What is the future of one of medicine's oldest and possibly most iconic art? Can you imagine a world in which physicians do not have stethoscopes? Or will the digital revolution propel it for 200 more years of clinical practice?

The rest of this article is organized as follows. In Section 2, we review a state of the art of the auscultation procedure and the evolution of stethoscopes. We discuss the new challenges of digital auscultation, namely electronic health records, telemedicine and the clinical decision support systems Section 3. The state of the art of the teaching of auscultation is reviewed on Section 4, and novel perspective discussed, contextualized by one of our own case studies. A final discussion and conclusions are addressed in Sections 5 and 6, respectively.

2. BACKGROUND OF CLINICAL AUSCULTATION

2.1. The Importance of Auscultation: Lost Art, Difficulties (302 de 300)

The stethoscope is the oldest cardiovascular diagnostic instrument in clinical use. However, cardiac auscultation is in decline and the lack of ability to either hear or interpret a cardiac abnormality starts with medical students and continues through to physicians of different ages (Pelech, 2004).

By auscultating the heart we have an understanding of the heart rate and rhythm, the sound of the closing and, sometimes, the opening of valves, and anatomical abnormalities such as congenital or acquired defects. Heart sounds are caused by turbulent blood flow, while laminar flow is silent. Cardiac auscultation is a valuable and inexpensive tool. When used properly the stethoscope often enables physicians to make a rapid and an accurate diagnosis without any additional studies.

Why is the auscultation becoming a lost art? The reasons for the decline in physicians' cardiac examination skills are numerous. High reliance on ordering diagnostic tests (Simel, 2006), conducting teaching rounds away from the bedside (Collins, Cassie, & Daggett, 1978; LaCombe, 1997), time constraints during residency (Shankel & Mazzaferri, 1986; Simel, 2006), and declining cardiac examination skills of faculty members themselves (Vukanovic-Criley et al., 2006) all may contribute to the diminished cardiac examination skills of residents. Residents, who themselves identify abnormal heart sounds at alarmingly low rates, play an ever-increasing role in medical students' instruction (Mangione & Nieman, 1997; Vukanovic-Criley et al., 2006) exacerbating the problem (Criley, Keiner, Boker, Criley, & Warde, 2008).

Later, for physicians, more elaborate and expensive technological advances, the fear of a litigious environment during the practice of medicine, along with sophisticated noninvasive and invasive diagnostic tests, are all reasons for considering the cardiac auscultation a lost and difficult art. We see often that the stethoscope around the practitioner´s neck is more of a decorative ornament than a diagnostic tool, with a growing perception among some practitioners that cardiac auscultation is old-fashioned. However, despite the current emphasis on technology, the stethoscope, when used properly, remains a valuable and cost-effective clinical skill that often establishes the diagnosis and severity of heart disease, with the added benefit of contribution to the creation of a stronger personal bond with the patient, privileging their doctor-patient relationship.

2.2. Evolution of Stethoscopes

The earliest description of the heart sounds comes from William Harvey´s De Motu Cordis (Mangione, Nieman, Gracely, & Kaye, 1993) in 1628, in which he compared the heart sounds to "two clacks of a water bellows to raise water". In 1816, Laennec proposed the use of "a cylinder of wood, perforated in its center longitudinally, by a bore three lines in diameter, and formed so as to come apart in the middle" (Laennec, 1819); this he termed the cylinder or stethoscope.

Traditional stethoscopes depend solely on acoustics to amplify and transmit the heart sounds to the physician. The concept of electronic stethoscope arrived when electronic components were first used to amplify, filter and transmit the sound (Durand & Pibarot, 1995). We can thus think of digital stethoscopes as an evolution of the later, since we exploit the advantages of converting the audio signal to the digital domain, whether these are storage, transmission, analysis or simply visualization. Bredesen and Schmerle (Bredesen & Schmerler, 1993) have patented an intelligent stethoscope designed for performing auscultation and for automatically diagnosing abnormalities by comparing digitized sounds to reference templates using a signature analysis technique. Several other electronic stethoscopes have been developed and described in the literature (Brusco & Nazeran, 2006; Hedayioglu, Mattos, Moser, & de Lima, 2007; Morton E Tavel, Brown, & Shander, 1994).

3. HEALTH CARE BENEFITS OF THE DIGITAL AUSCULTATION

3.1. Complete the Electronic Health Record with Auscultation

Cardiovascular disease is universally considered as an important underlying or direct cause of death and morbidity that impacts quality of life, medical procedures, and healthcare costs (Roger et al., 2011). Important clues of heart disease may be detected during clinical cardiovascular examination, and despite of technological advances such as the echocardiography, cardiac auscultation skills have been the central clinical tool for the screening and diagnosis of the main heart diseases.

A digital stethoscope auscultation is able to provide a documentation of cardiac sounds, displaying visual sonograms of heart sounds and murmurs. Future analyses of such recordings and second opinions facilitate the distinction between innocent and pathological sounds, and the teaching of cardiac auscultation.

The technique used for auscultation of heart sounds with the digital systems is the same as used in the routine cardiac examination: with the patient in the sitting and reclined positions, and afterwards in the left lateral decubitus, the recording sounds are obtained from the same classic areas of auscultation. Proper identification and classification of audible systolic murmurs, collected by the stethoscope enables health professionals to identify their mechanism and likely source, for example (M. E. Tavel, 1996).

Other important point to highlight is that the digital storage system allows an electronic register of heart sounds during medical assistance. Since subsequent reassessment of auscultation is often required, it is now possible and simple to replay the auscultation, also allowing a better tracking of these sounds' changes, or subsequent progress after medical interventions. This input could be a revolutionary enhancement of the quality of current electronic health records.

Case Study 1 now follows that illustrates the potential of storing and including these sounds in electronic health records. Pregnancy is a particularly interesting situation given the almost weekly changes in a woman's heart and its associated sounds. Results confirmed the suspicion of this usefulness, with several situations in which the comparison with heart sounds from previous weeks led to better clinical descriptions and decisions for some individual cases.

Case Study 1, Belo Horizonte, Brazil, 2014: In a cross-sectional study, heart auscultation was recorded with a digital stethoscope and Doppler echocardiography tests were performed in 29 pregnant women, in the second trimester of pregnancy and 27 non-pregnant women, all healthy. The digital heart auscultation of healthy pregnant subjects was able to detect frequent physiologic changes of pregnancy, confirming the importance of actions involving medical training and scientific studies to analyze beeps and heart images of pregnant women (Araújo et al., 2013).

3.2. Telemedicine

The World Health Organization (Organization, 1998) defines telemedicine as the delivery of health care services, where distance is a critical factor, by all healthcare professionals using information and communication technologies for the exchange of valid information for diagnosis, treatment and prevention of disease and injuries, research and evaluation, and for the continuing education of health care providers, all in the interests of advancing the health of individuals and their communities.

Auscultation fits naturally into telemedicine scenarios since these typically involve locations in which both equipment and human resources are limited, and in which the needs are typically population screening and patient follow-up. The simplicity and portability of the stethoscope examination, its adequacy as the first stage of cardiac screening, and the need of a specialist opinion for high effectiveness, creates a strong incentive for digital auscultation and its ability to both transmit or store heart sounds in situations where remote access to specialized clinical facilities is available, either immediately (tele-consultation) or sometime afterwards (EHR completion in a field scenario).

As an example, a recent study has shown that real-time tele-stethoscopy, together with a videoconference system that allows a remote specialist to oversee the auscultation, may be a very helpful tool in rural areas of developing countries (Foche-Perez et al., 2012).

The DigiScope Sharing is a good example of a technology that can bridge this gap, combining wireless digital stethoscopes with common smartphones to create a highly simple and portable platform for digital auscultation and transmission on the field. Besides recording the heart sound, it can be easily connected into the microphone socket of any computer (thus integrating any sound transmission software such as Skype) or, if available, transmit the sound to other electronic stethoscopes nearby.

Case Study 2 now follows that illustrates a collaboration between the University of Porto and the Non-Governmental Organization (NGO) Circulo do Coração, to develop, deploy and test in the field technologies for telemedicine. An evolved version of this technology will be present in Caravana do Coração 2015, in which algorithms for detecting heart sounds, murmurs and screening pulmonary hypertension are already integrated.

Case Study 2, Pernambuco-Paraíba, Brazil, 2014: In October 2011, the state of Paraíba in cooperation with the largest hospital in northeast Brazil, Real Hospital Português, in Pernambuco, launched a large-scale pediatric cardiology telemedicine initiative to screen nearly 20.000 neonates per year. Various digital auscultation experiments were performed during these activities, namely Caravana do Coração 2014, a 13 day journey throughout 13 cities in Paraíba in which 1019 children and pregnant women were screened for cardiac pathologies and their heart and lung sounds integrated in the resulting EHR using digital auscultation technology (Gomes, Frade, Castro, Cruz-Correia, & Coimbra, 2015). Furthermore, the Digiscope Sharing technology has been deployed in João Pessoa, one of the main hubs of this telemedicine network, with which various auscultations signals have been transmitted and discussed successfully with Pernambuco (see Figure 1).

3.3. Clinical Decision Support Systems (671 de 750 Palavras)

The use of the electronic auscultation has brought the ability to store and reproduce the phonocardiogram (PCG) not only for telemedicine, but also for patient follow-up in an electronic health record (Gomes, Frade, Castro, Cruz-Correia, & Coimbra, 2015). Although these are already great benefits, early the potential for signal processing and decision support systems has been recognized (Cathers, 1995), especially since it is common knowledge that auscultation is a hard skill to master, and that young or

Figure 1. a) Digital auscultation technology (Gomes, Frade, Castro, Cruz-Correia, & Coimbra, 2015) being used in Paraíba, Brazil, to record and integrate into an EHR the heart sounds of 1019 patients during the Caravana do Coração 2014 initiative; b) Dra. Sandra Mattos and Dra. Juliana Soares using the Digiscope Sharing technology to stream a newborn auscultation sound via Skype between the neighboring Brazilian states of Paraíba and Pernambuco

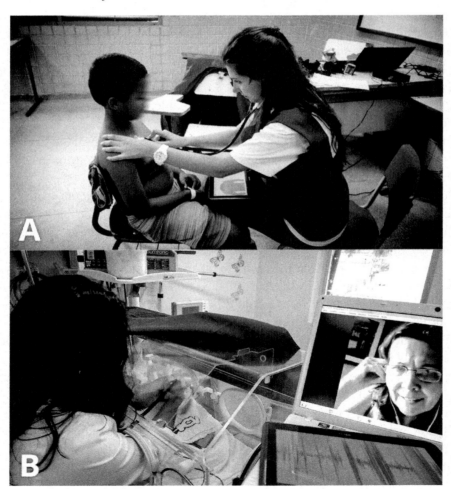

inexperienced professionals may disregard important events such as the presence of murmurs in an auscultation (Mangione & Nieman, 1997).

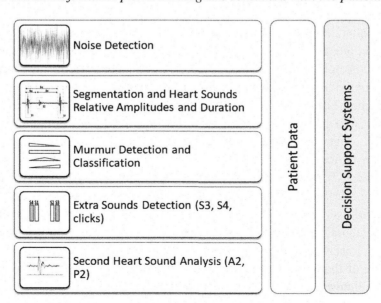

Researchers have recently explored the information contained in the PCG in the search of objective, reproducible systems that may aid in the detection of alarming events in the signals, and in the quantification of these events in terms of severity (Chauhan, Wang, Sing Lim, & Anantharaman, 2008; DeGroff et al., 2001; Smith & Ventura, 2013). This is however difficult to obtain due to the nonstationary signal characteristics (Xu, Durand, & Pibarot, 2001) and harsh collection environments where ambient noise and other physiological signals, such as respiration, may reduce signal quality (J Hadjileontiadis & M Panas, 1998; Tang, Li, & Qiu, 2010; Tsalaile, Sameni, Sanei, Jutten, & Chambers, 2009). Research in this field has focused in few mainstreams schematically represented in Figure 2: noise detection and filtering (J Hadjileontiadis & M Panas, 1998; Tang et al., 2010; Tsalaile et al., 2009); heart sound components segmentation (S1, systole, S2, and diastole), relative amplitude and duration analysis (Castro, Vinhoza, Mattos, & Coimbra, 2013; Choi & Jiang, 2008; Naseri & Homaeinezhad, 2013); murmur detection and classification in terms of location in the heart cycle, duration, intensity, and shape (Chauhan et al., 2008; Vepa, 2009; Wang, Lim, Chauhan, Foo, & Anantharaman, 2007); extra sound detection (S3, S4, clicks) (Hult et al., 2005); second heart sound morphology and its relation to systemic and pulmonary circulation blood pressure (hyperphonesis, intensity, and split) (Castro, Mattos, & Coimbra, 2014; Xu et al., 2001). More recently the modeling of the electrical and mechanical events of the heart, and their relations to other cardiovascular variables such as the blood pressure (Sola, Proença, et al., 2013), arterial stiffness, or cardiac output (Paiva et al., 2009) have also been analyzed, in the search of noninvasive beat-to-beat estimations of these variables, that usually require invasive measurements, a prominent field of research (Zheng et al., 2014).

The first challenge in PCG analysis is the noise detection, especially taking into account the harsh environment of data collection. Work in this field has includes the detection of signal patterns, such as the cardiac and respiratory cycles (J Hadjileontiadis & M Panas, 1998), multi-band noise detection (Falk

Figure 2. Schematic representation of a decision support system's structure with the signal processing blocks, and features extracted from the phonocardiogram combined with the patients' data

& Chan, 2008), and similarity analysis (Tsalaile et al., 2009). These techniques take advantage of the knowledge of spectral characteristics of the contaminating noise sources such as respiration sounds, that exhibit higher frequency components, and on its cyclic nature, to detect and remove noise interference. Following it is necessary to segment the heart cycle, which may seem a simple problem to answer, since systole and diastole have quite different durations, however for higher heart rates, such as in children, this does not hold, and more robust techniques taking into account the individual heart sound characteristics need to be applied (Castro et al., 2013; Choi & Jiang, 2008; Naseri & Homaeinezhad, 2013; Oliveira, Castro, & Coimbra, 2014). Typical PCG of healthy subjects is characterized by two main sounds: the first heart sound, corresponding mainly to the closure of the atrioventricular valves, is low in pitch and relatively long-lasting; the second heart sound results from the aortic and pulmonary valves closure at the end of the systole, a rapid snap since these valves close rapidly, and the surroundings vibrate for a short period. In pathological cases heart sound might exhibit further components such as the S3 and S4. The lung-thorax system has high impact on the determination of amplitude and frequency distribution of the externally acquired heart sounds (Sava & McDonnell, 1996). Depending on the auscultation site, relative amplitudes of heart sounds vary, and the second heart sound usually presents higher tone when compared to the first heart sound (Bickley & Szilagyi, 2012). The adequate identification of first and second heart sounds is of paramount importance since the localization of the features, namely for heart murmurs, strongly affects diagnostic accuracy. Different cardiovascular pathologies are associated to murmurs, and its correct identification is highly dependent on the site of auscultation and localization within the heart cycle (systole / diastole) (Bickley & Szilagyi, 2012). Heart murmurs detection and classification has a variety of proposed features in the time and frequency domains, perceptual analysis, and nonlinear and chaos based approaches (Chauhan et al., 2008; Pedrosa, Castro, & Vinhoza, 2014; Vepa, 2009; Wang et al., 2007), with relative good results in comparison to the usual clinical detection rate (Ferreira et al., 2013; Mangione & Nieman, 1997), making these a promising clinical aid.

An accurate segmentation is also important for the analysis of the first and second heart sounds' characteristics. Heart sounds are related to the mechanical processes of blood flow and turbulence, and the second heart sound is a combination of these mechanical phenomena, including the closure of the aortic and pulmonary valves. It has been demonstrated that the resonant frequency of P2 is proportional to the pulmonary blood pressure (Longhini et al., 1991), and a similar hypothesis was demonstrated for the aortic pressure (Bartels & Harder, 1992). Separation of the aortic and pulmonary components of the second heart sound, and the extraction of features from this component have been used to estimate pulmonary blood pressure (Tsalaile et al., 2009; Xu et al., 2001), and the systemic blood pressure (Castro et al., 2014). Separation of the two second heart sound components is still an issue, since these components overlap in the time and frequency domains (Xu et al., 2001).

The described research issues (*Case Study 3*) lacked the existence of an open realistic research dataset, in which researchers could apply their algorithms and compare the results obtained. This has motivated the creation of a public dataset, that will be subsequently described, and has since been used for numerous publications from authors all around the world.

Case Study 3, London-Porto, UK-Portugal, 2011: One of the major hurdles of this research field is the lack of relevant public datasets of real auscultation signals obtained during real clinical practice. Most published algorithms' performance does not translate well between the high-quality heart sounds gathered in research laboratory environments to the noisy, incomplete and highly variable real-world conditions, which is precisely where these systems can have impact. Digital auscultation was fundamental to the creation of one of the most relevant public heart sound datasets today, the PASCAL "Classifying Heart Sounds Challenge", co-organized by University College London and the University of Porto, in which a set of manually annotated pediatric auscultations obtained during real clinical practice are provided freely for researchers with the purpose of measuring the performance of both segmentation and classification algorithms (Bentley, Nordehn, Coimbra, & Mannor, 2011).

4. LEARNING/TEACHING

4.1. Evolution of Auscultation Teaching Methods

Traditionally, cardiac auscultation has been taught best at the bedside during clinical undergraduate training and in preparation for postgraduate membership examinations. It is an essential component of the clinical examination, but like most clinical skills requires repetition (Barrett, Lacey, Sekara, Linden, & Gracely, 2004) and clinical experience to make an accurate diagnosis. The traditional clinical teacher will defend that there is no substitute for clinical bedside teaching, while the modern educationalist will opt for multimedia applications, audio files and patient simulators (Karnath, Frye, & Holden, 2002; Karnath, Thornton, & Frye, 2002).

However, as many as three-quarters of USA interns and two-thirds of cardiology trainees no longer receive formal teaching in cardiac auscultation (Mangione et al., 1993). Several studies have reported an apparent lack of ability of interns to correctly diagnose a cardiac murmur (Alam, Asghar, Khan, Hayat, & Malik, 2010) and this decline in competency in cardiac auscultation spreads across the board, from medical students to practicing physicians (Vukanovic-Criley et al., 2006).

If this decline is related to the lack of clinical exposure and deficiencies in current teaching methods, maybe this can be rectified by proposing new methodologies, approaches and solutions. Recent studies encourage this possibility, showing that the use of computer based teaching increases the ability and confidence in detecting cardiac murmurs and added heart sounds (Ostfeld et al., 2010), auscultation skills (Stern et al., 2001), knowledge of cardiac auscultation (Vukanovic-Criley, Boker, Criley, Rajagopalan, & Criley, 2008) and general improvement in auscultation (Criley et al., 2008; Tuchinda & Thompson, 2001).

4.2. Auscultation Teaching Using Electronic Stethoscopes

Besides early attempts to use electronic stethoscopes for computer assisted decision, some studies have shown that the cardiac auscultation skills of undergraduate medical students were not negatively influenced by the use of an electronic sensor-based stethoscope (Høyte, Jensen, & Gjesdal, 2005; Sverdrup, Jensen, Solheim, & Gjesdal, 2010). The effect of using electronic stethoscopes has been evaluated either by comparing with acoustic performance (Abella, Formolo, & Penney, 1992; Ertel, Lawrence, & Song, 1969; Kindig, Beeson, Campbell, Andries, & Tavel, 1982) or by registering clinicians' self-reported preferences (Grenier MSc, Gagnon, Genest Jr, Durand BEng, & Durand PhD, 1998; Philip & Raemer, 1986). Their effect on diagnostic precision has been examined in one study with only 12 observers (Iversen et al., 2005), which did not show a significant difference between one acoustic and one electronic stethoscope. The effect of teaching and training has been evaluated in only one clinical study, which suggested a beneficial effect of training and teaching on auscultatory accuracy (Favrat, Pecoud, & Jaussi, 2004). The study was however non-randomized, and included only 10 observers examining the same patients before and after teaching. Other studies used recordings of cardiac murmurs, which do not necessarily correlate well with bedside skills, and showed only minimal or no effect of training on auscultatory performance (Barrett et al., 2004; Clair, Oddone, Waugh, Corey, & Feussner, 1992; Mahnke,

Nowalk, Hofkosh, Zuberbuhler, & Law, 2004; Mangione & Nieman, 1997). All of this reinforces our belief that this learning could then benefit from a system that includes an electronic stethoscope, if an adequate interactive solution is studied, implemented and deployed (de Lima Hedayioglu, Coimbra, & da Silva Mattos, 2009).

4.3. Physical Patient Simulators

The first appearance of patient simulators was the "Harvey Simulator" in 1968. This sophisticated mannequin is able to display a number of cardiovascular indices including blood pressure (by auscultation), jugular venous pulse waveforms and arterial pulses, precordial impulses and auscultatory findings in the four classic areas (synchronized with the pulse and varying with respiration) (Cooper & Taqueti, 2004). Harvey underwent rigorous testing as an educational model with pilot studies first reporting promising results in 1980 (Gordon et al., 1980), in 1987 (Ewy et al., 1987). It has since undergone several modifications and remains an important learning resource for healthcare professionals and trainees. Several other simulators have followed the advent of Harvey like Ausculation Trainer with SmartScope (Scientific, 2015), Cardiology Patient Simulator "K" ver.2 (Kagaku, 2015), SimPad Sounds Trainer (Laerdal, 2015). An important limiting factor for the widespread usage of this technology was its very high purchase and maintenance costs, which prevented it from achieving its promised education impact.

A number of recent review articles have exalted the virtues of high-fidelity patient simulation for learning many skills related to clinical medicine, from relatively simple skills such as the recognition of heart sounds to complex skills of crisis management (Barry Issenberg, McGaghie, Petrusa, Lee Gordon, & Scalese, 2005; Bradley, 2006; Maran & Glavin, 2003). Some enthusiasm appears justified because high-fidelity simulations have a number of potential advantages over actual patient experiences: they can provide standardized and graded experiences; they can reduce the use of faculty staff instructor time, and they can provide opportunities for contact with rare or life-threatening situations in a low-risk environment. Furthermore, it would seem that high-fidelity simulations that feature many aspects of a 'real' patient represent a genuine advantage over less realistic simulations. This is mainly true in assessment situations, in which a candidate's competence test should resemble the situation in which the competence will actually have to be used (Schuwirth & Van der Vleuten, 2003). In another trial that tested modern equipment like electrophonograms and infrared stethoscopes (Woywodt et al., 2004), the authors concluded that such equipment is a valuable supplement to conventional bedside training.

Although many reports attest to the value of using teaching devices for auscultation training, studies usually compare such training with no additional training (Horiszny, 2001; Woywodt et al., 2004). It is still unclear whether teaching programs with technical devices facilitate learning skills because they are more effective, or if the benefits merely are due to more time spent on the subject.

4.4. Virtual Patient Simulators

Without easy access to real patients and to forbiddingly expensive physical simulators, a medical student can only resort to passively listening to libraries of sounds that are usually synthesized or collected in unrealistic environments. Would it be possible to explore novel interaction technologies to produce virtual patient simulators, that can reach a compromise between these two approaches?

The Digiscope Learning (DsLearning) is a virtual patient simulator designed for tablet devices that allows students to auscultate a virtual torso with a real digital stethoscope, listening to real auscultations gathered from real patients in a variety of real environments (Pereira et al., 2013) (Figure 3). Heart

Figure 3. (a) Picture of a medical student using the virtual simulator "Digiscope Learning"; (b) 2D torso with four sounds ready for auscultation; (c) Zoomed 2D torso and a depiction of the phonocardiogram of the sound that is being sent and played by the digital stethoscope

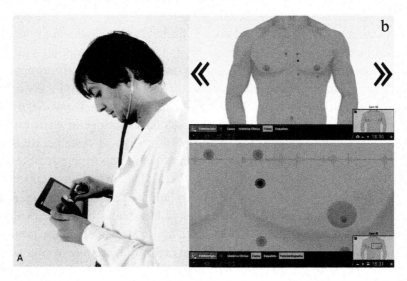

sounds libraries can provide students with a rich and realistic set of sounds, but still fail to mimic the required mechanical gestures and stethoscope positioning of a real auscultation exam. The DsLearning takes advantage of digital stethoscopes and the rich touch interaction available in most portable devices to simulate the touch of the stethoscope with the torso of the patient. When the student touches the screen with the stethoscope tip, a sound is sent the stethoscope corresponding to the one that he would be listening in a real body, training muscular memory and visual positioning. The combination of this virtual environment with a library rich in real auscultations provides the students with personal and portable simulators that will increase their number of training hours as well as the number of different signs a medical student will hear during his training.

After the development of the prototype we have begun a new evaluation phase with the objective of measuring the technological acceptance and robustness of this type of solution. Our *Case Study 4*, describes this experience, reassuring us with very good perspectives about a positive impact and usefulness of this technology in the teaching of auscultation.

Case Study 4, Porto, Portugal, 2014: The most advanced validation effort made so far the DsLearning technology was that a simplified version of this technology has been used very successfully by Prof. Ovídio Costa to teach an auscultation b-learning course for 100 nursing and sports medicine students at FMUP, with very high satisfaction from both the lecturer and the students, especially the interactive exploration of individual cases in a group discussion format.

5. DISCUSSION

The inclusion of sounds (e.g. heart, lungs) in EHR may rise legal and integration issues. By storing auscultations the health professional performance can be evaluated, whilst currently there is no way to know what he/she actually ears. Regarding the integration, the attachment of such sounds is technically very easy in terms of file upload, central storage and file format, but very hard in designing a sequence of steps that health professionals should take to associate a particular auscultation and the EHR of that patient. This is due to the fact that the digital stethoscope still does not have an interface to input a patient identifier, and therefore depends on the such association to be performed on a later moment, increasing the possibility of mistakes.

The use of auscultation in telemedicine sessions is probably less challenging, mainly due to the fact that existing telemedicine platforms can be used to guarantee that the sounds go from the origin of the auscultation to the remote health professional. A simple Internet connection is probably enough to send it to a specialist, allowing a quick and cheap tele-diagnosis. Theoretically, a well trained person is enough to manipulate the digital stethoscope in a way the remote health professional can make a diagnosis, further opening the possibilities of decreasing the health professionals shortage in some regions.

Regarding research to achieve effective clinical decision support systems, digital auscultation offers the possibility to store and analyze the PCG with objective and reproducible algorithms for the extraction of clinically relevant features (Gomes et al., 2015). Due to the harsh collection environments, interindividual variability, and intricate physiological relations, signal processing of an auscultation is far from being settled (Pedrosa et al., 2014). Several studies address this issue with promising results (Sola, Proenca, et al., 2013; Wang et al., 2007; Xu et al., 2001), especially in the noninvasive estimation of cardiovascular signals such as the pulmonary arterial pressure (Smith & Ventura, 2013), that usually require invasive procedures with risks for the patient and high costs. Decision support systems for the digital auscultation already present significant results in the detection and classification of murmurs and estimation of pulmonary blood pressure, combining features extracted from the PCG and patient data (Ferreira et al., 2013).

Many factors are considered to limit adequate teaching and maintenance of cardiac auscultation skills. Indeed the requirements and expectations of junior doctors, with regard to auscultation, are much lower now than in previous generations. While technological advancements, such as echocardiography, may well have contributed to the demise of cardiac auscultation, interactive technologies incorporating digital auscultation may well revive its place in clinical medicine.

6. CONCLUSION

The authors feel that it is important to fight the idea that cardiac and pulmonary auscultation will become a lost art soon. It still remains a very economic way to perform health care, with few misdiagnoses when done properly.

The inclusion of auscultation sounds in EHR has a great potential for health care, namely by allowing the evaluation of a patient's evolution, the establishment of second opinions and the creation of realistic sound libraries for research purposes.

Telemedicine provides answers to health needs related to the extension of life, especially in regions where health care is insufficient for the demand for care populations. By incorporating auscultations in telemedicine platforms, remote diagnosis of cardiovascular and pulmonary pathologies becomes easier. Given the current technological viability of this incorporation, it should be considered immediately, as the successful experiences in Paraíba clearly hint at.

Computer-assisted auscultation (CAA) provides objectivity to a traditionally subjective clinical skill. As an objective diagnostic support tool, it may improve the number of appropriate cases of murmurs that are referred for echocardiography from primary care. It may provide a decision support tool for mid-level and community health workers, with linkage to central expertise and training through telemedicine. Although we are still far from having robust CAA tools, the potential return clearly justifies the investment in this line of research.

Regarding the teaching of health professionals in the art of patient auscultation, the possibilities are many. Examples include using these sounds in traditional classes to demonstrate clinical cases, integrating these cases into existing e-learning solutions, the creation of tools for self-study, allowing multiple persons (eg teacher and many students) to simultaneously auscultate one particular patient, or to perform automatic student evaluation of auscultation capabilities. The success of these tools, is essential to the education of new auscultation specialists.

ACKNOWLEDGMENT

This work was partially funded by the Fundação para a Ciência e Tecnologia (FCT, Portuguese Foundation for Science and Technology) under the references Heart Safe PTDC/EEI-PRO/2857/2012 and SFRH/BD/80650/2011; Project I-CITY - ICT for Future Health/Faculdade de Engenharia da Universidade do Porto, NORTE-07-0124-FEDER-000068, funded by the Fundo Europeu de Desenvolvimento Regional (FEDER) through the Programa Operacional do Norte (ON2) and by national funds through FCT/MEC (PIDDAC); Project NanoSTIMA, "NORTE-01-0145-FEDER-000016" that is financed by the North Portugal Regional Operational Programme (NORTE 2020), under the PORTUGAL 2020 Partnership Agreement, and through the European Regional Development Fund (ERDF); and FCT grant SFRH/BD/80650/2011.

REFERENCES

Abella, M., Formolo, J., & Penney, D. G. (1992). Comparison of the acoustic properties of six popular stethoscopes. *The Journal of the Acoustical Society of America, 91*(4), 2224–2228. doi:10.1121/1.403655 PMID:1597610

Alam, U., Asghar, O., Khan, S. Q., Hayat, S., & Malik, R. A. (2010). Cardiac auscultation: An essential clinical skill in decline. *Br J Cardiol, 17*(1), 8–10.

Araújo, M. M., Reis, Z. S. N., Porto, R. B., Freire, C. M. V., Goulart, V. B., Fernandes, F. A.,... Cruz-Correia, R. (2013). *Auscultatory changes identified through digital stethoscope and echocardiographic findings associated with healthy pregnancy.* Paper presented at the 1st International Congress on Cardiovascular Technologies, CARDIOTECHNIX 2013, Vilamoura, Algarve.

Barrett, M. J., Lacey, C. S., Sekara, A. E., Linden, E. A., & Gracely, E. J. (2004). Mastering Cardiac MurmursThe Power of Repetition. *CHEST Journal, 126*(2), 470–475. doi:10.1378/chest.126.2.470 PMID:15302733

Barry Issenberg, S., McGaghie, W. C., Petrusa, E. R., Lee Gordon, D., & Scalese, R. J. (2005). Features and uses of high-fidelity medical simulations that lead to effective learning: A BEME systematic review*. *Medical Teacher, 27*(1), 10–28. doi:10.1080/01421590500046924 PMID:16147767

Bartels, A., & Harder, D. (1992). Non-invasive determination of systolic blood pressure by heart sound pattern analysis. *Clinical Physics and Physiological Measurement, 13*(3), 249–256. doi:10.1088/0143-0815/13/3/004 PMID:1424474

Bentley, P., Nordehn, G., Coimbra, M., & Mannor, S. (2011). *The PASCAL Classifying Heart Sounds Challenge 2011 (CHSC2011) Results*. Academic Press.

Bickley, L., & Szilagyi, P. G. (2012). *Bates' guide to physical examination and history-taking*. Lippincott Williams & Wilkins.

Bradley, P. (2006). The history of simulation in medical education and possible future directions. *Medical Education, 40*(3), 254–262. doi:10.1111/j.1365-2929.2006.02394.x PMID:16483328

Bredesen, M. S., & Schmerler, E. D. (1993). *Intelligent stethoscope: Google Patents*. Academic Press.

Brusco, M., & Nazeran, H. (2006). Development of an intelligent PDA-based wearable digital phonocardiograph. Paper presented at the Engineering in Medicine and Biology Society, 2005. IEEE-EMBS 2005. 27th Annual International Conference of the.

Castro, A., Mattos, S., & Coimbra, M. (2014). *Noninvasive Blood Pressure and the Second Heart Sound Analysis*. Paper presented at the IEEE EMBC 2014, Chicago, IL.

Castro, A., Vinhoza, T. T., Mattos, S. S., & Coimbra, M. T. (2013). *Heart sound segmentation of pediatric auscultations using wavelet analysis*. Paper presented at the Engineering in Medicine and Biology Society (EMBC), 2013 35th Annual International Conference of the IEEE. doi:10.1109/EMBC.2013.6610399

Cathers, I. (1995). Neural network assisted cardiac auscultation. *Artificial Intelligence in Medicine, 7*(1), 53–66. doi:10.1016/0933-3657(94)00026-O PMID:7795716

Chauhan, S., Wang, P., Sing Lim, C., & Anantharaman, V. (2008). A computer-aided MFCC-based HMM system for automatic auscultation. *Computers in Biology and Medicine, 38*(2), 221–233. doi:10.1016/j.compbiomed.2007.10.006 PMID:18045582

Choi, S., & Jiang, Z. (2008). Comparison of envelope extraction algorithms for cardiac sound signal segmentation. *Expert Systems with Applications, 34*(2), 1056–1069. doi:10.1016/j.eswa.2006.12.015

Clair, E. W. S., Oddone, E. Z., Waugh, R., Corey, G. R., & Feussner, J. R. (1992). Assessing housestaff diagnostic skills using a cardiology patient simulator. *Annals of Internal Medicine, 117*(9), 751–756. doi:10.7326/0003-4819-117-9-751 PMID:1416578

Collins, G. F., Cassie, J. M., & Daggett, C. J. (1978). The role of the attending physician in clinical training. *Journal of Medical Education, 53*(5), 429–431. PMID:660609

Cooper, J., & Taqueti, V. (2004). A brief history of the development of mannequin simulators for clinical education and training. *Quality & Safety in Health Care, 13*(suppl 1), i11–i18. doi:10.1136/qshc.2004.009886 PMID:15465949

Criley, J. M., Keiner, J., Boker, J. R., Criley, S. R., & Warde, C. M. (2008). Innovative web-based multimedia curriculum improves cardiac examination competency of residents. *Journal of Hospital Medicine, 3*(2), 124–133. doi:10.1002/jhm.287 PMID:18438809

de Lima Hedayioglu, F., Coimbra, M. T., & da Silva Mattos, S. (2009). *A Survey of Audio Processing Algorithms for Digital Stethoscopes*. Paper presented at the HEALTHINF.

DeGroff, C. G., Bhatikar, S., Hertzberg, J., Shandas, R., Valdes-Cruz, L., & Mahajan, R. L. (2001). Artificial neural network–based method of screening heart murmurs in children. *Circulation, 103*(22), 2711–2716. doi:10.1161/01.CIR.103.22.2711 PMID:11390342

Durand, L.-G., & Pibarot, P. (1995). Digital signal processing of the phonocardiogram: review of the most recent advancements. *Critical Reviews™ in Biomedical Engineering, 23*(3-4).

Ertel, P., Lawrence, M., & Song, W. (1969). How to test stethoscopes. *Medical Research Engineering, 8*(1), 7. PMID:5765901

Ewy, G. A., Felner, J. M., Juul, D., Mayer, J. W., Sajid, A. W., & Waugh, R. A. (1987). Test of a cardiology patient simulator with students in fourth-year electives. *Academic Medicine, 62*(9), 738–743. doi:10.1097/00001888-198709000-00005 PMID:3625738

Falk, T. H., & Chan, W.-Y. (2008). *Modulation filtering for heart and lung sound separation from breath sound recordings.* Paper presented at the Engineering in Medicine and Biology Society, 2008. EMBS 2008. 30th Annual International Conference of the IEEE. doi:10.1109/IEMBS.2008.4649547

Favrat, B., Pecoud, A., & Jaussi, A. (2004). Teaching cardiac auscultation to trainees in internal medicine and family practice: Does it work? *BMC Medical Education, 4*(1), 5. doi:10.1186/1472-6920-4-5 PMID:15056393

Ferreira, P., Vinhoza, T. T., Castro, A., Mourato, F., Tavares, T., Mattos, S.,... Coimbra, M. (2013). *Knowledge on heart condition of children based on demographic and physiological features.* Paper presented at the Computer-Based Medical Systems (CBMS), 2013 IEEE 26th International Symposium on. doi:10.1109/CBMS.2013.6627808

Foche-Perez, I., Ramirez-Payba, R., Hirigoyen-Emparanza, G., Balducci-Gonzalez, F., Simo-Reigadas, F.-J., Seoane-Pascual, J., & Martinez-Fernandez, A. et al. (2012). An open real-time tele-stethoscopy system. *Biomedical Engineering Online, 11*(1), 1–17. doi:10.1186/1475-925X-11-57 PMID:22917062

Gomes, P., Frade, S., Castro, A., Cruz-Correia, R., & Coimbra, M. (2015). *A proposal to incorporate digital auscultation and its processing into an existing electronic health record.* Paper presented at the HEALTH-INF - International Conference on Health Informatics, Lisbon, Portugal. doi:10.5220/0005222901430150

Gordon, M. S., Ewy, G. A., Felner, J. M., Forker, A. D., Gessner, I., McGuire, C., & Waugh, R. et al. (1980). Teaching bedside cardiologic examination skills using "Harvey", the cardiology patient simulator. *The Medical Clinics of North America, 64*(2), 305. PMID:6155573

Grenier, M.-C., Gagnon, K., Genest, J., Durand, J., & Durand, L.-G.Grenier MSc. (1998). Clinical comparison of acoustic and electronic stethoscopes and design of a new electronic stethoscope. *The American Journal of Cardiology, 81*(5), 653–656. doi:10.1016/S0002-9149(97)00977-6 PMID:9514471

Hadjileontiadis, , L., & Panas, S. (1998). A wavelet-based reduction of heart sound noise from lung sounds. *International Journal of Medical Informatics, 52*(1), 183–190. doi:10.1016/S1386-5056(98)00137-3 PMID:9848415

Hedayioglu, F., Mattos, S., Moser, L., & de Lima, M. (2007). Development of a tele-stethoscope and its application in pediatric cardiology. *Indian Journal of Experimental Biology, 45*(1), 86. PMID:17249332

Horiszny, J. A. (2001). Teaching cardiac auscultation using simulated heart sounds and small-group discussion. *Family Medicine-Kansas City, 33*(1), 39–44. PMID:11199907

Høyte, H., Jensen, T., & Gjesdal, K. (2005). Cardiac auscultation training of medical students: A comparison of electronic sensor-based and acoustic stethoscopes. *BMC Medical Education, 5*(1), 14. doi:10.1186/1472-6920-5-14 PMID:15882458

Hult, P., Fjällbrant, T., Hildén, K., Dahlström, U., Wranne, B., & Ask, P. (2005). Detection of the third heart sound using a tailored wavelet approach: Method verification. *Medical & Biological Engineering & Computing, 43*(2), 212–217. doi:10.1007/BF02345957 PMID:15865130

Iversen, K., Greibe, R., Timm, H. B., Skovgaard, L. T., Dalsgaard, M., Hendriksen, K. V., & Hrobjartsson, A. (2005). A randomized trial comparing electronic and conventional stethoscopes. *Am J Med, 118*(11).

Kagaku, K. (2015). *Cardiology Patient Simulator "K"ver.2*. Retrieved 01-06-2015, 2015, from https://www.kyotokagaku.com/products/detail01/mw10.html

Karnath, B., Frye, A. W., & Holden, M. D. (2002). Incorporating simulators in a standardized patient exam. *Academic Medicine, 77*(7), 754–755. doi:10.1097/00001888-200207000-00046 PMID:12114178

Karnath, B., Thornton, W., & Frye, A. W. (2002). Teaching and testing physical examination skills without the use of patients. *Academic Medicine, 77*(7), 753. doi:10.1097/00001888-200207000-00044 PMID:12114177

Kindig, J. R., Beeson, T. P., Campbell, R. W., Andries, F., & Tavel, M. E. (1982). Acoustical performance of the stethoscope: A comparative analysis. *American Heart Journal, 104*(2), 269–275. doi:10.1016/0002-8703(82)90203-4 PMID:7102511

LaCombe, M. A. (1997). On Bedside Teaching. *Annals of Internal Medicine, 126*(3), 217–220. doi:10.7326/0003-4819-126-3-199702010-00007 PMID:9027273

Laennec, R. T. (1819). *De l'auscultation médiate: ou traité du diagnostic des maladies des poumons et du coeur* (Vol. 2). Academic Press.

Laerdal. (2015). *SimPad Sounds Trainer*. Retrieved 01-06-2015, 2015, from http://www.laerdal.com/doc/250/SimPad-Sounds-Trainer

Longhini, C., Baracca, E., Brunazzi, C., Vaccari, M., Longhini, L., & Barbaresi, F. (1991). A new non-invasive method for estimation of pulmonary arterial pressure in mitral stenosis. *The American Journal of Cardiology, 68*(4), 398–401. doi:10.1016/0002-9149(91)90840-H PMID:1858684

Mahnke, C. B., Nowalk, A., Hofkosh, D., Zuberbuhler, J. R., & Law, Y. M. (2004). Comparison of two educational interventions on pediatric resident auscultation skills. *Pediatrics, 113*(5), 1331–1335. doi:10.1542/peds.113.5.1331 PMID:15121949

Mangione, S., & Nieman, L. Z. (1997). Cardiac auscultatory skills of internal medicine and family practice trainees: A comparison of diagnostic proficiency. *Journal of the American Medical Association, 278*(9), 717–722. doi:10.1001/jama.1997.03550090041030 PMID:9286830

Mangione, S., Nieman, L. Z., Gracely, E., & Kaye, D. (1993). The teaching and practice of cardiac auscultation during internal medicine and cardiology training: A nationwide survey. *Annals of Internal Medicine, 119*(1), 47–54. doi:10.7326/0003-4819-119-1-199307010-00009 PMID:8498764

Maran, N., & Glavin, R. (2003). Low-to high-fidelity simulation–a continuum of medical education? *Medical Education, 37*(s1), 22–28. doi:10.1046/j.1365-2923.37.s1.9.x PMID:14641635

Naseri, H., & Homaeinezhad, M. (2013). Detection and boundary identification of phonocardiogram sounds using an expert frequency-energy based metric. *Annals of Biomedical Engineering, 41*(2), 279–292. doi:10.1007/s10439-012-0645-x PMID:22956159

Oliveira, J., Castro, A., & Coimbra, M. (2014). *Exploring Embedding Matrices and the Entropy Gradient for the Segmentation of Heart Sounds in Real Noisy Environments.* Paper presented at the IEEE EMBC 2014, Chicago, IL. doi:10.1109/EMBC.2014.6944314

Organization, W. H. (1998). A Health Telematics Policy in Support of WHO's Health for All Strategy for Global Health Development: Report of the WHO Group Consultation on Health Telematics, 11-16 December, Geneva 1997. World Health Organisation.

Ostfeld, R. J., Goldberg, Y. H., Janis, G., Bobra, S., Polotsky, H., & Silbiger, S. (2010). Cardiac auscultatory training among third year medical students during their medicine clerkship. *International Journal of Cardiology, 144*(1), 147–149. doi:10.1016/j.ijcard.2008.12.201 PMID:19195724

Paiva, R., Carvalho, P., Aubert, X., Muehlsteff, J., Henriques, J., & Antunes, M. (2009). *Assessing PEP and LVET from heart sounds: algorithms and evaluation.* Paper presented at the Engineering in Medicine and Biology Society, 2009. EMBC 2009. Annual International Conference of the IEEE. doi:10.1109/IEMBS.2009.5332572

Pedrosa, J., Castro, A., & Vinhoza, T. (2014). *Automatic Heart Sound Segmentation and Murmur Detection in Pediatric Phonocardiograms.* Paper presented at the IEEE EMBC 2014, Chicago, IL. doi:10.1109/EMBC.2014.6944078

Pelech, A. N. (2004). The physiology of cardiac auscultation. *Pediatric Clinics of North America, 51*(6), 1515–1535. doi:10.1016/j.pcl.2004.08.004 PMID:15561171

Pereira, D., Gomes, P., Mota, É., Costa, E., Cruz-Correia, R., & Coimbra, M. (2013). *Combining a Tablet and an Electronic Stethoscope to Create a New Interaction Paradigm for Teaching Cardiac Auscultation. In HCI International 2013-Posters' Extended Abstracts* (pp. 206–209). Springer.

Philip, J. H., & Raemer, D. B. (1986). An electronic stethoscope is judged better than conventional stethoscopes for anesthesia monitoring. *Journal of Clinical Monitoring, 2*(3), 151–154. doi:10.1007/BF01620547 PMID:3746368

Roger, V. L., Go, A. S., Lloyd-Jones, D. M., Adams, R. J., Berry, J. D., Brown, T. M., & Ford, E. S. et al. (2011). Heart disease and stroke statistics—2011 update a report from the American Heart Association. *Circulation, 123*(4), e18–e209. doi:10.1161/CIR.0b013e3182009701 PMID:21160056

Sava, H. P., & McDonnell, J. T. (1996). Spectral composition of heart sounds before and after mechanical heart valve implantation using a modified forward-backward Prony's method. *IEEE Transactions on Bio-Medical Engineering, 43*(7), 734–742. doi:10.1109/10.503181 PMID:9216145

Schuwirth, L. W., & Van der Vleuten, C. P. (2003). The use of clinical simulations in assessment. *Medical Education, 37*(s1), 65–71. doi:10.1046/j.1365-2923.37.s1.8.x PMID:14641641

Scientific, B. (2015). *Ausculation Trainer with SmartScope*. Retrieved 01-06-2015, 2015, from https://www.3bscientific.es/auscultation-trainer-and-smartscope,p_148_4991.html

Shankel, S. W., & Mazzaferri, E. L. (1986). Teaching the resident in internal medicine. Present practices and suggestions for the future. *Journal of the American Medical Association, 256*(6), 725–729. doi:10.1001/jama.1986.03380060051024 PMID:3723771

Simel, D. L. (2006). TIme, now, to recover the fun in the physical examination rather than abandon it. *Archives of Internal Medicine, 166*(6), 603–604. doi:10.1001/archinte.166.6.603 PMID:16567596

Smith, R., & Ventura, D. (2013). A general model for continuous noninvasive pulmonary artery pressure estimation. *Computers in Biology and Medicine, 43*(7), 904–913. doi:10.1016/j.compbiomed.2013.04.010 PMID:23746733

Sola, J., Proença, M., Ferrario, D., Porchet, J., Falhi, A., Grossenbacher, O.,... Sartori, C. (2013). *Noninvasive and non-occlusive blood pressure estimation via a chest sensor*. Academic Press.

Sola, J., Proenca, M., Ferrario, D., Porchet, J.-A., Falhi, A., Grossenbacher, O., & Sartori, C. et al. (2013). Noninvasive and nonocclusive blood pressure estimation via a chest sensor. *Biomedical Engineering. IEEE Transactions on, 60*(12), 3505–3513.

Sverdrup, Ø., Jensen, T., Solheim, S., & Gjesdal, K. (2010). Training auscultatory skills: Computer simulated heart sounds or additional bedside training? A randomized trial on third-year medical students. *BMC Medical Education, 10*(1), 3. doi:10.1186/1472-6920-10-3 PMID:20082701

Tang, H., Li, T., & Qiu, T. (2010). Noise and disturbance reduction for heart sounds in cycle-frequency domain based on nonlinear time scaling. *Biomedical Engineering. IEEE Transactions on, 57*(2), 325–333.

Tavel, M. E. (1996). Cardiac auscultation. A glorious past--but does it have a future? *Circulation, 93*(6), 1250–1253. doi:10.1161/01.CIR.93.6.1250 PMID:8653848

Tavel, M. E., Brown, D. D., & Shander, D. (1994). Enhanced auscultation with a new graphic display system. *Archives of Internal Medicine, 154*(8), 893–898. doi:10.1001/archinte.1994.00420080097010 PMID:8154952

Tsalaile, T., Sameni, R., Sanei, S., Jutten, C., & Chambers, J. (2009). Sequential blind source extraction for quasi-periodic signals with time-varying period. *Biomedical Engineering. IEEE Transactions on, 56*(3), 646–655.

Tuchinda, C., & Thompson, W. R. (2001). *Cardiac auscultatory recording database: delivering heart sounds through the Internet*. Paper presented at the AMIA Symposium.

Vepa, J. (2009). *Classification of heart murmurs using cepstral features and support vector machines*. Paper presented at the Engineering in Medicine and Biology Society, 2009. EMBC 2009. Annual International Conference of the IEEE. doi:10.1109/IEMBS.2009.5334810

Vukanovic-Criley, J. M., Boker, J. R., Criley, S. R., Rajagopalan, S., & Criley, J. M. (2008). Using virtual patients to improve cardiac examination competency in medical students. *Clinical Cardiology, 31*(7), 334–339. doi:10.1002/clc.20213 PMID:18636531

Vukanovic-Criley, J. M., Criley, S., Warde, C. M., Boker, J. R., Guevara-Matheus, L., Churchill, W. H., & Criley, J. M. et al. (2006). Competency in cardiac examination skills in medical students, trainees, physicians, and faculty: A multicenter study. *Archives of Internal Medicine, 166*(6), 610–616. doi:10.1001/archinte.166.6.610 PMID:16567598

Wang, P., Lim, C. S., Chauhan, S., Foo, J. Y. A., & Anantharaman, V. (2007). Phonocardiographic signal analysis method using a modified hidden Markov model. *Annals of Biomedical Engineering, 35*(3), 367–374. doi:10.1007/s10439-006-9232-3 PMID:17171300

Woywodt, A., Herrmann, A., Kielstein, J., Haller, H., Haubitz, M., & Purnhagen, H. (2004). A novel multimedia tool to improve bedside teaching of cardiac auscultation. *Postgraduate Medical Journal, 80*(944), 355–357. doi:10.1136/pgmj.2003.014944 PMID:15192171

Xu, J., Durand, L.-G., & Pibarot, P. (2001). Extraction of the aortic and pulmonary components of the second heart sound using a nonlinear transient chirp signal model. *Biomedical Engineering. IEEE Transactions on, 48*(3), 277–283.

E-Mental Health:
Contributions, Challenges, and Research Opportunities from a Computer Science Perspective

Dennis Becker
Leuphana Universität Lüneburg, Germany

INTRODUCTION

E-mental health is the fusion of computer science and mental health, where the computer science aims at supporting the work of the physicians. It is a recently emerged research field that utilizes information and communication technologies to support and improve mental health. Furthermore, it is an interdisciplinary research topic that contributes to the welfare of society. The use of social media, online and smartphone applications helps to close the large gap between the need and actual treatment for mental disorders (Kohn, 2004). In addition, it aims at the reduction of costs for the society that arises from the direct treatment and the indirect costs, due to the loss of productivity or even the workplace (Fiscal, 2005; Harwood, 2000).

E-Mental health inherits the problems and benefits of clinical mental health, and many research results from mental health also apply to e-mental health. Interventions, screening and assessment for the treatment of mental disorders can effectively be delivered with Internet-based software. The adherence in therapy and dropout are problems that are linked to the design and implementation of the e-mental health software as well as the provided treatments and interactions with the guiding therapist. Therefore, the development of these applications requires guidelines to guarantee its quality and success.

During the process of treatment, a huge amount of data is collected that contain information that can be unraveled with data mining. Data mining algorithms are useful for the support of the physicians work, because it can provide predictions of the client's recovery based on previous patients. In addition, it can be used to extract the mood of the client from written text or record the activity profile using a mobile phone. Despite the amount of conducted research many questions are still unanswered. Accordingly, this chapter discusses the contribution of computer science to e-mental health, and suggest directions for further research.

FROM COMPUTERIZED THERAPY TO MACHINE LEARNING

The efficacy of a computerized cognitive behavioural therapy were demonstrated (McCrone, 2004), and online interventions are proven effective for a variety of different mental diseases such as depression (De Graaf et al., 2009), anxiety (Andrews, Cuijpers, Craske, McEvoy & Titov, 2010), eating disorders (Dölemeyer, Tietjen, Kersting & Wagner 2013) and they can be used to improve the medication adherence (Linn, Vervloet, Dijk, Smit & Van Weert 2011).

In the beginning of e-mental health the quality and success of the e-mental health applications were questionable, because this field was lacking of development and style guides, which led to a variety of different applications with low user adherence and the results were hardly comparable. This was mostly

DOI: 10.4018/978-1-4666-9978-6.ch071

due to the lack of user involvement in the design of e-mental health applications and missing collaboration between software developers and health service researchers (Pagliari, 2007).

Another major concern was the usability and safety of the clients. The potential of medical errors within the applications has to be minimized, to increase the client's safety. This goal goes hand in hand with the usability of the software and adherence in therapy, because a user unfriendly software can lead to rejection by the customer and is prone to possible medical mistakes (Karsh, 2004). Nowadays still privacy concerns and doubt about the effectiveness of online treatment remain barriers for many patients (Musiat et al., 2014).

Besides the early troubles, currently, many commercial treatment offers exist and even more research studies are conducted within this field. Additionally, many countries invested significantly into the eHealth sector, which enforced the need for development guidelines. This led raise to different proposed frameworks. The suggested frameworks are aiming at including the clients, medical researchers and stakeholders into the development of the application, to improve the impact and the integration in the health sector (Van Gemert-Pijnen et al., 2013).

Apart from the development of software, the conduction of research studies in this field is under research and about to change. The online technologies develop that quickly, that there is the possibility that when a result of a randomized trial is published, the newly studied intervention is already dated and unappealing. To prevent that clients use outdated interventions that are less effective, suggestions to speed up and improve the impact of studies were made (Baker, Gustafson & Shah, 2014).

Another problem within online treatment is early drop-out of therapy. Ineffective treatments or a lack of usability are reasons for a client to drop out of therapy, which endangers their remission. The dropout rate in mental health is a severe problem because the adherence of the clients to the therapy is essential for their remission, and the same applies to e-mental health. The adherence to computerized treatment is even significantly lower than regular treatment (So et al., 2013), and the dropout rate in e-mental health is even higher compared to regular face to face treatment (Melville, Casey & Kavanagh, 2010). This poses challenges on e-mental health, that are yet to research and conquer (Stegemann, Weg, Ebenfeld & Thiart 2012).

Ways to keep the client engaged in the online therapy are under research and fundamental for the success of e-mental health and the remission of the client symptoms. The use of a simple monthly reminder email has already shown to improve the maintenance in therapy (Gill, Contreras, Muñoz & Leykin, 2014). Since mobile phones are widely used and integrated into daily life, mobile applications are extremely useful to deliver mental-health service directly to the customer.

The use of an SMS or a reminder function can also increase the adherence to the therapeutic application and increase the engagement in the overall therapy (Whittaker, Borland & Bullen, 2009). Another benefit of using mobile applications is that they are steadily available. Especially disorders where the symptoms can appear quickly like anxiety, panic disorder or nicotine dependence can be treated effectively with mobile applications because the applications can be used whenever they are needed.

Therapeutic mobile phone applications can also be delivered as a game. The process of transforming an medical interventions into a game is called gamification. Within the gamification of an intervention, the interventions are modified in a way that they require interactions typically found in games. A recent study demonstrated that gamification of an attention-bias modification training leads to reduction of stress and anxiety (Dennis & O'Toole, 2014). Although, the effect of serious games has already been researched, there is still a lack of serious games for additional treatment of mental disorders (Fernández-Aranda et al., 2012). This is a new area of research, where the effectiveness has initially been demonstrated, but the topic still requires more research and still poses unanswered questions.

Despite the effort to improve the clients' condition a deterioration of the client symptoms is possible. Negative side effects of psychotherapy are known, but have just recently been researched for the online therapeutic counterpart (Boettcher, Rozental, Andersson & Carlbring, 2014). It is yet unknown what causes the deterioration of the symptoms and what type of clients are affected. Therefore, an early identification of these clients is necessary to prevent their dropout and prevent further deterioration of the symptoms.

MACHINE LEARNING AS SUPPORTING TOOL

A therapist is likely to supervise many different clients, which makes it nearly impossible to take equality care of each client. Therefore, computer science can provide a useful tool to assist the physicians in therapy. This tool is called machine learning. Machine learning uses methods from math and statistics, to identify patterns in previously observed client's data to make predictions for new clients. These predictions can be of various types: the course the disease, the therapy outcome of the individual patient, a recommended therapy, or the identification of a disease.

One is inclined to know the outcome of the therapy beforehand, but the first available data are the demographic data of the client. An outcome prediction from this data is inconclusive and does not allow the prediction of the overall outcome of the therapy. With the beginning of the therapy more and more data of the client is collected that can be used for the assessment of the client and outcome prediction. Usually, an early response to the therapy (Van et al., 2008), the relation to the therapist and special outcome questionnaires (Schibbye, Ghaderi & Ljótsson, 2014) are used for the outcome prediction.

Outcome questionnaires, which can be used for early outcome prediction, can also be used to track the clients improvement. The measurement of the outcome questionaire allows the estimation of the current state of the therapy for the client and a prediction of the therapy outcome based on previously observed clients (Knaup, Koesters, Schoefer, Becker, & Puschner, 2009). This property can be used to build an early warning system that compares the expected recovery patterns of the client and notifies the supervising therapist about the current recovery rate (Lueger, 1998). Computer science aids in automatically analyzing the data and proving the therapist a recommendation for each client based on previously collected data and therapy outcomes. By proving these kind of information to the therapist, the adherence and outcome results of the clients can be improved (Lambert & Whipple, 2003). In addition, this should make the work of the physicians more efficient, so that they can focus on clients prone to drop-out and therapy failure.

All these analyses can only indicate the direction of improvement or suggest clients for further review. The final judgment of the therapist is always required because the therapist might have more insight into the current situation of the client than the computer system. Nonetheless, the identification of clients that does not respond to the therapy or even deteriorate, reduces costs for treating them in an unsuited therapy and these clients can attend another more appropriated therapy, which improves his conditions, earlier.

This leaves the question how could a computer estimate a beneficial treatment for the client.

A method that can be used for the estimation of a beneficial therapy for an individual client is a virtual patient model. Virtual patient is a technology that simulates real-life clinical scenarios that is mainly used for education. A virtual patient system allows the student to train his skills by interviewing the system, making physical exams, diagnostic and therapeutic decisions. Usually this training is done with actors that are trained to portray and report symptoms associated with a certain condition (Hubal & Kizakevich, 2000). However, the virtual patient provides standardized feedback and unlimited repetitions. In the context of the client assessment a virtual patient model can be used to model the course of a therapy beforehand to estimate the therapy with the highest benefit (Both & Hoogendoorn, 2011).

A problem within e-mental health is the lack of visual and audio information in contrast to face to face treatment of the client. Therefore, in the case of online treatment sentiment detection could be a useful tool for the therapist to get additional information about the client's mood and condition.

During the last years, the methods of text analysis are constantly improving and have proven quite powerful. Sentiment detection can be used to extract the emotions out of text or speech samples (Chang, Fisher & Canny, 2011). These tools can assist the physician to obtain the current mood of the client out of text samples from email or chat conversation. Especially, when a diary is used within the therapy, it is sheer impossible for the therapist to read all entries for all the clients. This is where automated text analysis becomes in very handy. All the text samples from the client can be processed automatically. If the system recognizes a deterioration or an abnormality, the system would notify the therapist for further review of this client.

The methods of text analyses has also been used on suicide notes to estimate if the writer is inclined to commit another suicide attempt. The system was able to distinguish between suicide notes from suicide completers and suicide notes from a healthy control group as accurate as mental health professionals (Pestian & Nasrallah, 2010). Methods like these would be useful for the screening of writings from depressive clients.

Mobile phones and machine learning can be used to collect more subtle information about the client's behaviour like its activity profile throughout the day. The identification of the daily activities of a client can be of huge benefit for its assessment because many diseases are linked to physical inactivity. The use of activity recognition has been researched for many diseases such as cardiovascular disease, hypertension, diabetes mellitus and depression (Preece et al., 2009). States of depressions are often correlated with a lack of activity. Therefore, mobile phones can be used for activity recognition and tracking of the clients daily activity level. For this measurement, the accelerometers of a mobile phone are used to recognize the current activity of a person. The activities of walking, jogging, ascending and descending of stairs, sitting and standing activities can be successfully recognized (Kwapisz, Weiss & Moore, 2011). By monitoring and processing this type of information, the therapist would have one more detail to assess the recovery process of the client.

After the successful treatment of the mental disorder, the prediction of future relapse is profitable for the estimation of the required aftertreatment. Relapse is a problem, especially in clients with partial remission and residual symptoms. The data of a 1-year follow-up survey was used with machine learning methods to predict the risk of depressive episodes in the future (Voorhees, Van & Paunesku, 2008). It is suggested that the clients with a low risk continue with an internet based behavioural therapy, whereas the clients with a high risk require further face-to-face counselling.

All these methods are of great benefit for the therapist, that has to supervise many different clients. If the system provides appropriate feedback and additional information such as the mood development and daily activities, the therapist could have a clearer view on the client's condition. All these algorithms are no guarantee to prevent drop-out or deterioration of a client, but it would definitely improve the overall treatment and alleviate the work of the physicians.

DIRECTIONS FOR FURTHER RESEARCH

Based on the previous section we can define four possible categories for further research: application design, pre-treatment, treatment, relapse prevention.

These different categories are not distinct they are interconnected. Application design phase focuses on the design of e-mental health applications. This incorporates the planning and implementation. Just like in software planning, the provided functionality has to be defined. This encompasses the front end and back end. Besides the used technologies the back end incorporates the used screenings and interventions, as well as machine learning algorithms. The frond end provides the functionality to the therapists and clients. As mentioned in the previous section the usability has to prevent mistakes by the users.

If the focus lies on the per-treatment phase, there algorithms for the identification of mental illness, outcome and dropout prediction can be researched. For example, text analysis can be used to assist the diagnosis of a patient's disorder based on text samples. The usage of words in a text provides information about a possible disease, like for the diagnosis of schizophrenia (Song & Diederich, 2014). When one plans to incorporate and research such a method within the e-mental health application, one has to go back to application design to incorporate this functionality and feedback to the therapist. The therapist might make better decisions based on the diagnostic help and provide the clients with a more suited treatment, which would require further research.

Now, where we introduced the connection between these different categories, we continue with the treatment phase. The treatment phase might be the most interesting phase because this phase has the highest interaction with the client and the most data is collected. Research studies mainly focus on the approval of a certain therapy type for a certain disease. This neglects the possibility of machine learning algorithms and the individuality of the clients' needs. One therapy design is applied to all clients, this neglects individuality. One could argue that face-to-face treatment provides more individual treatment based on the fact, that human therapists will adapt to the client. But why should an online treatment not also adapt to the requirements of the individual client. One might also argue, that this would endanger the cost-effectiveness and the treatment of more clients, but machine learning and adequate feedback to the physicians could counter this problem. Research has stated that feedback improves the adherence and improvement of the clients (Lambert 2010). Clearly, this also requires the incorporation of the application design phase, and the cooperation of the clients, therapists and financial stockholders, since each one pursues different objectives.

Moving on to the relapse prevention phase. After a successful treatment, the client requires after-care to prevent relapse. The same as in the previous treatment phase applies for the relapse prevention phase, but in addition this phase also requires some of the results of the pre-treatment and treatment phase. Because typically after-care prediction relies on the initial symptom severity, demographic features and the symptom severity after the active treatment(Domino et al., 2005; Farren et al., 2013; Pedersen & Hesse, 2009; Voorhees, Van & Paunesku, 2008).

Finally, after research on one topic has been conducted the results have to be incorporated into the mental-health application by entering the application design phase again.

The main research opportunity is in successfully incorporating diagnosis support, drop-out, outcome, and relapse prediction into online treatment. Continues assessment of the client with provided feedback for the therapist has been realized in the past (Miller et al., 2006), but it is not established as a standard. By using these techniques, the treatment of the clients could be more individualized regarding their needs.

One could also incorporate these tools into self-help applications and provide the feedback to the clients, to aid the clients to steer their therapy. The effect of such methods is yet to research.

After providing such functionality one could incorporate more fine grained measures of the clients. Usually questionnaires are used to assess the client, but as mentioned earlier, mobile phones can be used to capture the clients activity and condition without the client even noticing. These more fine grained measures can further improve the quality of the predictions and could be applied to individualize the treatment.

CONCLUSION

In summary, all the discussed research topics within e-mental health require further research. This can be within the field of developing guidelines for the implementation of e-mental health applications in general, the gamification of existing interventions, the development of new intervention or even the way how research is conducted within this field.

Dropout, engagement in therapy or deterioration of symptoms are problems of e-mental health likewise in clinical mental health. Their solution is essential for the success of mental health and the wellbeing of the clients. Even though, these phenomena are known and well researched, the results are inconclusive and in the case of symptom deterioration due to psychotherapy are not fully understood, as well as the phenomenon that some patients improve more rapidly than others during therapy. Research has shown that a reminder email or SMS improves the adherence, but there might be more ways to keep the client engaged into therapy and to increase the frequency of interaction with the application.

The prediction of the outcome of the overall therapy for the client is closely linked to these problems. Strategies on the measurement of the clients outcome are the satisfaction of the client, engagement, relation to the therapist and the use of outcome questionnaires. All these topics are from clinical mental health, but they also apply to e-mental health where some have just recently been researched in the context of e-mental health.

Text analysis can be used to gain information about the mood of the client from text or voice samples, to compensate for missing face to face treatments. The use of mobile phones allows activity recognition to record the daily activity profile of the client. These are just two examples of a variety of possibilities for the screening of clients to observe their improvement.

Technologies are constantly evolving and paving the way for better treatment possibilities.

E-mental health is a young research topic that requires much more research, to become an accepted and effective treatment for mental disorders. The interdisciplinarity makes it a thrilling topic that poses great benefits, but needs the cooperation of the medical and technical staff to become successful.

REFERENCES

Andrews, G., Cuijpers, P., Craske, M. G., McEvoy, P., & Titov, N. (2010). Computer therapy for the anxiety and depressive disorders is effective, acceptable and practical health care: A meta-analysis. *PLoS ONE*, *5*(10), e13196. doi:10.1371/journal.pone.0013196 PMID:20967242

Baker, B. T., Gustafson, H. D., & Shah, D. (2014). How Can Research Keep Up With eHealth? Ten Strategies for Increasing the Timeliness and Usefulness of eHealth Research. *Journal of Medical Internet Research*, *16*(2), e36. doi:10.2196/jmir.2925 PMID:24554442

Boettcher, J., Rozental, A., Andersson, G., & Carlbring, P. (2014). Side effects in Internet-based interventions for Social Anxiety Disorder. *Internet Interventions*, *1*(1), 3–11. doi:10.1016/j.invent.2014.02.002

Both, F., & Hoogendoorn, M. (2011). Utilization of a virtual patient model to enable tailored therapy for depressed patients. *Neural Information Processing*, 700–710. Retrieved from http://link.springer.com/chapter/10.1007/978-3-642-24965-5_79

Chang, K., Fisher, D., & Canny, J. (2011). Ammon: A speech analysis library for analyzing affect, stress, and mental health on mobile phones. *Proceedings of PhoneSense*. Retrieved from http://www.cs.berkeley.edu/~jfc/papers/11/AMMON_phonesense.pdf

De Graaf, L. E., Gerhards, S., Arntz, A., Riper, H., Metsemakers, J. F. M., Evers, S. M. A. A., & Huibers, M. J. H. et al. (2009). Clinical effectiveness of online computerised cognitive-behavioural therapy without support for depression in primary care: Randomised trial. *The British Journal of Psychiatry*, *195*(1), 73–80. doi:10.1192/bjp.bp.108.054429 PMID:19567900

Dennis, T. a., & O'Toole, L. J. (2014). *Mental Health on the Go: Effects of a Gamified Attention-Bias Modification Mobile Application in Trait-Anxious Adults*. Clinical Psychological Science; doi:10.1177/2167702614522228

Dölemeyer, R., Tietjen, A., Kersting, A., & Wagner, B. (2013). Internet-based interventions for eating disorders in adults: A systematic review. *BMC Psychiatry*, *13*(1), 207. doi:10.1186/1471-244X-13-207 PMID:23919625

Domino, K. B., Hornbein, T. F., Polissar, N. L., Renner, G., Johnson, J., & Alberti, S., & Hankes. (n.d.). Effectiveness of a web-based intervention for problem drinkers and reasons for dropout: Randomized controlled trial. *Journal of Medical Internet Research*, *12*(4).

Farren, C. K., Snee, L., Daly, P., & McElroy, S. (2013). Prognostic Factors of 2-year Outcomes of Patients with Comorbid Bipolar Disorder or Depression with Alcohol Dependence Importance of Early Abstinence. *Alcohol and Alcoholism (Oxford, Oxfordshire)*, *48*(1), 93–98. doi:10.1093/alcalc/ags112 PMID:23059424

Fernández-Aranda, F., Jiménez-Murcia, S., Santamaría, J. J., Gunnard, K., Soto, A., Kalapanidas, E., & Penelo, E. (2012). Video games as a complementary therapy tool in mental disorders: PlayMancer, a European multicentre study. *Journal of Mental Health (Abingdon, England)*, *21*(4), 364–374. doi:10.3 109/09638237.2012.664302 PMID:22548300

Fiscal, I. (2005). *President's budget request for NIMH*. Bethesda, MD: National Institute of Mental Health.

Gill, S., Contreras, O., Muñoz, R. F., & Leykin, Y. (2014). Participant retention in an automated online monthly depression rescreening program: Patterns and predictors. *Internet Interventions*, *1*(1), 20–25. doi:10.1016/j.invent.2014.02.003 PMID:25045623

Harwood, H. (2000). *Updating estimates of the economic costs of alcohol abuse in the United States: Estimates, update methods, and data*. The Lewin Group for the National Institute on Alcohol Abuse and Alcoholism.

Hubal, R., & Kizakevich, P. (2000). *The virtual standardized patient. Medicine Meets Virtual*. Retrieved from http://spectra.rti.org/pubs/Patient.PDF

Karsh, B.-T. (2004). Beyond usability: Designing effective technology implementation systems to promote patient safety. *Quality & Safety in Health Care*, *13*(5), 388–394. doi:10.1136/qshc.2004.010322 PMID:15465944

Knaup, C., Koesters, M., Schoefer, D., Becker, T., & Puschner, B. (2009). Effect of feedback of treatment outcome in specialist mental healthcare: Meta-analysis. *The British Journal of Psychiatry*, *195*(1), 15–22. doi:10.1192/bjp.bp.108.053967 PMID:19567889

Kwapisz, J., Weiss, G., & Moore, S. (2011). Activity recognition using cell phone accelerometers. *ACM SigKDD Explorations....* Retrieved from http://dl.acm.org/citation.cfm?id=1964918

Lambert, M. (2010). Yes, it is time for clinicians to routinely monitor treatment outcome. *Monitoring Treatment Outcome*, 239–266. doi:10.1037/12075-008

Lambert, M., & Whipple, J. (2003). Is it Time for Clinicians to Routinely Track Patient Outcome? A Meta-Analysis. *Clinical Psychologist*, 288–301. doi:10.1093/clipsy/bpg025

Linn, A. J., Vervloet, M., van Dijk, L., Smit, E. G., & Van Weert, J. C. M. (2011). Effects of eHealth interventions on medication adherence: A systematic review of the literature. *Journal of Medical Internet Research*, *13*(4), e103. doi:10.2196/jmir.1738 PMID:22138112

Lueger, R. J. (1998). U*sing feedback on patient progress to predict the outcome of psychotherapy. Journal of Clinical Psychology, 54*(3), 383–393. doi:10.1002/(SICI)1097-4679(199804)54:3<383::AID-JCLP7>3.0.CO;2-Q PMID:9545173

McCrone, P. (2004). Cost-effectiveness of computerised cognitive-behavioural therapy for anxiety and depression in primary care: Randomised controlled trial. *The British Journal of Psychiatry*, *185*(1), 55–62. doi:10.1192/bjp.185.1.55 PMID:15231556

Melville, K. M., Casey, L. M., & Kavanagh, D. J. (2010). Dropout from Internet-based treatment for psychological disorders. *The British Journal of Clinical Psychology*, *49*(4), 455–71. doi:10.1348/014466509X472138

Miller, Scott D., Duncan, Barry L., Brown, Jeb, Sorrell, Ryan, & Chalk, Mary Beth, Miller, S. D., Sorrell, R. (2006). Using Formal Client Feedback to Improve Retention and Outcome: Making Ongoing, Real-time Assessment Feasible. *Journal of Brief Therapy*, *5*(1), 5–22.

Musiat, P., Goldstone, P., & Tarrier, N. (2014). Understanding the acceptability of e-mental health--attitudes and expectations towards computerised self-help treatments for mental health problems. *BMC Psychiatry*, *14*(1), 109. doi:10.1186/1471-244X-14-109 PMID:24725765

Pagliari, C. (2007). Design and Evaluation in eHealth: Challenges and Implications for an Interdisciplinary Field. *Journal of Medical Internet Research*, *9*(2), e15. doi:10.2196/jmir.9.2.e15 PMID:17537718

Pedersen, M. U., & Hesse, M. (2009). A simple risk scoring system for prediction of relapse after inpatient alcohol treatment. *The American Journal on Addictions*, *18*(6), 488–493. doi:10.3109/10550490903205983

Pestian, J., & Nasrallah, H. (2010). Suicide note classification using natural language processing: A content analysis. *Biomedical ...*, *2010*(3), 19–28. Retrieved from http://www.ncbi.nlm.nih.gov/pmc/articles/PMC3107011/

Preece, S. J., Goulermas, J. Y., Kenney, L. P. J., Howard, D., Meijer, K., & Crompton, R. (2009). Activity identification using body-mounted sensors--a review of classification techniques. *Physiological Measurement*, *30*(4), R1–R33. doi:10.1088/0967-3334/30/4/R01 PMID:19342767

Schibbye, P., Ghaderi, A., Ljótsson, B., Hedman, E., Lindefors, N., Rück, C., & Kaldo, V. (2014). Using Early Change to Predict Outcome in Cognitive Behaviour Therapy: Exploring Timeframe, Calculation Method, and Differences of Disorder-Specific. *PLoS ONE*, *9*(6), e100614. doi:10.1371/journal.pone.0100614 PMID:24959666

Scott, E. R., & Mars, M. (2013). Principles and Framework for eHealth Strategy Development. *Journal of Medical Internet Research, 15*(7), e155. doi:10.2196/jmir.2250 PMID:23900066

So, M., Yamaguchi, S., Hashimoto, S., Sado, M., & Furukawa, T. A., & McCrone, P. (2013). Is computerised CBT really helpful for adult depression?-A meta-analytic re-evaluation of CCBT for adult depression in terms of clinical implementation and methodological validity. *BMC Psychiatry, 13*, 113. doi:10.1186/1471-244X-13-113 PMID:23587347

Song, I., & Diederich, J. (2014). Speech Analysis for Mental Health Assessment Using Support Vector Machines. *Mental Health Informatics.* Retrieved from http://link.springer.com/chapter/10.1007/978-3-642-38550-6_5

Stegemann, S., Weg, R., Ebenfeld, L., & Thiart, H. (2012). Towards measuring user engagement in internet interventions for common mental disorders. *Ewic.bcs.org.* Retrieved from http://ewic.bcs.org/upload/pdf/ewic_hci12_pcp_paper7.pdf

Van, H. L., Schoevers, R., Kool, S., Hendriksen, M., Peen, J., & Dekker, J. (2008). Does early response predict outcome in psychotherapy and combined therapy for major depression? *Journal of Affective Disorders, 105*(1-3), 261–265. doi:10.1016/j.jad.2007.04.016 PMID:17521743

Van Gemert-Pijnen, E. W. C. J., Nijland, N., van Limburg, M., Ossebaard, C. H., Kelders, M. S., Eysenbach, G., & Seydel, R. E. (2011). A Holistic Framework to Improve the Uptake and Impact of eHealth Technologies. *Journal of Medical Internet Research, 13*(4), e111. doi:10.2196/jmir.1672 PMID:22155738

Van Velsen, L. (2013). Designing eHealth that matters via a multidisciplinary requirements development approach. *JMIR Research, 2*(1), e21. doi:10.2196/resprot.2547 PMID:23796508

Van Voorhees, B., Paunesku, D., Gollan, J., Kuwabara, S., Reinecke, M., & Basu, A. (2008). Predicting future risk of depressive episode in adolescents: The Chicago Adolescent Depression Risk Assessment (CADRA). *Annals of Family Medicine, 6*(6), 503–511. doi:10.1370/afm.887 PMID:19001302

Whittaker, R., Borland, R., & Bullen, C. (2009). Mobile phone-based interventions for smoking cessation. . . . . *Database Syst Rev, 11*(4), CD006611. doi:10.1002/14651858.CD006611.pub3 PMID:19821377

KEY TERMS AND DEFINITIONS

Activity Recognition: Uses methods from machine learning to identify a person's current activity.

Data Mining: Basically the same as machine learning.

Framework: Describes how the software has to be constructed.

Gamification: Treatments are modified and programmed as a game. The game aims on alleviating the symptoms of the client as the regular intervention would do.

Machine Learning: Algorithms that allow to identify patterns in data to make predictions on new data based on old data.

Outcome Prediction: Data from previous clients and machine learning is used, to predict the outcome of the therapy for new clients.

Sentiment Detection: Subfield of machine learning and natural language processing that tries to identify the emotions within a text or speech sample.

The European Union Legal Framework on E-Health, Telemedicine, and Privacy

Pedro Pina
Polytechnic Institute of Coimbra, Portugal

INTRODUCTION

The practice of medicine, both in the phase of diagnosis and treatment, necessarily involves the activity of collecting and processing personal data concerning health and genetics of patients. According to the European Union's legislation, such kind of personal data is included in the scope of the patient's fundamental right to informational and communicational self-determination, where it is qualified as sensitive data, therefore deserving greater protection when compared to non-sensitive data. Indeed, personal health data relate to nuclear, inalienable and indispensable dimensions of human dignity privacy or integrity of the person concerned.

Traditionally and in the analog world, the patient rights to privacy and to health data were sufficiently guaranteed by the imposition of duties of professional secrecy on doctors and medical collaborators. In fact, since the origins of the profession, the special relationship of trust that needs to exist between patient and physician has been recognized as one of the main important dimensions of the exercise of medical professions, and the need for doctors to keep confidential any information disclosed to them is codified in the Hippocratic Oath (Whiddett, Hunter, Engelbrecht & Handy, 2007, p. 534).

However, with the growing use of information and communication technologies (ICT), especially the internet, in the practice of medicine, medical informatics and, in particular, telemedicine revealed an enlargement of the circle of people with access to the collected medical data beyond the traditional physician - patient relationship.

Although there is no specific sectorial legislation on the protection of privacy in telemedicine, the European Union has sought to differentially regulate the activity of collecting and processing clinical and health data, through (a) the Directive 95/46/EC of the European Parliament and Council, imposing special requirements for obtaining a special title for collection and treating health data and also the obligation of implementing technical security measures to prevent, among others, the access by unauthorized persons; and (b) also by the Directive 2002/58/EC of the European Parliament and of the Council, on privacy and electronic communications, where it is imposed the adoption of technical measures assuring the inviolability electronic communications.

More than a decade after the approval of the referred directives, technological developments provided the globalization of data flows, the popularization of cloud computing and easy retrieval of massive information through search engines, making it absolutely necessary to update the terms of the legal protection. Considering this necessity, in March 2014, the European Parliament approved a data protection package reinforcing privacy rights in a digital context.

The present chapter aims to expose the rationale for the protection of health data, to describe its particular vulnerability in the context of electronic communications and telemedicine in particular, and to analyze the terms of the current and the proposed European Union legal regime on the matter.

DOI: 10.4018/978-1-4666-9978-6.ch072

ELECTRONIC HEALTH SERVICES AND DATA PRIVACY

Telemedicine, e-health, telehealth or health telematics are terms often used as synonyms which were coined to describe the provision of healthcare and medical services at a distance. According to the World Health Organization's broad definition of telemedicine, such activities consists in the

delivery of health care services, where distance is a critical factor, by all health care professionals using information and communication technologies for the exchange of valid information for diagnosis, treatment and prevention of disease and injuries, research and evaluation, and for the continuing education of health care providers, all in the interests of advancing the health of individuals and their communities. (1998, 10)

However, in a narrow sense, the term 'telemedicine' regards only the provision of clinical services at a distance by the use of medical information exchanged from one site to another through electronic communications regarding the improvement of a patient's clinical health status. The terms e-health and health-telematics are umbrella concepts that cover all the activities involving the provision of remote health care services, clinical or not – like the ones carried out by nurses, social workers or therapists –, tele-education for health or telematics for health services management or health research.

Although the delivery of health care services at a distance is not a new phenomenon, since in the past, in a limited way, some services could be provided by radio, by telephone or by mail, the development of ICT has dramatically increased the possibilities of the use of telemedicine and e-health, putting in evidence their benefits. With the use of ICT, it is possible to provide health care services to patients living in isolated communities and remote regions, home or abroad, to reduce waiting times in health care systems, to monitor chronically ill patients without in-person meetings, or to professionals to easily exchange clinical information without a physical reunion. Electronic health services may consist: (a) in interactive services, where patients and health professionals have real time interactions; (b) in remote monitoring, where physicians are enabled to remotely monitor their patients through the exchange of network-monitoring data; (c) in storing and forwarding data such as diagnostic images or videos with patient data for later evaluation offline.

Regardless the type of e-health or telemedicine, acquiring, recording and transmitting patient's clinical data are their core technological activities.

As it is recognized by the Commission of the European Communities (2008),

privacy and security related aspects are also major components of building trust and confidence in telemedicine systems. The respect of rights and fundamental freedoms, like the fundamental rights to private life and to the protection of personal data, must be guaranteed during the collection and processing of personal data, in particular when relating to health. As any other transmission of personal health-related data, telemedicine can pose a risk to data protection right (in the sense that disclosure of a medical condition or diagnosis could adversely affect an individual's personal and professional life). Data privacy aspects should be systematically assessed whenever telemedicine services are provided.

Maintaining the secrecy of the data is no longer a burden only of the physician or of other clinical professional, but also of all the persons that, in the data network, beyond the relationship clinical professional-patient, directly or indirectly contact with such data, transmitting it, receiving it, assuring its integrity or preventing unauthorized access.

N

Protection of clinical data and medical records is no longer treated only as a question of professional and medical secrecy. In fact, data digital transmission and communication can be easily observed, collected and controlled, considering the electronic trail that online users leave. As a result, "safeguards against the treatment and misuse of computerized personal data are becoming increasingly important [since] their tense relationship with various fundamental rights, freedoms and guarantees (development of the personality, personal dignity, private life) is unquestionable" (Canotilho & Moreira, 2007, pp. 550-551).

THE RIGHT TO COMMUNICATIONAL AND INFORMATIONAL SELF-DETERMINATION

In the European Union, data protection and privacy have overcome the borders of the defensive mere right to privacy as some Constitutions predicted the right to communicational and informational self-determination as a fundamental right with a larger scope of protection. The term was first used in a seminal 1983's decision of the Germany Federal Constitutional Court (BVerfGE, 1983) ruling that

in the context of modern data processing, the protection of the individual against unlimited collection, storage, use and disclosure of his/her personal data is encompassed by the general personal rights constitutional provisions. This basic right warrants in this respect the capacity of the individual to determine in principle the disclosure and use of his/her personal data.

The right to communicational and informational self-determination was then defined as "the authority of the individual to decide himself, on the basis of the idea of self-determination, when and within what limits information about his private life should be communicated to others".

The new conceptualization of the individual's right over personal data took it from a mere guarantee of the right to privacy to a true fundamental right with an independent meaning, conceived

for the protection of new facets of personality – it is a right of personality – and consisting in the recognition of the freedom to control the use of information respecting to it (if it is personal), and in the protection against attacks arising from the use of such information. (Castro, 2005, pp. 65 ss)

The right to communicational and informational self-determination displays two inseparable but autonomous dimensions. The first one, built as a negative right, has a defensive nature, similar to the guarantee for the secrecy of correspondence and of other means of private communication, and protects the holder against interference by the State and by individuals or corporations who are responsible for processing digital or analogical data or others. The second dimension reveals a positive right and a true fundamental freedom, "a right to dispose of your own personal information, a power of controlling it and from which exercise you may determine what others can, at every moment, know about your respect" (Castro, 2006, p. 16).

This conception goes beyond the traditional understanding, dominant in the USA law, of the right to privacy as "the right to be left alone" (Warren & Brandeis, 1890), imposing only opacity to the others. As a consequence, in the traditional American conception of privacy, there is an individual's right to act only in cases of commitment of tortious acts. In fact, according to the Restatement (second) of torts § 652a (1977), invasion of privacy means one of the following invasions: intrusion upon the seclusion of another or his private affairs or concerns; appropriation to his own use or benefit of the other's name or likeness; publicity to a matter concerning the private life of another when the matter publicized is of a kind that would be highly offensive to a reasonable person, and is not of legitimate concern to the public (Garcia, 2005, pp. 1238-1239).

This reactive solution is defended by those who support that market regulation of privacy is more efficient than State regulation. In the USA, where that conception prevails, apart from the government regulation of specific sectors like the protection of children online, the procedures for collecting, keeping or transferring consumer's data are left to the industry self-regulation. The Federal Trade Commission (FTC), an independent agency of the USA government, whose main mission is the promotion of consumer protection, has an important role on promoting fair privacy policies. Besides that, the FCT only has the power

to prosecute firms whose practices are at variance with their policy disclosures for engaging in a deceptive trade practice. However, Web sites are not required to post any disclosures, and without a posted privacy policy, the FTC has no basis for acting under its current authority. (Culnan, 2000, p. 25)

In the aforementioned conception of privacy, in the absence of public regulation imposing duties to the industry, online consumers may not have the power to obtain information on who is using their data or the powers to control what personal information is collected, how it is collected, how it will be used, if it will be disclosed or transferred to third parties, amongst other usages.

On the contrary, the right to communicational and informational self-determination gives an individual the power to control at any time all the possible usages of his/her personal data. There is philosophical background that supports the mentioned view, as the right is based on the protection of the personality of the individual. Following the legal tradition in civil law jurisdictions based on the protection of the dignity of the human person, personality rights have a specific normative and legal meaning as they are constructed to guarantee the protection of human dignity and the right to freely develop one's personality. Such rights recognize and protect the individual's life, moral and physical integrity, autonomy and free will and impose a general duty of abstention from interfering in the protected field. Furthermore, in the core matters of protection, personality rights are non-transmissible and non-renounceable rights and, therefore, kept outside the possibilities of legal trade.

The right to communicational and informational self-determination is recognized in the European Union as a true fundamental right, connected to the development of the personality of each individual, in article 8 of the European Union Charter of Fundamental rights, where it is foreseen that

1. *Everyone has the right to the protection of personal data concerning him or her.*
2. *Such data must be processed fairly for specified purposes and on the basis of the consent of the person concerned or some other legitimate basis laid down by law. Everyone has the right of access to data which has been collected concerning him or her, and the right to have it rectified.*
3. *Compliance with these rules shall be subject to control by an independent authority.*

Article 16(1) of Treaty on the Functioning of the European Union, as introduced by the Lisbon Treaty, also establishes the principle that everyone has the right to the protection of personal data concerning him or her.

The Charter and the Treaty were influenced by the European Convention on Human Rights and by the jurisprudence from the European Court of Human Rights. In fact, more than a matter of no trespassing or of abstaining from interfering with individuals' privacy, the State also has "to provide individuals with the material conditions needed to allow them to effectively implement their right to private and family life. In other words, […] States are under the obligation to take all appropriate measures in order to protect fundamental rights of the individuals including against infringements by other non-state parties" (Rouvroy & Poullet, 2009, pp. 51-52).

On the European Union derivative law level, two directives can be highlighted: Directive 95/46/EC of the European Parliament and of the Council of 24 October 1995 on the protection of individuals with regard to the processing of personal data and on the free movement of such data; and Directive 2002/58/EC of the European Parliament and of the Council of 12 July 2002 concerning the processing of personal data and the protection of privacy in the electronic communications sector (Directive on privacy and electronic communications).

The right to the protection of personal data concerning patients' health is also recognized in Directive 2011/24/EU of the European Parliament and of the Council of 9 march 2011on the application of patients' rights in cross-border healthcare. As it is foreseen in Recital 25, these personal data should be able to flow from one Member State to another, but at the same time the fundamental rights of the individuals should be safeguarded. Therefore, the provisions of Directive 95/46/EC should also apply in the context of cross-border healthcare.

From the above mentioned directives, where personal data is considered as

any information relating to an identified or identifiable natural person ('data subject'); an identifiable person is one who can be identified, directly or indirectly, in particular by reference to an identification number or to one or more factors specific to his physical, physiological, mental, economic, cultural or social identity,

it can be concluded that, in the European Union, the activity of electronic collecting and computer processing of personal data is regulated according to standards that embody the following principles: (a) the principle of lawful collecting, according to which collecting and processing of data constitute a restriction on the holder's informational self-determination and are only permitted within the parameters of the law and, particularly, with the holder's knowledge and consent, (b); the finality principle, meaning that the data collection and the data processing can only be made with a clear, specific and socially acceptable finality that must be identifiable right at the moment of the gathering; (c) the principle of objective limitation, as the use of the collected data must be restricted to the purposes that were communicated to the holder in the moment of the collection, and must respect the ideas of proportionality, necessity and adequacy, (d) the principle of temporal limitation, meaning that data shall not be kept by more than the time needed to achieve the justificative finality (e) the principle of data quality, according to which the collected data must be correct and up to date, (f) the principle of the free access to data by its subject, who must be able to know the existence of the collection and the storage of his/her personal data and to rectify, erasure or block the information if incomplete and inaccurate; (g) the security principle, under which the controller must implement appropriate technical and organizational measures to protect personal data against accidental or unlawful destruction or accidental loss, alteration, unauthorized disclosure or access, in particular where the processing involves the transmission of data over a network; (h) the confidentiality principle, meaning that confidentiality of communications and the related traffic data by means of a public communications network and publicly available electronic communications services shall be ensured, as it is prohibited to listening, tap, store or other to perform other kinds of interception or surveillance of communications and the related traffic data by persons other than users, without the consent of the users concerned, except when legally authorized to do so (Pina,

2011, p. 247). The respect for the aforementioned principles shall be monitored by national independent and regulatory data protection public agencies.

In what concerns health and clinical data in particular, such matter is characterized by the European Union's legislation as a special category of personal data because of their special sensitive nature and essentiality for the protection of human personality. By default, it is prohibited the processing of sensitive data. It is excepted, however, from the prohibition the processing of data required for the purposes of preventive medicine, medical diagnosis, the provision of care or treatment or the management of health-care services, where those data are processed by a health professional subject under national law or rules established by national competent bodies to the obligation of professional secrecy or by another person also subject to an equivalent obligation of secrecy. Nevertheless, only the general prohibition of processing of sensitive data is legally excluded, since the general rules regarding the need for obtaining previous and informed consent for collecting, treating or exchanging data are maintained.

THE 2014 EUROPEAN PARLIAMENT DATA PROTECTION PACKAGE REINFORCING PRIVACY RIGHTS IN A DIGITAL CONTEXT

The Data Protection Reform Package

On the 12th of March 2014, the European Parliament approved the European Commission's data protection reform to strengthen online data protection rights and tackle the challenges of globalization and new technologies like cloud computing, meaning that more and more data is being stored on remote servers instead of personal computers, and the astounding intensification of the scale of data sharing and collecting. The data protection reform package consists of two draft laws: a general regulation updating the principles established by Directive 95/46/EC and covering the central aspects of personal data processing in the European Union and a directive on processing data to prevent, investigate, detect or prosecute criminal offences or enforce criminal penalties.

Although the legislative intervention of the European Union´s institutions regards mainly economic facets and the strengthen of the digital single market where data is the currency of digital economy by making it easier for companies to move across the European Union, it is recognized that such objective must be combined with a high level of protection of fundamental rights of natural persons like the right to the protection of personal data.

The Proposed New Legal Solutions

In the approved proposal, the Commission and the European Parliament recognized that the absence of common rules would create the risk of different levels of protection in the Member States and create restrictions on cross-border flows of personal data between Member States with different standards and also that there are practical challenges to enforcing data protection legislation and a need for co-operation between Member States and their authorities, which needed to be organized at European Union level to ensure unity of application of Union law. Considering the economic concern, the Regulation foresees one one-stop shop mechanism where, for the treatment of data in all the European Union's territory, controllers or processors, those who process personal data on behalf of the formers, only have to deal with the supervisory authority of the Member State in which they have its main establishment.

Article 5 of the Regulation sets out the general principles relating to personal data processing, which correspond fundamentally to those already foreseen in Article 6 of Directive 95/46/EC added by the transparency principle requiring that any information addressed to the public or to the data subject should be easily accessible and easy to understand, and that clear and plain language is used.

Processing of personal data shall be lawful only if the data subject has given consent to the processing of their personal data for one or more specific purposes, or if it is necessary for the performance of a contract to which the data subject is party or in order to take steps at the request of the data subject prior to entering into a contract; for compliance with a legal obligation to which the controller is subject; in order to protect the vital interests of the data subject; for the performance of a task carried out in the public interest or in the exercise of official authority vested in the controller or for the purposes of the legitimate interests pursued by a controller, except where such interests are overridden by the interests or fundamental rights and freedoms of the data subject which require protection of personal data, in particular where the data subject is a child.

The Regulation maintains the general prohibition of processing of sensitive personal data such as those revealing race or ethnic origin, political opinions, religion or beliefs, trade-union membership, and of the processing of genetic data or data concerning health or sex life or criminal convictions or related security measures. Particularly regarding health personal data, the prohibition is not applicable if the processing of data is done on the basis of Union law or Member State law providing for suitable and specific measures to safeguard the data subject's legitimate interests, and is necessary for the purposes of preventive or occupational medicine, medical diagnosis, the provision of care or treatment or the management of health-care services, and where those data are processed by a health professional subject to the obligation of professional secrecy or another person also subject to an equivalent obligation of confidentiality under Member State law or rules established by national competent bodies.

The Regulation seminally introduces in a legislative document the data subject's right to be forgotten and the obligation of the controller which has made the personal data public to inform third parties on the data subject's request to erase any links to, or copy or replication of that personal data. Notwithstanding, the main changes brought by the Regulation are related to the strengthening of the obligation of responsibility of the controller (or of joint controllers) and its extension to processors to comply with of the law and to the definition of obligatory procedures that data controllers will have to follow.

Article 33 imposes the obligation of controllers and processors to carry out a data protection impact assessment prior to operations that present specific risks, such as the ones related to the evaluation of natural person's health situation. The assessment shall contain at least a general description of the envisaged processing operations, an assessment of the risks to the rights and freedoms of data subjects, the measures envisaged to address the risks, safeguards, security measures and mechanisms to ensure the protection of personal data and to demonstrate compliance with the Regulation, taking into account the rights and legitimate interests of data subjects and other persons concerned.

Article 23 foresees the obligations of the controller arising from the principles of data protection by design and by default. Continuously taking into consideration the state of the art and the cost of implementation, the controller shall, both at the time of the determination of the means for processing and at the time of the processing itself, implement appropriate technical and organizational measures and procedures in such a way that the processing will ensure the protection of the rights of the data subject. Moreover, the controller shall implement mechanisms for ensuring that, by default, only those personal data are processed which are necessary for each specific purpose of the processing and are especially not collected or retained beyond the minimum necessary for those purposes, both in terms of the amount of the data and the time of their storage, ensuring, in particular, by means of those mechanisms that, by default, personal data are not made accessible to an indefinite number of individuals.

Article 30 obliges not only controllers but also processors to implement appropriate measures for the security of processing, extending that obligation, when compared to the one imposed by Article 17(1) of Directive 95/46/EC, to processors, irrespective of the contract with the controller.

Based on personal data breach notification foreseen in Article 4(3) of the e-privacy Directive 2002/58/EC, articles 31 introduces an obligation of controllers and processors to notify personal data breaches to the supervisory authority, no later than 24 hours after having become aware of it. According to Article 32, when the personal data breach is likely to adversely affect the protection of the personal data or privacy of the data subject, the controller shall, after the notification referred to in Article 31, communicate the personal data breach to the data subject without undue delay.

Article 35 introduces a mandatory data protection officer for the public sector, and, in the private sector, for enterprises employing 250 persons or more or where the core activities of the controller or processor consist of processing operations which require regular and systematic monitoring. The data protection officer shall be entrusted at least with the following tasks: to inform and advise the controller or the processor of their obligations pursuant to the Regulation and to document this activity and the responses received; to monitor the implementation and application of the policies of the controller or processor in relation to the protection of personal; to monitor the implementation and application of the Regulation, in particular as to the requirements related to data protection by design, data protection by default and data security and to the information of data subjects and their requests in exercising their rights; to maintain documentation of all processing operations under its responsibility; to monitor the documentation, notification and communication of personal data breaches; to monitor the performance of the data protection impact assessment by the controller or processor and the application for prior authorization or prior consultation; to monitor the response to requests from the supervisory authority, and, within the sphere of the data protection officer's competence, co-operating with the supervisory authority at the latter's request or on the data protection officer's own initiative; to act as the contact point for the supervisory authority on issues related to the processing and consult with the supervisory authority.

FUTURE RESEARCH DIRECTIONS

The Regulation's substantive and adjective solutions follow the European Union's recognition of personal data, especially sensitive data like health records, as fundamental rights. The main problems that arise in this field are related to the challenges brought by the Internet: how to enforce rights on digital information like e-health records, considering the geographical distribution of its users stressing the rules of territoriality and State's sovereignty, the intangible nature of informational contents and the free flow of information that ICT potentiate. If the system may work in a harmonized single market, international flow of personal health data to countries with a low level of protection may endanger data subject's rights. Despite the prohibition of transferring personal data to third countries with low level of protection, the enforcement of such right remains a practical problem, considering that Member States' jurisdictions lack the executive means to do so. The Regulation recognizes that its ambitious scope of protection have the appointed Achilles's heel and, in relation to third countries and international organizations, urges the European Commission to promote international co-operation for the protection of personal data, in particular in the cases where the Commission has decided that third countries' supervisory authorities ensure an adequate level of protection.

Compliance with data protection rules by third countries' controllers or processors becomes not only a matter of respect of data subject's rights but also of international trade law, since the market for telemedicine and e-health will only flourish at the international level if trust and security are assured. In the next years, international legal instruments will certainly be created in the field of personal data protection, particularly in the sub-area of telemedicine and e-health, most probably under the auspices of the World Trade Organization and not of the World Health Organization.

CONCLUSION

The development of telemedicine and e-health and the creation of an efficient market of online health-care services constitute a ground of common interests between States, corporations and individuals. The referred activities necessarily involve collecting, processing and transferring personal health data of patients. European Union's legislation recognizes the right to private life and to the protection of personal data as a fundamental right, including the protection of sensitive data related to the health situation of natural persons within the scope of the right to informational self-determination. Trust and security related to collecting, storing and processing health and medical records are, therefore, essential for telemedicine and e-health systems.

The *acquis communautaire* on personal data protection, especially of sensitive data like health and medical records, reveals European union's leading role in the matter, recognizing data subjects the right not only to defend from informational trespass but also to dispose of his/her own personal information and the power of controlling it and to discern what others can, at every moment, know about data his/her respect. The proposal of Regulation contained in the European Parliament data protection package reinforcing privacy rights in a digital context strengthens the protection, adapting the previous legislation to the challenges of the continuous development of ICT and laying down detailed rules related to the prevision and exercise by controllers and processor of demanding duties. The digital nature of the informational content and the global distribution of users defies the content of the Regulation, especially in the cases of unauthorized transfer or access to personal data, considering the limitations of sovereignty and territoriality. European Union's rules on protection of personal data are fully enforceable within its borders. So that they can be more than merely normative outside the European Union, a strong effort has to be made to promote international co-operation for the protection of personal data, and to potentiate trust and security particularly of transnational telemedicine and e-health systems.

From the individual's point of view, one traditional problem that may be identified in this field is the lack of awareness of his/her rights and of the activities that may infringe them. Strong educative and information campaigns must take place to grant effectiveness to the legal recognition of the right to informational and communicational self-determination.

REFERENCES

BVerfGE. (1983). *1BVerfGE 65, 1 – Volkszählung Urteil des Ersten Senats vom 15. Dezember 1983 auf die mündliche Verhandlung vom 18. und 19. Oktober 1983 - 1 BvR 209, 269, 362, 420, 440, 484/83 in den Verfahren über die Verfassungsbeschwerden*. Retrieved October 13, 2014, from http://www.servat.unibe.ch/dfr/bv065001.html

Canotilho, J. J. G., & Moreira, V. (2007). *Constituição da República Portuguesa Anotada*. Coimbra: Coimbra Editora.

Castro, C. S. (2005). O direito à autodeterminação informativa e os novos desafios gerados pelo direito à liberdade e à segurança no pós 11 de Setembro. In *Estudos em homenagem ao Conselheiro José Manuel Cardoso da Costa, II*. Coimbra: Coimbra Editora.

Castro, C. S. (2006). *Protecção de dados pessoais na Internet, Sub Judice, 35*. Coimbra: Almedina.

Commission of the European Communities. (2008). *689: Communication from the Commission to the European Parliament, the Council, the European Economic and Social Committee and the Committee of the Regions on telemedicine for the benefit of patients, healthcare systems and society*. Retrieved October 13, 2001, from http://eur-lex.europa.eu/legal-content/EN/TXT/?uri=CELEX:52008DC0689

Culnan, M. J. (2000). Protecting Privacy Online: Is Self-Regulation Working? *Journal of Public Policy & Marketing, 19*(1), 20–26. doi:10.1509/jppm.19.1.20.16944

Pina, P. (2011). Digital Copyright Enforcement: Between Piracy and Privacy. In C. Akrivopoulou & A. Psygkas (Eds.), Personal Data Privacy and Protection in a Surveillance Era: Technologies and Practices (pp. 241-254). Hershey, PA: Information Science Reference.

Rouvroy, A., & Poullet, Y. (2009). The right to informational self-determination and the value of self-development. Reassessing the importance of privacy for democracy. In Reinventing Data Protection? (pp. 45-76). Berlin. Springer. doi:10.1007/978-1-4020-9498-9_2

Warren, S., & Brandeis, L. (1890). The Right to Privacy. *Harvard Law Review, 4*(5), 193–220. doi:10.2307/1321160

Whiddett, R., Hunter, I., Engelbrecht, J., & Handy, J. (2007). Privacy and Access to Electronic Health Records. In M. Quigley (Ed.), *Encyclopaedia of Information Ethics and Security* (pp. 534–541). Hershey, PA: Information Science Reference. doi:10.4018/978-1-59140-987-8.ch079

World Health Organization. (1998), *A health telematics policy in support of WHO's Health-For-All strategy for global health development: report of the WHO group consultation on health telematic*. Retrieved October 13, 2014, from http://apps.who.int/iris/handle/10665/63857

KEY TERMS AND DEFINITIONS

Data Concerning Health: Any information which relates to the physical or mental health of an individual, or to the provision of health services to the individual.

E-Health: Umbrella concept that covers all the activities involving the provision of remote health care services, clinical or not – like the ones carried out by nurses, social workers or therapists –, tele-education for health, telematics for health services management or health research.

Health Professional: A doctor of medicine, a nurse responsible for general care, a dental practitioner, a midwife or a pharmacist, or another professional exercising activities in the healthcare sector which are restricted to a regulated profession, or a person considered to be a health professional according to the legislation of the Member State of treatment.

N

Healthcare: Health services provided by health professionals to patients to assess, maintain or restore their state of health, including the prescription, dispensation and provision of medicinal products and medical devices.

Informational Self-Determination: The capacity of the individual to determine the disclosure and the use of his/her personal data, to control and to determine what others can, at every moment, know about his/her respect.

Medical Records: All the documents containing data, assessments and information of any kind on a patient's situation and clinical development throughout the care process.

Telemedicine: The delivery of clinical services at a distance by the use of medical information exchanged from one site to another through electronic communications regarding the improvement of a patient's clinical health status.

An Investigation into Doctors' Perceptions of Internet Informed Patients

Rajesh Chandwani
Indian Institute of Management Ahmedabad, India

Iris Reychav
Ariel University, Israel

INTRODUCTION

Traditionally, health professionals have been the primary source of health information for patients and their relatives, the other important 'offline' sources of health information being friends and relatives, and other persons/ families suffering from similar ailments. However, the increasing penetration of Internet has allowed patients to search the net to obtain health information. Studies have shown that health related information is one of the most frequently sought issues while browsing the Internet (Fuerts et al., 2007). According to the Pew Internet and American Life Project, 82 percent of the adult American population uses the Internet and of that, 72% of users have looked up health related information in the last year on the net (Rice, 2006). Even in developing countries like India, there has been an increase in Internet use to seek health related information (Akerkar et al., 2005; Bakshi, 2012).

Patients may access the Internet before consulting with a doctor to gain information about their symptoms and/or disease, as well as after the consultation process, to validate and verify the information provided by the doctor (Mcullan, 2006). Policy makers have emphasized that this increasing use of Internet for health information can be tapped to educate the patient, and hence foster patient empowerment (Edejer, 2000). Patient empowerment refers to the process of facilitating self directed behavioural change in patients, in order to ensure the delivery of 'patient centered' healthcare service (Anderson and Funnel, 2010). The term 'empowerment', as described by Paulo Freire, underlines the importance of education.

...There is no such thing as a neutral education process. Education either functions as an instrument which is used to facilitate the integration of generations into the logic of the present system and bring about conformity to it, or it becomes the 'practice of freedom', the means by which men and women deal critically with reality and discover how to participate in the transformation of their world. (Freire, 2014: 34)

The Internet allows patients to access health information at the convenience of a click, ensures anonymity, and also enables people to reach out to support groups, and as such, is becoming an important source of health information seeking. Scholars have argued that internet based health information can, potentially, enhance patients' understanding of their disease and self management capabilities (Sommerhalder et al, 2009). Thus, potentially, Internet can act as a medium to 'educate' the patient about his/ her illnesses, and can result in patient empowerment as described above. However, the process of empowerment and delivery of patient centred care should be understood in the context of the interface between the patient and the healthcare system (Johns, 2006). The fulcrum of the patient's connect with the healthcare system is the doctor-patient interaction.

DOI: 10.4018/978-1-4666-9978-6.ch073

Arguably, the use of Internet based health information would result in a change in the manner in which patients interact with their doctor, and hence, impact the way in which physicians deal with such patients. In other words, Internet health information seeking by the patients may affect the dyadic process of doctor-patient interaction (Fuertes et al., 2007), which is one of the most important determinants of the quality of healthcare. The majority of the studies have analyzed the impact of the use of Internet based health information only from the patient's perspective (Sommerhalder et al., 2009). The investigation of the issue from a physician's perspective has been limited (McMullan, 2006). Drawing upon the Structuration theory, this chapter attempts to analyze the effect of Internet health information seeking on doctor-patient interactions, more specifically, from the perspective of doctors.

BACKGROUND

An effective doctor-patient relationship enables effective healthcare delivery and has been positively linked to outcome measures such as patient satisfaction, treatment adherence and treatment outcomes (Fuertes et al., 2007). The doctor-patient interaction attempts to balance the doctor's concerns about the hard biomedical science and the patient's subjective experiences. While former relates to the aspects of disease, such as the cause, treatment options and prognosis; the latter related to illness, such as how will it constrain one's socio-economic life and lifestyle. Doctor-patient interactions which form the building blocks of a doctor-patient relationship are thus instrumental in bridging the potential gap between hard biomedical facts and the softer subjective dimensions. Patient information and awareness is seen as an important aspect that facilitates doctor-patient interaction, especially in chronic diseases which have a protracted and complicated course of progression, and when the therapy involves the active participation of the patient and their relatives, entailing significant changes in their lifestyle for example in patients having diabetes or hypertension. The concept of 'patient empowerment' emphasizes that the educated and informed patient who understands the implications of his/ her illnesses and treatment will engage in a participatory decision making process with the doctor. The use of internet for accessing health information is therefore, regarded as facilitating patient empowerment.

However, survey studies of physicians have reported mixed perceptions about the impact of Internet based health information on the doctor-patient relationship (McMullan, 2006). Murray et al. (2003) conducted a survey amongst 1050 physicians in the US to examine their perceptions about internet informed patients. They reported that only 38 % of the physicians believed that Internet health information has a beneficial effect on the doctor-patient relationship; 54 % reported no effect; and 8 % claimed that they were 'challenged' by such patients, which can potentially worsen the doctor-patient interactions. Potts et al (2002) conducted a survey of 800 web literate physicians and corroborated the above findings. They reported that while web based information seeking results in more benefits than problems for patients, physicians reported more problems than benefits. The above findings warrant a detailed analysis of the problem faced by the doctors in interacting with these patients, and the perception of the doctors about the Internet informed patient. Using structuration theory, this chapter presents a detailed account of the processual aspects of physicians' perceptions about the access of Internet based health information by the patients and its effect on doctor-patient interaction, Understanding the physicians perspective is highly essential, as the process of patient empowerment and delivery of patient centred care involves a dyadic relationship, of which the physician is an integral part. Therefore, it is critical to comprehensively understand the phenomenon of how physicians are experiencing and managing the altered doctor-patient interaction.

Most of the studies examining patient's health information access over Internet have been carried out in the context of the developed world (Fuertes et al., 2007), where awareness about health information and the penetration of Internet has been high. Doctor-patient interaction and relationship depend upon the socio-cultural dimensions of the context (Johns 2006; Kim et al., 2000). Extant studies have used western developed country samples where power distance is low (Hofstede, 1991) and participatory decision making is seen as a norm, rather than an exception. In this chapter, we explore the context of a developing country like India, characterized by a high-power distance culture (Hofstede, 1991), where the idea of patient participation at a wider level is uncommon. In the Indian context, the doctor-population ratio is extremely low, which in turn increases physicians' workload and they might have limited capacity to engage with patients over lengthy interactions (Abraham and George, 2015). But developing countries are rapidly changing due to the penetration and use of Internet by a fast growing educated and literate middle class. Indeed, studies have shown that developing countries like India too are witnessing the phenomenon of patients and their relatives accessing Internet for medical information, especially in urban areas (Akerkar et al., 2005). However, the 'structures' invoked by the doctors and patients about the changing socio-cultural norms determining doctor patient interaction, hence, would be drastically different in the context of developing world. Thischapter attempts to provide a detailed analysis of physicians' perspectives about Internet information seeking by patients in a rapidly changing developing economies context.

Structuration Theory

By conceptualizing the 'use of technology' as a contextually embedded phenomenon, we draw upon tenets of Structuration theory to examine the phenomenon. Structuration theory is a "general theory of social organization... explaining the relationship between individual and society" (Jones and Karsten, 2008: 129). Giddens posits that "human agents draw on social structures in their actions, and at the same time these actions serve to produce and reproduce social structure." According to Giddens (1979), human technology interaction is guided by structures which refer to the existing mental schemas in the human mind. It is these structures that determine the rules and norms that govern action. Though actions tend to reproduce and reinforce the structures, these structures themselves are dynamic, as they are subject to the recursive interpretation of actions by human agency. Structuration theory thus attempts to achieve a balance between determinism and agency. Conceptualizing technology use in terms of structures invoked by actors embedded in the socio-cultural context is opportune, insofar as it sheds light on the emerging processes and perceptions, for example how doctors and patients will perceive the phenomenon of Internet health information access and how the relationship between the doctor and patient will be affected because of engagement with a new technology (Jones and Karsten, 2008).

From the perspective of structuration theory, the use of Internet for health information access by the patients occurs in a situated context of structures that are determined by existing healthcare system and relationships. The perception about patients' access to Internet health information is determined by the respective interpretation and use by the actors (doctors and patients). Doctors and the patients can, potentially, ascribe diverse perspectives to the meaning of Internet health information access, which can influence the doctor patient interaction. The Internet health information access and doctor-patient interaction can be viewed from the three dimensions introduced by Giddens, systems of meaning, forms of power relations and sets of norms. The doctor-patient interaction depend upon the interplay of the structures invoked by the actors: for example, the doctors might view Internet health information access as challenge to their authority while patients may see it as an option to take a second opinion. Similarly the power relations in the doctor patient relationship and the norms about an interaction could be re-inforced or challenged by the use of technology depending upon the structures invoked by the actors.

As the phenomenon of Internet access by patients is a relatively nascent one in the Indian context, the structures can be assumed to be evolving. The objective of this chapter is to understand the physicians' interpretation of patients accessing health information over the Internet by exploring the three dimensions of structuration theory, namely the meanings ascribed by the actors, the affect of power dynamics and influence on the existing socio-cultural norms. More specifically, the study explores how Internet access for health information would be perceived by doctors and patients along the above three dimensions, and further posits how doctors might respond to the phenomenon.

MAIN FOCUS OF THE CHAPTER

Perception about Internet Health Information: A Structuration Perspective

From the perspective of structuration theory, the use of the Internet to access health information occurs in a situated context of structures that are determined by the existing doctor patient relationships and the socio-cultural norms that govern such a relationship. Hence, while Internet facilitated patient education might aim to empower the patient in such a way that the interaction becomes more patient centric, the evolution of technology, its use by actors and perceptions about technology in turn determines how the interaction unfolds. These diverse actors can, potentially, ascribe different perspectives to the meaning of Internet health information, which can influence the doctor patient interaction. The table below (table 1) describes the structurational analysis (c.f. Walsham, 2002) of the phenomenon of Internet health information access by the patient in terms of three dimensions: *meanings* ascribed to the phenomenon, *influence* on power dynamics and the *socio-cultural norms*. On the basis of the analysis, we describe different types of perception that a doctor can attribute.

More specifically, the chapter considers the context of developing countries like India in carrying out structuration analysis. The developing countries are characterized by high power distance between the doctor and the patient and the resulting doctor-patient relationship is of a 'paternalistic' nature (Fochsen et al., 2006). These relationships are characterized by high trust that patient places on the doctors to take a decision about his/ her well being. Further, the doctor population in these contexts is generally low, leading to doctors being busy and overworked. The increasing penetration of the Internet as in the developed world, is leading many patients to access health related information over the Internet (Akerkar et al., 2005; Bakshi, 2012).

One of the important aspects of online health information that concerns both patients and doctors is the authenticity of the information available and the perceived credibility of the information. In the following subsection, we examine the issues related to perceived credibility as these issues would have implications for the changing role of doctors in the era where many patients access health information on the internet.

Credibility of Online Health Information

Lack of requirement of stringent quality control such as editorial boards, reviewers along with easy and affordable publishing process entails flooding of Internet with information without strict publication standards (Fiksdal et al., 2014). Thus the Internet provides access to huge amount of unfiltered information. Studies have shown that though most of adult population places more trust on health information

Table 1. Structurational analysis of Internet health information access by the patient

Structurational Dimension	Doctors' and Patients' Perceptions
Meaning	*Patients may consider Internet channels as a means of accessing information about their symptoms, diseases, treatment protocols etc. They might view the Internet as a medium for education and empowerment. Education, however, may result in raising their curiosity about different options available for treatment, the side effects of the drug they are being prescribed etc. It is precisely this awareness that forms the core of patient empowerment, enabling them to be engaged in participatory decision making.* *Doctors on the other hand, may view Internet health information in multiple ways. Their perception may align with that of patients, where the 'educated' patient is aware of the importance of self management of disease, especially in chronic diseases like diabetes, which involves substantial lifestyle modifications. Here the doctors may view the Internet as 'facilitating' their consultation process by decreasing the time required to explain the self management processes and in motivating the patients.* *However, doctors may also view the Internet as hindering their consultancy process, as the 'Internet informed' patients tend to be more inquisitive and ask more questions, thus straining their already extremely busy schedules. The doctors may feel that patients who seek Internet medical information 'ask too many irrelevant questions'. This may be especially the case where the doctor is largely involved in acute care delivery and is dealing with long OPD queues.* *Further, the perception about the accuracy and validity of the information available over the Internet has been repeatedly questioned. For example the NHS has issued special directives for patients who are accessing health related information over the net. Doctors, in particular, may question the reliability of the information available on uncontrolled media such as the Internet, and also the validity of the inferences drawn by patients from that information.*
Power	*In the context of developing countries, the knowledge gap between the doctor and patient is the principle reason for high power distance between the two. Patient access to information through the Internet may decrease the perceived gap. In other words, doctors may perceive that patients may use the Internet based knowledge to challenge the knowledge based authority of the doctors, thus altering the perceived power dynamics between the two key actors. Doctors with such conceptualization might believe that many of the questions asked by Internet informed patients will be directed to test the knowledge of the doctors rather than to clear the doubts. Thus, the doctors may view Internet informed patients as 'challenging the authority of doctors'. Further, in an era of increasing litigation over doctors, the doctors may perceive Internet informed patients to be potential litigators.* *Thus, Internet health information may affect the perceived power dynamics in the doctor patient interaction in the developing country context characterized by high power distance between the two*
Norms	*As highlighted above, Internet health information may question a basic norm about the trust in the doctor patient relationship. The lack of trust is especially relevant in developing countries like India, where the poor awareness about health related issues attaches greater importance to the trust established between the doctor and patient.* *As explained above, the doctors may consider that Internet informed patients would be more likely to take the 'litigation' route in case of adverse outcomes. Thus, doctors may perceive that the patients who seek Internet health information before coming for the consultations lack trust on their doctors. Arguably, the perception of lack of trust can adversely affect the doctor-patient relationship which primarily involves building trust between the healthcare provider and healthcare seeker.* *Doctors who consider that information provided over the Internet is usually faulty and opinionated may further consider that the incorrect or incomplete knowledge may also perpetuate lack of trust in the doctor's advice.*

provided by their doctors, they visit access online information first (Hessey et al., 2005) Largely, people trust the online information available and use this information as a basis of their discussion with the doctors (Newnham et al., 2006). Structurational analysis of the Internet health information access reveals that doctors may emphasize the inaccuracy of the available health information online and use this pretext to discourage online information access, The questionable accuracy and authenticity of health information may be more important in contexts such as India where the phenomenon is a relatively recent ones and regulations governing internet information availability are not fully evolved.

SOLUTIONS AND RECOMMENDATIONS

The increasing access to Internet and a rapidly expanding literate middle class in developing countries like India has enabled access to extensive medical information for patients. Many of the patients, even in rural and semi urban areas access health related information before and after meeting the doctors (Akrekar et al., 2005; Bakshi, 2012). Invoking the structuration theory, the above chapter analyzes the doctor's perception of patients accessing health information over Internet, and examines how the doctors may respond to such patients.

Most studies have shown that physicians perceived that Internet-informed patients had better knowledge about their diseases, and therefore, it was easier to interact with them. Indeed many physicians not only encourage patients to access online health information but also use social media for sharing health related information (McGowan et al., 2012). However, the structurational analysis of Internet health information seeking reveals that doctors and patients may ascribe different interpretations to the phenomenon affecting the power dynamics of the doctor-patient interaction and challenging the existing socio-cultural norms regarding the interactions. In the context of developing countries like India, where the power distance between the health care provider and the healthcare seeker is high, and the relationship between them is largely trust based, Internet health information seeking may be viewed negatively by some doctors

The doctor's perceptions about 'Internet informed patients, in turn, may affect the behaviour of doctors while dealing with such patients. For example if doctors perceive that such patients challenge the authority of the doctor or are potential litigators, the doctors may take a cautious approach in revealing information, thus inhibiting the free flow of information between the doctor and patient. Further, if the patient is perceived to be a 'litigator', the doctor-patient relationship with such patients may be characterized by lack of trust. Thus, Internet access on the part of patients may adversely affect the doctor-patient relationship, which, paradoxically, could result in constraining the flow of information between the healthcare provider and healthcare seeker. However, the doctors who view the Internet as facilitating their consultation process by enabling the process of motivating the patient for self management of chronic illnesses might appreciate the role of Internet in creating knowledgeable patients, as it becomes easy for them to communicate regarding the disease.

In the above analysis, we contribute to the existing discourse on the 'digital divide'. Critics have highlighted the existence of a 'digital divide' which emphasizes that the increasing penetration of Internet may not benefit certain sections of the population (Compaine, 2001). Cammaerts (2008) observe that dominant discourses regarding the digital divide represent concerns about unequal access to technology resulting in differential capabilities, whereas not having access automatically leads to socio-cultural, political and/or economic exclusion. Scholars have highlighted the existence of digital divide in the domain of online health information (Wyatt et al., 2005). By using the structuration theory, this chapter presents another dimension of the digital divide- that of differential perceptions about technology by two key stakeholders, namely the doctor and patient, which can affect doctor patient interaction, and hence the delivery of healthcare services. The perception of doctors that there is a 'lack of trust' in the doctor-patient relationship and that Internet informed patients are potential litigators can, potentially, limit the spontaneity and openness in communication between the doctor and the patient. In other words, rather than 'empowering' the patients, Internet information seeking can adversely affect the evolution of the relationship between the doctor and patient itself, which in turn can affect the flow of information between the healthcare provider and healthcare seeker.

To provide insights on the role of doctors in the internet information era, we draw upon Bakardjieva's conceptualization of 'warm expert'–a person well versed with technical capabilities and who is in a position to help a new Internet user. A warm expert plays the role of mediation between the specialized knowledge and skills necessary to gain advantage of the technology and the specific contextual aspects of the 'novice'. Bakardjieva (2001) found that warm experts, who were personally engaged with the novice internet users, played a crucial role in learning and appropriation of the technology. The concept of warm expert emphasizes the value of informal learning (Stewart, 2003; Sørensen and Stewart, 2002). The above study emphasizes that 'patient empowerment' through Internet health information will be realized when both doctor and patient engage in a participatory decision making process. As the information available over the Internet is overwhelming and de-contextualized, it is important for the doctor to play a role of a 'warm expert', by enabling the patient to access authentic information and also to make sense of the information according to his/her personal condition. The doctor in the role of a warm expert will enable the meanings ascribed to the use of Internet for health information by both stakeholders, namely the doctor and patient to be aligned. Indeed, authors have posited that in the Internet era, physician s should proactively help the patients to understand the relevance of Internet health information.

The role of 'warm expert' can be further comprehended through the concept of disintermediation and apomediation (Eysenbach, 2007). Traditionally, patients have turned to experts such as doctors, nurse managers and/or their social network (friends, family members, community members) for seeking health related information and solving their queries. Internet health information can lead to disintermediation, making the role of human intermediaries redundant in health information seeking process. However, as the availability of health information on the net is overwhelming, unregulated and non-contextual, doctors need to act as apo-mediators (supporting patients in the search process) rather than inter-mediators (situating themselves between the patient and information). As an apomediator, the doctor can enable the patient to interpret and contextualize the information available.

FUTURE RESEARCH DIRECTIONS

While the health information seeking over the Internet has potential to enhance patient's awareness about diseases in developing countries like India, physicians might be slow to respond to the changed dynamics of the doctor-patient relationship. In a related work Chandwani and Kulkarni (2016) empirically examine the doctors' perspectives about internet informed patient in Indian context. Future researchers should examine the issue in more detail in similar contexts. The doctor patient relationship is related to the broader socio-cultural context. For example, the doctor's response may be entirely different in a context where there is significant power distance between the doctor and patient. The above chapter presents a structurational analysis of physician's perspective about Internet informed patients. Future researchers are urged to empirically explore the phenomenon both qualitatively and quantitatively to discern the important variables which can enable the researchers to understand the phenomenon. More specifically, exploring the doctor's perspective is important in developing an understanding of the possible role of doctors in facilitating the change from an authoritative interaction to a more participatory one.

Doctors may need support and encouragement to adapt to their role in dealing with Internet-informed patients as facilitators who can use the Internet literacy to bridge the gap between patient's access to information and doctor's expertise. Further studies are thus required to understand the designing and implementation of such initiatives and then to assess the impact of the interventions. A comprehensive exploration of the phenomenon will require researchers to take a multi-stakeholders perspective, illuminating both patient's as well as doctor's concern about the phenomenon, while also considering the contextual nuances. The above study highlights the importance of taking an interdisciplinary approach to examining the effect of health information seeking over the Internet, involving researchers from the fields of Information science, technology, sociology and health

N

CONCLUSION

There is no doubt that the Internet is bringing fundamental changes to the medical profession, as patients become more informed, more participatory, and consequently, more empowered. This chapter takes an embedded view of technology, arguing that Internet information can affect the 'interaction' between the doctor and patient, which in turn, is dependent upon socio-cultural norms of the context. From the perspective of structuration theory, doctors and patients may ascribe different meanings to the health information in the Internet, which in turn, will determine their perception of the phenomenon. For the Internet to enable patient empowerment, doctors should play the role of 'warm experts', actually enabling the patients to make sense of the information available and also guiding the behavioural changes accordingly. In the Indian context, doctors may need support and encouragement to adapt to their role in dealing with Internet-informed patients.

REFERENCES

Abraham, G., & George, T. K. (2015). Rethinking the Postgraduate Teaching Program and Examinations in Today's India. *The Journal of the Association of Physicians of India*, 63. PMID:26731837

Akerkar, S. M., Kanitkar, M., & Bichile, L. S. (2005). Use of the Internet as a resource of health information by patients: A clinic-based study in the indian population. *Journal of Postgraduate Medicine*, *51*(2), 116–118. PMID:16006703

Anderson, R. M., & Funnell, M. M. (2010). Patient empowerment: Myths and misconceptions. *Patient Education and Counseling*, *79*(3), 277–282. doi:10.1016/j.pec.2009.07.025 PMID:19682830

Bakardjieva, M. (2001). Becoming a domestic Internet user. *Proceedings of the 3rd International Conference on Uses and Services in Telecommunications*, (pp. 12-14).

Bakshi, S. M. H. (2012). Assessment of Internet Use and Effects amongst General Practitioners in Non Metro Cities of Hyderabad and Secunderabad. *Middle East Journal of Family Medicine*, *7*(10), 44.

Cammaerts, B. (2008). Critiques on the participatory potentials of Web 2.0. *Communication, Culture & Critique*, *1*(4), 358–377. doi:10.1111/j.1753-9137.2008.00028.x

Chandwani, R., & Kulkarni, V. (Forthcoming). Who's the doctor? Physicians' perception of internet informed patients in India. Accepted for publication- Computer Human Interaction, ACM CHI conference proceedings 2016

Compaine, B. M. (2001). *The digital divide: Facing a crisis or creating a myth?* MIT Press.

Edejer, T. T. (2000). Disseminating health information in developing countries: The role of the Internet. *BMJ (Clinical Research Ed.)*, *321*(7264), 797–800. doi:10.1136/bmj.321.7264.797 PMID:11009519

Eysenbach, G. (2007). From intermediation to disintermediation and apomediation: New models for consumers to access and assess the credibility of health information in the age of Web2. 0. *Studies in Health Technology and Informatics*, *129*(1), 162. PMID:17911699

Fiksdal, A. S., Kumbamu, A., Jadhav, A. S., Cocos, C., Nelsen, L. A., Pathak, J., & McCormick, J. B. (2014). Evaluating the process of online health information searching: A qualitative approach to exploring consumer perspectives. *Journal of Medical Internet Research, 16*(10). PMID:25348028

Fochsen, G., Deshpande, K., & Thorson, A. (2006). Power imbalance and consumerism in the doctor-patient relationship: Health care providers' experiences of patient encounters in a rural district in India. *Qualitative Health Research, 16*(9), 1236–1251. doi:10.1177/1049732306293776 PMID:17038755

Freire, P. (2014). *Pedagogy of the oppressed 30th Anniversary Edition*. Bloomsbury Publishing USA.

Fuertes, J. N., Mislowack, A., Bennett, J., Paul, L., Gilbert, T. C., Fontan, G., & Boylan, L. S. (2007). The physician–patient working alliance. *Patient Education and Counseling, 66*(1), 29–36. doi:10.1016/j.pec.2006.09.013 PMID:17188453

Giddens, A. (1979). *Central problems in social theory: Action, structure, and contradiction in social analysis*. Univ of California Press. doi:10.1007/978-1-349-16161-4

Hesse, B. W., Nelson, D. E., Kreps, G. L., Croyle, R. T., Arora, N. K., Rimer, B. K., & Viswanath, K. (2005). Trust and sources of health information: the impact of the Internet and its implications for health care providers: findings from the first Health Information National Trends Survey. *Archives of Internal Medicine, 165*(22), 2618–2624. doi:10.1001/archinte.165.22.2618 PMID:16344419

Hofstede, G. (1991). *Cultures and organizations*. London: McGraw-Hill.

Johns, G. (2006). The essential impact of context on organizational behavior. *Academy of Management Review, 31*(2), 386–408. doi:10.5465/AMR.2006.20208687

Jones, M. R., & Karsten, H. (2008). Giddens's structuration theory and information systems research. *Management Information Systems Quarterly, 32*(1), 127–157.

Kim, M., Klingle, R. S., Sharkey, W. F., Park, H. S., Smith, D. H., & Cai, D. (2000). A test of a cultural model of patients' motivation for verbal communication in patient-doctor interactions. *Communication Monographs, 67*(3), 262–283. doi:10.1080/03637750009376510

McGowan, B. S., Wasko, M., Vartabedian, B. S., Miller, R. S., Freiherr, D. D., & Abdolrasulnia, M. (2012). Understanding the factors that influence the adoption and meaningful use of social media by physicians to share medical information. *Journal of Medical Internet Research, 14*(5), e117. doi:10.2196/jmir.2138 PMID:23006336

McMullan, M. (2006). Patients using the Internet to obtain health information: How this affects the patient–health professional relationship. *Patient Education and Counseling, 63*(1), 24–28. doi:10.1016/j.pec.2005.10.006 PMID:16406474

Murray, E., Lo, B., Pollack, L., Donelan, K., Catania, J., Lee, K., & Turner, R. (2003). The impact of health information on the Internet on health care and the physician-patient relationship: National U.S. survey among 1.050 U.S. physicians. *Journal of Medical Internet Research, 5*(3), e17. doi:10.2196/jmir.5.3.e17 PMID:14517108

Newnham, G. M., Burns, W. I., Snyder, R. D., Dowling, A. J., Ranieri, N. F., Gray, E. L., & McLachlan, S. A. (2006). Information from the Internet: Attitudes of Australian oncology patients. *Internal Medicine Journal, 36*(11), 718–723. doi:10.1111/j.1445-5994.2006.01212.x PMID:17040358

Potts, H. W., & Wyatt, J. C. (2002). Survey of doctors' experience of patients using the Internet. *Journal of Medical Internet Research, 4*(1), e5. doi:10.2196/jmir.4.1.e5 PMID:11956037

Rice, R. E. (2006). Influences, usage, and outcomes of Internet health information searching: Multivariate results from the Pew surveys. *International Journal of Medical Informatics, 75*(1), 8–28. doi:10.1016/j.ijmedinf.2005.07.032 PMID:16125453

Sommerhalder, K., Abraham, A., Zufferey, M. C., Barth, J., & Abel, T. (2009). Internet information and medical consultations: Experiences from patients' and physicians' perspectives. *Patient Education and Counseling, 77*(2), 266–271. doi:10.1016/j.pec.2009.03.028 PMID:19411157

Sørensen, K. H., & Stewart, J. (2002). *Digital divides and inclusion measures: A review of literature and statistical trends on gender and ICT.* Senter for teknologi og samfunn, Institutt for tverrfaglige kulturstudier, Norges teknisk-naturvitenskapelige universitet-NTNU.

Stewart, J. (2003). The social consumption of information and communication technologies (ICTs): Insights from research on the appropriation and consumption of new ICTs in the domestic environment. *Cognition Technology and Work, 5*(1), 4–14.

Walsham, G. (2002). Cross-cultural software production and use: A structurational analysis. *Management Information Systems Quarterly, 26*(4), 359–380. doi:10.2307/4132313

Wyatt, S., Henwood, F., Hart, A., & Smith, J. (2005). The digital divide, health information and everyday life. *New Media & Society, 7*(2), 199–218. doi:10.1177/1461444805050747

KEY TERMS AND DEFINITIONS

Doctor Patience Interaction: The doctor-patient interplay, which comprises the social as well as clinical aspects of a confidential relationship shared by physician and patients.

Health Information: Any information, whether oral or recorded in any form or medium, that is related to the past, present, or future physical, social or mental health or condition of any individual."

High Power Distance: Power distance is one of the dimensions of Hofstede's cultural dimensions theory. High power distance cultures are characterized by societal members being deferential to figures of authority and generally accepting an unequal distribution of power.

Patient Centered Care: A model of healthcare delivery in which healthcare providers partner with patients and their families to identify and satisfy patient needs and preferences while providing professional care.

Patient Empowerment: A process designed to facilitate self-directed behavior change by designing and delivering health care services which enables citizens to take control of their health care needs.

Structuration Theory: Giddens' structuration theory suggests there is a social structure (traditions, institutions and moral codes) that guide human behaviour. However, these structures themselves can be modified by human agency, for example by reproducing them differently or interpreting them differently or replacing them.

Issues in Telemedicine Service:
Acceptance and Willingness

Noorliza Karia
Universiti Sains Malaysia, Malaysia

INTRODUCTION

The knowledge-based economy, health quality, rapid technology progress, green innovation and digital society have inspired the Malaysian government and Ministry of Health to acknowledge telemedicine blueprint since 1997 (Ministry of Health, 1997). However, the original push on telemedicine to promote lifelong wellness has not led to a large-scale telemedicine sector in Malaysia due to poor infrastructure (limited availability of broadband Internet), premature funding and low public acceptance (Maarop and Than, 2012). Most healthcare providers have greater interest in using Health Information Technology (IT) to implement electronic health records and reduce administrative costs rather than in using these technologies to make more healthcare-related services extensively available.

The purpose of this chapter is to tackle one of the most important and challenging trends in healthcare and health-related service namely telemedicine. It is currently the most necessary and demanding trend in healthcare industry. It aims for lifelong wellness enrichment where each individual is accountable for the supervision of his/her own health. The investment in innovation of health care and health-related services is aimed at producing a nation with healthy society through telemedicine (health service system) that is efficient, technologically appropriate, and environmentally adaptable and consumer friendly with prominence and eminence on quality, innovation and value of health. Thus, this chapter regards telemedicine as an innovation service offered by innovative healthcare providers which offer service portfolios such as healthcare advice, instruction and monitoring by healthcare service (HCS) for patients. For example, telemedicine facilitates a patient when he/she wishes to consult with the doctor or nurses or vice versa when the doctor or nurses need to supervise the patient at certain times within a given day.

The increasing number of telemedicine services is in response to customer demand and competitive pressure. This chapter discusses a comprehensive practical introduction to the shift towards health service system or telemedicine of healthcare service providers from the users' perspective. The main concept of telemedicine is explained with the intention of establishing a common understanding and usage of the terminology among the wider audience. The chapter focuses primarily on telemedicine implementation that explores users' willingness to accept it. Hence, this chapter will emphasize on individuals' worldviews on telemedicine such as evaluation, perception and decision on accepting and rejecting telemedicine.

BACKGROUND

There is no definite universal definition of telemedicine. Telemedicine is a term used to describe the health service system, often interchangeable with terms such as telecare, tele monitoring, telehealth, e-health or Health Information Technology (HIT) related issues (Lankton, 2007; Liu, 2009; Peeters et al., 2012; Huang, 2013). Hein (2009) states that the American Telemedicine Association (ATA) defines telemedi-

DOI: 10.4018/978-1-4666-9978-6.ch074

cine as the use of medical information exchange from one site to another via electronic communications to improve patients' health status. Telemedicine is a tool or solution to improve and/or sustain healthcare delivery and/or patient health performance by using IT. Dyk (2014) demonstrates the relationship between e-health, telehealth, telemedicine, telecare and m-health. In general e-health covers telehealth that relates to a broader set of activities including patient and provider solution whereby telemedicine is a subset of telehealth that has a narrow focus on curative, preventive and promotive aspects. Telecare refers to continuous, automatic and remote monitoring of real time emergencies or a preventive health application. Further, m-health may be regarded as e-health applications that use mobile technologies.

Telemedicine comprises products and services (Hein, 2009; Peeters et al., 2012) ranging from medical devices to delivery system. Examples of telemedicine products are medical devices which are capable of collecting and electronically transmitting information (either immediately or in the future) which can be digitized to be used in telemedicine applications e.g. blood glucose meters, pulse oximeters, blood pressure cuffs, CT scanners, and MRI machines. They include devices targeted for home healthcare and the needs of patients' interest in monitoring health status closely and devices for facilitating information between hospitals, clinics and physicians. Examples of telemedicine-related services include store-and-forward technology for documents and images, remote monitoring of a patient's vital signs, secure messaging; e-mail exchange of data, alerts and reminders between physicians and patients and having a specialist remotely available by video conference to observe and diagnose a patient's condition and recommend treatment. Other services are electronic exchange of prescription information between physicians, pharmacies and consumers; or transmission of information to alert communities about pandemics and other widespread health threats.

One of the few unearthed research areas in telemedicine sector in Malaysia is the development and competitiveness of HCSs (Maarop et al., 2011; Maarop and Than, 2012). Initially HCSs have invested in IT for processing records, keeping health information and transmitting data rather than use these technologies to create more healthcare-related services. For example, electronic health records can be used by patients, physicians, nurses, hospitals and clinics; these health information can be exchanged or used to detect trends of public health and to determine patients' history (Hashim, 2003; Huang, 2013). There are studies on telemedicine which investigated willingness to use telemedicine or telemedicine acceptance (Werner and Karnieli, 2003; Klein, 2007; Kowitlawakul, 2008; Liu, 2009; Templeton, 2010; Peeter et al., 2012; Huang 2013). However, none of these has tackled the means for HCSs to develop and achieve competitiveness.

ISSUES IN TELEMEDICINE

What Is Telemedicine?

Telemedicine is a form of self-health management via self-service technology. Telemedicine has become an essential necessity in the world of HCSs. It had been seen as a prime prospect for enriching the nation's standard of health quality and advancement of lifelong wellness via internet communications technology or the latest telecommunications technology. Innovations in internet communication such as availability of cheaper bandwidth and higher bandwidth speed have expanded internet communication capabilities and provide more accessible and strong platform for telemedicine implementation (Hein, 2009; Huang, 2013). Consequently, telemedicine can be viewed as an innovation of the provision of healthcare and health-related services using telecommunications, information and multimedia technologies to link the participants in the healthcare system.

Nevertheless, telemedicine is still regarded as a challenging venture. Knowledge in healthcare industry on what telemedicine entails and how it can be accomplished and succeeded in practice is still sparse. Given the significance for HCSs, human nature law provides the framework for accessing the feasibility of adopting the telemedicine orientation.

Why Is Telemedicine?

The growth of natural life span and population have intensified the demand for the nation's health care service providers. Telemedicine can be a great option for facilitating communication and relationship between patients and practitioners for evaluating, diagnosing and treating patients remotely and gaining numerous benefits. Research indicates that the use of telemedicine results in numerous positive outcomes. For example, it reduces the number of visits and travels to receive healthcare, enables practitioners to monitor discharged patients and track their recovery, reduces cost related to regular hospitals visits, manages chronic conditions and helps faster recovery (Templeton, 2010; Kowitlawakul, 2008; Klein, 2007). According to Eikelboom and Atlas (2005), thirty two percent of audiology patients, especially men who have previously heard of telemedicine and used the internet for health-related matters, are willing to use telemedicine as it reduces the waiting time and cost.

Despite advances in healthcare, high stress and unhealthy lifestyles among people have resulted in greater episodes of chronic diseases such as diabetes, heart disease and hypertension which all demand continuous lifelong care. Sixty per cent of all deaths worldwide are due to chronic diseases and 80% of these deaths are in low to middle income countries (Piette et al., 2010), leading many chronic patients to obtain an effective chronic illness care. Ongoing, proactive monitoring and self-management support is essential for effective chronic illness care. As chronic conditions require the patient to consistently obtain health care support for medication and management, health care costs are increasing while financial resources remain limited. Therefore, the increasing frequencies of chronic illnesses are associated with the continuous lifelong care which in turn will increase the significant demand for telemedicine practices.

A greater use of telemedicine is crucial to manage self-health management effectively. Telemedicine adoption will allow vital sign information and monitoring to be gathered frequently, not only during periodic physician visits. Messages can be simultaneously transmitted to the treatment team allowing for possible early intervention (a physician or hospital visit) if a patient's condition deteriorates. In addition, chronic diseases (e.g. diabetics, congestive heart failure and obstructive pulmonary disease) necessitate long-term treatment and use of multiple specialists all of which involve high costs. The use of telemedicine is also significant for improving care of elderly and physically challenged patients. Telemedicine adoption will reduce the frequency of visits to physician offices and hospitals which in turn will offer greater convenience and compliance for elderly and home-based patients. Physicians may monitor remotely and timely patient intervention before acute treatment. Thus, telemedicine adoption offers benefits, satisfaction and positive consequences to patients.

Further, telemedicine is a critical tool for empowering patients to directly monitor their medicines and report basic health to their physicians. Each individual is accountable for supervising his/her health. Self-health management increases the patients' responsibility level to facilitate improvement in health. Patients will more likely comply with treatment protocols leading to faster recovery. Another advantage of telemedicine is that it can help reduce deaths and injuries caused by treatment and medication errors arising from inaccurate patient information. Furthermore, it can reduce exposure to illness from other patients by limiting the number of visits to hospital and reduce errors in dispensing medicines by eliminating error and/or handwritten prescription.

Telemedicine is vital to extend the utilization of HCSs by providing, improving and addressing healthcare services in a nation. The widespread use of telemedicine services will extend the use of healthcare professionals and specialists offering timely healthcare delivery without any obstacles and reducing operation and transportation costs to both urban and rural areas. Telemedicine helps to address the possible future shortages of healthcare professionals by enabling remote consultations by physicians and nurses for patients located in remote areas (Deitenbeck, 2011). Ultimately, telemedicine helps to improve the level of community and population health by electronic sharing of information between public health services.

It is therefore necessary for the nation's healthcare to integrate information and multimedia technologies for telemedicine implementation in order to encounter the overwhelming demand of standard quality of HCS. However, the number of HCSs that have implemented telemedicine is still limited and even fails to attract and satisfy all users with the services offered. Despite of growing demand for the standard quality of HCSs, there are still many HCSs challenged with constraint resources and capabilities and operating at high cost. What HCSs or telemedicine industry call for are strategies and solutions for telemedicine that will enhance their growth by assessing the cause for high acceptance rate in telemedicine from users' worldview and developing the co-creation of telemedicine value.

Impact of Technology, Telemedicine, and Human Nature

Telemedicine is an innovation tool to enhance efficiency in delivery of healthcare service that leads to green economy and environmental improvement. It is a significant mechanism of modern economy, facilitating the provision of healthcare and health related services by using telecommunications, information and multimedia technologies to link to the public in the healthcare system. Indeed the need for telemedicine may increase due to shortage of healthcare professionals, lack of specialists and health facilities, greater incidence of chronic conditions, need for efficient care of the elderly, home-bound and physically challenged patients and rising healthcare cost. Furthermore the emerging improvements in medical care may enhance the life expectancy and patients' self-management capacity which in turn increase the demand for innovation healthcare services from providers. The advance of Health IT increases the frequency and usage of technology driven for remote monitoring and consulting to treat patients. The availability of innovative medical products and/or services can enhance the application of telemedicine.

Telemedicine highly depends on online communication using the latest information and communications technologies (ICT) such as by using health IT applications such as electronic health records, administrative billing applications and store and forward image transfer software. Such technology resources involve design, development, implementation and maintenance of an array of information system used in the healthcare industry. Advancements in these health IT systems help to reduce medical costs, improve efficiency and provide better patient cares and services.

In short, telemedicine has made distance HCS and lifelong care possible, practical and profitable. However, the extent of an individual's belief and confidence of the ability of the system and its benefits for them will determine the effect on their acceptance to use telemedicine. Hence, it is crucial for HCSs to assess users' acceptance and willingness to use such ICT particularly in adopting telemedicine practices.

The main objective of this chapter is to explore whether telemedicine can be implemented as practice. It is also crucial to explore the dominant factors of telemedicine acceptance. Hence, the extent to which individuals perceive, understand and think about the new practice (telemedicine) will determine telemedicine adoption or rejection.

How Is Telemedicine Viewed?

Human nature is always new; it is a norm. People always wish a simple and an easy life for them to perform and accept a practice. Some may be innovative and willing to adopt telemedicine but some may ignore or resist changing due to a norm of human aspects. Telemedicine is regarded as a new practice or an innovation of healthcare which requires a diverse process of human participation, perception and thought before an individual can accept or reject telemedicine. People's willingness to accept or reject telemedicine depends upon many aspects of human nature such as thinking (knowledge), feeling, soul, attitude (behavior) and other influential environmental factors such as society, rules and regulation, education and experience. To know about telemedicine is to understand about self. Once self is known, then self-understanding towards telemedicine is increased. Once telemedicine is understood, self will be disregarded and self-service technology will be appreciated.

In logic, the human nature law should be considered as a crucial variable for initiating a theory or hypothesis. In any scenario, we would usually practice what we know will benefit us. When life is difficult or uneasy, we would have the tendency to dislike a practice, ignore it or sometimes give it up. Typically we can enhance or move further if we already have the fundamental of practice, value or belief. We also believe that performing work without knowledge is worse than performing work without practice and experience. Further, we normally accept something when we know their rewards or benefits or we believe and accept/ are satisfied with the given thing after knowing the results from someone who has already seen or received it. On the whole, people can easily stimulate a person's behavior because of self-tendency of belonging or truth even though it may not necessarily be good or bad. However, there are still those who would not practice or accept something with or without hesitation, insecurity, vagueness and uncertainty.

A user's worldview towards telemedicine is definitely associated with this human nature law. Normally, the user's worldview has been constructed based on the extent of his/her confidence level based on knowledge, observation and proven true of certainty in telemedicine. The following gives three different stages of confidence level of telemedicine acceptance and further explains elements driving the acceptance of telemedicine or innovation.

1. **Knowledge of Certainty:** It is limited when an individual knows telemedicine through knowledge only which is based on knowledge and information from others or society. There are many ways in which an individual may be constructed by society including social power and technology concern.
   a. **Social Power:** The extent to which an individual is constructed by society to accept telemedicine. Telemedicine that is adapted as a normal life by society tends to increase an individual's willingness to adopt telemedicine. The strong society power in influencing the compliance behavior of an individual will determine the telemedicine acceptance.
   b. **Technology Concern:** The extent to the feeling of secure and comfort while users practice telemedicine. An individual may know from others that telemedicine is good but those who have experienced trauma, phobia or hardship of using telemedicine tend to resist their willingness to adopt telemedicine. An individual's uneasiness, apprehension or anxiety about the use of telemedicine may lead to the rejection of telemedicine.

2. **Observation of Certainty:** This is when an individual is able to see telemedicine with certainty. An individual, will be confident with telemedicine if he/she can see the benefits of telemedicine with his/her own eyes. Individuals who could see the benefits of telemedicine will be more confident than those who know telemedicine based on knowledge or theory only. For instance:

   a. **Benefit:** The extent to which telemedicine is perceived as benefits, better than the previous or typical healthcare. Telemedicine that has an unambiguous advantage over the previous approach will be more easily adopted and implemented. If telemedicine is awarding benefits, the user will be more likely to adopt it.

   b. **Simplicity:** The extent to which telemedicine is perceived as easy, effortless to understand and smooth to use. Telemedicine that is user friendly, straightforward and easy to use will not easily be resisted. If telemedicine is not difficult to use, the user will be more likely to adopt it.

3. **Proven True of Certainty:** This is acknowledged when an individual has been encountering telemedicine. An individual who has gone through telemedicine by himself /herself as a patient, monitors his/her own health every day without commuting to the hospital tends to have a high confident level on the telemedicine. For instance:

   a. **Consequence:** The extent to which the outcomes of telemedicine are visible by users. The easier it is for users to see the outcomes, results, benefits or impact of telemedicine, the more likely they intend to adopt the telemedicine.

   b. **Satisfaction:** The extent to which telemedicine can suit and match with user present values, past and concrete experiences and needs of potential adopters and can be assimilated into an individual's life. If telemedicine is able to satisfy the user's desires, the user will be more likely to adopt it.

   c. **Trial:** The extent to which telemedicine can be simulated, be piloted or be experimented. Those who have received and trained in telemedicine simulation will approach telemedicine easily. If telemedicine is given a chance or trial before acceptance, the user will be more adaptive to telemedicine.

Telemedicine can be viewed in terms of four main constructs: (1) innovation - the perception of innovation has a great influence on telemedicine; (2) knowledge - the tacit and explicit understanding will construct decision; (3) period - time has a great influence on decision from the first encounter until formed decision; and (4) social value - the value of telemedicine is socially constructed. Telemedicine can be viewed through mind process of decision making. The state of the human mind during decision making process involves four cycle or stages: starting from (1) knowledge - evaluate and learn about telemedicine; (2) formation - develop the perception towards telemedicine; (3) action - decide whether to accept or reject telemedicine; (4) implementation - execute and confirm the decision on telemedicine.

TELEMEDICINE PRACTICES

Telemedicine service acceptance has been acknowledged to be slow in real healthcare setting (Rho et al., 2014). Little is known about the predictive factors influencing physicians' willingness (Rho et al., 2014; Dunnebeil et al., 2012;) and patients' willingness (Maarop and Than, 2012) to use telemedicine. Therefore it is essential to explore the significant factors in various healthcare providers and patients' intention to use telemedicine services. As various telemedicine services are in their early stage, the findings of most studies may not be generalizable to other countries and contexts. However general factors of opinions, attitudes and knowledge such as standardization, IT utilization, information security, process orientation, documentation (e.g. accessibility of medical records), the telemedicine or e-health related knowledge and individual factors (e.g. self-efficacy) could be applied as significant drivers for accepting telemedicine practices. As telemedicine is regarded with innovation, the theory of innovation diffusion and technology of acceptance model have been applied in most studies (Jung and Loria, 2010).

The telemedicine project is a new medical technology in Malaysia; hence it takes a lot more work to change the paradigm and requires careful assessment of the real value of time and understanding of the users, health professionals and patients. Malaysian health professionals and patients do have a positive attitudes towards the use of the telemedicine concept and found it to be useful (Ibrahim et al., 2010; Maarop and Than, 2012). Most of health professionals indicated that computers are important for the profession such as in areas of medicine and health care and they have a high inclination towards using computers and IT machines (Ibrahim et al., 2010). Meanwhile, German physicians in ambulatory care show that the perceived importance of standardization and IT utilization are the most significant drivers for accepting electronic health services in their practices (Dunnebeil et al., 2012). Korean physicians in medical centers and hospitals show that the accessibility of medical records and of patients directly have a positive impact on the perceived usefulness (PU) of telemedicine. Also, self-efficacy has a positive impact on both the perceived ease of (PEU and PU) telemedicine, and perceived incentives are important for their intention to use telemedicine practices (Rho et al., 2014). The PU of telemedicine is believed to have a positive impact on behavioral intention to use telemedicine practices, and the PEU of telemedicine is believed to have a positive impact on both the PU and the behavioral intention.

Opinions from public users are necessary to take into consideration in exploring telemedicine acceptance (Hashim, 2003; Maarop and Than, 2012). There is an abundance of verifications of the telemedicine implementation in practice from the users' perspective in Malaysia. The interview findings from the public users revealed that most of them were working; either male or female; married or single; age above 21 years old with at least a high school education. They agreed that telemedicine can be implemented in practice and perceived that benefit, simplicity, satisfaction, trial, consequence, technology concern and social power are explanatory factors of telemedicine acceptance. The following are factors driving the acceptance and/or need for telemedicine from the public users.

- **Benefit:** Users accepted telemedicine because it is more useful than the existing healthcare delivery because it helps them to get access to the hospital or doctors at any time and place as they require, and it takes better care of their health. They perceived that telemedicine allows them to require a nurse or doctor and family members less often to look after them if they are suffering from a long term medical condition that requires regular checkup. Telemedicine allows doctors to remotely diagnose, monitor and recommend treatment for patients located in remote areas. Lack of accessibility to health care professionals could be an obstacle to the benefits of telemedicine. For example, some users gain benefits from telemedicine, but due to limited resources and capabilities (nurses and expert doctors) other users have experienced disadvantages.
- **Simplicity:** Users accepted telemedicine because it would be easy for them to seek medical advice and interact with their doctors or nurses at their convenient time and place. They also perceived that telemedicine facilitates them to monitor their condition. For example, patients with a chronic heart disease are monitored and observed by distance. Lack of user friendliness to use telemedicine could be an obstacle for users to accept telemedicine. For example, difficulty to communicate interfaces with an expert doctor to discuss their problem via telemedicine may lead patients to

perceive higher complexity to use telemedicine. Users tend to have negative experience due to difficulty to understand and use the system of telemedicine.

- **Satisfaction:** Users accepted telemedicine because it can satisfy, please, match or suit with their current life style and/or regular background. In particular, telemedicine is consistent with how they want to continue to seek for healthcare. For example, patients perceived that telemedicine allows them to monitor their healthcare consistently without disturbing their busy activities, thus greatly enhancing their willingness to use telemedicine. In addition, telemedicine can limit patients' exposure to infections by eliminating or limiting the need to visit a physician's office for healthcare services. If telemedicine demands a lot more time for medical advice and consultation than normal healthcare, then users will ignore telemedicine services. The compatibility of innovative medical products and/or services of existing products and/or services can enhance the application of telemedicine.

- **Trial:** Users accepted telemedicine because they have used and knowledge in using technology to seek and keep contact with their nurses and doctors. They also perceived that telemedicine is easy and useful after trial telemedicine projects coupled with training and education of ICT. For example, users who are given a trial to stimulate the reality for a certain period of time will be more experienced and adaptive to telemedicine. Lack of knowledge and experience about operating telemedicine could be an obstacle for users to accept it.

- **Consequence:** Users accepted telemedicine because they can have more free time, independent and increase self-health management. They perceived that telemedicine has positive impact on patients such as saving in commuting time to hospital and cost and enhancing the level of convenience. Lack of flexibility and benefits of telemedicine as compared to typical healthcare could be an obstacle for users to adopt telemedicine. For example, patients with chronic condition can have frequent information of their basic personal information such as glucose level, pulse rate and heart rate remotely which in turn can lead to improved health for many patients. In addition, the patients are able to manage their health after getting advice from doctors and at the same time have more time to handle their family and work.

- **Technology Concern:** Users accepted telemedicine because they are comfortable using technology to communicate and share thoughts and feelings with nurses and doctors. They also feel secure when using telemedicine. The patients are not afraid to use technology and are happy with self-service technology to connect to their personal doctor. For example, patients' innovativeness enhances their willingness to practice telemedicine. A high level of apprehension would reduce the user's perceived value on telemedicine and reduces the potential of telemedicine adoption.

- **Social Power:** Users accepted telemedicine because people who are important to them have positive feeling and encourage them to use telemedicine. Furthermore their society has also influenced and encouraged them to use it. User behavior is constructed by society. For example, the interest of society, social forces and peer group perform a significant role on a user's adoption of telemedicine. Users might even comply with certain behaviors that they did not necessarily agree with as long as it is well received by their peer group.

The above verifications show that users have the intention for accepting telemedicine together with their willingness to adopt telemedicine mainly in the emerging advances in technology. Based on these main elements of innovation (benefit, simplicity, satisfaction, trial, consequence, technology concern and social power) this chapter initiates a theory and hypothesis that may be used as explanatory factors of willingness to adopt telemedicine. However, we are still yet to uncover which elements and how these elements can lead to the best outcomes. Hence, this chapter offers some thoughts, views and arguments for enhancing telemedicine acceptance. Perhaps some HCSs have failed to attract users due to lack of the above aspects. Thus, telemedicine that are provided by HSCs did not facilitate willingness for individuals to adopt it.

Although this chapter discovers crucial elements of willingness to adopt telemedicine, there are indications suggesting that most users are struggling to accept these elements. The users stated that they found it very hard to accept telemedicine since it requires investment of time and funds to learn to accept and adopt it. There is also evidence signifying that most users of telemedicine were under stress during learning and understanding telemedicine which sometimes made it difficult for them to understand and apply telemedicine.

RECOMMENDATIONS

The chapter provides practical strategies for implementing telemedicine. HCSs compete by offering diverse services and improving value-added services to their patients. By implementing telemedicine, HSCs may achieve good profit growth since it is highly demanding and challenging for users' healthcare. This chapter ascertains that telemedicine can be implemented in practice and further verifies that benefit, simplicity, satisfaction, trial, consequence, technology concern and social power are crucial elements of telemedicine acceptance. Consequently, HCSs should enhance their strategies towards such acceptance elements for telemedicine. Furthermore, HCSs need to provide a wide variety of resources and capabilities so that they may continue to expand and develop.

CONCLUSION

The chapter claims novelty in the attempt to consolidate and formalize the knowledge of telemedicine to date, so that opportunities can be widely accessed by a large number of health care services. Further, the chapter lays an important foundation in the field of telemedicine. However, it might leave the reader with the impression that it is still work in progress, which could be partially attributed to the novelty of the field.

Overall, this chapter discusses what telemedicine is, why it is important and its impact on HCSs is. Since telemedicine is a new practice, HCSs should focus more on the process of users' understanding, perception and thinking towards telemedicine. The evidence gathered indicate that there are associations between elements of telemedicine acceptance and willingness to adopt telemedicine. Users perceived that telemedicine is awarding benefits, satisfaction, and consequences to patients. If they are given ample time, awareness, knowledge, training and education about telemedicine, then most would be willing to accept telemedicine concept and practice. Some accept telemedicine due to their social interest or peer group and other external forces such as government and regulation, patient chronic illness and time factors.

REFERENCES

Deitenbeck, B. A. (2011). *Technology infrastructures for healthcare access to rural residents*. (Master dissertation). Avaiable from ProQuest Dissertations and Theses database. (UMI No. 864276924).

Dunnebeil, S., Sunyaev, A., Blohm, I., Leimeister, J. M., & Krcmar, H. (2012). Determinants of physicians technology accceptace for e-health in ambulatory care. *International Journal of Medical Informatics*, *81*(11), 746–760. doi:10.1016/j.ijmedinf.2012.02.002 PMID:22397989

Dyk, L. V. (2014). A review of telehealth service implementation framework. *International Journal of Environmental Research and Public Health*, *11*(2), 1279–1298. doi:10.3390/ijerph110201279 PMID:24464237

Eikelboom, R. H., & Atlas, M. D. (2005, December 1). Attitude to telemdicine and willingness to use it in audiology patients. *Telemed Telecare*, *11*(2), 22–25. doi:10.1258/135763305775124920

Hashim, A. (2003). Overview Of Malaysia's integrated telehealth project. *International Medical Journal*, *12*, 1–14.

Hein, M. A. (2009). *Telemedicine: An Important Force in the Transformation of Healthcare*. International Trade Specialist, US Department of Commerce, International Trade Administration, Manufacturing and Services, Office of health and Consumer Goods. Retrieved from http://ita.doc.gov/td/health/telemedicine_2009.pdf

Huang, J. C. (2013). Innovative health care delivery system—a questionnaire survey to evaluate the influence of behavioral factors on individuals' acceptance of telecare. *Computers in Biology and Medicine*, *43*(4), 281–286. doi:10.1016/j.compbiomed.2012.12.011 PMID:23375377

Ibrahim, M. I. M., Phing, C. W., & Palaian, S. (2010). Evaluation of knowledge and perception of Malaysian health professionals about telemedicine. *Journal of Clinical and Diagnostic Research*, *4*, 2052–2057.

Jung, M. L., & Loria, K. (2010). Acceptance of Swedish e-health services. *Journal of Multidisciplinary Healthcare*, *3*, 55–63. PMID:21289860

Klein, R. (2007). Internet-based patient-physician electronic communication applications: Patient acceptance and trust. *e-Service Journal*, *5*(2), 27–51. doi:10.2979/ESJ.2007.5.2.27

Kowitlawakul, Y. (2008). *Technology acceptance model: predicting nurses' acceptance of telemedicine technology (eICU)* (Doctoral of dissertation). Available from Mason Electronic Theses and Dissertations. (http://hdl.handle.net/1920/3058)

Lankton, N. K., & Wilson, E. V. (2007). Factors influencing expectations of e-health services within a direct-effects model of user satisfaction. *e-Service Journal*, *5*(2), 85–111. doi:10.2979/ESJ.2007.5.2.85

Liu, J. J. (2009). *Pervasive telemonitoring for patients living with chronic heart failure: A quantitative study of telemedicine acceptance* (Doctoral dissertation). Available from ProQuest Dissertations and Theses database. (UMI No. 305166705).

Maarop, N., & Than Win, K. (2012). The interplay of environmental factors in the acceptance of teleconsultation technology: A mixed methods study. *Open International Journal of Informatics*, *1*, 46–58.

Maarop, N., Win, K. T., Masrom, M., & Hazara-Singh, S. (2011). Exploring factors that affect teleconsultation adoption: in the case of Malaysia. *PACIS 2011: 15th Pacific Asia Conference on Information Systems: Quality Research in Pacific* (pp. 1-12). Queensland: Queensland University of Technology.

Ministry of Health. (1997). *Malaysia Telemedicine Blueprint*. Author.

Peeters, J. M., de Veer, A. J., van der Hoek, L., & Francke, A. L. (2012). Factors influencing the adoption of home-telecare by elderly or chronically ill people: A national survey. *Journal of Clinical Nursing, 21*(21-22), 3183–3193. doi:10.1111/j.1365-2702.2012.04173.x PMID:22827253

Piette, J.D., Mendoza Avelares, M.O., Miltan, E.C., Lange, I., & Fajardo, R. (2010). Article. *Telemedicine and e-health Journal, 16*(10), 1030-1041.

Rho, M. J., Choi, I. Y., & Lee, J. (2014). Predictive factors of telemedicine service acceptance and bahviroal intention of physicians. *International Journal of Medical Informatics, 83*(8), 559–571. doi:10.1016/j.ijmedinf.2014.05.005 PMID:24961820

Templeton, J. R. (2010). *Trust and trustworthiness: A framework for successful design of telemedicine* (Doctoral dissertation). Avaiable from ProQuest Dissertations and Theses database. (UMI No. 755017524).

Werner, P., & Karnieli, E. (2003). A model of the willingness to use telemedicine for routine and specialized care. *Journal of Telemedicine and Telecare, 9*(5), 264–272. doi:10.1258/135763303769211274 PMID:14599329

Opportunities and Challenges for Electronic Health Record:
Concepts, Costs, Benefits, and Regulation

Marc Jacquinet
Universidade Aberta, Portugal

Henrique Curado
Escola Superior de Tecnologia da Saúde do Porto, Instituto Politécnico do Porto, Portugal

INTRODUCTION

The emergence of electronic health record (EHR) in recent decades and its deepening and broadening has triggered either heated debates or highly technical discussions, and all this, not only but significantly, across the academic literatures of medicine, public health, governance, management, public policy, law and legal studies. Those issues present both opportunities and challenges. The process is gaining momentum, still limited to OECD countries however, but spreading fast, and its future shape will depend on the changes under way and the interaction of different users, actors, institutions, public policies, legislations and networks as much as the globalization and diffusion processes under way. The present chapter aims at giving a description of the recent evolution, the main characteristics and the challenges ahead. The history is recent, still debated, and most studies focus on recent trends, namely the last decade, and evidence is still lacking on many issues (Black et al., 2011; Greenhalgh, Hinder, Stramer, Bratan, & Russell, 2010; Greenhalgh, Potts, Wong, Bark, & Swinglehurst, 2009; Olson et al., 2014; Sidorov, 2006).

The literature on e-health –and more specifically on electronic health record–, in a period of little more than a decade, is now vast and the present discussion is limited to selected themes such as legal issues, governance, privacy, public interest, cost and benefits and prospects. The Electronic Health Record (EHR) is one of the most controversial elements of the concept of ehealth and its role in current reforms. It is at the centre of the transformation of professional and organizational structure of health care system under way in the last decade and for the proximate future.

The aim of this entry is to define some concepts about electronic health record and clarify their context in today's literature and giving an overview of the recent debates and dimension in recent history as well as its promises, processes and achievements.

CONCEPTS AND BACKGROUND

In this section, after a brief history, the issue of definition and several dimensions of electronic health records will be tackled. If the first known medical records can be traced to Hippocrates and the goals he attributed to these records were to describe accurately the course of a disease and gives a probable cause of it; the electronic dimension of these records can be traced back to the 1960s in some hospitals

DOI: 10.4018/978-1-4666-9978-6.ch075

that started a more systematic recording and use of patients' data by services and doctors. But it is still more recently, in the 1990s, with the ever wider use of internet and online databases that the electronic health record emerged as a new tool in the public health systems of OECD countries.

There are different definitions of electronic health record, depending on the theoretical perspective or even the main user or the political point of departure taken in the implementation process. Even so, here and in the literature on the subject, the electronic health record has become and is the generic term. Other focuses like electronic medical record (or registry) and the electronic patient record are based on either the perspective of the user or the subject of the information. All these expressions are part of the general move from traditional management of health and medicine to electronic health and medicine or e-health (written more and more frequently ehealth as its use spreads across countries and within national health and health care systems).

To settle the record straight, the definition of the Electronic Health Record that can serve as a consensus for the current exposition as well as a starting point for further research is the one given by the International Standards Organization (document ISO/TR 20514:2005) as a "repository of information regarding the health status of a subject of care, in computer processable form" (ISO 2005, p.2).

Electronic health record has become a formal tool or formal system (Berg, 1997) to get rid of the papers and dispersed information and to concentrate the information in one or very few places and to create the "paperless ward", in much the same hope and biased perception as the paperless office. This formal tool is not just limited to move toward a paperless ward or more globally a paperless world. It is also a tool for control, governance, and, following Foucault, surveillance, and also, a path to governmentality (Foucault, 2010) or, in other words, regulation. Governmentality can be defined as a "particular rationality for governing the population which has become ubiquitous in modern societies" (Villadsen, 2011, p. 125).This is a bridge for setting the stage of the problem of power and electronic record of health data of individuals and citizens.

This challenge of governance and governmentality is related to the issues of regulation and the transformations of the role of the state, of values in society, and of the legal, economic and social norms. The governance is related to the issue of promoting benefits, controlling or reducing costs as discussed in the next paragraph. There are other issues that must be tackled such as the imposed or negotiated order, the role of networks and social online networks, the risk and uncertainty around EHR and its use, its relationship with medical technology and innovation, surveillance and management and managerialism in health care systems.

The hopes and intentions about the EHR are well described in an editorial of the Bulletin of the World Health Organization by Richard Alvarez, President and Chief Executive Officer, Canada Health Infoway: "Information technology, which has empowered most parts of our daily lives, is woefully absent from health care. Clearly the application of e-health technologies will pay huge dividends in improving the quality of health care for all" (Alvarez 2005, 323). This situation about a decade ago has drastically changed in the OECD countries and it will change for the other countries in the years to come. The question that the next section tackles is exactly the benefits and costs of the introduction of information technology for the use and control of health information and the digitalization of whole areas of the administrative management of health care interventions.

The research on the subject of electronic health record is still lacking clear cut conclusions. However, it is important to have more evidence-based reports and studies on the subject and to follow a more systematic research on the subject, for example through general reviews and meta-analyses. Following Black, Car, Pagliari and co-authors (2011, 1), a distinction of eHealth technologies as well as electronic health record can be made and the following categories can help identify the main areas of change: first, the storing, managing and transmission of data, second, the clinical decision support (which is what the electronic medical registry is all about), and third, the "facilitating care from distance" (Black et al., 2011). The evidence so far suggests that "the success of those relatively few solutions identified to improve quality and safety [...] has yet to be established" (Black et al., 2011, 1).

COSTS, BENEFITS, AND REGULATION

After a brief conceptual discussion and a general setting it is important to focus on the main challenges of the electronic health record that go much beyond the information and big data debates currently under way in systems of information and data management. The themes retained are, on the one hand, costs and benefits, often associated to the early hopes in the sector of public health, and, on the other hand, the regulatory issue of its legal and social aspects. After all, management is a social endeavour (Witzel 2012, 4).

Between the costs and benefits associated with the implementation of electronic health record (EHR) lies the necessary balance between privacy and public interest, even if it refers mainly to an individual interest, i.e., an anonymous citizen. Among the different benefits, the celerity of access to the personal information of a patient allows a faster decision process as well as minor costs of access to the relevant information. Those two aspects are particularly significant in situations of emergency and absence or lack of consciousness of the patient given that very electronic health record allows to characterize the health state and history of the citizen, adapted to the specificity of the health care in every moment of her or his life-cycle (ACSS, 2010, p. 9-10). Several studies argue that expected costs reductions are lower than actually realized. There is a gap between the political and technical discourses based on mere opinions and expectations and evidenced based programs (Black et al., 2011; Blumenthal & Tavenner, 2010; Greenhalgh et al., 2009; Sidorov, 2006). After all, this literature suggests that benefits, in global terms, are lower than expected.

On the other hand, there is a collective benefit emerging from the electronic health record that traduces itself in the empowering of the mission and actions within the ambit of public health (ACSS, 2009, p 1) like the monitorization of the health state of the population, the research activity, the vigilance and control, and the epidemiological studies, among others. The possibility of sharing information for the purpose of research advancement is often underscored. This research activity is particularly relevant not only at the level of the treatment of diseases but also at the level of the technological and pharmacological development. It is important to note that health, beyond obvious aspects of individual nature, constitutes a public good. This requires the intervention of the State not only in the provision of healthcare but also in the coordination of the different systems, guaranteeing not just the universality and generality of the provision of the health care but also that the benefits of learning in the treatment and care given at the individual level that translates into a common good.

The reverse of this situation is the inherent costs associated to the loss of privacy, construed as a public good in itself or through the effects associated to it such as the possibility of undue access from third parties that pretend to retain a benefit from that very information. Access to data of health situation and history of individuals is a clear illustration of that problem in the case of insurance companies or employers trying to get relevant information about the health situation of clients or employees. This access can have implications for the negotiation or not of contracts and for prohibiting the access to specified places. The dangers of the intrusion in the private lives of people can be amplified by the EHR given that the process occurs without the use of microphones or cameras and allows little tractability of the retrieval of available pieces of information from that same repository or record (Doneda, 2000).

Recent changes that appear at that level translate in different countries through the implementation of electronic health records, looking to foresee different aspects highlighted as conflicting and presupposes a redefinition of the legal framework. This definition of the legal aspects has to guarantee the equivalence between the health record on physical support and those in digital format (material or physical processes and dematerialized processes). It has also to promote the clarification of the necessity of medical mediation in the access for the citizen to their health data and contributes to build a normative distinction in the access by the providers of health care in the context of ambulatory situations in cases of emergency and the internment in health units (ACSS, 2009, p. 32-33). Other relevant questions of practical nature are related to the necessity of consent of the citizen on a piecemeal basis limited to the access in ambulatory situations or by third parties as well as to the possibility of informed consent being provided on electronic or digital support.

Obviously, the challenges in terms of privacy presuppose a response not just a normative component but a technical one, enabling the security of the information not only through anti-abuse norms and predictability of the duty of secret, but also technical guarantees of the security of the information. At this level the possibilities are diverse, as highlighted by the Portuguese Central Administration for health or Administação Central do Sistema de Saúde (ACSS, 2010).

Accordingly, in the definition of equilibrium between privacy and public interest, if the notion of freedom imposes the maximum level of protection of the personality, some restriction has to be made to privacy determined by the necessity of treatment of personal data in order to guarantee that the health that each one claims for herself or himself as a value to preserve and to protect by the society be shared, therefore constituting a public good. The singularity of the individual does not prevent from presupposing a casuistic evaluation of the weighting of interests, responding to the necessity of its weighting with regard to social and moral values existing in any given epoch (Greco & Braga, 2012, p. 153-163).

In this sense, the guarantee of privacy exists associated to the security of information, at the legal and technical levels and not only for not sharing health data relevant to the common good. Acensão has made a good argument (1995) when, in relation to the exclusive tutelage of privacy, he refers that the "right of personhood" is being transformed into rights of private egoisms. This goes against what should be its fundamental basis, considering the person. The person is acquaintanceship or sociability and society. No consideration of intimacy can be stronger than this essential aspect of the personality.

The conception of the electronic health record, beyond normative questions, presupposes the construction of a model whose efficiency must underlie not only the prosecution of the public interest but also the maintenance of the most genuine private interest and protecting privacy, always on the basis that the patient is the titular of the right to information (ERS, 2009). In so far as its gathering and treatment depend on informed, free and enlightened decision, it consists also in the right to informational privacy that is simultaneously a right of guarantee to the reserve preservation of private life and a fundamental right that is translated into the faculty of the individual to determine and control the use of her or his personal data (Moniz, 2002, p 246). In this domain, it matters to take the option of hosting information on a single server or alternative if based on various interconnected servers related between them through the delimitation of different types of access.

The definition of the model of information has to consider, beyond the definition of the data to include in the record, the distinctions of the different types of access, for the health care provider, for the data shared by different users as well the data that are not specifically about the health of the patients or the users the health care system but about common and generic information for all individuals such as the name, address and civil identity data. The definition of different levels of responsibility and risk in face of the access to available information and of the responsibility in its use is related to the structure of the model of information that goes beyond the organization of the data of the EHR.

The mentioned conception and delimitation of an efficient system presuppose that the legal be determinant not just of the system of guarantee of privacy in legal terms – criminal and civil – but also of the approbation of a model managing sensitive data, i.e., in the definition of the software application and technological architecture.

Finally, the EHR is also related to the problem of risk, governance and regulation. Hopes and investment are dedicated to the use of electronic health registries to tackle issues of epidemics and the control of diseases. These hopes are related to the reduction of costs, the supply of new services, the answering of professional and patients' needs, the improvement in the quality of health care services and the providing of better access to information about patients and the control of epidemics. The regulation issues are divided into two realms, as described above, on the one hand the protection of privacy and, on the other hand, the promotion of the public interest, i.e. the collect of information of diseases, such as Ebola and other ones, that can threaten in several countries the status quo of public health to the point of provoking local or regional collapse of health care systems.

CONCLUSION

The electronic health record is part of the general transformation of the health care system and the emergence of the concept of electronic health or ehealth.

Having some notions of the limitations of the progress reached so far, it is important to keep in mind the current situation and what are the changes and trends observed. First, there is a clear increase in investment and implementation of electronic health record systems, not just in the OECD countries, but also beyond. Second, there is an integration, under the overall umbrella of ehealth, of different processes, like use of information technologies (e.g., the use of SMS for information of Ebola and prevention of the disease in countries such as Senegal) and the electronic health record. This integration is synonymous of deepening of the use and application of this formal tool. Third, the EHR is also activated in control policies and situations of emergency, such as the Ebola outbreak in West Africa and across countries affected by its spread through travelling. Fourth, there are a lot of applications of EHR that are not documented in many countries, not to say of methodologically sound research reports. Five, mixed results will continue given the different interest and the policy changes under way. This is especially true about legal and regulatory challenges and narrow technological solutions.

REFERENCES

ACSS - Administação Central do Sistema de Saúde - ACSS. (2009). *A. C. do S. de S.* Lisboa: RSE – Registo de Saúde Electrónico - Orientações para Especificação Funcional e Técnica do Sistema de RSE.

ACSS - Administação Central do Sistema de Saúde - ACSS. (2010). *A. C. do S. de S.* Lisboa: RSE – Registo de Saúde Electrónico - Plano de Operacionalização.

Ascensão, J. O. (1995). Teoria Geral do Direito Civil. Lisboa: Faculdade de Direito.

Berg, M. (1997). Of Forms, Containers, and the Electronic Medical Record: Some Tools for a Sociology of the Formal. *Science, Technology & Human Values, 22*(4), 403–433. doi:10.1177/016224399702200401

Black, A. D., Car, J., Pagliari, C., Anandan, C., Cresswell, K., Bokun, T., & Sheikh, A. et al. (2011). The impact of eHealth on the quality and safety of health care: A systematic overview. *PLoS Medicine*, *8*(1), e1000387. doi:10.1371/journal.pmed.1000387 PMID:21267058

Blumenthal, D., & Tavenner, M. (2010). The "Meaningful Use" Regulation for Electronic Health Records. *The New England Journal of Medicine*, *363*(6), 501–504. doi:10.1056/NEJMp1006114 PMID:20647183

Doneda, D. C. M. (2000). *Considerações iniciais sobre os bancos de dados informatizados e o direito à privacidade*. Academic Press.

Entidade Regulatora da Saúde - ERS. (2009). *E. R. da S*. Consentimento Informado.

Foucault, M. (2010). Birth of Biopolitics (Michel Foucault: Lectures at the College De France). *International Journal of Cultural Policy*, *16*, 368.

Greco, R., & Braga, R. R. P. (2012, January). Da principiologia penal ao direito à intimidade como garantia constitucional. *Direito E Desenvolvimento*.

Greenhalgh, T., Hinder, S., Stramer, K., Bratan, T., & Russell, J. (2010). Adoption, non-adoption, and abandonment of a personal electronic health record: Case study of HealthSpace. *BMJ (Clinical Research Ed.)*, *341*(nov16 1), c5814. doi:10.1136/bmj.c5814 PMID:21081595

Greenhalgh, T., Potts, H. W. W. W., Wong, G., Bark, P., & Swinglehurst, D. (2009). Tensions and Paradoxes in Electronic Patient Record Research: A Systematic Literature Review Using theMeta-narrative Method. *The Milbank Quarterly*, *87*(4), 729–788. doi:10.1111/j.1468-0009.2009.00578.x PMID:20021585

ISO. (2005). *Health Information and Management Systems Society. EHR: electronic health record*. International Standards Organization. Retrieved from http://www.himss.org/ASP/topics_ehr.asp

Moniz, H. (2002). *Os problemas jurídico-penais da criação de uma base de dados genéticos para fins criminais* (C. Editora, Ed.). Revista Portuguesa de Ciência Criminal.

Olson, J. E., Bielinski, S. J., Ryu, E., Winkler, E. M., Takahashi, P. Y., Pathak, J., & Cerhan, J. R. (2014). *Biobanks and personalized medicine. Clinical Genetics*. Blackwell Publishing Ltd.

Sidorov, J. (2006). It Ain't Necessarily So: The Electronic Health Record And The Unlikely Prospect Of Reducing Health Care Costs. *Health Affairs*, *25*(4), 1079–1085. doi:10.1377/hlthaff.25.4.1079 PMID:16835189

Villadsen, K. (2011). Governmentality. In *Key Concepts in Critical Management Studies*. London: Sage. doi:10.4135/9781446289013.n30

KEY TERMS AND DEFINITIONS

eHealth or E-Health: A concept comprising all applications used at the level of information technology, including the Internet, to enable more efficient patient care, thereby improving access and the quality of management of clinical processes. The Electronic Health Record is part of this set of tools.

Electronic Health Record (EHR and also Electronic Health Registry): See also electronic patient registry, medical electronic record. This is the creation of digital information, its storing, management, transmission, access, modification and use across a health care unit, several units or even a whole system of health care. In its basic generic form, the definition of EHR, according to the document ISO/TR 20514:2005 of the ISO – International Standards Organization, can be stated as followed: "repository of information regarding the health status of a subject of care, in computer processable form" (ISO 2005).

Governmentality: This concept is coming from Foucault as being a "particular rationality for governing the population which has become ubiquitous in modern societies" as defined by Villadsen (2011, 125).

Health: Health, according to the World Health Organization, is a state of complete physical, mental and social well-being and not merely the absence of disease or infirmity.

Health Information: This concept means all kinds of information (present or future) directly or indirectly linked to a person's health, or clinical and family history, whether that person is alive or deceased.

Patient Information: It is the same as *Health information.*

Privacy: Means a personnel right inherent to human dignity. Includes intimacy, private life and honor people. Consequently individuals have the right to informational self-determination, that is, individuals have the right to determine and control the use of your personal data.

Technical Definition of Electronic Health Record: "The Electronic Health Record (EHR) is a longitudinal electronic record of patient health information generated by one or more encounters in any care delivery setting. Included in this information are patient demographics, progress notes, problems, medications, vital signs, past medical history, immunizations, laboratory data and radiology reports. The EHR automates and streamlines the clinician's workflow. The EHR has the ability to generate a complete record of a clinical patient encounter—as well as supporting other care-related activities directly or indirectly via interface—including evidence-based decision support, quality management, and outcomes reporting" taken from the Health Information and Management Systems Society. EHR: electronic health record. http://www.himss.org/ASP/topics_ehr.asp. Accessed February 15, 2011.

Opportunities and Threats for E-Health on an Ageing Society

Ana Pinto Borges
ISAG - European Business School, Portugal & Lusíada University – North, Porto, Portugal

Claudia Cardoso
Polytechnic Institute of Cávado and Ave, Portugal

INTRODUCTION

E-health includes tools for health professionals and for patients (personalized health systems), enabling the promotion of patient's autonomy (raising the involvement of patients and responsibility for their own health). This autonomy, associated with a communication system capable of providing, timely, specific information to the patients, can be a possible way to reduce costs in the health sector.

This chapter is driven by the following evidence: the population is ageing (in 2013, life expectancy on average across OECD countries exceeded 80,5 years); information and communication technologies (ICTs) have an increasingly key role on health sector (for example, 60% of the countries, that respond to the 2009 Global Survey on e-health conducted by the World Health Organization (WHO), offered some form of teleradiology; and near 30% of those countries use some form of patient monitoring by mobile technology); the weight of health expenditures grew (despite the deceleration since 2009, the weight of health expenditure on GDP, on OECD countries, increased from 7,8%, in 2000, to 8,9% in 2013). We intend to correlate these three dimensions by demonstrating that e-health could help controlling the expenditures with the health of the elders and improve their quality of life. However, there are many obstacles for good results in the short term.

The use of ICTs in health can be organized into three axes: e-health; health information systems; and, media and communication in health. The growing computerization of clinical practice places important challenges to practitioners and health institutions, but it also presents significant opportunities. The objective of the use of the ICTs for health professionals is not to reduce human contact in the provision of care, but mainly to improve the medical procedure to create the conditions so that patients can have a better quality of life, staying independent and active. Also, the development of the Internet can be considered as an opportunity and, simultaneously, a challenge for health professionals. Patients have easy access to a large volume of health information. In addition, Internet allows the exchange of experiences and views between the patients. The great challenge for patients is to select and decode the information on the Internet.

The increase in the elderly population is forcing the healthcare market to offer senior-friendly products and services related to long-term care, health and wellbeing. ICTs and specifically e-health have notables' technological advances covering health services such as teleconsultation, telemonitoring, telecare, e-prescription and e-referral. These advances allow to support the ageing and ill population in maintaining independence and mobility for as long as possible. Despite the evolution of ICTs, the senior population is still info-excluded in many ways. This may inhibit them to fully extract its advantages, restricting the results of the use of e-health tools.

DOI: 10.4018/978-1-4666-9978-6.ch076

This chapter intends to demonstrate that despite the opportunities of usage of e-health on treatment and accompaniment of the senior patients, there are financial, educational and social constraints setting obstacles for e-health to be the solution for controlling health expenditure, in the short run.

IMPACT OF POPULATION AGEING ON HEALTH AND HEALTHCARE

The developed and emerging economies witnessed a significant improvement in overall health status across populations, which was reflected in improvement on living conditions, a reduction of certain risk factors (e.g., smoking rates) and progress in health care (OECD, 2013).

The reasons behind these improvements are not consensual among researchers. There are some authors who argue that the improvement verified in populations' health status was achieved due to technical developments in medicine. Others authors defend that such phenomenon were due to social advances verified in the living conditions of populations (McKeown and Lowe, 1974). However, marginal gains on population health eventually reached a threshold, paving the way for technological innovation, including ICTs, in healthcare, as the main catalyst for future development in the sector. In addition, little is known about what will be the consequences in terms of age structure or in terms of health status of the population or the best way to provide health care.

In reality the life expectancy on average across OECD countries exceeded 80 years, an increase of ten years since 1970. Switzerland, Japan and Spain lead a large group of over two-thirds of OECD countries in which life expectancy at birth now exceeds 80 years. A second group, including the United States, Chile and a number of central and eastern European countries, has a life expectancy between 75 and 80 years (OECD, 2015). In the case of the 28 EU countries, the overall size of the population is projected to be slightly larger by 2060 but much older than it is now. The EU population is projected to increase (from 507 million in 2013) up to 2050 by almost 5%, when it will peak (at 526 million) and will thereafter decline slowly (to 523 million in 2060). The life expectancy at birth for males is expected to increase by 7.1 years over the projection period, reaching 84.8 in 2060. For females, it is projected to increase by 6.0 years, reaching 89.1 in 2060 (European Commission, 2015).

Population ageing is a sign of economic and social progress however, in developed countries, can also be a sign of increase in healthcare spending (Reinhardt, 2003; Reinhardt and Oliver, 2015). Even though some studies confirm the positive and significant influence of ageing on healthcare spending (Jönsson and Eckerlund, 2003; Schulz *et al.*, 2004; Breyer and Felder, 2006, Breyer *et al.*, 2010; European Commission, 2015); there are others that estimate a residual or insignificant influence (Barros, 1998; Gerdtham and Jönsson, 2000; Stearns and Norton, 2004; Ginsburg, 2008; Kingsley, 2015); and others that reveal a mix effect, i.e., ageing increases spending on health until a certain age level and then its effect decreases (Bains, 2003).

However, the contribution of the ageing population to the growth in healthcare spending is much lower than is commonly perceived. Some studies defend that it is not age per se that enhances the increase in healthcare spending but it is the proximity of death (Moïse, 2003; Seshamani and Gray, 2004a),b); Serup-Hansen *et al.*, 2002; Stearns and Norton, 2004; Schulz *et al.*, 2004; Breyer and Felder, 2006; Arora, 2015).

Along with the increase in life expectancy, the rise in the complexity of medical procedures and the emergence of new chronic diseases created a pressure on health systems budgets, revealing the need to reduce health costs. Because of ageing, accompanied by chronic diseases and the change of family structures, we also observe the rise on long-term care (Knapp and Somani, 2009; Guerzoni and Zuleeg, 2011). In fact, the *European Commission 2009 Ageing Report* estimates that the number of people relying on informal care will increase by 84% between 2007 and 2060, while in the same period the number of people receiving formal care will grow by 151% (home care) and 185% (institutional care). On the *European Commission 2012 Ageing Report*, public expenditure on long-term care, for the EU27, is projected to increase by more than 80%. In percentage points, the projected increase amounts to 1.6 p.p. of GDP on average for the EU27, i.e. from 1.8% in 2010 to 3.4% in 2060.

Despite the possible predisposition of an ageing population to incur higher levels of healthcare spending, there are several others factors that play an even more important role in driving up healthcare spending. Empirical research suggests that health technology has been a major driver of expenditures and others factors, as income *per capita*, private insurance, physician induced demand, drug consumption, and "gatekeepers" also contribute for this phenomenon. Actually, the weight of health expenditures grew, despite the deceleration since 2009, the weight of health expenditure on GDP, on OECD countries, increased from 7,8%, in 2000, to 8,9% in 2013 (OECD, 2015).

In essence, ensuring the sustainability of health systems and the growing demand for healthcare with more quality at affordable prices are engrained necessities, eventually pressing governments to effectively and efficiently manage the health sector, not only in qualitative and safety terms but also at the level of resources utilized. The challenge of this moment is to demonstrate that e-health could help controlling the expenditures with the health of the elders and improve their quality of life.

THE ROLE OF E-HEALTH

The use of the ICTs, and specifically e-health, as a strategic tool in the promotion of safer and more adequate healthcare, enables the health professionals to spend more time with their patients and to adapt healthcare to individual needs using available resources more efficiently and effectively. ICTs have an increasingly key role on health sector. The *e-health Strategies* final report (Stroetmann *et al.*, 2011) revealed an important evolution, on European Union (EU), on the national level activities toward the implementation of e-health tools, between 2006 (data from the e-health European Research Area (ERA) study[1]) and 2010 (data from the *e-health Strategies* study).

The EHR (Electronic Health Record) Patient Summary was the only aspect that was already a concern on all the 27 countries, in 2006. In fact, the EHR is the base for the majority of e-health instruments. The EHR can be used to detect patterns and build a story towards a better understanding of the patient.

Table 1. National level activities in the EU27 countries

E-Health Activities	Countries That Reported Activities		Variation
	2006	**2010**	
Legal Activities	14	22	+57%
Evaluation	5	21	+320%
EHR Patient Summary	27	27	0%
ePrescription	16	26	+63%
Tele-health	23	27	+17%
Patient ID	24	26	+8%
Standards (Technical/semantic)	19	27	+42%

Adapted from Stroetmann et al. (2011).

It can also be used as an auxiliary memory of the doctor and as a way of data transmission in medicine. Therefore, ICTs are used to feed the EHR (using information provided by the patient, the health professionals or electronic devices, as, for example, a blood pressure meter) and also to channel the data to the right users.

Other instruments, like the electronic prescription (ePrescription), are much more efficient if used combined with the EHR. In fact, the main advantage of the ePrescription is to be complete and perfectly readable: it only uses accurate vocabulary and abbreviations; it may have alerts of incomplete forms, forcing the doctor to write all the prescription items; and it can incorporate information from medical leaflets or guidelines, alerting to abnormal situations. Additionally, when combined with the EHR, all the prescriptions are automatically recorded on the clinic story of the patient. A complete system of ePrescription would include three elements: the electronic prescription, itself, that could result on an electronic file or a paper prescription; the electronic transfer, if the prescription file is automatically transferred to a pharmacy; and the electronic dispensation, if from the dispensation on the pharmacy results an electronic file that is transferred again to the EHR of the patient. The majority of the European countries only had available the first part of the system (Stroetmann *et al.*, 2011).

Tele-health (or telemedicine) was also a well spread activity on the EU. This included the provision of health services at a distance (consultations, complementary exams or the monitoring of surgeries or other medical acts) but also the monitoring of patients at home. The 2009 Global Survey on e-health conducted by the WHO showed that 60% of the 114 respondent countries offered some form of tele-medicine; and near 30% of those countries use some form of patient monitoring by mobile technology (WHO, 2010 and 2011). Solving the issue of distance is important to guarantee equity on the provision of health services despite the location of the patient, but also to provide professional health services without taking away the patients from their homes.

We also assist to an improvement on institutional activities on EU countries, namely, improving legislation, evaluation, identification systems and standards. In fact, the novelty of many ICT tools on health and their challenges demand for institutional answers to guarantee confidentiality and integrity of data (Cheng and Huang, 2006), access to the services or interchangeability of data.

The growing computerization of clinical practice places important challenges to practitioners and health institutions, but it also presents significant opportunities. The objective of the use of the ICTs for health professionals is to create the conditions so that patients can have a better quality of life, staying independent and active. Also, the development of the Internet can be considered as an opportunity since patients have easy access to a large volume of health information.

However, two barriers may emerge here: i) the level of health literacy in the population, and ii) the use of new technologies. In terms of health literacy, nearly 9 out of 10 adults have difficulty using the everyday health information that is routinely available in health care facilities, retail outlets, media, and communities in the United States (Nielsen-Bohlman *et al.*, 2004; Kutner *et al.*, 2006; Rudd *et al.*, 2007). These results were not expected on countries with high levels of literacy. Also, we observe that typically older adults have low Internet literacy. For example, in the EU27 countries, in 2014, only 44% of the age group of 65 to 74 years used the computer in the last three months, contrasting with the percentage of 77% of total individuals (PORDATA, 2015). It is also observed that individuals who used the Internet on average at least once a week, as a percentage of total individuals by age group, from 2004 to 2014, increased by 40 percentage points in individuals between 55 and 64 years, and 22 percentage points in individuals between 65 to 74 years. Despite the growth, the latter age group displays only a percentage of 39% (PORDATA, 2015).

In this scenario, making use of online health information can be especially challenging for people lacking these skills, as frequently occurs with older adults (Xie, 2011; de Veer et al., 2015). However, Oh *et al.* (2005) defend that the increasing use of ICT in healthcare presents opportunities and challenges for improving health literacy. Thus, the two barriers are revealed simultaneously opportunities to improve information in the provision of health care.

European policymakers are investing heavily in e-health developments, but e-health implementation is not always successful (Hage *et al.*, 2013). E-health is known to have adoption problems not only within organizational settings (Boonstra and van Offenbeek, 2010), but also in context of e-health in rural communities (Hage *et al.*, 2013) or isolated communities (Scharwz *et al.*, 2014). This last issue is important because those communities may have greater need for e-health services, not only because the ageing process increases health care demand, but also because of local scarcity of alternative health services and personnel (Hage *et al.*, 2013).

E-HEALTH TOOLS FOR SENIOR PATIENTS

The increase in the elderly population is forcing the healthcare market to offer senior-friendly products and services related to long-term care, health and wellbeing. ICTs and specifically e-health have notables' technological advances covering health services such as teleconsultation, telemonitoring, telecare, e-prescription and e-referral. These advances allow to support the ageing and ill population in maintaining independence and mobility for as long as possible.

But what are the challenges for e-health tools for the elderlies? Despite the evolution of ICTs, the senior population is still info-excluded in many ways. This may inhibit them to fully extract its advantages, restricting the results of the use of e-health tools. The senior population also faces more language barriers. In addition, the elderlies are commonly reluctant to admit the lack of internet skills. All this constrains obliges e-health tools for the elderlies to be more user friendly than other instruments for other consumers. For example, Page (2014) showed that elderlies considered touchscreens to be easier to use than systems which are generally perceived as more 'simple' systems such as keypads on a mobile phone. When difficulties are insuperable for the elderly patient, the tools may be used by caregivers (which are expected to be younger and more likely to use these technologies) or by health professionals. A literature review showed that the focus of research is computer-based technology designed to be used by health professionals and not by elderlies themselves (Teixeira and Suomi, 2014). Since the complexity of technology and databases is many times unavoidable, another way to overcome the problem is to use programmable tools where the elderly have minimal intervention.

Brignell *et al.* (2007) reviewed the literature about the application of telemedicine to geriatric medicine. They found evidence that telemedicine can be applied effectively and safely in geriatric medicine, like consultation or triage for some health services, especially when the contact is between health professionals (for example, a home nurse and the hospital doctor). However, authors held that there is a lack of evaluation of telemedicine on the care of senior patients.

Physical limitations associated with ageing put also obstacles to the use of ICTs. Mainly, two types of limitations have been under analysis: limitations of hearing and vision.

The Senior Watch Study 2007 (European Commission, 2007), a survey conducted in EU and applied to citizens with 50 years and plus, reported that 44.9% of the inquired have interferences between the hearing aid systems and telephone handsets. Also, among the respondents who reported several visual restrictions, only 27.2% use visual assistive technology, such as programs that turn text into voice, special keyboards or printers for Braille output.

But physical limitations are not reduced to hearing and vision. ICTs use decreases significantly with greater limitations in physical capacity and greater disability. Memory limitations were associated with lower likelihood of technology use (Gell *et al.*, 2013). The Senior Watch Study 2007 also reported that one of the reasons for the elderly to stop using internet is severe hand impairment (22% of the ex-users of the internet).

All these factors reinforce the need to develop specific products for the elderly. The need to integrate the senior patients when developing new e-health products (and to attend to their needs and expectations) is important to improve the products itself and its acceptance. (Planinc and Kampel, 2013)

Senior patients will benefit from every e-health tools that are used for the population in general. However, the health status associated with ageing makes some tools more necessary at this age. Preschl *et al.* (2011) pointed the relevance of e-health interventions for depression, anxiety disorder, dementia, and other disorders in older adults. Their review indicated that tools, as Ambient-Assisted Living (AAL) and smart phones, game-based applications and training programs, are important to improve wellbeing of those patients.

One of the main problems associated with ageing is the decline in ability to perform tasks of everyday life. There are already robots that perform household tasks. However, opportunities for use of robots to perform difficult tasks for the elderly are numerous (such as help in taking medication, daily hygiene, physical training, clinical indicators monitoring, etc.). These robots can improve the autonomy and consequently the well-being of elderly people, enhancing their health status (Broadbent *et al.*, 2009). Research and development activities on care robotics constantly increased since the late 1970s, with the main role played by the Japanese universities and firms (Goeldner *et al.*, 2015).

Also, the isolation of many elderlies contributes to a sense of helpless in case of a health emergency. Therefore, devices of automatic alarm in case of distress may help. The results from the Senior Watch Study 2007 showed that, among European citizens with 50 years and plus, the use of community alarm services was still low (near 5%, and within this group the majority of the respondents had 80 years and plus).

Briefly, the tools of e-health for the elderly, to be effective, have to overcome the specific difficulties and health problems of this group. Often, the technology used by the general population won't have any usefulness in this group of the population.

ECONOMIC IMPACT OF E-HEALTH FOR SENIOR PATIENTS

The efforts applied on the improvement of health care quality and safety have grown increasingly over the years. From a social perspective, the questions that arise are: improving quality will reduce costs for patients, hospitals and funders?; the added value of this quality justifies more expense in care? As the expected growth of demand for health care by the ageing population will demand for the resources available, some form of prioritization should occur. This involves making choices about what to fund in order to achieve financial and economic sustainability in the health sector.

In a context of adoption of e-health for senior patients, evaluation must be done using health technology assessments (HTA), which compare the net benefit of an innovation relative to options of treatment. Actually, economists and managers of health, society and politicians have been pressured to implement more cost effective technologies and reject inefficient technologies.

The health technology is generally believed to be the principal factor of health care spending. Recent estimates suggests that medical technology explains 27 to 48% of health care spending growth since 1960 (Smith *et al.*, 2009).

E-health, and specifically tele-health applications, has been shown to offer significant socio-economic benefit, to patients and families, health-care providers and the health-care system. The main benefits identified were: increased access to health services, cost-effectiveness, enhanced educational opportunities, improved health outcomes, better quality of care, better quality of life and enhanced social support (Jennett *et al.*, 2003). Any e-health technology that displays similar results and is cost-effective should be adopted to increase access to health care and reduce spending.

CONCLUSION

This chapter proposes to demonstrate that e-health could help controlling the expenditures with the health of the elders and improve their quality of life. However, there are many obstacles for good results in the short term. To promote the use of e-health on an aging society, opportunities and threats should be clearly identified. To develop health programs and policies to improve the health of ageing society, special attention should be given to the current socio-economic context and cultural factors, to the extent that affects the health status of this population. And lastly, should promote the education of the elderly population on the rights to health and the requirements for using e-health.

In fact, as the rest of the population, the elderly can benefit, in terms of health, from ITCs. We have seen that there are a set of tools that can help overcome or reduce problems that are more common in the elderly. When technology can improve the autonomy and well-being at a reasonable price, there is a real individual and social gain. There are already many products on the market and there has been an increasing interest in the e-health on the part of public health services. However, the difficulties with the use of technology on the part of the elderly, physical disabilities and sometimes the high costs of implementing innovative technologies (even with a net gain in the long run) can be barriers to a complete utilization of these.

Furthermore, the economic results of the adoption of new health technology are not certain and rigorous health technology assessments should be applied to all the e-health tools to be used by the elderly population. Although it was not the main purpose of this article, future research should focus on the analysis of opportunities and threats for e-health on an ageing society on the different national health systems.

Table 2. Opportunities and threats for e-health on an ageing society

Opportunities	Threats
To improve patient's autonomy, mobility and well-being	Select and decode the information on the Internet
To reduce patient's isolation	Financial, educational and social constraints
To improve preventive health care	Low levels in some countries of health literacy
To accelerate the access to acute care	Low levels of Internet literacy of the elderlies
Reduction of costs in the health sector	The lack of technological skills by the elderlies
To expand the flow of reliable information from patient to doctor	Physical limitations of the elderlies

REFERENCES

Arora, S. (2015). Aging in Healthcare Policy. In The Transitions of Aging (pp. 157-182). Springer International Publishing. doi:10.1007/978-3-319-14403-0_9

Bains, M. (2003). Projecting future needs. Long-term projections of public expenditure on health and long-term care for EU member states. In *A disease-based comparison of health systems. What is best and at what costs.* Academic Press.

Barros, P. P. (1998). The Black Box of Healthcare Expenditure Growth Determinants. *Health Economics, 7*(6), 533–544. doi:10.1002/(SICI)1099-1050(199809)7:6<533::AID-HEC374>3.0.CO;2-B PMID:9809710

Boonstra, A., & Van Offenbeek, M. (2010). Towards consistent modes of e-health implementation: Structurational analysis of a telecare programme's limited success. *Information Systems Journal, 20*(6), 537–561. doi:10.1111/j.1365-2575.2010.00358.x

Breyer, F., Costa-Font, J., & Felder, S. (2010). Ageing, health, and health care. *Oxford Review of Economic Policy, 26*(4), 674–690. doi:10.1093/oxrep/grq032

Breyer, F., & Felder, S. (2006). Life Expectancy and Healthcare Expenditures: A new Calculation for Germany using the Costs of Dying. *Health Policy (Amsterdam), 75*(2), 178–186. doi:10.1016/j.healthpol.2005.03.011 PMID:15893848

Brignell, M., Wootton, R., & Gray, L. (2007). The application of telemedicine to geriatric medicine. *Age and Ageing, 36*(4), 369–374. doi:10.1093/ageing/afm045 PMID:17449535

Broadbent, E., Stafford, R., & MacDonald, B. (2009). Acceptance of healthcare robots for the older population: Review and future directions. *International Journal of Social Robotics, 1*(4), 319–330. doi:10.1007/s12369-009-0030-6

Cheng, V., & Hung, P. (2006). Health Insurance Portability and Accountability Act (HIPAA) complaint access control model for web services. *International Journal of Healthcare Information Systems and Informatics, 1*(1), 22–39. doi:10.4018/jhisi.2006010102

de Veer, A. J., Peeters, J. M., Brabers, A. E., Schellevis, F. G., Rademakers, J. J., & Francke, A. L. (2015). Determinants of the intention to use e-Health by community dwelling older people. *BMC Health Services Research, 15*(1), 103. doi:10.1186/s12913-015-0765-8 PMID:25889884

European Commission. (2007). *Seniorwatch 2 Assessment of the Senior Market for ICT Progress and Developments, SMART 2006/0062.* Retrieved October 29, 2014, from http://ec.europa.eu/information_society/newsroom/cf/newsletter-item-detail.cfm?item_id=4286

European Commission. (2012). *The 2012 Ageing Report: Economic and budgetary projections for the 27 EU Member States (2010-2060). European Economy 2/2012.* Retrieved October 29, 2014, from http://ec.europa.eu/economy_finance/publications/european_economy/2012/pdf/ee-2012-2_en.pdf

European Commission. (2015). *The 2015 Ageing Report: Economic and budgetary projections for the 28 EU Member States (2013-2060), European Economy 3/2015.* Retrieved July 10, 2015, from http://ec.europa.eu/economy_finance/publications/european_economy/2015/pdf/ee3_en.pdf

Gell, N. M., Rosenberg, D. E., Demiris, G., LaCroix, A. Z., & Patel, K. V. (2013). Patterns of Technology Use Among Older Adults With and Without Disabilities. *The Gerontologist*. PMID:24379019

Gerdtham, U. G., & Jönsson, B. (2000). International comparisons of health expenditure: theory, data and econometric analysis. Handbook of Health Economics, 1, 11-53.

Ginsburg, P. B. (2008). High and rising healthcare costs: Demystifying U.S. healthcare spending, *Research Synthesis Report*, 16.

Goeldner, M., Herstatt, C., & Tietze, F. (2015). The emergence of care robotics—A patent and publication analysis. *Technological Forecasting and Social Change*, 92, 115–131. doi:10.1016/j.techfore.2014.09.005

Guerzoni, B. & Zuleeg. F. (2011). *Working away at the cost of ageing: the labour market adjusted dependency ratio*. European Policy Council Issue Paper, 64.

Hage, E., Roo, J. P., van Offenbeek, M. A., & Boonstra, A. (2013). Implementation factors and their effect on e-Health service adoption in rural communities: A systematic literature review. *BMC Health Services Research*, 13(1), 19. doi:10.1186/1472-6963-13-19 PMID:23311452

Jennett, P. A., Affleck Hall, L., Hailey, D., Ohinmaa, A., Anderson, C., Thomas, R., & Scott, R. E. et al. (2003). The socio-economic impact of telehealth: A systematic review. *Journal of Telemedicine and Telecare*, 9(6), 311–320. doi:10.1258/135763303771005207 PMID:14680514

Jönsson, B., & Eckerlund, I. (2003). Why do different countries spend different amounts on health care. In *A Disease-Based Comparison of Health Systems: What Is Best and at what Cost*, (pp. 107-119). Academic Press.

Kingsley, D. E. (2015). Aging and Health Care Costs: Narrative Versus Reality. *Poverty & Public Policy*, 7(1), 3–21. doi:10.1002/pop4.89

Knapp, M., & Somani, A. (2009). Health financing: Long term care, organization and financing. In Health systems policy, finance, and organization. Academic Press.

Kutner, M., Greenberg, E., Jin, Y., & Paulsen, C. (2006). *The Health Literacy of America's Adults: Results From the 2003 National Assessment of Adult Literacy (NCES 2006-483)*. National Center for Education Statistics.

McKeown, T., & Lowe, C. R. (1974). *An Introduction to Social Medicine*. Oxford, UK: Blackwell.

Moïse, P. (2003). The technology-health expenditure link. *A Disease-based Comparison of Health Systems*, 195.

Nielsen-Bohlman, L., Panzer, A. M., & Kindig, D. A. (Eds.). (2004). *Health Literacy: A Prescription to End Confusion*. Washington, DC: National Academies Press.

OECD (2013). *Health at a Glance 2013: OECD Indicators*. OECD Publishing. doi:10.1787/health_glance-2013-en

OECD. (2015). *OECD Health Statistics 2015*. Available at: http://www.oecd.org/health/health-data.htm

Oh, H., Rizo, C., Enkin, M., & Jadad, A. (2005). What is e-health? A systematic review of published definitions. *World Hospitals and Health Services*, 41(1), 32–40. PMID:15881824

Page, T. (2014). Touchscreen mobile devices and older adults: A usability study. *International Journal of Human Factors and Ergonomics, 3*(1), 65–85. doi:10.1504/IJHFE.2014.062550

Planinc, R., & Kampel, M. (2013). E-health System Development based on End User Centered Design. In *eTELEMED 2013, The Fifth International Conference on e-health, Telemedicine, and Social Medicine,* (pp. 83-86).

Preschl, B., Wagner, B., Forstmeier, S., & Maercker, A. (2011). E-health interventions for depression, anxiety disorders, dementia and other disorders in older adults.A review. *Journal of Cyber Therapy and Rehabilitation, 3*(4), 371–385.

Reinhardt, R., & Oliver, W. J. (2015). The Cost Problem in Health Care. In K. Soyez (Ed.), *Challenges and Opportunities in Health Care Management* (pp. 3–13). Springer.

Reinhardt, U. E. (2003). Does the aging of the population really drive the demand for health care? *Health Affairs, 22*(6), 27–39. doi:10.1377/hlthaff.22.6.27 PMID:14649430

Rudd, R. E., Anderson, J. E., Oppenheimer, S., & Nath, C. (2007). Health literacy: An update of public health and medical literature. *Review of Adult Learning and Literacy, 7,* 175-204.

Scharwz, F., Ward, J., & Willcock, S. (2014). E-Health readiness in outback communities: An exploratory study. *Rural and Remote Health, 14*(2871). PMID:25190566

Schulz, E., Leidl, R., & König, H. (2004). The Impact of Ageing on Hospital Care and Long-Term Care – The example of Germany. *Health Policy (Amsterdam), 67*(1), 57–74. doi:10.1016/S0168-8510(03)00083-6 PMID:14726007

Serup-Hansen, N., Wickstrøm, J., & Kristiansen, I. S. (2002). Future Healthcare Costs – Do Healthcare Costs During the Last Year of Life Matter? *Health Policy (Amsterdam), 62*(2), 161–172. doi:10.1016/S0168-8510(02)00015-5

Seshamani, M., & Gray, A. (2004a). Ageing and health-care expenditure: The red herring argument revisited. *Health Economics, 13*(4), 303–314. doi:10.1002/hec.826 PMID:15067669

Seshamani, M., & Gray, A. (2004 b). A Longitudinal Study of the Effects of Age and Time to Death on Hospital Costs. *Journal of Health Economics, 23*(2), 217–235. doi:10.1016/j.jhealeco.2003.08.004 PMID:15019753

Smith, S., Newhouse, J. P., & Freeland, M. S. (2009). Income, insurance, and technology: Why does health spending outpace economic growth? *Health Affairs, 28*(5), 1276–1284. doi:10.1377/hlthaff.28.5.1276 PMID:19738242

Stearns, S. C., & Norton, E. C. (2004). Time to Include Time to Death? The Future of Healthcare Expenditure Predictions. *Health Economics, 13*(4), 315–327. doi:10.1002/hec.831 PMID:15067670

Stroetmann, K. A., Artmann, J., Stroetmann, V. N., & Whitehousee, D. (2011). European countries on their journey towards national eHealth infrastructures. *Final European Progress Report,* 1-47.

Teixeira, J., & Suomi, R. (2014). *A Literature Review on Information Systems Supporting the Physical Wellbeing of Elderly People.* arXiv:1406.2863

WHO – World Health Organization. (2010). *Telemedicine: opportunities and developments in Member States: report on the second global survey on e-health 2009*. Global Observatory for e-health Series, 2. WHO.

WHO – World Health Organization (2011). *mHealth: new horizons for health through mobile technologies: second global survey on e-health*. Global Observatory for e-health Series, 3. WHO.

Xie, B. (2011). Older adults, e-health literacy, and collaborative learning: An experimental study. *Journal of the American Society for Information Science and Technology, 62*(5), 933–946. doi:10.1002/asi.21507

An Overview and a Future Perspective in Health Information Systems in Portugal

Sandra Vilas Boas Jardim
Polytechnic Institute of Tomar, Portugal

António Cardoso Martins
Sectra Medical Systems S.L., Spain

INTRODUCTION

The activity of providing health care is a complex task, which stems from several factors, among which it can be highlighted the complexity of the information flow, particularly in clinical processes, the wide variety and different clinical data formats, the ambiguity of the concepts used, the inherent uncertainty in medical diagnosis, the large structural variability of medical records and the organizational and clinical practice cultures of the different institutions (Rouse & Serban 2014). There are growing needs for information at point of care, intended to be complete, homogeneous, accurate, current and of interest to clinical decision (Bath, 2008). Several studies show that information systems can cause a positive effect on quality of care (Lenz & Reichert, 2007), as well as being presently unquestionable their potential economic benefits (Uslu & Stausberg, 2008). One of the main advantages of using computational systems in the health care activity comes from their ability to provide useful information for decision making to health professionals. Thus, their main purpose is to increment the quality and efficiency of health care delivery. In order to achieve these purposes, Health Information Systems (HIS) must fulfil interoperability standards, quality, security, scalability, reliability and timeliness in data storage and processing terms. One of the main problems in this area is that, the large amounts of data produced by health care organizations (which can be of different types, shapes and nature) are stored in several databases with different management platforms and often differ in the architectural levels, which have been developed over the years, in order to support specific needs of certain services or sectors coexisting in the same organization, which may have a large number of heterogeneous and spread systems (Kitsiou, Matopoulos, Manthou & Vlachopoulou, 2007). On the other hand, a large number of health informatics applications do not share information, and when they do, they do it at a very basic level. When communication between different HIS exists, it is mainly achieved through proprietary integration solutions.

In Portugal, several projects were developed in an effort to implement an Electronic Medical Record (EMR) based on the many repositories of information available, but limitations in the existing HIS have prevented this goal to become a reality in a significant extent. To allow a health professional to view the entire medical history of a patient, he must have access to a significant number of documents, which may be spread over many different systems. To make this practical and useful, the user would view all the information from a single system (EMR) that previously received all the information from several other systems (centralized architecture). Alternatively, a more distributed solution may exist, where the user would access other systems besides the EMR. This EMR would contain a set of pointers

DOI: 10.4018/978-1-4666-9978-6.ch077

to remote systems, which store and present the information related with the patient in the study. This is the solution implemented in Portugal through the *Plataforma de Dados da Saúde* – PDS (Health Data Platform) (Saude, 2014d).

Regardless of the EMR scenario using centralized information, decentralized or even a mixed solution, there are certain minimum assumptions in information format and communication that must be met so that an EMR can arise with reliable and accessible information that can be maintained over time. One of the major difficulties is the lack of good and standardized interoperability among information systems. One of the most important might be the lack of a common unique identifier for each patient. In Portugal there is a project, named *Registo Nacional de Utentes* – RNU (Patient National Registry) (Saude, 2010), to overcome this problem, but it currently only solves the problem for the applications developed by the Health Ministry. This solution does not present integration mechanisms regarding patient's identification numbers for non-Government applications. Without a precise relationship in patient's identification through the different health care systems and their information, it won't be possible to effectively gather all the existing information of a single patient. One of the ways to overcome this difficulty would be the adoption of already developed standards for the patient information cross reference like the Integrating the Healthcare Enterprise (IHE) Patient Information Cross-referencing and Patient Demographics Query (PIX/PDQ) (Enterprise, 2010; Trotter & Uhlman, 2011) profiles and the adherence of current systems to those standards. This would require the creation of a system that can manage all the identifiers for a single patient in different systems (domains) playing a central role in the query and distribution of updated patient identifiers. Assume there can be only one unique identifier common to all health care systems is infeasible, as there will always be restrictions on the patient identifiers in the applications, legacy systems with older identifiers and the will to broaden health care information to bigger enterprises, regions or even countries that surely have their own identifiers already.

This paper aims to present the state of art in interoperability among Portuguese HIS and to propose an approach to overcome the inexistence of some structural systems that would promote interoperability and therefore an increase in the information available to an EMR.

HEALTH INFORMATION SYSTEMS

Progress in information technology is a real and unavoidable fact, it plays an important role in the health care sector regarding its final goal – treating patients more effectively. In this sector, his scope of action covers various areas such as the HIS, Telemedicine, Biological Signal Processing (in which is included the Medical Image Processing), Health Informatics Security, etc..

Information and Communication Technologies (ICT) increased use in health care organizations presents a pattern that is similar to what happened in major companies that rely in a well developed Information Technologies (IT) infrastructure. The use of web technologies, database systems, and network infrastructures are some initiatives that affect both the practice and management of health care market (Jardim, 2013).

Regarding the evolution of information and communication technologies in health care organizations, there is a strong resistance to the adoption of e-health systems - the use of the so-called Electronic Medical Records (EMR). With the use of patient data information systems, information goes from a paper record to electronic format in the form of files, thus allowing easier and more effective management.

The concept of HIS emerges from Health Information and Communication Technologies (HICT), constituting one of the three main lines along which they are organized (Saude, 2012). HIS are frequently described as the interaction between individuals, processes and technology in order to support fundamental information operations, management and availability, so that health care services can be improved (Almunawar & Anshari, 2011). Similarly to other sectors, the nature of the health sector has changed over time from a relatively stable activity to a dynamic backdrop. HIS whose evolution is based on several different technologies, can be described as those who, through data processing, provide information and enhance the knowledge creation in health care environments (Winter et al., 2011). Giving more detail to this definition we can say that an Hospital Information System can be defined as a mechanism for storing, processing, analysing and transmitting information required for planning, organization, execution and evaluation of health services.

The main goal of HIS is to contribute to an efficient and high quality health care (Almunawar & Anshari, 2011). These systems should also promote the development, rationalization and improvement of its management. Besides the fulfilment of interoperability standards, quality, security, scalability, reliability and timeliness in data storage and processing terms requirements, they should ensure efficiency and security of information flows, eliminating duplicate actions, namely diagnoses, and simultaneously enhance the speed, efficiency and proximity of health information. Also note that these systems should have not only clinical features, as well as management ones, which should share information through interoperability, allowing access to data needed for performance monitoring and correlation of the one needed for economic evaluation of studies, case-mix consolidation and data mining to support the providers procurement, health planning, greater accountability, better decision-making and evidence-based policies and reorganization of logistics and supply flows.

Health Information Systems in Portugal

In Portugal there are ~104 public hospitals and 875 primary care units (427 health care centers and 448 family health units) Saude (2014a). The governmental organization *Serviços Partilhados do Ministério da Saúde* - SPMS (Health Ministry Shared Services, formerly called ACSS) develops and manages around 34 IT projects that fall inside the HIS Saude (2014b). Those systems are in use in public health care units distributed along the whole country, some of them are listed in Table 1 due to their relevance or number of institutions in which they are installed.

The systems SONHO and SINUS were the first ones, adopted by most public hospitals and primary care units since the 90s, mostly because they are centrally promoted, installed and supported by SPMS with a presumably low total cost of ownership (TCO) for the Health Ministry. Others followed the same path and some are even mandatory for public hospitals in Portugal. The functions of SONHO/SINUS are mostly administrative, being its original purpose, the reimbursement of health care providers by the Government (through the use of DRG's) (Saude, 2014b; Saude, 2014e).

Besides the already described systems, public health care units usually have systems for the management of many departments, mainly the Radiology (PACS systems), Laboratory Information System (LIS) as well as applications that manages parts of departments like the emergency, cardiology, dermatology, gynaecology/obstetrics and ophthalmology. IT solutions for other departments exist, but are less frequent. These are usually provided by different manufacturers, either global or local companies. There are some examples where specialized solutions are locally developed.

Private hospitals or other care providers cannot use SPMS's systems. However, since they provide services for the government, they must provide related information to public systems (usually managed by SPMS) in order to be refunded by the government. Sometimes, this information must be manually

Table 1. Governmental HIS use in Portuguese health care institutions (Saude, 2014b)

Acronym	System Name	Purpose
sClínico	*Sistema de Informação Clínica Hospitalar* (Hospital Clinical Information System (EMR))	Information system that manages clinical information relevant for performing patient appointments. Used by medical professionals, nurses, nutritionists and other health professionals, is evolutional software that joins the systems SAM (*Sistema de Apoio ao Médico* – Medical Support System) and SAPE (*Sistema de Apoio à Prática de Enfermagem* – Nurse Practice Support System), in order to exits a common application for all health professional. The supporting database is shared with SONHO.
PDS	*Plataforma de Dados da Saúde* (Health Data Platform)	Web platform that provides a central system for recording and sharing of clinical information in accordance with the requirements of the National Commission for Data Protection. The platform provides access to information for citizens who have a patient number of the National Health Service (NHS) and for healthcare professionals in various parts of the NHS (hospitals, emergency, primary care, national network of continuous care), without displacing them from the safe place where they are kept. (Saude, 2014d)
PEM	*Prescrição Eletrónica Médica* (Electronic Medical Prescription)	Information system for electronic prescription of medications and home respiratory care based on centralization and data security, which enables the recording of information on conditions that benefit those involved in the prescription process: users, doctors and NHS. (Saude, 2014c)
GID	*Gestão Integrada da Doença* (Integrated Management of Disease)	Information system for the registration of treatment hemodialysis and peritoneal dialysis (Martins, 2014)
SISO	*Sistema de Informação para a Saúde Oral* (Oral Health Information System)	Information system with a set of services that fully support all information generators and receivers processes.
RENTEV	*Registo Nacional de Testamento Vital* (Living Will National Register)	Information system that receives, stores, organizes and maintains information and documentation relating to the advance directives document of the will and power of attorney for health care.
SONHO	*Sistema Integrado de Informação Hospitalar* (Patient Administration System (PAS))	Patient Administration System (PAS) for hospitals that works as a fundamental pillar of patients and episodes referencing in health care institutions that use it. From a functional point of view, the main objective of this system is to control the flow of hospital patients. (Teixeira & Brochado, 2005; Saude, 2014e)
SINUS	*Sistema de informação para unidades de saúde primárias* (Primary Care Information System)	Patient Administration System (PAS) for primary care, managing encounters in consultation, emergency and immunization.
RNU	*Registo Nacional de Utentes* (Patient National Registry)	Provides information of NHS users to the different organizations in the Ministry, as well as other entities authorized to access the data. Serves the same purpose as a Master Patient Index, but only for the SPMS's systems, using fully proprietary integrations.
RCU/RCU2	*Resumo Clínico Único* (Unique Clinical Summary)	Digital document with the Patient Summary - Summary of patient key clinical aspects (connected with the epSOS/EXPAND European project). The first project where HL7 and IHE profiles have been used, result of European interoperability requirement.

typed in SPMS's systems independently of how the private organization manages that information, in other cases it is automatically transferred using proprietary interfaces specially developed by the private sector IT provider and SPMS in order to provide technical interoperability.

INTEROPERABILITY ISSUES IN HEALTH INFORMATION SYSTEMS IN PORTUGAL

In general, each system referred in the previous section has its own data repository, which results in some relevant data that should be shared in order for the remaining systems and users to benefit from. Integrations rarely use interoperability standards or best practices in workflows and patient demographic information does not flow, as well as any other clinical information. Basic media like paper or CD's are commonly used to transport information across health enterprises, but that information is simply viewed, not integrated in the other systems, as they present too many different formats, information is unstructured and ambiguous in order to be merged into the destination systems. This fact entails, beyond the increased cost inherent to the frequent changes of information systems, great difficulties concerning the extraction of reliable information, capable of supporting decisions of different actors leading to knowledge creation.

Perhaps the most important problem arises from the fact that SONHO and SINUS (PAS) used in some 99 public hospitals, are not prepared to share information with other systems (non-SPMS), mainly the patient identification for which they assume to be the assigning authority in their domain. Over the years, the IT solutions from various other manufacturers that were introduced in the Portuguese health care market, implemented specially developed mechanisms to enable the access to the most relevant information related to the identification of patients in these existing systems. These integrations were developed with ad-hoc methods, very simple, non scalable, inflexible, and the communication is not based on events, but in unreliable polling methods.

Nowadays, many applications use the SONHO's database primary key know as the "sequential number" as the unique patient identification number, (not a Nationally unique number) others use another SONHO database column named *numero de processo*, a kind of Medical Record Number that allowed NULLS (also not a Nationally unique number). Some of the other systems include a prefix or a suffix to these identifiers, some simply disregard all these numbers and have only their own (but these simply do not integrate with anything).

Patient demographic updates or patient merges are rarely implemented, resulting in serious consistency problems. It's true that many goals have been achieved as a result of these integrations, like the avoidance of re-typing of patient's demographic information, or the recording of performed procedures for later billing/reimbursement.

When SPMS's SAM and SAPE were developed (nowadays sClinico) with similar functions to those of an EMR, the need to share information with the SONHO and SINUS emerged. It was then decided by an implicit and unstructured sharing. These applications began to share database tables to enable information sharing. This was only possible because they all had been developed by the same organization. Other third party applications did not had the same opportunity because sharing database tables with SONHO and SINUS would be infeasible and could cause serious disruptions in applications designed and managed by different entities. Yet, there are some SONHO and SINUS tables that can be read or written by third party systems.

The information isolation within the systems, lack of standards integrations and data sharing motivated most health applications manufacturers to not share their own information since SPMS does not support it in their applications nor they really promote it.

As the government legislated for the creation of a National Health Number, SPMS developed the RNU (Unique National Registry) project with the goal of reconciling the demographic information of patients in some ~ 400 instances of SINUS (which have since then been merged into a smaller number, the result of merges of hospitals and primary health care institutions in Hospital Centers or Local Health Units). Once again, a proprietary method of integration was chosen, that did not follow the recommendations of the Integrating the health care Enterprise (IHE) with actors and responsibilities on information distribution clearly defined, using HL7 messages triggered by events. To achieve this goal, the NHS number should be used. Unlike the "sequential number", the NHS number is Nation-wide unique. One of the initial problems was that many patients with a "sequential number" lacked the correspondent NHS number in order to promote the relationship. Assuming the existence of the NHS number, it would be possible to link many "sequential number" from different health care providers.

Recently, the requirement for inter-provider information sharing has become a requirement to which the Government responded with the PDS. This platform allows the connection of multiple sources of relevant clinical information in a distributed information architecture, having a common point of connection, the RNU identification number. If there is no record of the RNU number, there is no way to interconnect the different SPMS applications.

Additionally, the PDS will not be able to call an application that does not use the RNU number as patient unique identification number, which occurs with most applications, which over the years have been adopting the SONHO/SINUS sequential number.

Certainly it will always be possible to "invent" an intricate relationship of patient identifiers, through an entirely proprietary integration, which, apparently have lower initial costs, but serious management problems and end-up in a very high TCO.

PEM is a recent application that has been developed by SPMS with some interoperability in mind. It allows for 150.000 drug prescriptions a day (Saude, 2014c). Everyday all the prescriptions must be sent to a National central prescription database. There are a few applications from third-party vendors that also allow the prescription of drugs. For them, SPMS released a number of guidelines relating the integration with RNU for patient identification and central prescriptions database.

It is common to find systems like PACS, RIS and LIS developed by worldwide companies, that would normally use interoperability standards to communicate with the remaining systems in the organizations, but since they cannot use these standard processes because the "core" systems do not support them, they are not really implemented but in turn some proprietary solutions come into production.

Guidelines to Solve Interoperability Issues in Health Information Systems

Many solutions could be presented to help solve the interoperability issues that are present in the health care IT, either in Portugal as well as other countries. The most important ones are the ones related to motivation and distribution of knowledge for the use of health care standards, like HL7 or the adoption of IHE profiles.

- **Promote Use of Standards and Vocabularies:** There is still a lack of understanding that implementing a complex solution based on standards instead of developing a simple process to meet a small requirement may turn out to be much more costly in the long term. This is mostly due to the lack of reports and statistics that can testify the results achieved by some initiatives. Standards in health care are broad, rich and flexible, which means that an implementation using them will have the same characteristics. There is much more documentation regarding an integration using standards than the same proprietary integration.

- **Train Health Care IT Developers in the Use of Standards:** Besides knowledge, training can significantly reduce difficulties in trying to make sense out of long health care standards.

- **Promote the Start of a National "HL7" Organization:** HL7 was founded in 1987 and has now18 affiliates in Europe. An HL7 country affiliate would represent his countries needs at HL7 international, would also participate in the standards development process, but most importantly would promote and educate about the relevance of HL7.

- **Deploy Health IT Infrastructure Services:** There are some minimal required infrastructure services that should be provided. In Portugal, health care is mostly a public service. SPMS is not only the entity that regulates the use of IT in this sector, but also the organization that owns the software in use in most of the production PAS and EMR systems in the primary and secondary health care organizations. Private organizations should also adhere because the government is the co-payer in most of the services provided. The following services should be deployed as part of the referred infrastructure:

  - *Redefine, distribute and maintain a set of definition files* that are unique in that particular country. Tables like Portuguese districts, cities, health care providers, health care professionals, lab test definition file, exam code definition file, charge file for government reimbursement purposes. In Portugal, these lists are distributed by the government, but have not been adapted for IT use and consequently they have no codes like an Organizationally Unique Identifier (OID) (IEEE, 2014) that would guarantee the uniqueness of each value and are not electronically distributed and maintained. IHE has the Sharing Value Sets profile (SVS) profile, part of the IT infrastructure profiles, that describes this process, using HL7 version 3, XML and web services.

  - *Deploy a National Patient Identification Registry,* also called Master Patient Index (MPI). The linking among the multiple patient identifier of the same person in different domains will allow linking clinical and administrative information from different health IT systems that is now separate. Systems will have to share their information using interoperability standards and using these identifiers. IHE has the PIX/PDQ profile that describes how different systems with patient identifiers valid in their own domain must communicate with a patient identifier cross-reference manager (MPI) in order to identify a patient across organizations. In Portugal, the logical would be to improve the RNU to embody the MPI features, but many systems, mainly the SONHO and SINUS (PAS) would have to be changed to cooperate in this integration. All other public or private health care IT systems would be able to participate in the patient identification as long as they support the IHE PIX/PDQ profile.

  - *Deploy Centralized Audit Record Repositories.* User accountability is provided through audit trail. Nowadays, traceability of user activities is almost impossible, as they are not recorded, or when it does, it is local to each system and very difficult to inspect. Instead of having one audit repository per system, this repository should be deployed at the organization level, increasing security and facilitating the work of a security officer as well as the domain security policies. IHE has the Audit Trail and Node Authentication (ATNA) profile, that addresses this need. Although this is not an enabler of interoperability between systems, it's an important requirement for each of them, increasing security and awareness of Patient Health

Information (PHI) access. In the USA, PHI information access is enforced by the Health Insurance Portability and Accountability Act (HIPAA) and systems must comply. Having a central audit repository would be part of the requirement, but not all.

- **Issue Regulation That Defines the Minimum Set of Interoperability Standards Systems Must Comply:** In Portugal there is a lack of technical regulations regarding the use of standards. This is true for the patient data, the integrations between systems and even the vocabularies like observations, procedures and others. Even if this would apply only for public health care providers, it would set a baseline of requirements the systems must have in order to be acquired and used.

- **Certify Applications and/or Integration:** In order ease the procurement process and maintain a certain level of freedom of choice for the IT managers in the health care organizations, the regulator could periodically certify a set of applications for the market, that comply with the minimum set of requirements regarding the expected features but also the kind of standards and protocols they use for integrations with other systems, security aspects, user authentication, logging, vocabularies used and other aspects.

- **Monitor the Evolution of the Solutions in Health Care IT and Issue Reports:** Periodically, the regulator should issue reports that reflects the current state of art in health care applications and use. These reports would provide the required feedback in order to continue to improve the systems as well as provide good directions where to make further recommendations regarding some aspects of the systems and use.

FUTURE TRENDS

Information systems will become wiser and more effective providing the information users needs in order to treat patients with more quality. This will be related to the increased number of systems sharing information among them, with more integrations. HL7 version 3 will overcome version 2 (the most used standard for health information interchange nowadays), but that has not yet happened because of big challenges that are hard to overcome, mostly because they deal with users and the way they interact, more than cost or lack of IT solutions or standards to support it.

The move from the technical interoperability (where two or more systems are capable of communicating and exchanging data) to the semantic one (the systems can automatically interpret the information exchanged meaningfully and accurately in order to produce useful results) will require that complex vocabularies specific to specialties and context are efficiently used across communicating systems, allowing one observation to have the exact same meaning through all of them. The Common Terminology Services (CTS) will provide the required infrastructure in order to share standard vocabularies like SNOMED-CT, ICD9/10, CPT, HCPCS, LOINC, RxNorm, UMLS and others.

When that day arrives, health IT systems will be able to provide the health care professional with guidance and insight on reminders, drug-allergies and inference between apparently disparate information that the user would otherwise not notice, with the information displayed and formatted in the "language" each user better understands in his specialty. These are some of the features that an Electronic Medical Record system (EMR) will display.

CONCLUSION

HIS interoperability problems are present in all countries. The United States had taken a clear political decision and emphasis regarding interoperability in the US Federal Health Information Technology for Economic and Clinical Health (Government, 2009). The main motivation is to provide better services through the use of a real EMR, while increasing value for money invested. Austria has developed a project called ELGA since 2006 to promote the implementation of a nationwide Electronic Health Record (Duftschmid, 2009). Some other countries are much more quieter around this subject.

In Spain, there are many autonomous communities, each of them with their own unique interoperability policies and patient identification numbers. As in Portugal, if they do not have a common set of standards for integration of health information, they will not be able to share information through infrastructures from different communities.

Sweden is a very different country. They have had a unique patient identification through the whole country for a long time. Still, they face interoperability problems among different applications. As they are part of the European Union, they will are gradually involved in providing and consuming patient information generated elsewhere in the European Union. That information, surely will comply with the best practices developed by communities of experts, like the IHE that for some time now have been releasing integration profiles for many health care areas.

The current setting in Portugal calls for a change in mindset, mostly from the SPMS's side, as they develop a very important part of the health care IT applications and have a very big market segment in the PAS and EMR market segment. Recently, SPMS has promoted some events for the adoption of SNOMED-CT and HL7, which denotes their recent awareness for these standards.

SPMS is a governmental organization that depends on National politics. Decision makers have moving agendas. Structural changes in Health IT are usually difficult to implement and have their major effect only on mid to long term. This makes many strategic projects come to an end sooner than they can produce visible effects.

The private health sector in Portugal depends greatly on the governmental demands for quality, compliance for standards and IT innovation. If there are no strict requirements on interoperability, the private sector will not take initiatives to implement them.

In the end, having a complete country using the same basic set of health IT systems is an advantage that is only obscured by the slow rhythm of innovation, typical when there is no competition in players for a market segment.

It's always important to see the "present" of others in order to design our "future". Like this document that describe the "present" experiences in Portugal, other countries experiences should be learned and taken as a basis for the development of the health care interoperability and EMR challenges in a country. Each country has many problems already solved by the standards of that area, as well as a few that might be unique, probably worth of being discussed and solved within the communities that publish best practices in health care IT, like IHE or HL7.

REFERENCES

Act of 2009. (n.d.). Retrieved March, 15, 2015 from https://standards.ieee.org/develop/regauth/tut/oid.pdf

Almunawar, M. N., & Anshari, M. (2011). Health Information Systems (HIS): Concept and Technology. In *Proceedings of the International Conference on Informatics for Development*. Yogyakarta, Indonesia: Academic Press.

Bath, P. A. (2008). Health informatics: Current issues and challenges. *Journal of Information Science*, *34*(4), 501–518. doi:10.1177/0165551508092267

Duftschmid, G., Dorda, W., & Gall, W. (2009). *The ELGA initiative: A plan for implementing a nationwide electronic health records system in Austria*. Section on Medical Information and Retrieval Systems (MIAS), Medical University of Vienna. Retrieved March, 15, 2015 from http://www.meduniwien.ac.at/msi/mias/papers/Duftschmid2009a.pdf

Enterprise, I. H. (2010). Patient Identifier Cross-Reference HL7 V3, (PIXV3) and Patient Demographic Query HL7 V3 15 (PDQV3). *IHE IT Infrastructure Technical Framework Supplement*. Retrieved September, 25, 2014 from http://www.ihe.net/technical_framework/upload/ihe_iti_suppl_pix_pdq_hl7v3_rev2-1_ti_2010-08-10.pdf

IEEE. (2014). *S. A*. Object Identifier. Retrieved from American Recovery and Reinvestment.

Jardim, S. V. B. (2013). The Electronic Health Record and its Contribution to Healthcare Information Systems Interoperability. In *Proceedings of International Conference on Health and Social Care Information Systems and Technologies* (pp. 940-948). Lisbon, Portugal. doi:10.1016/j.protcy.2013.12.105

Kitsiou, S., Matopoulos, A., Manthou, V., & Vlachopoulou, M. (2007). Evaluation of integration technology approaches in the healthcare supply chain. *International Journal Value Chain Management*, *1*(4), 325–343. doi:10.1504/IJVCM.2007.015091

Lenz, R., & Reichert, M. (2007). IT support for healthcare processes – premises, challenges, perspectives. *Journal of Data & Knowledge Engineering*, *61*(1), 39–58. doi:10.1016/j.datak.2006.04.007

Martins, H. (2014). SPMS - Os Compromissos com Melhor Saúde. In *Proceedings of Conference As TIC e a Saúde no Portugal de 2013*. Lisbon, Portugal: Academic Press.

Rouse, W. B., & Serban, N. (2014). *Understanding and Managing the Complexity of Healthcare*. The MIT Press.

Saude, A. C. (2012). *National Health Plan 2012 – 2016*. Retrieved September, 19, 2014 from http://pns.dgs.pt/nhp-in-english/

Saude, D. G. G. (2010). Registo Nacional de Utentes (RNU). *Diretório de Informação em Saúde*. Retrieved September, 25, 2014 from http://dis.dgs.pt/2010/07/08/registo-nacional-de-utentes-rnu/

Saude, S. P. M. (2014a). *Prestadores de serviços de saúde*. Retrieved September, 15, 2014 from https://servicos.min-saude.pt/utente/portal/paginas/Prestadorescuidadossaude%E2%80%93pesquisa.aspx?MenuContext=33

Saude, S. P. M. (2014b). *Projetos SPMS*. Retrieved September, 15, 2014 from http://spms.min-saude.pt/projetos-spms/

Saude, S. P. M. (2014c). *PEM em todos hospitais SAM*. Retrieved September, 15, 2014 from http://spms.min-saude.pt/blog/2014/01/31/pem-em-todos-hospitais-sam/

Saude, S. P. M. (2014d). *PDS – Plataforma de Dados da Saúde*. Retrieved September, 15, 2014 from http://spms.min-saude.pt/blog/2013/11/01/pds-plataforma-de-dados-da-saude/

Saude, S. P. M. (2014e). *SONHO*. Retrieved September, 15, 2014 from http://portalcodgdh.min-saude.pt/index.php/SONHO

Teixeira, A. A., & Brochado, A. M. (2005). Quando o SONHO se torna realidade...: Avaliação estatística do impacto das tecnologias de informação nos serviços de consulta externa hospitalar. *Revista Portuguesa de Saude Publica*, *23*(2), 43–55.

Trotter, F., & Uhlman, D. (2011). *Hacking Healthcare: A Guide to Standards, Workflows, and Meaningful Use*. O'Reilly Media Inc.

USA Government. (2009). *American Recovery and Reinvestment Act*. United States of America. Retrieved March, 25, 2015 from http://www.gpo.gov/fdsys/pkg/BILLS-111hr1enr/pdf/BILLS-111hr1enr.pdf

Uslu, A. M., & Stausberg, J. (2008). Value of the Electronic Patient Record: An Analysis of the Literature. *Journal of Biomedical Informatics*, *41*(4), 675–682. doi:10.1016/j.jbi.2008.02.001 PMID:18359277

Winter, A. (2011). *Health Information Systems*. Springer. doi:10.1007/978-1-84996-441-8

KEY TERMS AND DEFINITIONS

Electronic Medical Record (EMR): Systematic collection of electronic health information about an individual patient or population; a record in digital format capable, theoretically, of being shared across different health care settings.

Health Information System: Any system that captures, stores, manages or transmits information related to the health of individuals or the activities of organisations that work within the health sector.

Master Patient Index (MPI): An electronic medical database that holds information on every patient registered at a health care enterprise.

Patient Information Cross-referencing (PIX): Supports the cross-referencing of patient identifiers from multiple Patient Identifier Domains (transmitting patient identity information from an identity source to the Patient Identifier Cross-reference Manager and providing the ability to access the list(s) of cross-referenced patient identifiers either via a query/response or via an update notification).

Semantic Interoperability: The ability of different information technology systems and software applications to, automatically, interpret the information exchanged meaningfully and accurately in order to produce useful results.

Technical Interoperability: The ability of different information technology systems and software applications to communicate and exchange data.

Vocabularies, Terminologies, or Coding Systems: Structured list of terms which together with their definitions are designed to describe unambiguously the care and treatment of patients. Terms cover diseases, diagnoses, findings, operations, treatments, drugs, administrative items, etc.

Rethinking ICTs and E-Health:
A Focus on Issues and Challenges

Bolanle A. Olaniran
Texas Tech University, USA

Yan Zhang
Texas Tech University Health Sciences Center, USA

INTRODUCTION

A major driver of e-health involves the significant advances in information communication technologies (ICTs). These advances allow for information collection, dissemination, and general use or application by healthcare providers, patients and or consumers. Collectively, this phenomenon has led to a new buzzword or terminology referred to as e-health. Despite the technology advances and enthusiasm about what e-health can do to improve quality of healthcare at large, the enthusiasm should be tempered with caution, because without careful planning and systematic consideration in policy, e-health may not achieve its lofty expectations and goals (see Viswanath & Kreuter, 2007).

BACKGROUND

Furthermore, e-health creates a race to digitize health information in an easily accessible digitized format or platform (e.g., Online). This paper presents theoretical arguments about factors affecting e-health adoption and usage. Specifically, we plan to explore the nature of e-health and factors that makes it attractive while exploring other factors that pose challenges to e-health.

MAIN FOCUS OF THE ARTICLE

We argue that while e-health may help with issue of efficiency, such as cost-cutting, and instant access to healthcare information and records, its adoption and effectiveness is not as clear cut and may threaten the survival of certain medical practices (i.e., complementary or alternative medicine [CAM] that characterizes some of the non-western medical or health care services). In order to explore issues relating to adoption and use of e-health, we looked at the dimension of cultural variability (i.e., Hofstede, 1996, 2001) as a general framework given its wide appeal and established record in literature, especially in the adoption of an innovation such as e-health. In particular, the collectivism and individualism dimension of cultural variability is useful in exploring the difference between oral tradition and digital tradition cultures in terms of how they might adopt and use e-health. Specifically, we argued that the disparity between oral tradition and digital traditional cultures is such that information in oral tradition culture simply cannot be easily translated into written or digital one because of the art form implied within the

DOI: 10.4018/978-1-4666-9978-6.ch078

oral tradition. Hence, the failure to recognize this important challenge may very well makes oral tradition cultures and their embedded medical practices extinct and consequently may hinder adoption and usage decision. This problem is not limited to e-health consumers, but may impact e-health practices altogether (Olaniran, 2012). First, however, it is necessary to provide an overview of e-health.

Overview of E-Health

e-health represents a method by which health information is collected and disseminated through information communication technologies (ICTs). More importantly, e-health allows for storage and exchange of health information among consumers, providers, government and other entities (Dominguez-Mayo, et al., 2015). In the U. S. A., the race to comply with government mandated e-health policy is at a feverish pace. As healthcare providers might miss out on incentives for compliance and in certain situations can be penalized for noncompliance. Thus, the mandate to reshape healthcare infrastructure crystallized a commitment by the United States to make patients' medical records universally available through ICTs further fueling the growth of e-health and its capabilities (US Department of Health and Human Services, 2004).This idea is not unique to U. S. A., as other governments around the globe are also pushing to join the race in e-health. Some see e-health as way to address the needs of the underserved, or to reach individuals in rural areas where access to established medical centers may not be possible. Some see e-health as a way to bridge the disparities in the quality of healthcare services for different population groups (e.g., Obasola, Mabawonku, & Lagunju, 2015, Wald, Dube, & Anthony, 2007).

At the same time, certain e-health platforms such as web available information (e.g., medical forums, WebMD) offer advantages that include assisting patients in making informed health care choices. It also offers healthcare providers the opportunity to collaborate with other providers (Scholl & Olaniran, 2013) and/or patients in a team environment either by supplementing physician provided information or engaging in an online support groups along with providers who have access to patient medical records (Dominguez-Mayo, et al., 2015; Wald, et al., 2007). E-Health also promise safe storage of information along with accuracy of information that safeguards against error while promising increase efficiency and effectiveness of healthcare (Dominguez-Mayo et al., 2015). On the other hand, e-health is compounded by certain factors that may impact the extent which e-health promises are attained. For instance, there is greater level of information and misinformation due to information found on the Internet, along with possible exacerbation of socioeconomic health disparities, and the shifting nature of the traditional physician–patient relationship in terms of *medical authority* (Visnawath & Kreuter, 2007; Wald, et al., 2007). Specifically, Visnawath and Kreuter (2007) points to the fact that not all providers have the ability to install new technologies to foster their e-health goals and their operational needs. These authors also questioned whether making the investments in these technologies are worthwhile or cause organizations to shift limited resources from other important areas and whether the deployment and use of the technologies can be sustained given the required recurring expenditures. At the same time, when e-health hardware is universal, the use and content of the programs may pose a barrier to certain user groups (Abel & Obeten, 2015; Visnawath & Kreuter, 2007).

Dominguez-Mayo et al (2015) discuss the *interoperability* challenge-which refers to ability of two or more different platforms to exchange information or communicate (see also, Shiferaw & Zolfo, 2012). Similarly, majority of the websites or portals aiding e-health in spite of being designed for easy navigation still require certain level of literacy (i.e., for individuals with above an 8th grade education reading level) and language proficiency which may further creates divide in access, information processing, and overall competency of the e-health system in what is now known as digital illiteracy (Obasola et al.,

2015; Shiferaw & Zolfo, 2012; Visnawath & Kreuter, 2007). Others have pointed to the role of culture and cultural differences in how people attend to their healthcare needs (e.g., Chang & Gibbons, 2008; Kreuter & McClure; Visnawath & Kreuter, 2007) especially in terms of how individuals process and use ICTs. Given that this is an area that is not always taken into consideration in e-health, it is important to look at the impact of these cultural differences on e-health because it is designed to cater to people regardless of different cultural backgrounds. However, culture influences effectiveness of any innovation and in particular pervasive E-Heath. Thus, the next section will look at the culture along with a theoretical premise and its application to e-health.

Culture and Theoretical Underpinning for E-Health

No technology transfer or application outside of the culture of origin to another can be completed without an unforeseen cultural implication in the adopting culture or contexts (Neuhauser & Kreps, 2003; Olaniran, 2007). From this premise, it is important to understand the importance of culture in e-health. Hofstede's 'dimensions of cultural variability' (1980, 2001) offer a useful theoretical approach. Hofstede's dimensions of cultural variability present a general framework for where and how a particular culture from a certain region of the world can be categorized along 4 to 5 dimensions. The dimensions of cultural variability initially consisted of four spectrum of cultures namely, 'power distance', 'uncertainty avoidance', 'individualism-collectivism', and 'masculinity-femininity'; later, however, a fifth dimension (i.e., 'time orientation') was added (Hofstede, 1996; see also Dunn & Marinetti, 2002; Olaniran, 2007 for overviews of cultural value orientations and cultural dimensions).

Power distance, which is explained as "the extent to which the less powerful members of institutions and organizations accept that power is distributed unequally" (Hofstede & Bond, 1984, p. 418). *Uncertainty avoidance* describes "the extent to which people feel threatened by ambiguous situations and have created beliefs and institutions that try to avoid these" (Hofstede & Bond, 1984, p. 419). *Individualism-collectivism* acknowledges the fact that in individualistic cultures, "people are supposed to look after themselves and their family only." However, in collectivistic cultures, "people belong to in-groups or collectivities which are supposed to look after them in exchange for loyalty" (Hofstede & Bond, 1984, p. 419). *Masculinity-Femininity* is where masculinity focuses on cultures "in which dominant values in society are success, money and things," whereas femininity refers to cultures "in which dominant values are caring for others and quality of life" (Hofstede & Bond, 1984, p. 419-420). One of the challenges to dimensions of cultural variability is that comparisons are relative and restricted to two objects (e.g., cultures, regions, countries etc.). The last dimension is time orientation which focuses on the degree to which a given culture emphasizes short vs. long term view.

There has been extensive critique of Hofstede's dimensions as being too simplistic for exploring complex intercultural interaction (see Ess & Sudweeks, 2006; Martin & Cheong, 2007; MacFadyen, 2008). MacFadyen (2008) also points to the challenge of viewing a culture from the standpoint of nationality or ethnicity and thus recommends the need to include other factors such as age and gender. In spite of these criticisms, Hofstede's dimensions offer a general and useful framework, especially when one takes into account other variables such as socioeconomic development, and social relationships, among other things. The dimensions of individualism-collectivism and power distance are particularly useful when exploring cultural impacts in e-health adoption and use. First, the dimensions of individualism-collectivism and power distance directly influence how one communicates or interacts with people using ICTs (Olaniran, 2004, 2007; Kifle, Payton, Mbarika, & Meso, 2010; Rocker, Ziefel, & Holzinger, 2014). Second, both dimensions have implication for how members of cultural groups may be open or resistant to certain changes (Smith, 2002). For instance, regardless of economic changes that might have moved individuals from collectivistic cultures toward individualistic tendencies (e.g., accumulation of things and material wealth), people still strive to hold on to their sociocultural identity, retain traditional norms that guide perception of e-health (Olaniran, 2007; Smith, 2002).

Specifically, culture allows one to understand peoples' use of technology – and perhaps the adoption/selection of technology, which is responsible for the resulting social consequences. Specifically, advances in ICTs and Internet capabilities have allowed individuals from U. S. A. and elsewhere in the Western hemisphere to use these technologies to cater to their cultural tendencies and needs that tend to lean towards individualistic cultural approach. To this extent, e-health is not only a possibility but rather an avenue to broaden the reach of healthcare specialists beyond doctor-patients and the confine of office visits to consumers. Hence, consumers in such environments take control over how they consume or participate in their own health care and thus, e-health is seen as beneficial for all involved (Alagoz, et al., 2010; Neuhauser & Kreps, 2003; Rocker et al., 2014). On the other hand, not everyone is from individualistic cultures, meaning certain individuals belong to cultures on the opposing extreme of individualism (i.e., collectivism). Those individuals who identify with collectivistic culture tend to focus more on the relationship developed along the lines of families, groups among others. At the same time, collective cultures sometimes exhibit the power distance dimension (e.g., Japanese) where individuals tend to defer their own power to those with higher status within the collectives. This could be supervisor, parents and expert professionals such as healthcare givers. We contend that these differences would play a role in whether people embrace E-Health. For instance, Rocker et al (2014) indicate that there are differences within users in a particular culture (intracultural such as age and gender differences) and that the difference is more pronounced when comparing other cultures (intercultural). The impact of collectives on health decisions has been recognized by the health belief model which stresses the importance of larger social contexts as central to health actions taken, rather than strict emphasis on individuals as primary decision maker (e.g., Kifle, et al., 2010; Neuhauser & Kreps, 2003; Rocker et al., 2014; Wilkowska, Ziefle, & Alagoz, 2012). This effects such things as the extent that individuals may seek to take or not undertake preventive actions for an underlying illness or disease and how they use e-health to seek information about their conditions. One such example, involves the belief known as *fatalism* – which address the idea that disease are divinely ordained and as such there is nothing anyone can do about it but to accept it. Fatalism has been found to be rampant among African Americans and other ethnic groups (Kressin & Petersen, 2001). Fatalism among these group has been linked to the consideration that *seeking help for hypertension* is a sign of weakness (Gibbons, 2005; Rose, Kim, Dennison, & Hill, 2000). These beliefs, however are also considered as partially responsible for the non-compliance to medication as prescribed and inadequate self-monitoring of blood pressure among African-Americans as well (Chobanian et al., 2003). It needs to be said that fatalism is not an outcome of e-health but such a belief will hinder how people view and seek information about their health and thus impact attitude toward e-health.

More specific to e-health however, is the fact that, the distinction in cultural world view has been found in conformance to standards of electronic health records between Americans and Chinese. Specifically, Xu, et al., (2011) compared the level of conformity in American and Chinese electronic health records (EHR) to the international standards (i.e., ISO/TS 18308) and found that the Chinese standard conform at a lower rate (77%) than the Americans (89.5%). Consequently, the study concluded that the Chinese EHR standards should focus on addressing issues such as privacy, security and relationship attributes in data characteristics. This findings, is not necessarily surprising given that societies view issues of privacy and security among other variables differently depending on how the concepts are operationalized (e.g., Olaniran, 2008). Perhaps more telling is Xu et al., (2011)'s recommendation that future investigations should take a closer look at relational attributes of data itself. This is more evident in the observation that e-health data, when taken out of context is otherwise meaningless. For example, part of the EHR architecture provide guidelines for medical record governing three different scenarios for the Chinese (again focusing on the context) 1. Modern medicine, 2. Traditional Chinese Medicine (TCM), and 3. Integration of modern medicine with TCM also known as CAM. Thus, if care is not taken to discern which of these three contexts along with specific details such as history of the patients, any such data with be meaningless. Dominguez-Mayo et al (2015) discuss this idea when addressing the issue of regulatory compliance in e-health. Furthermore, Xu et al (2011) indicate that "the explicit expression of relationship among information cannot only help clinicians to rebuild and understand the clinical context and make informed decisions, but also facilitates semantic retrieval" (p. 559). The next section examines the aspect of CAM and implication for e-health.

E-Health and Alternative/Complementary Medicinal Practice

An area of concern is the increase in popularity and use of alternative medical practice. According to an estimate, more than 70% of the developing world's population still rely on complementary and alternative systems of medicine (Shaikh & Hatcher, 2005). Also contributing to this trend is the fact that cultural beliefs and practices along with proximity to healthcare facilities often lead individuals to seek out self-care or home remedies and consultation with alternative healers especially for those living in rural areas (Imogie, Agwubike, & Aluko, 2002; Shaikh & Hatcher, 2005). CAM practitioners often play dual or multiple roles including clergyman, faith and spiritual healers (Shaikh & Hatcher, 2002). If indeed alternative medicine plays such a big role in the general healthcare for many people in the developing world we belief it may impact e-health in terms of whether people are able to get CAM information through it. Similarly, these cultural beliefs may impact the level of trust in such systems along with perceived safety (Dominguez-Mayo et al., 2015). For instance, some evidence based CAM suggests that alternative medicine are the first choice for individuals with health problems including *infertility, epilepsy, psychosomatic troubles, depression and even in child birth* (Imogie, et al., 2002; Obasola et al., 2015; Shaikh & Hatcher, 2005).

Notwithstanding, the role of culture cannot be overstated in delivery of care within alternative medicine. For instance, significant number of cultures tend to be collectivistic when compared to some developed Western cultures and hence these collectivistic cultures lean more to oral traditions and not necessarily written traditions which is more tenable for digitizing information. This discrepancy is noted in a study comparing 925 health websites in Gulf cooperation council countries (GCC), which found that in spite of large immigrant workers in the region that speaks Hindi, Tamil, and Tagalog only one website is available in language other than Arabic and English (Weber, Verjee, Rahman, Ameerudeen & Al-Baz, 2015). CAM also involve the mixing of herbs and/or mind-body approaches that have been known to show medical benefits (NIH, 2009). Others have found that CAM is a way for older Chinese immigrants in U.S.A. to connect with their culture of origin, perform their social roles, and a way to hang on to values within that society just as Hofstede dimension of culture predicted (see Kong & Hsieh, 2012). Those who are involved in CAM know the need to customize treatment to each patient. In other words, CAM is quite contrary to the western medicinal practice of *one size fits all* that tends to dominate prescription for ailment. Rather, attention to overall mind-body wellbeing and what herbs do along with the quantity and quality for different patients is just as important in the effectiveness of the treatment or prescription (Ergil, Kramer, & Ng, 2002). This dynamic factor creates a challenge in digitizing such information indiscriminately to the extent that one can argue that CAM is both an art and science form. For instance, taking the concept of TCM's acupuncture, one of the mind-body approaches, there are different variations and techniques depending on how healthcare practitioners perceive the patient symptoms (Bishop, Amos, Yu, & Lewith, 2012; Lewin, 1974; Veith, 1973).

The educational structure for mastering alternative medicinal practices are mostly based on apprenticeship. As such, the relationship between the conventional allopathic physicians and alternative medicine practitioners are contentious because orthodox medicine has rarely been in favor of alternative medicine (Fink, 2002; Imogie, et al., 2002; Shaikh & Hatcher, 2005). Hence, alternative medicine is vigorously denounced as nothing but unproven and antiscientific procedure not worthy of devoting time to and the practitioners are sometimes misconceived as nothing but quacks. More recently, however, the boundaries between complementary and conventional medicine overlap and change with time. For example, guided imagery and massage, both once considered complementary or alternative, are used in some hospitals to help with pain management (Bishop, et al., 2012).

On the other hand, due to the apprenticeship nature of traditional medicine and the fact that they are mostly practiced by local and indigenous people, no formal repository mechanism exists for gathering and storing of information either as a way to verify or prove their effectiveness (Shaikh & Hatcher, 2005). At the same time, the lack of storage or digitizing data about alternative medicines also points to the threats of their continued sustainability and impending eradication altogether. Again, these problems underscore the challenge for e-health with alternative medicines when one weighs the difference between oral tradition and written tradition, or digital cultures, as information preservation are passed orally and often generationally rather than through centralized system such as e-health.

While conventional and alternative medicines do have their disagreements, it needs to be emphasized that the faith of clients or consumers in CAM is nonetheless real. Similarly, culture and traditions that underlie CAM use cannot be easily dismissed and should be addressed. For instance, Imogie et al., (2002) presents the case of the traditional birth attendants (TBAs) health care in Nigeria. They found that preference for TBAs by rural dwellers have both cultural and economic precedence. TBAs are seen by patrons as members of their extended family (a view aligning with collectivistic dimension) who can communicate or speak same language and are perceived as being trustworthy (see also Abel & Obeten, 2015). It is however unknown how the same level of trust can be conveyed using e-health, given that people have come to develop trust based on the relationship they build with individuals they know.

In the developed countries, the average 12-month prevalence of CAM use was 41.1% and the average lifetime prevalence was 51.8% in UK (Posadzki, Watson, Alotaibi, & Ernst, 2013), and estimates of 12-month prevalence of CAM use (excluding prayer) showed remarkable stability in Australia (49%, 52%, 52%; 1993, 2000, 2004) and USA (36%, 38%; 2002, 2007) (Harris, Cooper, Relton, & Thomas, 2012). The issue may not be so much e-health platforms and apps cannot be used to deliver life-saving information or aid CAM use as much as getting people to change to adopting e-health technology. A study in Sub-Sahara Africa found that e-health cannot replace health workers and more importantly, that health workers are crucial for e-health success and adoption (Obasola et al., 2015).

Furthermore, from culture perspective, the concepts of *universals and particulars* also underscore the notion of oral knowledge and a shift to written knowledge (Veltman, 2004). Universals focus on the attempt to standardize information possibly for multiple users. Particulars, on the other hand, focus on the nature of information for specific contextual use. There is tension between universals and particulars that creates challenge for e-health. For instance, different herbs may serve a similar purpose given that plants availability are geographically located and hence digitizing such information from e-health may offer little help. This may raise the question of how valuable is e-health when information offer through it may be unable to address user's need and especially with CAM?

Linguistic Challenges in E-Health

The language in which electronic medical record is kept creates another area of concern for e-health. Although, English has been dubbed as the *de facto* language of the Internet and Internet commerce (Kayman, 2004) it needs to be said that English is not always the language in which medical or electronic records are kept and this poses a challenge for non-English speakers from different standpoints. One reason entails the inability of indigenous people to comprehend and use technologies because of a language barrier is vivid (Olaniran,, 2007; Olaniran & Edgell, 2008; Kawachi, 1999). From a different standpoint is also the fact that inability to comprehend information directly limits adoption and usage of a technology or innovation (Kawachi, 1999; Olaniran & Edgell, 2008) like e-health (Abel & Obeten, 2015; Obasola et al., 2015). Consequently, language hindrances prevent the accomplishment of the potential socio-economic benefits from ICTs in less economically developed countries (LEDCs) (Kazakan & Dada, 2008; Olaniran, 2008; Omojola, 2009).

Since the majority of Internet content is in the English language, this threatens nations whose primary language is not English making them feel that their languages need protection. The problem with English as a primary language of communication also emanates from the issue of identity (Olaniran, Rodriguez, Olaniran, & Olaniran, 2013). There are countries that believe English as part of their colonial heritage and are trying to move away from it (Kayman, 2004). Furthermore, some view an increase in the use of English within communication technology that creates a divide that widens the gap between the "haves" and the "have-nots" (Crystal, 2003; Kayman, 2004). Kayman (2004) went on to argue that the association of English with communication technology that reinforces its claim as the primary medium of globalization branded as the language of interaction. Universally, the reliance on the English language as the vehicle of global communication creates difficulty—especially among those individuals with little competence in the English language. One could make the arguments that there are web based e-health platforms and phone apps that could allow conversion from English to other languages. Unfortunately, this is not the case for all languages and language conversion apps cannot take into account localized expressions (Obasola et al., 2015). Consequently this fact also restricts some countries' resistance to adopt technologies and specifically, e-health.

Furthermore, language is viewed as the most important element of a culture (Omojola, 2009; Salawu, 2006). When one looks at the power distance dimension of cultural variability it can be argued that language embodied this dimension. For instance, it has been suggested that African countries with diverse indigenous languages are presented with a colonial legacy of acculturation where they are forced to communicate in a second language (e.g., English or French). As a result, their primary language is subjugated to a secondary category and in some cases no position at all (Mbagwu & Obiamalu, 2009; Omojola, 2009). For example, Nigeria has over 360 languages and dialects, yet individuals are compelled to communicate in English or some version of English which categorizes English speakers to the elite group (i.e., powerful) while non-fluent speakers are simply categorized as illiterates (i.e., less powerful).

Similarly, the power distance pronouncement can be seeing in how *Microsoft office*, which is offered in over 27 languages, was offered in Italian, which is spoken by 60 million people located in Italy, Switzerland, and Croatia. On the other hand, other languages that come close to, or exceeded, this figure are not given the same treatment (Omojola, 2009). A case in point is Hausa spoken by over 70 million, Swahili, by 100 million and even Yoruba spoken by another 40 million are not given the same level of recognition when compared to English or French (Loubser, 2010; Omojola, 2009; Olaniran, 2012). Computer keyboard design and letters on computers make it difficult to write some words in local languages thereby rendering some languages as irrelevant or extinct. This is not unique to Nigeria or Africa, but rather around the globe. Similarly, the oral tradition of Nigerian and African cultures hinders e-health adoption and consequent use, given that e-health requires and favors digitization or written cultures (Olaniran, 2008). In essence, the elite group, or fluent English speakers, are advantaged in accessing information from e-health. However, access to technology is directly determined by knowledge of the foreign language that in most cases people may not understand. Hence, individuals especially in the LEDCs may be hesitant in adopting new technologies such as e-health as another agent of globalization to spread Western values across the world (Omojola, 2009; Yau, 2004). Consequently, indigenous cultures are considered insignificant with ICTs. Therefore, this relegates some of these cultures into irrelevance in which they appear as non-consequential in the grand scheme (Omojola, 2009; Salawu, 2006).

Other Factors

Internet/Infrastructure

The issue of access to ICTs and subsequently e-health was raised earlier. In order for E-Health to serve users, there must be opportunity to access it. While there is an explosion in the growth of mobile phones one needs to understand that not everyone can afford one and also the fact that not all mobile phones are able to connect to the Internet. Yet most e-health applications require the need to be on some form of internet networks. However, data from internetworldstats (see Table 1) indicate disparities across regions of the world in this area. For instance, less than a third (i.e., 27.5%) of people in Africa have access to or use the internet. The figure in Asia is not much better either as approximately 1/3 (34.8) of the people have internet access. Put in another way, regions with 71.5% of the world population have less than a quarter (23.7%) of its people as internet users. In essence, there is a digital divide which will also impact adoption and use of E-Health. Aside from disparity in internet access, there are other infrastructure that can hinder or promote E-Health use. Mobile telephone or computer use needs to be powered by electricity a factor that is often taken for granted. However most developing nations suffer from frequent power outage or what has been termed as *epileptic power* that could further hinder access to e-health information (Abel & Obeten, 2015; Idowu, Cranford, & Bastin, 2008; Obasola, et al., 2015).

Table 1. Regional internet usage statistics as a percentage of population

Regions	Population	Users (% of Population)
Africa	1,158,353,014	27.5
Asia	4,032,654,624	34.8
Europe	827,566,464	70.4
Middle East	236,137,235	48.1
North America	357,172,209	86.9
Latin America	615,583,127	52.4
Oceania/Australia	37,157,120	72.1
World Total	7,264,623,793	42.4%

Based on December 31, 2014 data. Obtained from www.internetworldstats.com

Age

Age is another factor affecting adoption of ICTs. Most technological innovations such as e-health is believed to be targeted by designers at young adults or millennials, and males in the middle and upper class of western nations (Rocker, et al., 2014; Rogers, 2009; Ziefle & Jakobs, 2010). Thus, older adults who traditionally are less technically competent in the use of ICTs may be disadvantaged with e-health possibilities in terms of its adoption and use. The disadvantage is believed to not be limited to *cognitive and sensory* capacity but also in terms of the technology acceptance (Heart & Kalderon, 2011; Kifle et al., 2010; Rocker et al., 2014). Similarly, educated older adults received their education at a time ICT are not ubiquitous (Rocker, 2014). Age is also an aspect of culture in particular the power distance dimension where the elderlies usually dictate or set the tones for what is acceptable and what is not and the youths are supposed to comply (Kifle, et al., 2010). Hence, if elderlies are the ones who are less technically inclined, it is doubtful that they will hold a positive view of ICTs or e-health and subsequently they may resist adoption of the technology.

Gender

Gender also seems to be another factor impacting ICT use. Consequently, gender is important in understanding acceptance of pervasive medical technologies (i.e., e-health) (Rocker, et al., 2014). Studies indicated that women reported lower levels of technology *self-efficacy* and anxiety when compare to men, which could negatively bias e-health acceptance and other pervasive medical technologies (Rocker et al., 2014; Wilkowska, Gaul, & Ziefle, 2010). Like age, gender treatment is also an aspect of culture that can be explained by the power distance dimension. In some collectivistic cultures, women do not enjoy the same treatment as men and are often refused education that could offer them technical literacy needed to use ICTs or e-health.

SOLUTIONS AND RECOMMENDATIONS

When e-health and other technologies are designed and implemented, the effects of people's attitudes and cultures are seldom taken into consideration. Consequently, emphasis appears to focus on what technology and e-health offers. Neuhauser and Kreps (2003) echoed this idea when they suggested that e-health technical promises may be effective only when the social reality of how different individuals accept them (see also, Wickramasinghe, Fadlalla, Geisler, & Schaffer, 2005). Similarly, ICTs have intended purposes, which can be positive or negative depending on how they are used (Olaniran, 2007). Also, the drive towards e-health may indirectly embed *hegemonic discrimination* against oral tradition and creates a dilemma for how different people view e-health even when these effects are unintentional (Olaniran, 2009; Rocker et al., 2014).

With pervasive medical technology such as e-health gradually entering personal spaces and *private spheres* it raises questions about control, risk, privacy, and reliability that are crucial for eventual adoption and use that must be addressed (Dominguez-Mayo, et al., 2015; Rocker, 2014). Furthermore, one must examine society attitudes toward e-health target groups in terms of the assumption about how we treat elderly, women, and others based on social classifications (Rocker et al., 2014). For example, the notion of false sense of inclusive reality seems applicable to e-health. If one assumes that e-health is the solution for reaching traditionally underserved people (rural, elderlies, women, illiterates, etc.,) when the reality is that e-health may further alienate these people either through digital divide or digital illiteracy.

As the push for e-health continues, there is a need to consider how to bridge the global digital divide locally and especially in LEDCs. A significant number of people around the globe still lives in rural communities and towns with no electricity and phones, it becomes increasingly difficult to take advantage of e-health even if they want to. To this end, accessibility and affordability poses a challenge for e-health implementation and eventual adoption especially when a choice must be made between meeting basic economic needs versus information needs (Kazakan & Dada, 2008; Olaniran, 2008; Omojola, 2009). Also, providing and using e-health in a culturally appropriate manner is pressing, in an attempt to adapt e-health to improve health needs of the disadvantaged people and those who live in rural communities.

e-health must help in avoiding the perception that befell other ICTs as a way to help commoditize Western culture ideals in LEDCs. There needs to be reciprocal exchange and cultural learning. One area for such learning and cultural exchange is the need for integration of traditional with contemporary medicinal practices. Integrative medicine has emerged to provide care that is patient centered, healing oriented, emphasizes the therapeutic relationship, and uses therapeutic approaches originating from conventional and alternative medicine. (Maizes, Rakel, & Niemiec, 2009) Such integration may also hold promise in fostering trust in health information and overall e-health

FUTURE RESEARCH DIRECTIONS

One area that future research can focus is the need to recognize that e-health makes its most contribution in allowing communication or health information to change from being passive to a more active and interaction driven (Neuhauser & Kreps, 2003; Rice & Katz, 2001). Hence, for e-health information to be effective, one must figure out a way to accomplish this level of engagement with users, but only by focusing on communication reality where e-health must address user attitudes in their own cultural contexts. Failure to acknowledge this reality would have a deleterious effect including abject resistance to the e-health.

There appears to be a mismatch in the rational assumption that technology innovation will survive in any environment as long as it is fulfilling a need by virtue of acculturation (Kifle et al., 2010). However, more and more studies are indicating that the technology acculturation assumption rarely holds. Thus it is recommended the need to account for the cultural contexts and/or social factors influencing technology such as e-health adoption and use. Thus it might be worthwhile for future research to explore perhaps how culture in particular collectivistic and power distance aspects of a culture can be used to get people to accept e-health. For example, can a power distant culture where submission to hierarchy is the norm succeed in mandating people to use a particular technology? Similarly it would be worthwhile to explore how poor LEDCs are circumventing the cost associated with e-health in an attempt to reach individuals in rural area without the necessary infrastructure needed to use e-health.

CONCLUSION

This article identifies challenges facing e-health especially from global standpoint. One area of focus is the role of culture and its impact on individuals' subsequent use of e-health. The artricle stresses the importance of culture by elucidating certain factors that impact and complicate e-health acceptance and adoption. Finally, the article identifies areas for future direction in e-health.

REFERENCES

Abel, E. E., & Obeten, E. (2015). Funding E-Health in Nigeria by NGOS/Multinational Organization: Overview and Perspectives. *International Journal of Computers and Applications, 111*(11).

Alagöz, F., Calero Valdez, A., Wilkowska, W., Ziefle, M., Dorner, S., & Holzinger, A. (2010). From cloud computing to mobile internet, from user focus to culture and hedonism: The crucible of mobile health care and wellness applications. *IEEE 5th International Conference on Pervasive Computing and Applications, 1*, 38–45.

Balch, D. C., & Tichenor, J. M. (1997). Telemedicine expanding the scope of health care information. *Journal of the American Medical Informatics Association, 4*(1), 1–5. doi:10.1136/jamia.1997.0040001 PMID:8988467

Bishop, F. L., Amos, N., Yu, H., & Lewith, G. T. (2012). Health-care sector and complementary medicine: Practitioners' experiences of delivering acupuncture in the public and private sectors. *Primary Health Care Research and Development, 13*(03), 269–278. doi:10.1017/S1463423612000035 PMID:22317950

Chang, S., & Gibbons, M. (2008). Healthcare System Factors in Healthcare Disparities. In M. Gibbons (Ed.), *e-health solutions for healthcare disparities* (pp. 30–38). Baltimore, MD: Springer. doi:10.1007/978-0-387-72815-5_4

Chobanian, A. V., Bakris, G. L., Black, H. R., Cushman, W. C., Green, L. A., & Izzo, J. L. Jr et al.. (2003). The seventh report of the joint national committee on prevention, detection, evaluation, and treatment of high blood pressure: The JNC 7 report. *Journal of the American Medical Association, 289*, 2560–2572. doi:10.1001/jama.289.19.2560 PMID:12748199

Crystal, D. (2003). *English as a global language* (2nd ed.). Cambridge University Press. doi:10.1017/CBO9780511486999

Domínguez-Mayo, F. J., Escalona, M. J., Mejías, M., Aragón, G., García-García, J. A., Torres, J., & Enríquez, J. G. (2015). A Strategic Study about Quality Characteristics in e-Health Systems Based on a Systematic Literature Review. *The Scientific World Journal.* PMID:26146656

Dunn, P., & Marinetti, A. (2002). *Cultural adaptation: necessity for global e-learning.* Retrieved March 10, 2014, from http://www.linezine.com

Ergil, K. V., Kramer, E. J., & Ng, A. T. (2002). Chinese herbal medicines. *The Western Journal of Medicine, 176*(4), 275–279. Retrieved from http://www.ncbi.nlm.nih.gov/pmc/articles/PMC1071750/ PMID:12208838

Ess, C., & Sudweeks, F. (2005). Culture and computer-mediated communication: Toward new understandings. *Journal of Computer-Mediated Communication, 11*(1), 179–191. Retrieved onJuly172006. doi:10.1111/j.1083-6101.2006.tb00309.x

Fink, S. (2002). International efforts spotlight traditional, complementary, and alternative medicine. *American Journal of Public Health, 92*(11), 1734–1739. doi:10.2105/AJPH.92.11.1734 PMID:12406796

Gibbons, M. C. (2005). Patient Factors in Healthcare Disparities. In M. Gibbons (Ed.), *eHealth solutions for healthcare disparities* (pp. 19–29). Springer.

Harris, P., Cooper, K., Relton, C., & Thomas, K. (2012). Prevalence of complementary and alternative medicine (CAM) use by the general population: A systematic review and update. *International Journal of Clinical Practice, 66*(10), 924–939. doi:10.1111/j.1742-1241.2012.02945.x PMID:22994327

Heart, T., & Kalderon, E. (2013). Older adults: Are they ready to adopt health-related ICT? *International Journal of Medical Informatics, 82*(11), e209–e231. doi:10.1016/j.ijmedinf.2011.03.002 PMID:21481631

Hofstede, G. (1996). *Cultures and organizations: Software of the mind.* New York: McGraw Hill.

Hofstede, G., & Bond, M. (1984). Hofstede's cultural dimensions: An independent validation using Rokeach's value survey. *Journal of Cross-Cultural Psychology, 15*(4), 417–433. doi:10.1177/0022002184015004003

Hofstede, G. H., & Hofstede, G. (2001). Culture's consequences: Comparing values, behaviors, institutions and organizations across nations. *Sage (Atlanta, Ga.).*

Imogie, A. O., Agwubike, E. O., & Aluko, K. (2002). Assessing the role of traditional birth attendants (TBAs) in health care delivery in Edo State, Nigeria. *African Journal of Reproductive Health, 6*(2), 94–100. doi:10.2307/3583135 PMID:12476721

Kawachi, P. (1999). *When the sun doesn't rise: Empirical findings that explain the exclusion of Japanese from online global education.* Retrieved on August 26, 2005 from http://www.ignou.ac.in/Theme-3/Paul%20%20KAWACHI.html

Kayman, M. (2004). The state of English as a global language: Communicating culture. *Textual Practice, 18*(1), 1–22. doi:10.1080/0950236032000140131

Kazakan, C., & Dada, J. (2008). Rural women's use of cell phones to meet their communication needs: A study from northern Nigeria. In African Women & ICTs: Investigating Technology, Gender, & Empowerment, (pp. 44-55). International Development Research Center.

Kifle, M., Payton, F. C., Mbarika, V., & Meso, P. (2010). Transfer and adoption of advanced information technology solutions in resource-poor environments: The case of telemedicine systems adoption in Ethiopia. *Telemedicine Journal and e-Health, 16*(3), 327–343. doi:10.1089/tmj.2009.0008 PMID:20406120

Kressin, N. R., & Petersen, L. A. (2001). Racial differences in the use of invasive cardiovascular procedures: Review of the literature and prescription for future research. *Annals of Internal Medicine, 135*(5), 352–366. doi:10.7326/0003-4819-135-5-200109040-00012 PMID:11529699

Kreuter, M. W., & McClure, S. M. (2004). The Role of culture in Health Communication. *Annual Review of Public Health, 25*(1), 439–455. doi:10.1146/annurev.publhealth.25.101802.123000 PMID:15015929

Lewin, A. J. (1974). Acupuncture and Its Role in Modern Medicine. *Western Journal of Medicine, 120*(1), 27–32. http://www.ncbi.nlm.nih.gov/pmc/articles/PMC1129299/?page=2]121`

Loubser, H. (2010, August 10). We speak your language. *Technet Blog.* Retrieved from http://blogs.technet.com/b/microsoft_on_the_issues_africa/archive/2010/08/10/we-speak-your-language.aspx

MacFadyen, L. (2008). The perils of parsimony: "National culture" as red herring? *Proceedings of the Sixth International Conference on Cultural Attitudes towards Technology and Communication.*

Maizes, V., Rakel, D., & Niemiec, C. (2009, September-October). Integrative medicine and patient-centered care. *Explore (New York, N.Y.), 5*(5), 277–289. doi:10.1016/j.explore.2009.06.008 PMID:19733814

Martin, J., & Cheong, P. (2007). Cultural Considerations of Online Pedagogy. In K. St.Amant & S. Kelsey (Eds.), *Computer-Mediated Communication across Cultures: International Interaction in Online Environments*. IGI Global.

Mbagwu, D. U., & Obiamalu, G. O. (2009). Documentation of African Languages: A Panacea for the Negative Effects of Globalization. *OGIRISI: a New Journal of African Studies*, 6(1), 86–92.

Neuhauser, L., & Kreps, G. L. (2003). Rethinking communication in e-health era. *Journal of Health Psychology*, 8(1), 7–23. doi:10.1177/1359105303008001426 PMID:22113897

NIH. (2009, March). *Traditional Chinese Medicine: An Introduction*. NCCAM Pub No. D428. Retrieved from http://nccam.nih.gov/health/whatiscam/chinesemed.htm

Olaniran, B. A. (2004). Computer-mediated communication in cross-cultural virtual groups. In *Dialogue among Diversities* (pp. 142–166). Washington, DC: NCA.

Olaniran, B. A. (2007). Challenges to implementing e-learning in lesser developed countries. In A. Edmundson (Ed.), *Globalized e-Learning Cultural Challenges* (pp. 18–34). Idea Group. doi:10.4018/978-1-59904-301-2.ch002

Olaniran, B. A. (2008). A proposition for developing trust and relational synergy in international e-collaborative groups. Handbook of research in electronic collaboration and organizational synergy, 2.

Olaniran, B. A. (2012). Culture and New Media: Exploring Cultural Challenges in E-Learning. In P. Cheong, J. Martin, & L. McFadyen (Eds.), *New Media and Intercultural Communication* (pp. 61–74). New York: Peter Lang.

Olaniran, B. A., & Edgell, D. (2008). Cultural implications of collaborative information technologies (CITs) in international online collaborations and global virtual teams. In P. Zemliansky & K. St-Amant (Eds.), *Handbook of Global virtual workspaces* (pp. 118–133). Hershey, PA: IGI Global. doi:10.4018/978-1-59904-893-2.ch010

Olaniran, B. A., Rodriguez, N. B., Olaniran, O. S., & Olaniran, O. O. (2013). Culture and Some Unintended Consequences of Computer-Mediated Communication (CMC) in Africa: Using Nigeria as a Case Study. In Handbook of Research on Discourse Behavior and Digital Communication: Language Structures and Social Interaction. Hershey, PA: IGI Global.

Omojola, O. (2009). English-oriented ICTs and ethnic language survival strategies in Africa. Global Media Journal-African Edition, 3(1), 33-45.

Posadzki, P., Watson, L. K., Alotaibi, A., & Ernst, E. (2013). Prevalence of use of complementary and alternative medicine (CAM) by patients/consumers in the UK: Systematic review of surveys. *Clinical Medicine*, 13(2), 126–131. doi:10.7861/clinmedicine.13-2-126 PMID:23681857

Rice, R. E., & Katz, J. E. (2001). Preface. In R. E. Rice & J. E. Katz (Eds.), *The Internet and health communication* (pp. xiii–xvi). Thousand Oaks, CA: Sage.

Röcker, C., Ziefle, M., & Holzinger, A. (2014). From computer innovation to human integration: current trends and challenges for pervasive Health Technologies. In *Pervasive Health* (pp. 1–17). Springer London. doi:10.1007/978-1-4471-6413-5_1

Rogers, Y. (2009). The Changing Face of Human-Computer Interaction in the Age of Ubiquitous Computing. In A. Holzinger & K. Miesenberger (Eds.), *Human Computer-Interaction and Usability for e-Inclusion. LNCS 5889* (pp. 1–19). Berlin: Springer. doi:10.1007/978-3-642-10308-7_1

Rose, L., Kim, M., Dennison, C., & Hill, M. (2000). The context of adherance for African-Americans with high blood pressure. *Journal of Advanced Nursing, 32*(3), 587–594. doi:10.1046/j.1365-2648.2000.01538.x PMID:11012800

Salawu, A. (2006). *Paradox of a milieu: Communicating in African indigenous languages in the age of globalisation. In Indigenous Language Media in Africa* (pp. 1–20). Lagos: CBAAC.

Scholl, J. C., & Olaniran, B. A. (2013). ICT Use and Multidisciplinary Healthcare Teams. In M. Cruz-Cunha, I. Miranda, & P. Gonçalves (Eds.), *Handbook of Research on ICTs for Human-Centered Healthcare and Social Care Services* (pp. 627–645). Hershey, PA: Medical Information Science Reference; doi:10.4018/978-1-4666-3986-7.ch033

Shaikh, B. T., & Hatcher, J. (2005). Complementary and alternative medicine in Pakistan: Prospects and limitations. *Evidence-Based Complementary and Alternative Medicine, 2*(2), 139–142. doi:10.1093/ecam/neh088 PMID:15937553

Shiferaw, F., & Zolfo, M. (2012). The role of information communication technology (ICT) towards universal health coverage: the first steps of a telemedicine project in Ethiopia. *Global Health Action, 5*.

Smith, P. B. (2002). Culture's consequences: Something old and something new. *Human Relations, 55*(1), 119–135. doi:10.1177/0018726702055001603

US Department of Health and Human Services. (2004). *Secretary Thompson, Seeking Fastest Possible Results, Names First Health Information Technology Coordinator. News Release.* Washington, DC: US Department of Health and Human Services.

Veith, I. (1973). Acupuncture in traditional Chinese medicine. An historical review. *California Medicine, 118*(2), 70–79. Retrieved from http://www.ncbi.nlm.nih.gov/pmc/articles/PMC1455171/?page=1 PMID:4573752

Veltman, K. H. (2004). Towards a semantic web for culture. *Journal of Digital Information, 4*(4), 3–15. http://jodi.ecs.soton.ac.uk/v04/v104

Viswanath, K., & Kreuter, M. W. (2007). Health disparities, communication inequalities, and e-health: A commentary. *American Journal of Preventive Medicine, 32*(5Suppl), S131–S133. doi:10.1016/j.amepre.2007.02.012 PMID:17466818

Wald, H. S., Dube, C. E., & Anthony, D. C. (2007). Untangling the Web—the impact of Internet use on health care and the physician–patient relationship. *Patient Education and Counseling, 68*(3), 218–224. doi:10.1016/j.pec.2007.05.016 PMID:17920226

Weber, A. S., Verjee, M., Rahman, Z. H., Ameerudeen, F., & Al-Baz, N. (2014). Typology and credibility of Internet health websites originating from Gulf Cooperation Council countries. *EMHJ, 20*(12).

Wickramasinghe, N. S., Fadlalla, A. M. A., Geisler, E., & Schaffer, J. L. (2005). A framework for assessing e-health preparedness. *International Journal of Electronic Healthcare, 1*(3), 316–334. doi:10.1504/IJEH.2005.006478 PMID:18048213

Wilkowska, W., Gaul, S., & Ziefle, M. (2010). A Small but Significant Difference – the Role of Gender on the Acceptance of Medical Assistive Technologies. In G. Leitner, M. Hitz, & A. Holzinger (Eds.), *HCI in Work and Learning, Life and Leisure USAB 2010, LNCS 6389* (pp. 82–100). Berlin, Heidelberg: Springer. doi:10.1007/978-3-642-16607-5_6

Wilkowska, W., Ziefle, M., & Alagoez, F. (2012). How user diversity and country of origin impact the readiness to adopt e-health technologies: An intercultural comparison. *Work (Reading, Mass.), 41*, 2072–2080. PMID:22317022

Xu, W., Guan, Z., Cao, H., Zhang, H., Lu, M., & Li, T. (2011). Analysis and evaluation of the electronic health record standard in China: A comparison with the American national standard ASTM E 1384. *International Journal of Medical Informatics, 80*(8), 555–561. doi:10.1016/j.ijmedinf.2011.05.003 PMID:21680236

Yau, Y. (2004). Globalisation, ICTs and the new imperialism: Perspective on Africa in the global electronic village. *Review of African Political Economy, 99*, 11–29. doi:10.1080/0305624042000258397

Ziefle, M., & Jakobs, E.-M. (2010). *New challenges in Human Computer Interaction: Strategic Directions and Interdisciplinary Trends*. 4th International Conference on Competitive Manufacturing Technologies, University of Stellenbosch, South Africa.

KEY TERMS AND DEFINITIONS

Complementary and Alternative Medicine: Focuses on the integration of traditional or alternative medicinal practices into contemporary medical practices.

Culture: Represents different value preferences that influence communication interaction and how people create meaning.

Dimensions of Cultural Variability: Shows or represents Cultural differences.

E-Health: Focuses on the provision and delivery of health information over electronic medium.

Information Communication Technologies: Electronic devices that aid in the transmission of information and interactions in terms of conveying messages.

Oral Tradition: Represents cultures whose main focus is in oral communication.

Written Tradition: Describes cultures who emphasizes textual information and hence makes information or messages suitable for digitizing.

The Role of Gender in Technology Acceptance for Medical Education

Laura Briz-Ponce
University of Salamanca, Spain

Juan Antonio Juanes-Méndez
University of Salamanca, Spain

Francisco José García-Peñalvo
University of Salamanca, Spain

INTRODUCTION

The history of women in Medicine dates to 3500 before common era (BCE). During a lot of years, women were actively discouraged from the practice of surgery (Wirtzfeld, 2009). Regulations for the practice of surgery were widely recognized and often barred women. For example, in 1313, women were not allowed to practice of surgery in Paris unless examined by a competent jury (Lipinska, 1930). However, women continued to practice without formal training or recognition for the next several centuries (Wirtzfeld, 2009).

A lot of years after that, woman started to rebel and wanted to have a formal training and have the opportunity for studying medicine. In 1847, Harriet Hunt was the first woman to apply to Harvard Medical School and her request was rejected ("A profile and history of Women in Medicine", 2013).

However, Elizabeth Blackwell was the first women in America to receive her medical degree (1849). She decided to be a doctor when a close friend who was dying suggested she would have been spared her worst suffering if her physician had been a woman ("Changing the Face of Medicine | Dr. Elizabeth Blackwell", n.d.). She applied to several Schools of Medicine but all of them rejected her request. There was a medical school, Geneva Medical College that decided not assume the sole responsibility for denying the request, so to justify their own decision, they asked the students thinking they would reject the proposal. On the contrary, the students themselves voted "yes", so Elizabeth was accepted to study medicine (Morantz-Sanchez, 2000). There were other women that were considered the first woman in their countries as Emily Jennings Stowe in Canada (Hacker, 1984) who graduated in 1867 or Dr. Aleu, the first Spanish woman who became a doctor in 1882 (López, 2007). In all those cases, it took them a great effort to become a physician and they were harshly criticized by the society. However, they achieved their goals and it was the beginning of a new hope for women.

Until 1970, women still were underrepresented considerably in the medical profession. Just fewer than 8% of US physicians were female. (A profile and history of Women in Medicine, 2013). However, this proportion was increasing steadily for the upcoming years as it is shown in Figure 1. This chart shows the percentage of female physicians since 1980 until 2013 for each country and it reveals that there has been a marked increase of the percentage each year reaching almost 50% in most part of the cases.

DOI: 10.4018/978-1-4666-9978-6.ch079

Figure 1. Percentage of female physicians in different countries
Source: Data obtained from OECD.StatExtracts Health Care Resources: Physicians by age and gender.

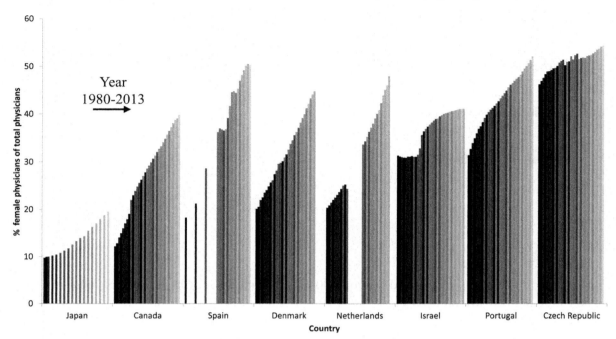

The woman incorporation into the workforce has encouraged the growth of number of woman in professions that used to be predominantly occupied by men. This culture change has impacted on Society, breaking the traditional rules imposed by them. Not only that, the woman are more employed in qualified jobs, opting for studying Social and HealthCare Sciences careers, whereas men are choosing to study more technical careers which it means a detriment to the other ones. This tendency is still growing, so for the last years, the students that signed up in Medical Schools are women in their majority. Approximately, since 1998, the proportion of female new students in Medical Schools in Spain is roughly 65%-71% (Estadística de Enseñanza Universitaria, 1998 a 2011).

In the EU7, the proportion of female physicians has increased between 1996 and 2006 in almost all Member States (41% of female physicians in 2006 compared with 35% in 1996) (Eurostat, 2009). According to Pololi (2010), the main reasons that they gave when they were asked were "they have loved Science in High School and College and wanted to use it to help people". Those figures reveal that women clearly impacted on Society, breaking the rules established by them and even defying them

On the other hand, the development of new technologies and its impact on Society are forcing changes on different sectors as Health and educational Area. According to Merriam-Webster, technology could be defined as "the use of science in industry, engineering etc to invent useful things or to solve problems". This is a general definition, but Merriam-Webster also considers technology as "the practical application of knowledge especially in a particular area" or " a manner of accomplishing a task especially using technical processes, methods, or knowledge". Burgelman, Christensen & Wheelwright, (2008) refers technology to "the theoretical and practical knowledge, skills and artefacts that can be used to develop products and services as well as their production and delivery systems". Other authors, as Pellisier (2008) does not consider technology as machines, but also as a concept related with human beings. This definition agreed with Simon (cited in Pellisier, 2008) that states that technology is "knowledge that is stored in millions of books, in hundreds of millions or billions of human heads, and, to an important ex-tent, in the artefacts themselves".

However, in the context of this paper, technology is not applied in a general way. This research is clearly focused in medical and educational area and how the doctors and teachers are incorporating mobile devices in their daily tasks or even the way they addressed to their patients or students respectively. These new technologies are allowing students to access information in a different way. Therefore, technologies could be remarked in this paper as any type of applications or devices used to access information any time anywhere.

Nowadays, practically most part of people owns a mobile device (Smartphone, tablet of both of them), what implies that the concept of accessing information is becoming more interactive and flexible. The potential that the new technologies offer in different contexts is already a reality. However, they are not yet widely and routinely used for work.

Because of that, the aim of this research is to make a first approach of Technology Acceptance in medical Education, considering that the incorporation of women to these sectors are becoming more and more a majority and we want to assess if this factor has exerted an impact on this sector.

Dillon and Morris (1998) defined technology acceptance as "the demonstrable willingness within a user group to employ information technology (IT) for the tasks it was designed to support "(p.5). Other authors (Hendrick and Brown, 1984) states technology acceptance as "an individual's psychological state with regard to his or her voluntary or intended use of a particular technology". Based on these definitions of technology acceptance, there are different models designed to measure the technological acceptance that contribute the methodology of this research. In this paper the method used is the Technology Acceptance Model proposed by Davis (1989)

This article is structured in this way. First, the paper gives a brief background of the situation of women in medical education. After that, the second section explains the methodology used for this research. This methodology includes an explanation of the process to collect data and the profile of the participants. The third section explains the results of this study. The study shows the comparison, on one hand between the acceptance of technology considering the different dimensions of the model and the gender and on the other hand between the score of the technology and the gender variable. Besides, this research explores the different factors that can influence of the acceptance of the technology. As part of the results and based on the analysis performed, a suggestion of pattern profile is explained. The next section exposes the future investigations that can complete more insights within this study. The last section draws the final conclusion on this investigation.

BACKGROUND

There were some researchers about the women in medicine and the role that they have had in the history. Some of them explain the differences that could exist in the attitude toward their technological abilities. The study findings published by Gefen & Straub (1997) suggested that researchers should include gender in IT diffusion models. In fact, it considered that gender has been generally missing from IT behavioral research. In this way, the gender is considered an engaging factor to assay in many researches.

For example (Hargittai & Shafer, 2006) analyzed the gender differences with respect to Internet-use ability. They tested how they self-perceived their abilities and how this may differ from gender. Their data suggested that overall men and women do not differ significantly in their online abilities. However, did also find that women are much more likely to have lower self-assessment regarding their web use skill and that may affect significantly the extent of their online behavior.

These findings are consistent with Correll's work (2001), which found that young women are less likely to perceive themselves as skilled in these domains. In the same way, another article examined the gender differences in computer attitudes and behaviors (Dambrot, Watkings-Malek, Silling, Marshall, & Garver, 1985). There were 944 students who agreed to take part in the study and they obtained that females were more negative in their attitudes toward computers.

Other research analyses the reasons of women to not become a scientific, and they claim that the culture determines the gender role in science and other traditionally male professions and it is created the psychological meaning of what it is to be male or female (Etzkowitz, Kemelgor, & Uzzi, 2000). Besides, there are some stereotypes since the primary school that make girls and then woman divert away from a scientific career. Similarly, Merrill (1991) suggested in his article that "males are more comfortable with new technologies than females", or Reinen & Plomp (1997) declared that females enjoy using the computer less than do male students.

There is one research conducted by Shaw and Marlow (1999) that makes an approach to evaluate students´ initial attitudes towards the use of Information and Communication Technology (ICT). They analyzed the data taking into account the gender and the age to find if there is any significant difference between them. The results reported considered that males feel more at ease with the new technology than females. By contrast, with Bonferroni's analysis, this significance disappears as Shaw and Marlow explained (1999). Besides, none other effect of gender was observed in the other dimensions described in the study.

Other study examined whether the technological innovation differentially affects men and women employees (Gutek & Bikson, 1985). They were also accord with the previous authors as they obtained that men are more familiar with computers than females but they added that women were more optimistic than men about the benefits of computer technology. However, Spennemann (cited in Shaw and Marlow, 1999) reported that females are less likely to own a personal computer.

This interpretation differs from that of Ory, Bullok & Burnaka (1997) who argued they did not find any significant gender differences from their use and attitudes about asynchronous learning networks (ALN) after one year of implementation in a university setting. They developed two surveys ("conferencing" and "web") and both of them were administered to 2151 students in different courses. Likewise, Mcdonald and Spencer (2000) designed a research to examine gender differences in web navigation and they obtained overall differences between male and female participants in efficiency were absent but they reported as well that males expressed higher degree of confidence in their web navigation skills than females.

There are different researches that analyze the different barriers for women to enter and take on professional roles on IT business (Ahuja, 2002; Danielsson & Slumpi, n.d). These articles may explain the reasons of those stereotypes. Ahuja for example proposed a model of barriers faced by women that affect their entry and performance in this field. She considered two types of factors that women have to deal with: social factors and structure factors. The first one is related with the self-view of women have of themselves and the expectations of society have for boys and girls and the second one is related with the stereotypes about women perceived to be family-oriented and unwilling to travel. Danielsson commented as well the main factors that Ahuja did but she also added the importance to understand of foundations of these barriers. She also discussed the barriers in terms of power, production, emotion and symbol.

The Table 1 shows a summary of the literature review mentioned above, but grouped on three categories: results based on differences of perception between males and females, differences based on behavior between males and females and results with no differences between males and females

Table 1. Summary of literature review and categorized the results on three categories

Category	Reference	Goal of the Study	Result
Results based on Perception	Gefen & Straub, 1997	Analysis of gender in IT	Gender is an engaging factor. Women and men differ in their perceptions but not use of email
	Ahuja, 2002	Barriers of women to take professional roles	Social and structured factors to consider as barriers
	Danielsson & Slumpi, n.i	Barriers to prevent women from taking professionals roles	Social and structural factors adding an analysis of the sources of the barriers.
	Clayton, 2006	Engaging of women in ICT careers	Perceptions of ICT impact
	Correll, 2001	Perception of abilities on technology	Women have lower self-assessment of web use ability than men. The greater they rate their mathematical competence, the greater the probabilities on taking a scientific profession.
	Dambrot, Watkings-Malek, Silling, Marshall & Garver,1985	Gender differences on computer attitude	Female participants were more negative in their attitude
	Etzkowitz, Kemelgor, & Uzzi, 2000	Reasons of women for not being a scientific	Mainly due to culture and stereotypes
Results based on Behavior	Merril, 1991	Reasons of women for not being a scientific	Male participants more comfortable with new technologies
	Reinen & Plomp, 1997.	Measure the knowledge of students about general information and simple computer skills	Female enjoy using computer less than do male student
	Shaw and Marlow, 1999	Evaluate initial attitude towards the use of ICT	Men feel more at ease with new technologies than women
	Gutek & Bikson, 1985	Analysis of technological innovation (computerized procedures) and how they affect men and women employees	Men are more familiar with computers than women but female are more optimistic of its benefits
	Spennemann cited in Shaw and Marlow	Use of computers	Women less likely to own a computer
	Hargittai & Shafer, 2006	Gender differences in Internet-use ability	No differences in online abilities. Perception of women about their skills, may affect their behavior.
Results with No differences	Ory, Bullok & Burnaka, 1997	Analysis of attitudes about asynchronous learning networks (ALN)	Not significance difference
	McDonald & Spencer, 2000	Gender differences in web navigation	No difference in efficiency, but males expressed more confidence in their skills

In summary, History has shown that female physicians are placed in a preference position in Medicine World. Cutting-edge technologies are becoming a reference in Health and Medical educational and the longstanding debate over whether females are not engaging in ICT careers continues to be contested (Clayton, 2006).Therefore, there are different theories about the underrepresented females in ICT and this paper wants to analyze whether gender variable could influence on technology acceptance in field with a majority proportion of women, i.e., if gender could influence on the use of new technologies and its acceptance.

METHODOLOGY AND RESULTS

The method used for the technology acceptance was a survey with 29 questions grouped in two sections. The first section included the first 19 questions related with demographic information in order to evaluate the profile of the participants and the second section included 10 items based on a Technological Acceptance model, TAM (Davis, 1989; Venkatesh, Morris, Davis & David, 2003). It included the different dimensions to evaluate the profiles: performance expectancy, effort expectancy, attitude toward using technology, social influence, self-efficacy, anxiety, and behavioral intention to use the system. In addition, two more dimensions were added in this study: reliability and recommendation (Briz-Ponce, Juanes-Méndez and García-Peñalvo, 2014a). This second section was formed by a "5-point Likert scale", where each category was mapped to a number. So, strongly disagree is mapped to number 1 and strongly agree mapped to number 5.

The survey was completely anonymous and the target population was undergraduate students from University of Salamanca and medical professionals from Salamanca, grouped in medical specialists, medical residents and medical teachers.

The total of participants was 124 and the data were collected from March 2014 to April 2014 (Briz-Ponce et al, 2014a).

There were 36,3% of male participants and 63,7% of female participants. The descriptive statistics on participant characteristics are described in (Briz-Ponce, Juanes-Méndez and García-Peñalvo, 2014b).

The figures reveal that there is major proportion of female students (63,7%) than male students (36,3%) This difference is also noticed in the student profile, as most part of them are women, whereas medical teachers are mainly male (33,3% and 3,8%). This could be explained because in the last years, the number of women students has been increased astoundingly as it was mentioned in the previous introduction section. Another difference that could be remarkable is that almost all of them own a mobile device, more male participants own both a Smartphone and a tablet than female participants (51,1% and 44,3% respectively).

Relationship between Technological Acceptance Dimensions and Gender

As mentioned before, a Technological Acceptance survey was carried out in the University of Salamanca. The analysis is performed to calculate if there is any significant difference between each dimension considered for the survey and based on the TAM model and the gender variable. It is important to note that previously to perform the variance test, it was necessary to test the normality assumption with the Kolmogorov-Smirnov method (Chakravarti, Laha, & Roy, 1967). Besides, the null hypothesis states that there is no relationship between each dimension and gender variable.

After performing the normality test, the results confirm that the variables do not have a normal distribution, so it is not possible to use parametric-methods, therefore non-parametric methods are employed. In fact, as one variable is qualitative and the other one is quantitative, the test used must be U Mann-Whitney (Vinacua, 2007)

Table 2 contains the results of the U Mann-Whitney to analyse the significant differences between the dimensions and the gender variables. In all cases, $\rho>0.05$, so at $\alpha=0.05$, the values reveal that there is no enough evidence to fail to reject the null hypothesis ($\rho>0.05$) that there is no relationship between both variables.

Table 2. *Results of descriptive statistics and U Mann-Whitney method*

Dimension	Male		Female		U Mann-Whitney Results	
	Md	SD	Md	SD	U Value	ρ-Value
Performance expectancy	2.977	1.3723	2.886	1.3680	1674.000	0.730
Effort Expectancy	4.227	0.9612	4.405	1.0193	1477.000	0.119
Attitude toward using technology	3.750	1.1023	3.397	1.3127	1476.000	0.187
Social Influence	2.295	1.2310	2.367	1.1343	1666.000	0.692
Facilitating conditions	3.047	1.4134	2.885	1.2272	1572.000	0.561
Self-efficacy	3.295	1.3044	3.266	1.3176	1709.000	0.875
Anxiety	3.386	1.2241	3.115	1.0809	1700.000	0.836
Behavioural intention to use the new technology	3.955	1.3460	3.949	1.0678	1441.000	0.126
Reliability	3.705	1.1529	3.354	1.1987	1597.000	0.502
Recommendation	3.0455	1.2380	3.000	1.2709	1444.000	0.110

Relationship between the Global Technological Acceptance Score and Gender

Besides, another variable was calculated based on the sum of all of scores that the participants assigned to each item. This new variable gives information of the final punctuation that the participants give to the acceptance of the technology. In this section, the degree and correlation of relationship between this variable of sum score and the gender is calculated. The null hypothesis attempts to show that there is no relationship between them.

The sum score variable was tested with the Kolmogorovo-Smirnov method (Chakravarti, Laha, & Roy, 1967) to confirm its normality. Besides, the p-value for Levene test was p=0.943>0.05, so it was possible to use t-test. After performing this method, the results are t=0.435, p=0.664>0.05, so at α=0.05, the values reveal that there is no enough evidence to fail to reject the null hypothesis (ρ>0.05) that there is no relationship between both variables.

Influential Factors in the Acceptance of Technology

As it is mentioned in the background section, there are some researchers who found gender differences between the attitudes towards technology, considering the new technologies easier to use for males. In order to deep more in detail about this theme, it could be interesting to evaluate how other variables may influence on the scores of the acceptance of technology. Until now, the research was focused, on one hand, on the relationship between dimension sectors and gender variables and on the other hand, on the relationship between the total score of the survey and gender variables. However, in this section, additional factors will be added to the study to calculate if they could influence in the score of the technology and, as a consequence, in the acceptance of technology. Those variables were selected previously and were included in the survey provided to the participants of University of Salamanca.

In this case, for the analysis, it is necessary to divide the results obtained in the survey in two groups: male and female results. Then, the statistical methods are fixed depending on the type of variables to analyse. Table 3 presents the outcome data and it also reveals the method performed to calculate the relationship between the two variables. The column Comparative conditions indicates the two variables

Table 3. Results for the relationship between different variables and the score of the acceptance of technology

Comparative Conditions	Method Used	Value	Female Value	Male Value	Conclusions
Experience and acceptance of Technology	Kruskal-Wallis	Val=22.749 P=0.000	Value=11.193 P=0.11	Value=18.069 P=0.000	Significance difference for male participants
Profile and acceptance of technology	One Way Anova Test	F=2.568 P=0.058	F=2.484 P=0.068	F=0.867 P=0.466	No significant differences
Age and Acceptance of technology	One Way Anova Test	F=2.142 P=0.080	F=1.511 P=0.208	F=0.929 P=0.457	No significant differences
Operating System for Smartphone and Acceptance of Technology	Chi-Square Method	Chi=13.446 P=0.001	Chi-square= 6.268 P=0.012	Chi-square=8.596 P=0.014	Significant differences for males and females.
Operating System for Tablets and Acceptance of Technology	One Way Anova test	F=7.342 P=0.000	F=2.312 P=0.066	F=9.293 P=0.000	Significance difference for male participants
Time of use for smartphones and Acceptance of Technology	Kruskal Wallis	Chi-square=13.472 P=0.009	Chi-square=6.204 P=0.184	Chi-square=8.889 P=0.031	Significance difference for male participants
Time of use for tablets and Acceptance of Technology	One Way Anova Test	F=9.199 P=0.000	F=3.023 P=0.055	F=10.341 P=0.000	Significance difference for male participants
Number of downloads for smartphones and Acceptance of Technology	One Way Anova Test	F=4.488 P=0.13	F=0.499 P=0.609	F=6.466 P=0.004	Significance difference for male participants
Number of downloads for Tablets and Acceptance of Technology	One Way Anova Test	F=12.431 P=0.000	F=6.175 P=0.003	F=14.585 P=0.000	Significant differences for males and females.
Payment and acceptance of technology	T test	T=3.414 P=0.001	T=-1.396 P=0.167	T=-3.856 P=0.000	Significance difference for male participants
Trust on applications and acceptance of technology	One Way Anova	F=0.059 P=0.942	F=0.019 P=0.981	F=0.070 P=0.933	No significant differences
Use of medicine applications and acceptance of technology	U-Mann Whitney	U=654 P=0.000	U=259.500 P=0.001	U=71.500 P=0.000	Significant differences for males and females.
Use of training medical applications and acceptance of technology	U-Mann Whitney	U=481 P=0.000	U=211.500 P=0.007	U=36.500 P=0.000	Significant differences for males and females.

that are considered for the null hypothesis. In all cases, as it happened before, the null hypothesis attempts to show that there is no relationship between them

The outcome data reveals that for the following variables: The experience for technology, operating system for tablets, the number of apps downloaded on Smartphones, the time of use for Smartphones and tablets, the payment of apps, at $\alpha=0.05$, there is enough evidence to fail to reject the null hypothesis ($\rho<0.05$) for male participants, so these variables could influence in the acceptance of technology depending on the gender.

The results also explain that these variables influence in the score of the acceptance but for women and men: operating system for Smartphones, number of downloads for tablets and the use of medicine apps and training medical apps.

However, for the rest of variables as the profile (student, teacher or professional), age and trust on apps are not variables that at $\alpha=0.05$, there is a significant difference between them, so the gender does not reveal any additional explanation.

PROFILE PATTERN BASED ON GENDER

Until now, within this research, the different variables have been analyzed following different statistical methods, obtaining the analytical results. Whereas other researches explain the attitude itself towards technology and consider if the gender attitude is different toward technology, this project moves beyond and considers interesting to represent the possible profile of the participants based upon the score of the acceptance of technology and the mobile devices that they own. It may allow creating a hypothesis comparing graphically the distribution between both sets of data.

From a practical standpoint, this graphic could give some general idea of the participants more active and proactive to the new technologies considering male and female interviewers.

The new median scores of the acceptance considering the ownership of the mobile devices should be calculated with the SPSS program. Due to the huge information that could be generated, there was only a small group of variables considered to include in this pattern. The median comparative test was used and repeated for each variable taking into account the values for both genders obtaining a new set of samples. As a result, Figure 2 and Figure 3 illustrate the comparative between both genders.

Comparing both results, male participants gave higher scores when they owned more mobile devices. The use of Smartphones was relatively low but they were active tablet users. Besides, they used both medical applications and training medical applications. The profile could be teachers, medical professionals but not students. Male participants with no mobile devices and no use of mobile apps provided the lowest scores. Besides, the results may suggest that the majority of participants that did not own a mobile device were teachers.

The medium score profile was divided within participants with two mobile devices or only a smartphone. They could be active or not active smartphone users but were active tablet users. They could use medical or training medical apps or not, obtaining better scores when they had downloaded any of them.

The graph shows a tendency where a successive increases in X-axis (the participants own more mobile devices), the Y-axis move further to higher scores. However, other variables could lead to lower scores.

Turning now to the women results, women participants gave higher scores when they owned both mobile devices or none of them. They are not active users of the smartphone or the tablet but they have downloaded medical apps. They are medical professionals in their majority, but not students or teachers.

Figure 2. Pattern for male participants
(Source: Made by author)

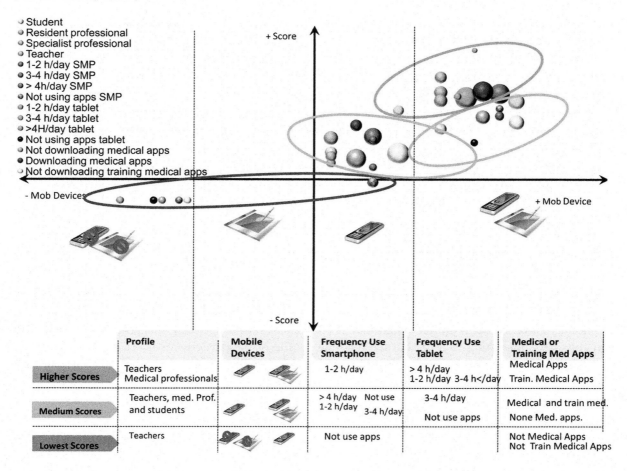

	Profile	Mobile Devices	Frequency Use Smartphone	Frequency Use Tablet	Medical or Training Med Apps
Higher Scores	Teachers Medical professionals		1-2 h/day	> 4 h/day 1-2 h/day 3-4 h</day	Medical Apps Train. Medical Apps
Medium Scores	Teachers, med. Prof. and students		> 4 h/day Not use 1-2 h/day 3-4 h/day	3-4 h/day Not use apps	Medical and train med. None Med. apps.
Lowest Scores	Teachers		Not use apps		Not Medical Apps Not Train Medical Apps

The medium profile was practically formed by medical professionals and students. They were also active users of the smartphone and the tablet downloading training medical applications. The lowest scores were formed surprisingly by users with one or two mobile devices, that used them very actively or they did not use them at all. In this case, as the male participants, teachers were the profile that gave lowest scores.

Taken together, these results suggest that there is an association between different variables and the scores that the participants provide to accept the new technologies.

The most striking result to emerge from the data was that the score for woman participants was steadily higher than man's score when they did not own a mobile device. As it was expected, the highest scores were found with both participants who own a smartphone and a tablet. The rest of the group revealed that the scores were very similar independently if the participant owned a mobile device or not.

Following this theme, woman did not need to be active users to provide higher scores whereas male participants did it. Medical professionals and students fall within medium scores profile, and the teachers gave the lowest scores in both cases.

Interestingly, when the participants have used a medical application or a training mobile application, they always gave higher scores.

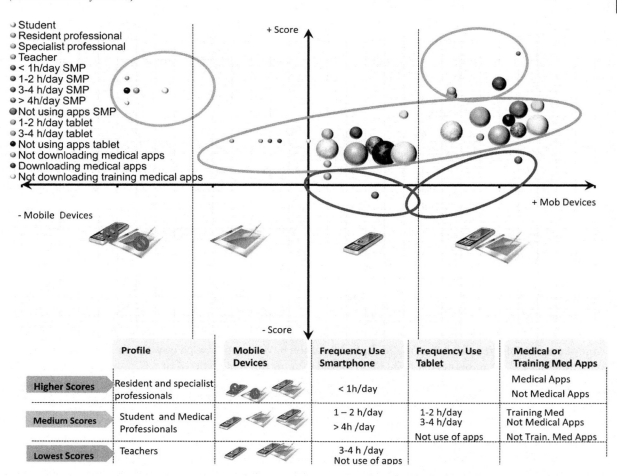

Figure 3. Pattern for female participants
(Source: Made by author)

	Profile	Mobile Devices	Frequency Use Smartphone	Frequency Use Tablet	Medical or Training Med Apps
Higher Scores	Resident and specialist professionals		< 1h/day		Medical Apps / Not Medical Apps
Medium Scores	Student and Medical Professionals		1 – 2 h/day / > 4h /day	1-2 h/day / 3-4 h/day / Not use of apps	Training Med / Not Medical Apps / Not Train. Med Apps
Lowest Scores	Teachers		3-4 h /day / Not use of apps		

FUTURE RESEARCH DIRECTIONS

The patterns obtained in this study provide some insights about the behavior of students, professionals and teachers in medical field. It classifies the type of person depending on its activity with mobile devices, if they are heavy users or not and determine if they are more proactive to the acceptance of technology. Besides, gender is also analyzed to make the study more completed providing two different patterns.

This initial research and the pattern results have an impact on two general important sectors: Society and Industry.

- Society, as it breaks the stereotypes of women not very proactive to the new technologies, as it was commented in the introduction of this paper. The pattern of behavior for women obtained in this research clearly shows how women really are.
- Industry, as the customers could be classified depending on their activity with mobile devices, make companies focus only on customers more proactive to adopt new technologies and, as a consequence, be more productive.

Therefore, this patterns could be very interesting to classify, understand and determine the type of students, physicians and students that our Society have and the study also highlight the importance of specific factors that could influence on the Acceptance of technology. However, Limitations of this study need to be noted. First, it is necessary to highlight that the research gathered data from only one university and the number of samples is enough to provide some insights in this field but it limits the generality of the results. According to Schulz (2004) it is possible to generalize if you make a comparative literature analysis and the results of the review is the same as the one obtained in your study. However, in this case, the results obtained could not be compared to any other. For this reason, Yin (2005) recommends to work with three to then single cases to generalize the results.

Second, this research discuss about the situation of woman in medical education and discuss about the role that they played in this environment and the different factors that could influence in the acceptance of technology. However, the number of factors analyzed is limited and it could be very interesting to add new factors or even compare patterns among different universities or countries.

CONCLUSION

This theme is very engaging to discuss as the historic stereotypes established by society make bring up some questions about the gender differences. These stereotypes have been changed according the different years, allowing women to integrate into the workforce, and in this case into the medicine World, overcoming the barriers of that moment. In fact, women have also provided new findings in the Medicine field, as there are 11 women that have been awarded with the Nobel Prize of Medicine, the first one in 1947 or the last one in 2014 (Zárate, Apolinar, Saucedo, & Basurto, 2015). These prizes also give women a new status in Science. They are not only women that want to be a physician; they also provide new ideas and advances to the Science, contributing to the development of Society, Industry and Economy.

Also, this research does not find any significance difference in the attitude towards technology based on the score given by the participants which also supports the findings of other authors (Ory, Bullok & Burnaka, 1997; McDonald & Spencer, 2000) who argued that they did not find any significance gender differences in their studies of the attitudes towards technology.

Different conclusion have drawn of a great variety of articles, exposing that there is no gender significance difference between the skills or the attitudes towards technology. However, they reported as well that the difference might be due to the lower self-assessment of the technical abilities from females, which may affect in their behavior.

This research reveals that there are some variables that may affect to the acceptance of technology in a different way if they are males or females. In fact, the experience of technology, the operating system used for tablets, the time of use of Smartphones and tablets, the number of apps downloaded for smartphone, and the use of paid applications are factors with a significance difference for male participants but not for female participants, so there are some gender significances in these factors influencing the acceptance of technology.

However, as a whole, this research suggests that there is no a relevant significance gender difference for the acceptance of technology and although the number of woman in medical education has been increased dramatically for the last years, it should not affect to the introduction of new technologies in medical education. In addition, the pattern profile obtained in this study may reveal that there are some variables that may influence in the scores of the acceptance of the technology. It also exposes that women encourage the new technologies and they are receptive to the introduction of new ways of learning, even they do not own a mobile device.

ACKNOWLEDGMENT

This research work is made within University of Salamanca PhD Programme on Education in the Knowledge Society.

REFERENCES

A profile and history of Women in Medicine. (2013). American Medical Association.

Ahuja, M. (2002). Women in the information technology profession: A literature review, synthesis and research agenda. *European Journal of Information Systems*, *11*(1), 20–34. doi:10.1057/palgrave. ejis.3000417

Briz-Ponce, L., Juanes-Méndez, J. A., & García-Peñalvo, F. J. (2014a). Analysis of certificated mobile application for medical Education purposes. In *Proceedings of the Second International Conference on Technological Ecosystem for Enhancing Multiculturality* (pp. 13-17). ACM New York. doi:10.1145/2669711.2669871

Briz-Ponce, L., Juanes-Méndez, J. A., & García-Peñalvo, F. J. (2014b). First approach of mobile applications study for medical Education purposes. In *Proceedings of the Second International Conference on Technological Ecosystem for Enhancing Multiculturality* (pp. 647-651). ACM New York doi:10.1145/2669711.2669968

Burgelman, R., Christensen, C., & Wheelwright, S. (2008). *Strategic Management of Technology and Innovation* (5th ed.). Boston: McGraw-Hill Education.

Chakravarti, Laha, & Roy. (1967). *Handbook of Methods of Applied Statistics*. John Wiley and Sons.

Changing the Face of Medicine | Dr. Elizabeth Blackwell. (n.d.). Retrieved from http://www.nlm.nih. gov/changingthefaceofmedicine/physicians/biography_35.html

Clayton, K. (2006). Attitudes Towards ICT in Australian High Schools. In Encyclopedia of Gender and Information Technology (pp. 44-49). Idea Group Inc. (IGI). doi:10.4018/978-1-59140-815-4.ch008

Correll, S. J. (2001). Gender and the Career Choice Process: The Role of Biased Self-Assessments. *American Journal of Sociology*, *106*(6), 1691–1730. doi:10.1086/321299

Dambrot, F. H., Watkings-Malek, M. A., Silling, S. M., Marshall, R. S., & Garver, J. A. (1985). Correlates of Sex Differences in Attitudes toward and Involvement with Computers. *Journal of Vocational Behavior*, *27*(1), 71–86. doi:10.1016/0001-8791(85)90053-3

Danielsson, U., & Slumpi, T. P. (n.d.). *Towards a deeper understanding of gender barriers in the IT business*. Academic Press.

Davis, F. D. (1989). Perceived Usefulness, Perceived Ease of Use, and User Acceptance of Information Technology. *Management Information Systems Quarterly*, *13*(3), 319. doi:10.2307/249008

Dictionary and Thesaurus | Merriam-Webster. (n.d.). Retrieved from http://www.merriam-webster.com/

Dillon, A., & Morris, M. (1998). Can they to will they: extending usability evaluation to address acceptance. In *Proceedings Association for information Systems Conference*. Baltimore, MD: Academic Press..

Estadística de Enseñanza Universitaria. (1998). In *Instituto Nacional de Estadística*. Retrieved from http://www.ine.es

Etzkowitz, H., Kemelgor, C., & Uzzi, B. (2000). *Athena Unbound: The Advancement of Women in Science and Technology*. Cambridge University Press. doi:10.1017/CBO9780511541414

Eurostat. (2009). *Proportion of female physicians, tertiary level academic staff and managers increasing* [Press Release]. Retrieved from http://epp.eurostat.ec.europa.eu/

Gefen, D., & Straub, D. W. (1997). Gender Differences in the Perception and Use of E-Mail: An Extension to the Technology Acceptance Model. *Management Information Systems Quarterly, 21*(4), 389–400. doi:10.2307/249720

Gutek, B. A., & Bikson, T. K. (1985). Differential experiences of men and women in computerized offices. *Sex Roles, 13*(3-4), 123–136. doi:10.1007/BF00287905

Hacker, C. (1984). *The Indomitable Lady Doctors*. Goodread Biographies.

Hargittai, E., & Shafer, S. (2006). Differences in Actual and Perceived Online Skills: The Role of Gender*. *Social Science Quarterly, 87*(2), 432–448. doi:10.1111/j.1540-6237.2006.00389.x

Hendrick, H., & Brown, O. (1984). *Human Factors in Organizational Design*. Amsterdam: North holland.

Lipinska, M. (1930). *Les femmes et le progrès des sciences medicales*. Paris: Masson.

López, M. (2007). Doctor Aleu, the first woman doctor in Spain. *Journal of Epidemiology and Community Health, 61*(Suppl 2), ii3–ii3. doi:10.1136/jech.2007.067215

Mcdonald, S., & Spencer, L. (2000). Gender Differences. In E. E. Balka & R. Smith (Eds.), Web Navigation (pp. 174–181). Springer, US: Women, Work and Computerization. Retrieved from http://link.springer.com/chapter/10.1007/978-0-387-35509-2_21

Merrill, M. D. (1991). Constructivism and instructional design. *Educational Technology, 31*(5), 45-53

Morantz-Sanchez, R. M. (2000). *Sympathy & Science: Women Physicians in American Medicine*. Univ of North Carolina Press.

Ory, J., Bullock, C., & Burnaska, K. (1997). Gender Similarity in the Use of and Attitudes About ALN in a University Setting. *Journal of Asynchronous Learning Networks, 1*(1), 39–51.

Pellissier, R. (2008). A Conceptual Framework for the alignment of innovation and Technology. *Journal of Technology Management and Innovation, 3*(3), 67-77. http://doi.org/<ALIGNMENT.qj></ALIGNMENT>10.4067/S0718-27242008000100007

Pololi, L. H. (2010). *Changing the Culture of Academic Medicine: Perspectives of Women Faculty*. UPNE.

Reinen, I. J., & Plomp, T. (1997). Information Technology and gender equality: A contradiction in terminis? *Computers & Education, 28*(2), 65–78. doi:10.1016/S0360-1315(97)00005-5

Schulz, R. (2004). *Meta Analysis: A comparison of Approaches*. Cambridge: Hogrefe & Huber.

Shaw, G., & Marlow, N. (1999). The role of student learning styles, gender, attitudes and perceptions on information and communication technology assisted learning. *Computers & Education, 33*(4), 223–234. doi:10.1016/S0360-1315(99)00020-2

Venkatesh, V., Morris, M. G., Davis, G. B., & David, F. D. (2003). User acceptance of information technology: Toward a unified view. *Management Information Systems Quarterly*, *27*(3), 425–478. Retrieved from http://www.jstor.org/stable/30036540

Vinacua, B. V. (2007). *Análisis estadístico con SPSS 14: estadística básica*. McGraw-Hill Interamericana de España S.L.

Wirtzfeld, D. A. (2009). The history of women in surgery. *Canadian Journal of Surgery*, *52*(4), 317–320. PMID:19680519

Yin, R. K. (2005). *Case Study Research: Design and Methods*. SAGE Publications.

Zárate, A., Apolinar, L. M., Saucedo, R., & Basurto, L. (2015). Article. *Gaceta Medica de Mexico*, *151*, 281–286. PMID:25946543

KEY TERMS AND DEFINITIONS

Anxiety Dimension: This is other dimension to describe the Technology Acceptance Model and it is related with the fears that the participants could feel using new technologies (as lack of information).

Mobile Application: This term is more common referred to as an app. It makes reference to the different programs that could be run out on Smartphones or tablets and provide additional services to the users (games, news, entertainment, chats, etc.).

Mobile Device: This term is the general name to call any device that could be used by people at different places. In this paper refers to smartphone and tablets.

Operating System: It describes the software of the smartphone. Nowadays, the most common operating systems are android (from Google), iOs (from apple) and Windows 8 (from Microsoft).

Reliability Dimension: This term refers to one of the dimensions explained in the chapter to describe the Technology Acceptance Model. It is related with the needed factors to generate trust to download an application.

Smartphone: It is a mobile phone that included more advanced features than the traditional phone (for example the touch screen).

Tablet Computer: Another type of mobile device similar to smartphone but it is larger than it. It is operated touching the screen. It is mainly used for Internet navigation.

The Role of Tailoring in E-Health and ICT-Based Interventions in Different Contexts and Populations

Cristina A. Godinho
Instituto Universitário de Lisboa (ISCTE-IUL), CIS-IUL, Portugal

Mário Rui Araújo
Faculdade de Psicológia, Universidade de Lisboa, Portugal

Maria-João Alvarez
Faculdade de Psicológia, Universidade de Lisboa, Portugal

INTRODUCTION

Developments in information and communication technologies (ICT's) have fostered the establishment of a new field at the intersection of healthcare practice, public health and business. This domain, supported by electronic processes, has been designated as electronic health or "e-health" (Eysenbach, 2001). In e-health, communication and information technologies may be used for healthcare provision and treatment, but also for health promotion and education, by delivering interventions to help individuals adopt healthier lifestyles and assisting them in their behavioural change processes. Amongst the advantages of the use of e-health interventions is the possibility they entail of providing individualized or "tailored" contents and formats, while having a potential high reach.

Tailoring is a strategy which sets out to increase the effectiveness of interventions by adapting them so that their contents, format, selected channel and/or message source is matched to the psychological, behavioural and demographic characteristics of individuals (Noar, Harrington, & Aldrich, 2009). Tailoring has been defined as "any combination of strategies and information intended to reach one specific person, based on the characteristics of that specific person, related to the outcome of interest, and derived from an individual assessment" (Kreuter, Strecher, & Glassman, 1999, p. 227). Tailoring offers a combination of high reach that was only previously possible through the use of undifferentiated mass health education interventions with personalization elements that are at the core of the clinical approach (Velicer, Prochaska, & Redding, 2006). Moreover, it has been shown to lead to greater efficacy in changing peoples' knowledge, attitudes, self-efficacy beliefs and health-related behaviours (Krebs, Prochaska, & Rossi, 2010; Lustria et al., 2013; Noar, Benac, & Harris, 2007; Portnoy, Schott-Sheldon, Johnson, & Carey, 2008).

Some authors have distinguished tailoring from a similar method, targeting, which is based on the identification of similarities in a group or sub-group of individuals and adapting communication to meet those characteristics (Noar et al., 2009). Others have situated tailoring and targeting in a continuum of message individualization (Hawkins, Kreuter, Resnicow, Fishbein, & Dijkstra, 2008; Kreuter, Farrell, Olevitch, & Brennan, 2000). This continuum varies from mass communication, directed at large audi-

DOI: 10.4018/978-1-4666-9978-6.ch080

ences, where virtually no audience segmentation or message customization are performed, to targeted communications where some degree of segmentation and customization is present according to the needs and preferences of a sub-group, to highly individualized, tailored health messages.

BACKGROUND: TAILORING IN E-HEALTH AND ICT INTERVENTIONS

In our global society, ICT's enable the provision of tailored information to a vast number of people in vital areas, including the health domain (Bacigalupe, 2011). Among US adults, 81% use the Internet, and among these users, 72% report having searched for health information online over the past year (Fox & Duggan, 2013). In Europe, several countries, namely, Denmark, Germany, Greece and Portugal, have shown a steady increase in the use of the Internet as a source for health information (Kummervold & Wynn, 2012). Moreover, the use of ICTs is not limited to Western societies. According to the International Telecommunication Union, mobile-cellular penetration rates stand at 96% globally, 121% in developed countries, 90% in developing countries, 89% in Asia and the Pacific, and 69% in Africa (ITC, 2014). The latter are the regions with the strongest mobile-cellular growth, despite lower penetration rates. Global penetration of mobile phones reveals higher access to them than to water and sanitation services worldwide.

The use of ICT's in health has also increased exponentially, bringing new possibilities and tools for healthcare professionals. Tailored health education programs are a good example, and can be used for health promoting activities, disease prevention, treatment, rehabilitation and chronic disease management (Kreps & Neuhauser, 2010). Many technologies (e.g., mobile smart-phones) are now used on a daily basis, so they can contribute in many health areas, from the management of chronic diseases to the promotion of healthy lifestyles (Qiang, Yamamichi, Hausman, Miller, & Altman, 2012). Additionally, these technologies may play an important role in decreasing the healthcare access gap among, for example, people in distant rural communities, hence contributing towards an increase in well-being and quality of life in such communities (Ruxwana, Herselman, & Conradie, 2010).

The biggest challenge for ICT and e-health is referred to by Ndiaye (2014), quoting InfoDev, 2007, p. 13: "ICT's are not simply neutral conduits of technical information, but require skilled and sensitive communicators to facilitate interactions". It's time to abandon the "one-size-fits-all" strategies and improve communication in a way that it fits the needs and characteristics of individuals, making use of feedback strategies and helping people in their urgent needs. In fact, research has shown that tailored interventions have increased odds of being read and remembered (Skinner, Strecher, & Hospers, 1994), being perceived as more relevant (Kreuter & Wray, 2003), interesting and engaging (Kreuter, Bull, Clark, & Oswald, 1999) and of being discussed with others (Brug, Steenhuis, van Assema, & de Vries, 1996). Furthermore, tailored interventions have also proved to be more effective in promoting changes in behaviours that have an impact on health, such as dietary behaviours, physical activity, smoking cessation and mammography screening (Krebset al., 2010; Lustria et al., 2013; Noaret al., 2007; Portnoy et al., 2008).

Advances in computer technology in the 90's were the first to make the development of individually tailored interventions possible (Harrington & Noar, 2012), but this first generation of computer-tailored interventions consisted mostly of print materials, which had several disadvantages such as a lack of interactivity, delayed feedback provision and cost (Brug, Oenema, & Campbell, 2003). The whole new world of ICT and e-health interventions thus encapsulates the potential to contribute towards the development and improvement of the second generation of tailored health communications that has progressively come to include gamification, videos and interactivity (Lustria et al., 2013). Before providing a review on e-health and ICT-based interventions at different levels and for different populations, ways by which they may be operationalized will first be explained.

HOW TO DEVELOP TAILORED INTERVENTIONS

Although tailoring is not restricted to computer-based interventions, the communication content is normally selected through a computer program/ software, hence commonly referred to as computer tailoring. The first step to develop a computer-tailored intervention is to identify and select the relevant psychosocial, behavioural and demographic variables that will serve as the basis for customizing the intervention. Secondly an algorithm, i.e., a non-ambiguous set of decision rules, must then be defined in order to attribute a specific intervention to the previously assessed individual parameters. These algorithms are generally defined through specific software that allow for multiple combinations of the evaluated variables. Furthermore, the creation of a database is necessary, containing all messages /intervention options that will correspond to each identified profile. Prior to the intervention, the individual has to be evaluated according to each selected variable, usually through answering a computerized / online questionnaire. Depending on individual answers to the questionnaire, a specific message / intervention is presented. Although the next section presents a summary of tailoring strategies and variables, interested researchers and practitioners may consult other sources for more detailed descriptions of this technique (e.g. Dijkstra & de Vries, 1999; Kreuter et al., 2000).

Tailoring Strategies

Several strategies have been used in order to tailor interventions to the individual level. Hawkins and colleagues (2008) have distinguished three types of strategies: 1) intervention personalization, 2) feedback provision and 3) matching the content to specific individual characteristics. Several communication tactics fall in the personalization category, such as: a) identifying the recipient by name or another unique identifier(s), b) making claims regarding how the information was selected with the recipient in mind, and c) presenting the information in the context of practices and values that are important to the individual (Hawkins et al., 2008). Feedback is also a commonly used strategy and can fall into three general categories: a) descriptive feedback, providing information about the individual, b) comparative feedback, providing information about the individual in comparison with others, and c) evaluative feedback, judging the desirability or suitability of what has been assessed about the individual. Content matching is often regarded as being at the core of tailoring (Hawkins et al., 2008) and consists of providing the information that is more likely to contribute to change in important behaviour change determinants and in behaviour itself (Kreuter & Skinner, 2000).

Although rarely mentioned in the context of tailoring, the authors contend that the choice of a specific frame is also worth considering. In fact, interventions may try to persuade individuals to change their behaviour by either stressing the benefits of performing the health behaviour, i.e., using a gain frame, or emphasizing the costs of failing to perform it, i.e., using a loss frame (Rothman & Salovey, 1997). Research has shown that, even when the underlying argument is the same, the way it is framed may have an impact on health behaviour change (Gallagher & Updegraff, 2012). Thus, besides the actual content of an intervention (i.e., *what* is said), how specific contents are framed (i.e., *how* it is said) should, in our view, also be considered.

Selection of Variables for Tailoring Interventions: Some Examples

Given that it is impractical and virtually impossible to assess all individual characteristics (Hawkins et al., 2008), the selection of variables that will be used for the tailoring of health interventions is of paramount importance. Despite the fact that interventions using constructs from behaviour change theories as a basis for tailoring are more effective (Noar et al., 2007), almost half of the studies included in recent meta-analyses do not explicitly report the theory behind the intervention (Lustria et al., 2013; Webb, Joseph, Yardley, & Michie, 2010). Studies reporting theory-driven interventions are mainly based on the Transtheoretical Model of Change, the Social Cognitive Theory and the Health Belief Model or Theory of Planned Behaviour (see Armitage & Conner, 2000), depending on the meta-analyses (e.g. Lustria et al., 2013; Noar, Harrington, Van Stee, & Aldrich, 2011; Webb et al., 2010). In the following section, two examples of theoretically-grounded variables, which the authors consider particularly relevant to be used as a basis for message tailoring, will be presented.

- **Stage of Change:** Stage models of health behaviour change, such as the Precaution Adoption Process Model (Weinstein, 1988) and the Health Action Process Approach Model (Schwarzer, 2008), postulate that health behaviour change is not a single event, but rather a process than unfolds over different phases, or stages. People at different stages are thought to be in different mindsets. Therefore, interventions should be stage specific, i.e., adjusted to the mindset of the individuals, given that different determinants are relevant at each stage transition and, consequently, people at different stages should require different types of information/ interventions in order to progress to the following stage (Weinstein, Rothman, & Sutton, 1998). For example, it has been suggested that individuals who are not yet motivated to change would best benefit from an intervention enhancing their risk perception (i.e., the belief that they are vulnerable to a certain health condition, which is considered to be severe), positive outcome expectancies (i.e., the anticipation of positive consequences from change) and self-efficacy (i.e., the belief that one is capable of changing) (Schwarzer, 2008). On the other hand, individuals who are already motivated to change would best benefit from a planning intervention that would stimulate them to think about when, where and how they can implement the intended changes, and to think about possible obstacles that may arise and hinder those plans, as well as on possible strategies that may be put into action to overcome such barriers. Besides planning, strengthening their self-efficacy beliefs is also important at this stage (Schwarzer, 2008).

Stage models, thus, offer a useful template for adapting interventions to individual needs, as they provide guidance for the selection of a parsimonious set of relevant determinants through which to tailor them (Godinho, Alvarez, & Lima, 2013). Additionally, although demographic variables such as gender, age, ethnicity and income are often used as a basis for tailoring, using stage is a more sophisticated approach, given that the psychosocial determinants are more proximal to health behaviour change (Slater, 1995). Previous experimental studies have demonstrated the superiority of stage-matched interventions for the promotion of different health behaviours such as physical exercise (Schwarzer, Cao, & Lippke, 2010), cervical cancer screening (Luszczynska, Goc, Scholz, Kowalska, & Knoll, 2011), fruit and vegetable intake (Godinho, Alvarez, Lima, & Schwarzer, 2015) and dental flossing (Schüz, Sniehotta, & Schwarzer, 2007).

- **Motivational Orientation:** One characteristic that impacts individuals' reactions to the message frame is their motivational orientation (Covey, 2014). Motivational orientation is related to differences in the end-points individuals tend to use in the regulation of their own behaviour, i.e., whether they primarily tend to regulate their behaviour in order to obtain gains or in order to avoid losses. Prior studies have shown that when the health message frame is congruent with individuals' motivational orientation, there is an increased chance of fostering changes in several health behaviours (Gerend & Shepherd, 2007; Godinho, Updegraff, Alvarez, & Lima, under review; Updegraff, Sherman, Luyster, & Mann, 2007). Thus, assessing individuals' motivational orientation and then providing them with tailored (i.e., congruently-framed) information may have a positive impact on health behaviour change.

TAILORING AT INDIVIDUAL, FAMILY, AND COMMUNITY LEVELS

Studies on the delivering of effective interventions have focused mainly on individuals, individualizing communication to create educational materials meeting the needs of a particular audience. Tailored interventions promoting individual health behaviour change have been mainly devoted to improving lifestyles (e.g., healthy eating, physical activity, smoking cessation and breast screening) or supporting/monitoring health conditions (e.g., arthritis, diabetes, hypertension). However, individuals do not change alone and research has shown that family engagement plays an important role in health behaviour, particularly when they are the only ones needing to do so within their close environment (Heimendinger et al., 2007).

Family-based intervention can be defined as the involvement of first or second-degree relatives, or those cohabiting under the same roof (McLean, Griffin, Toney, & Hardeman, 2003), or as an added component designed for another context, such as the school setting. Few interventions have been delivered in the home setting, despite the fact that it provides insights into family dynamics, potentialities and resources (Heimendinger et al., 2007). Interventions developed to involve the whole family are rare and the few family-based tailored interventions usually involve spouses or target a parent with a child (McLean et al., 2003). Participation of all family members may be a prerequisite for effective family-based interventions, at least for the adoption of some behaviours such as healthy eating (De Bourdeaudhuij, Brug, Vandelanotte, & Van Oost, 2002).

Any interactive communication and information technology, namely e-health services, can be used to enhance a community's quality of life (Hage, Roo, Van Offenbeck, & Boonstra, 2013). Thus, there are community e-health interventions, in addition to those geared towards individual or family health, although they are usually defined as targeted rather than tailored interventions. Community-based participatory approaches are advocated in the development and implementation of "tailored" interventions (e.g., Baker et al., 2002), whereby members of the community have an active role in the development of areas of interest, the process of dissemination and in the specific content and format of the technology materials. This participation is particularly important in digitally under-served populations due to researchers' misunderstandings and inexperience in community factors and communication needs (Chang et al., 2004).

TAILORED INTERVENTIONS WITH DIFFERENT POPULATIONS

N

Recent meta-analyses, exploring the efficacy of computer-tailored, web-based health behaviour change intervention on a wide range of health foci, have pointed to interventions addressing more adults than children or adolescents, more single than multiple behaviours and mainly physical activity, nutrition/diet and smoking cessation (Krebs et al., 2010; Lustria et al., 2013; Noar et al., 2011). To our knowledge, no systematic reviews of computer-tailored interventions for children are currently available. However, in a recent systematic review of school-based interventions for both physical activity and/or healthy eating in primary and secondary school children in Europe, computer-tailored personalized education proved to achieve better results than a generic classroom curriculum in adolescents (De Bourdeauhuij et al., 2010; Hamel & Robbins, 2013). Although Internet and e-health users tend to be young, more educated and confident with regard to computer use to search for health information, recent studies have found that older adults have now greater access to both technology and the Internet than in previous years, particularly respondents aged 65 years or over (e.g. Bujnowska-Fedak & Pirogowicz, 2014). It was mainly after 2005 that research on computer-tailored interventions with this population increased in the literature, and some studies have demonstrated the effectiveness of the interventions among adults over the age of 50 years (e.g., Hageman, Walker, & Pullen, 2005). A recent computer-tailored physical activity intervention comparing three age-groups between 19 and 89 years has shown an increase in physical activity in the oldest age-group (> 60 years) more than in the other two (Ammann, Vandelanotte, de Vries, & Mummery, 2013). This contrasts with former suggestions implying that older people might not be keen or skilled enough to use the Internet (Kaufman et al., 2006).

Furthermore, tailoring may also be refined by taking into consideration these age-graded factors. Despite the fact that many characteristics of tailoring that are appealing to adults have also been found to appeal to adolescents (e.g. personally tailored feedback) (Hamel & Robins, 2013), there is evidence that tailoring to age factors may increase the effectiveness of interventions. For instance, in children and adolescents, there are reasons to consider that social support may have even more of an impact on behaviour maintenance than in adults, since greater effectiveness has been found in school-based interventions, where support provided from teachers and participating classmates is available (Hamel & Robins, 2013). The immediacy of individually tailored feedback, its embeddedness in the high school curriculum, the provision of practical tips on how to change behaviour, and the use of social comparison with classmates or other adolescents, are all strategies that might improve tailoring for adolescent populations. Moreover, it is important for the messages provided to be short, and to convey new or relevant information. However, adapting these interventions, by adding parental support to the change of some health behaviours, has shown contradictory findings, thus requiring further research (Hamel, Robbins, & Wilbur, 2011; Mangunkusumo, Brug, Koning, van der Lei, & Raat,, 2007). For adults, additional features of tailoring may involve improvement of the usability of e-health applications, as they still prefer paper and pencil questionnaires to the online versions which enable tailored advice (e.g. van Beelen et al., 2013). Other characteristics might be suitable for older people such as website pages with little text and links, large visual objects, buttons and fonts, clear instructions, few questions on one single page, and a progress indicator (e.g. Ammann et al., 2013). In addition to focusing solely on intrapersonal determinants, tailoring addressing social and physical environmental determinants, such as presenting information about possibilities at home, in the neighborhood, and forums has proven to be promising, particularly with the elderly (e.g. van Stralen, de Vries, Bolman, Mudde, & Lechner, 2010).

DISCUSSION

New ICTs have made it easier and less costly to tailor the content and format of e-health interventions to individuals' characteristics and needs. We advocate that tailoring should be theory-driven and that behavioural science is in a privileged position to enhance the impact of these interventions, due to accumulated knowledge on the determinants of health behaviour and on the mechanisms involved and the conditions under which change likelihood is fostered. Hence, tailoring should not rely solely on the customization of intervention contents according to demographics, but should also capitalize on psychosocial and behavioural variables, which have empirically proven to be more proximal determinants of health behaviour change (Conner & Norman, 2005). Theories of health behaviour change can be very helpful for the choice of a specific set of variables to be used as a basis for tailoring, and contribute to increased intervention effectiveness (Noar et al., 2007). However, identifying the precise tailoring strategies that will work best in a specific setting, to change a given health behaviour, with a specific population, is still an empirical issue requiring further investigation.

An important form of adaptation to the individual's needs, central to the efficacy of e-health interventions, is the improvement of users' engagement. Engagement may be increased when content and persuasive arguments are matched to individuals' mindsets, such as their stage of change and their motivational orientation, besides risk factors and information needs. Indeed, stage-matched and congruently framed health interventions for the promotion of different health behaviours have been found to be far more effective (Covey, 2014; Schwarzer et al., 2010). Although framing issues have been more disregarded in the context of the literature on tailoring, the authors contend that both lines of research are very promising for the creation of personally relevant messages.

FUTURE RESEARCH DIRECTIONS

Tailoring research has, undoubtedly, increased over recent years. Interventions have improved on a number of levels, for instance, the point when feedback is provided, its adaptation not only to behavioural outcomes, levels of schooling and age, but also to psychosocial aspects and individuals' mindsets, and the addition of a social comparison element to the individual tailored feedback. However, research on the broad range of socio-demographic, psychosocial, biological, and clinical variables susceptible to tailoring should continue to be considered in order to determine those which are most relevant, so as to attain an optimal balance between extensive assessment and increased effectiveness of the intervention. Furthermore, the "added value" of different forms of tailoring (including graphs and other visual material) over and above that achieved by theoretical tailoring alone and of extending the characteristics used to tailor the interventions should be tested (e.g. Bannick et al., 2014; Noar et al., 2007).

In order to establish what does and does not work, researchers should be encouraged to provide better descriptions of their tailoring criteria and tactics used for message design, such as content and depth of tailoring, modes of delivery and intervention components (Harrington & Noar, 2012; Krebs et al., 2010). The greater elaboration of content that is hypothesized to follow tailoring can be more objectively measured with a neurophysiological assessment of brain wave activity using magnetic resonance imaging and eye-tracking analysis, for instance. Moreover, future studies should seek to include objective measures of behaviour change, such as pedometers in the case of physical activity and biomarkers in the case of dietary behaviours, besides self-reported measures. Long term outcomes and the cost-effectiveness of tailored interventions should also be established (Krebs et al., 2010; Noar et al., 2007).

Further research is also necessary to investigate the effects of individually tailored feedback on the health behaviours of children and adolescents. Some interventions with children induce minimal levels of change and draw attention to the need for more comprehensive interventions (e.g., Mangunkusumo et al., 2007), as well as the application of the same adolescents' web-based, tailored interventions in multiple settings such as the school and home (Bannick et al., 2014). It should be noted that contributing factors to the possible health divide must be acknowledged, particularly between the eldest members of the older population for whom the needs and abilities must be investigated to tailor and design meaningful health interventions for their particular context (Czaja et al., 2013).

CONCLUSION

The present chapter has provided an overview of tailored health education interventions, the development of which has been closely linked to the emergence of new ICT's and e-health tools. Nowadays, tailoring health interventions has become cheaper and easier to implement, enabling its widespread use. Although research is still needed on the psychological processes and on the precise circumstances behind tailoring effectiveness, the reviewed evidence supports that, when tailoring is theory-based, it may contribute towards maximizing health interventions' effectiveness, at individual, family and community levels and with different populations, including children, adults and older populations.

REFERENCES

Ammann, R., Vandelanotte, C., de Vries, H., & Mummery, W. (2013). Can a website-delivered computer-tailored physical activity intervention be acceptable, usable, and effective for older people? *Health Education Research*, *40*(2), 160–170. PMID:23077157

Armitage, C. J., & Conner, M. (2000). Social cognition models and health behaviour: A structured review. *Psychology & Health*, *15*(2), 173–189. doi:10.1080/08870440008400299

Bacigalupe, G. (2011). Is there a role for social technologies in collaborative healthcare? *Families, Systems & Health*, *29*(1), 1–14. doi:10.1037/a0022093 PMID:21417520

Baker, E., Kreuter, M., Homan, S., Starkloff-Morgan, S., Schonhoff, R., & Francioni, A. (2002). Using community-based participatory processes to bring health education technology to communities. *Health Promotion Practice*, *3*(1), 83–94. doi:10.1177/152483990200300110

Bannick, R., Broeren, S., Swanenburg, E., As, E., Looij-Jansen, P., & Raat, H. (2014). Use and appreciation of a web-based, tailored intervention (E-Health4Uth) combined with counseling to promote adolescents' health in preventive youth health care: Survey and log-file analysis. *JMIR Research Protocols, 3*(1), 1-16.

Brug, J., Oenema, A., & Campbell, M. (2003). Past, present, and future of computer-tailored nutrition education. *The American Journal of Clinical Nutrition*, *77*(4), 1028S–1034S. PMID:12663313

Brug, J., Steenhuis, I., van Assema, P., & de Vries, H. (1996). The impact of a computer-tailored nutrition intervention. *Preventive Medicine*, *25*(3), 236–242. doi:10.1006/pmed.1996.0052 PMID:8781000

Bujnowska-Fedak, M., & Pirogowicz, I. (2014). Support for e-health services among older elderly primary care patients. *Telemedicine Journal and e-Health*, *20*(8), 696–704. doi:10.1089/tmj.2013.0318 PMID:24359252

Chang, B., Bakken, S., Brown, S., Houston, T., Kreps, G., Kulafka, R., & Stavri, Z. (2004). Bridging the digital divide: Reaching vulnerable research population. *Journal of the American Medical Informatics Association*, *11*(6), 448–457. doi:10.1197/jamia.M1535 PMID:15299002

Colineau, M., & Paris, C. (2011). Motivating reflection about health within the family: The use of goal setting and tailored feedback. *User Model User-Adaptation International*, *21*(4-5), 341–376. doi:10.1007/s11257-010-9089-x

Conner, M., & Norman, P. (2005). *Predicting health behavior: Research and practice with social cognition models* (2nd ed.). Buckingham, UK: Open University Press.

Covey, J. (2014). The role of dispositional factors in moderating message framing effects. *Health Psychology*, *33*(1), 52–65. doi:10.1037/a0029305 PMID:22924446

Czaja, S., Sharit, J., Lee, C., Nair, S., Hernández, M., Arana, N., & Fu, S. (2013). Factors influencing use of an e-health website in a community sample of older adults. *Journal of the American Medical Informatics Association*, *20*(2), 277–284. doi:10.1136/amiajnl-2012-000876 PMID:22802269

De Bourdeaudhuij, I., Brug, J., Vandelanotte, C., & Van Oost, P. (2002). Differences in impact between a family versus an individual-based tailored intervention to reduce fat intake. *Health Education Research*, *17*(4), 435–449. doi:10.1093/her/17.4.435 PMID:12197589

De Bourdeauhuij, I., Cauwenberghe, E., Spittaels, H., Oppert, J.-M., Rostami, C., Brug, J., & Maes, L. (2010). School-based interventions promoting both physical activity and healthy eating in Europe: A systematic review within the HOPE project. *Obesity Reviews*, *12*(3), 205–216. doi:10.1111/j.1467-789X.2009.00711.x PMID:20122137

Dijkstra, A., & De Vries, H. (1999). The development of computer-generated tailored interventions. *Patient Education and Counseling*, *36*(2), 193–203. doi:10.1016/S0738-3991(98)00135-9 PMID:10223023

Eysenbach, G. (2001). What is e-health? *Journal of Medical Internet Research*, *3*(2), e20. doi:10.2196/jmir.3.2.e20 PMID:11720962

Fox, S., & Duggan, M. (2013, January 15). *Health online 2013*. Pew Internet and American Life Project. Retrieved from http://www.pewinternet.org/files/old-media//Files/Reports/PIP_HealthOnline.pdf

Gallagher, K. M., & Updegraff, J. A. (2012). Health message framing effects on attitudes, intentions, and behavior: A meta-analytic review. *Annals of Behavioral Medicine*, *43*(1), 101–116. doi:10.1007/s12160-011-9308-7 PMID:21993844

Gerend, M. A., & Shepherd, J. E. (2007). Using message framing to promote acceptance of the human papillomavirus vaccine. *Health Psychology*, *26*(6), 745–752. doi:10.1037/0278-6133.26.6.745 PMID:18020847

Godinho, C. A., Alvarez, M. J., & Lima, L. (2013). Formative research on HAPA model determinants for fruit and vegetable intake: Target beliefs for audiences at different stages of change. *Health Education Research*, *28*(6), 1014–1028. doi:10.1093/her/cyt076 PMID:23856178

Godinho, C. A., Alvarez, M. J., Lima, L., & Schwarzer, R. (2015). Health messages to promote fruit and vegetable consumption at different stages of change: A match-mismatch design. *Psychology & Health, 30*(12), 1410–1432. doi:10.1080/08870446.2015.1054827

Godinho, C. A., Updegraff, J. A., Alvarez, M. J., & Lima, L. (under review). *When is congruency helpful? Interactive effects of frame, motivational orientation, and perceived message quality on fruit and vegetable consumption.* Academic Press.

Hage, E., Roo, J., Van Offenbeck, M., & Boonstra, A. (2013). Implementation factors and their effect on e-health service adoption in rural communities: A systematic literature review. *BMC Health Services Research, 13*(1), 19. doi:10.1186/1472-6963-13-19 PMID:23311452

Hageman, P., Walker, S., & Pullen, C. (2005). Tailored versus standard internet-delivered interventions to promote physical activity in older women. *Journal of Geriatric Physical Therapy, 28*(1), 28–33. doi:10.1519/00139143-200504000-00005 PMID:16236225

Hamel, L., & Robbins, L. (2013). Computer and web-based interventions to promote healthy eating among children and adolescents: A systematic review. *Journal of Advanced Nursing, 69*(1), 16–30. doi:10.1111/j.1365-2648.2012.06086.x PMID:22757605

Hamel, L., Robbins, L., & Wilbur, J. (2011). Computer and web-based interventions to increase pre-adolescent and adolescent physical activity: A systematic review. *Journal of Advanced Nursing, 67*(2), 251–268. doi:10.1111/j.1365-2648.2010.05493.x PMID:21198800

Harrington, N., & Noar, S. (2012). Reporting standards for studies of tailored interventions. *Health Education Research, 27*(2), 331–342. doi:10.1093/her/cyr108 PMID:22156230

Hawkins, R. P., Kreuter, M., Resnicow, K., Fishbein, M., & Dijkstra, A. (2008). Understanding tailoring in communicating about health. *Health Education Research, 23*(3), 454–466. doi:10.1093/her/cyn004 PMID:18349033

Heimendinger, J., Uyeki, T., Andhara, A., Marshall, J., Scarbro, S., Belansky, E., & Crane, L. (2007). Coaching process outcomes of a family visit nutrition and physical activity intervention. *Health Education & Behavior, 34*(1), 71–89. doi:10.1177/1090198105285620 PMID:16740515

ITU (2014). The world in 2014. ICT facts and figures. Geneva: International Telecommunication Union. Retrieved from: http://www.itu.int/en/ITU-D/Statistics/Documents/facts/ICTFactsFigures2015.pdf

Kaufman, D., Pevzner, J., Hilliman, C., Weinstock, R., Teresi, J., Shea, S., & Starren, J. (2006). Redesigning a telehealth diabetes management program for a digital divide seniors population. *Home Health Care Management & Practice, 18*(3), 223–234. doi:10.1177/1084822305281949

Krebs, P., Prochaska, J., & Rossi, J. (2010). A meta-analysis of computer-tailored interventions for health behavior change. *Preventive Medicine, 51*(3-4), 214–221. doi:10.1016/j.ypmed.2010.06.004 PMID:20558196

Kreps, G. L., & Neuhauser, L. (2010). Editors' introduction Ehealth and the delivery of health care. *Journal of Computer-Mediated Communication, 20*(1). 364–366. doi: 10.1111/j.1083-6101.2010.01524.x

Kreuter, M. W., Bull, F. C., Clark, E. M., & Oswald, D. L. (1999). Understanding how people process health information: A comparison of tailored and nontailored weight-loss materials. *Health Psychology, 18*(5), 487–494. doi:10.1037/0278-6133.18.5.487 PMID:10519465

Kreuter, M. W., Farrell, D., Olevitch, L., & Brennan, L. (2000). *Tailoring health messages: Customizing communication with computer technology.* Lawrence Earlbaum Associates.

Kreuter, M. W., & Skinner, C. S. (2000). Tailoring: What's in a name? *Health Education Research, 15*(1), 1–4. doi:10.1093/her/15.1.1 PMID:10788196

Kreuter, M. W., Strecher, V. J., & Glassman, B. (1999). One size does not fit all: The case for tailoring print materials. *Annals of Behavioral Medicine, 21*(4), 276–283. doi:10.1007/BF02895958 PMID:10721433

Kreuter, M. W., & Wray, R. J. (2003). Tailored and targeted health communication: Strategies for enhancing information relevance. *American Journal of Health Behavior, 27*(1Supplement 3), S227–S232. doi:10.5993/AJHB.27.1.s3.6 PMID:14672383

Kummervold, P., & Wynn, R. (2012). Health information accessed on the internet: The development in 5 European countries. International Journal of Telemedicine and Applications, Article ID 297416, 3 pages. doi:10.1155/2012/297416

Lustria, M., Noar, S., Cortese, J., Van Stee, S., Glueckauf, R., & Lee, J. (2013). A meta-analysis of web-delivered tailored health behavior change interventions. *Journal of Health Communication, 18*(9), 1039–1069. doi:10.1080/10810730.2013.768727 PMID:23750972

Luszczynska, A., Goc, G., Scholz, U., Kowalska, M., & Knoll, N. (2011). Enhancing intentions to attend cervical cancer screening with a stage-matched intervention. *British Journal of Health Psychology, 16*(1), 33–46. doi:10.1348/135910710X499416 PMID:21226782

Mangunkusumo, R., Brug, J., Koning, H., van der Lei, J., & Raat, H. (2007). School-based internet-tailored fruit and vegetable education combined with brief counseling increases children's awareness of intake levels. *Public Health Nutrition, 10*(3), 273–279. doi:10.1017/S1368980007246671 PMID:17288625

McLean, N., Griffin, S., Toney, K., & Hardeman, W. (2003). Family involvement in weight control, weight maintenance and weight-loss interventions: A systematic review of randomized trials. *International Journal of Obesity, 27*(9), 987–1005. doi:10.1038/sj.ijo.0802383 PMID:12917703

Ndiaye, K. (2014). Highlighting the C in ICT: Key Communication and culture questions in ICT for health. *Journal of Health Communication, 19*(5), 529–531. doi:10.1080/10810730.2014.912547 PMID:24807041

Noar, S., Benac, C., & Harris, M. (2007). Does tailoring matter? Meta-analytic review of tailored print health behavior change interventions. *Psychological Bulletin, 133*(4), 673–693. doi:10.1037/0033-2909.133.4.673 PMID:17592961

Noar, S., Harrington, N., Van Stee, S., & Aldrich, R. (2011). Tailored health communication to change lifestyle behaviors. *American Journal of Lifestyle Medicine, 5*(2), 112–122. doi:10.1177/1559827610387255

Noar, S. M., Harrington, N. G., & Aldrich, R. S. (2009). The role of message tailoring in the development of persuasive health communication messages. *Communication Yearbook, 33*, 73-133.

Portnoy, D., Schott-Sheldon, L., Johnson, B., & Carey, M. (2008). Computer-delivered interventions for health promotion and behavioral risk reductions: A meta-analysis of 75 randomized controlled trials, 1988-2007. *Preventive Medicine, 47*(1), 3–16. doi:10.1016/j.ypmed.2008.02.014 PMID:18403003

Qiang, C. Z., Yamamichi, M., Hausman, V., Miller, R., & Altman, D. (2012). *Mobile applications for the health sector*. Washington, DC: World Bank.

Rothman, A. J., & Salovey, P. (1997). Shaping perceptions to motivate healthy behavior: The role of message framing. *Psychological Bulletin, 121*(1), 3–19. doi:10.1037/0033-2909.121.1.3 PMID:9000890

Ruxwana, N. L., Herselman, M. E., & Conradie, D. (2010). ICT applications as e-health solutions in rural healthcare in the Eastern Cape Province of South Africa. *Health Information Management Journal, 39*(1), 17–26.

Schüz, B., Sniehotta, F. F., & Schwarzer, R. (2007). Stage-specific effects of an action control intervention on dental flossing. *Health Education Research, 22*(3), 332–341. doi:10.1093/her/cyl084 PMID:16945985

Schwarzer, R. (2008). Modeling health behavior change: How to predict and modify the adoption and maintenance of health behaviors. *Applied Psychology, 57*, 1–29.

Schwarzer, R., Cao, D. S., & Lippke, S. (2010). Stage-matched minimal interventions to enhance physical activity in Chinese adolescents. *The Journal of Adolescent Health, 47*(6), 533–539. doi:10.1016/j.jadohealth.2010.03.015 PMID:21094429

Skinner, C. S., Strecher, V. J., & Hospers, H. (1994). Physicians' recommendations for mammography: Do tailored messages make a difference? *American Journal of Public Health, 84*(1), 43–49. doi:10.2105/AJPH.84.1.43 PMID:8279610

Slater, M. D. (1995). Choosing audience segmentation strategies and methods for health communication. In E. Maibach & R. L. Parrott (Eds.), *Designing health messages* (pp. 186–198). Thousand Oaks: Sage. doi:10.4135/9781452233451.n10

Updegraff, J. A., Sherman, D. K., Luyster, F. S., & Mann, T. L. (2007). The effects of message quality and congruency on perceptions of tailored health communications. *Journal of Experimental Social Psychology, 43*(2), 249–257. doi:10.1016/j.jesp.2006.01.007 PMID:18958299

van Beelen, M., Vogel, I., Beirens, T., Kloek, G., Hertog, P., & Raat, H. et al. (2013). Web-based e-health to support counseling in routine well-child care: Pilot study of E-health4Uth Home Safety. *JMIR Research Protocols, 2*(1), 1–13. doi:10.2196/resprot.1862 PMID:23611794

van Stralen, M., de Vries, H., Bolman, C., Mudde, A., & Lechner, L. (2010). Exploring the efficacy and moderators of two computer-tailored physical activity interventions: A randomized controlled trial. *Annals of Behavioral Medicine, 39*(2), 139–150. doi:10.1007/s12160-010-9166-8 PMID:20182833

Velicer, W. F., Prochaska, J. O., & Redding, C. A. (2006). Tailored communications for smoking cessation: Past successes and future directions. *Drug and Alcohol Review, 25*(1), 49–57. doi:10.1080/09595230500459511 PMID:16492577

Vodopivec-Jamsek, V., Jongh, T. D., Gurol-Urganci, I., Atun, R., & Car, J. (2012). Mobile phone messaging for preventive health care (Review). *Cochrane Database of Systematic Reviews, 12*. doi:.10.1002/14651858.CD007457.pub2

Webb, T., Joseph, J., Yardley, L., & Michie, S. (2010). Using the internet to promote health behavior change: A systematic review and meta-analysis of the impact of theoretical basis, use of behavior change techniques, and mode of delivery on efficacy. *Journal of Medical Internet Research, 12*(1), e4. doi:10.2196/jmir.1376 PMID:20164043

Weinstein, N. (1988). The precaution adoption process. *Health Psychology, 7*(4), 355–386. doi:10.1037/0278-6133.7.4.355 PMID:3049068

Weinstein, N. D., Rothman, A. J., & Sutton, S. R. (1998). Stage theories of health behavior: Conceptual and methodological issues. *Health Psychology, 17*(3), 290–299. doi:10.1037/0278-6133.17.3.290 PMID:9619480

Zurovac, D., Talisuna, A. O., & Snow, R. W. (2012). Mobile phone text messaging: Tool for malaria control in Africa. *PLoS Medicine, 9*(2), e1001176. doi:10.1371/journal.pmed.1001176 PMID:22363212

Smartphones:
Innovative Tools in Cancer Prevention

Nuno Ribeiro
Universidade do Porto, Portugal

Luís Miguel Nunes Silva Alves Moreira
Instituto Piaget, Portugal

Ana Margarida Pisco Almeida
Universidade de Aveiro, Portugal

Filipe Santos-Silva
Universidade do Porto, Portugal

INTRODUCTION

This chapter explores the potential of smartphones on cancer prevention. The acceptability of mobile health (mhealth) technologies as promoters of behavior change and the identification of desired features necessary to prototype a cancer prevention app were assessed in a target population.

It is estimated that, by the year 2030, cancer will affect more than 26 million people worldwide and over 17 million will die from this disease (IARC, 2008; Jemal, Bray, Ferlay, Ward, & Forman, 2011). More than half of cancer cases are due to unhealthy behavioral options (Colditz & Wei, 2012); if everyone adopt a healthier lifestyle, cancer incidence would fall dramatically (Colditz & Wei, 2012; Colditz, Wolin, & Gehlert, 2012). Research has shown that there is a link between knowledge and the adoption of healthy behaviors (Hawkins, Berkowitz, & Peipins, 2010; Keeney, McKenna, Fleming, & McIlfatrick, 2010; Niederdeppe & Levy, 2007). Still, exceptions remain, being smokers the most paradigmatic example: despite all the warnings and campaigns designed to promote smoking cessation, many people continue to smoke (International Union Against Cancer, 2004). Information campaigns are needed to increase cancer awareness but they simply are not enough to promote behavior change.

BACKGROUND

mHealth can be defined as all "medical and public health practice supported by mobile devices" (WHO, 2011, p. 6). mHealth solutions currently being developed could transform healthcare through patients' empowerment (reflected in a higher quality of life), while increasing healthcare systems efficiency and sustainability (European Commission, 2014). Presently, mHealth is being applied in most areas of medicine and healthcare, having made important contributions to research on cardiology, diabetes, obesity, smoking cessation, elderly care, and chronic diseases (Silva, Rodrigues, de la Torre Díez, López-Coronado, & Saleem, 2015; Steinhubl, Muse, & Topol, 2015). mHealth interventions can be used globally to target specific behaviors and prevent major diseases. For instance, the "Be He@lthy Be Mobile"

DOI: 10.4018/978-1-4666-9978-6.ch081

initiative uses mobile phones to tackle non-communicable diseases with nationwide interventions (e.g. mTobaccoCessation in Costa Rica or mCervicalCancer in Zambia) (ITU, 2014). mHealth has already generated much public interest: by the end of 2010, mHealth applications counted more than 200 million downloads and about 70% of worldwide citizens were interested in at least one mhealth application. This has led to a rapid expansion of available mhealth applications (there are more than 400,000 available in the U.S. Apple App Store alone) (Silva et al., 2015). But problems have arisen concerning the security, reliability, and quality of service of these applications. Several studies have already pointed out the need to regulate these applications in order to prevent potential hazards (Steinhubl et al., 2015).

CANCER PREVENTION USING SMARTPHONES

Population-wide measures targeting behaviors like inadequate sun exposure, smoking, excessive alcohol use, eating a poor diet, and physical inactivity could reduce overall cancer incidence in fifty per cent (Stein & Colditz, 2004). The European Code Against Cancer (Boyle et al., 2003) defines the following guidelines: (1) Do not smoke; (2) Avoid obesity; (3) Undertake some brisk physical activity every day; (4) Increase daily intake of vegetables and fruits (at least five servings per day); (5) Limit alcohol consumption to one or two drinks per day (women and men, respectively); (6) Avoid excessive sun exposure; (7) Enroll in cancer screening tests (cervical, breast and colorectal screening); (8) Participate in vaccination programs against hepatitis B virus and human papilloma virus; (9) Avoid exposure to known cancer-causing substances.

Individually, everyone should follow these cancer prevention guidelines to reduce their personal risk of cancer. But behavior change is a very hard task: people have generally favorable attitudes towards healthy behaviors, but they often lack the skills needed to maintain it as part of their daily routine (Kaptein, De Ruyter, Markopoulos, & Aarts, 2012). In many cases, cancer prevention involves changing several aspects of our lifestyles. Multiple behavior changes are difficult, but research suggests that it is possible. A study by Spring et al. (2012) showed that targeting diet and physical activity together seems to aid in the adoption and maintenance of healthy behaviors. It is argued that these two behaviors share physiological and behavioral mechanisms that, collectively, can impact energy balance, appetite and food choices (Mata et al., 2009). Physical activity is also recognized as a possible gateway to other health behavior changes (Kremers, De Bruijn, Schaalma, & Brug, 2004; Mata et al., 2009). By targeting multiple behaviors at once, one can promote a general sense of health that, in turn, might prompt other healthier behaviors with great benefits in the general health status.

According to Fogg (2009), behavioral changes occur when three elements converge in a given moment: motivation, ability and triggers. If one of these three elements is missing, change will not occur. This model clearly points out that motivation alone is not enough to induce a new behavior; the target behavior has to be simple enough to be performed by that person and a trigger has to be present to remind that person to perform that behavior (Stanford Persuasive Tech Lab, 2010). Fogg (2009) defines trigger as something that tells people to perform a behavior now. An effective trigger will remind and instigate people to perform the target behavior.

Fogg Behavior Model (Figure 1) predicts an action line that depends on the motivation and ability of individuals. This line determines whether a trigger will succeed or not. When a person is highly motivated to perform a behavior, a trigger might succeed even if the behavior is hard to do. When a behavior is easy to perform, even a person with low motivation will do it if prompted by the right trigger.

Figure 1. Fogg Behavior model
© *2007, BJ Fogg. Used with permission.*

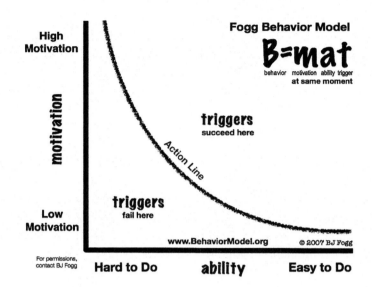

According to this model, behavior change is possible by motivating people, keeping the target behaviors simple and using the right trigger in the most appropriate moment.

Smartphones can be helpful aids in behavior change. Like all mobile phones, they are personal, portable and always connected. People carry them around and they are almost always turned on (Whittaker, Merry, Dorey, & Maddison, 2012). Smartphones are also becoming ubiquitous: it is estimated that by 2016 the number of smartphone users worldwide will surpass 2 billion and by 2018 they will represent more than half of all active mobile phone users (eMarketer, 2014). This allows extended behavior change interventions with relatively low implementation costs (Whittaker et al., 2012). Using the various built-in sensors, smartphones can "sense" time, location and even physical context in real time and induce behaviors adequate to the users immediate "needs". This presents a unique opportunity to use triggers to change, reinforce and reward the desired behaviors (Stanford Persuasive Tech Lab, 2010). Triggers can be adapted to specific moments of people's lives, merging behavior change interventions in people's routines (Fogg, 2009). Several studies have suggested that it is possible to change behavior using smartphones. They have been used successfully in several interventions ranging from smoking cessation, to weight loss and disease management (Bert, Giacometti, Gualano, & Siliquini, 2014; Fiordelli, Diviani, & Schulz, 2013; Klasnja & Pratt, 2012; Mosa, Yoo, & Sheets, 2012). Despite these encouraging results, the potential of smartphones in behavior change interventions hasn't yet been fully explored (Fiordelli et al., 2013).

There are several mhealth interventions targeting cancer with encouraging results (Davis & Oakley-girvan, 2014; ITU, 2014). But these solutions aren't without problems. A study concerning cancer-related applications (Pandey, Hasan, Dubey, & Sarangi, 2013) concluded that currently available applications lack scientifically supported data. The authors stated that only one-fourth of all applications were developed by health-care agencies. There is a need to ensure that valid and relevant information reaches the consumers and app developers should involve health-care agencies to ensure information quality. The majority of cancer-related applications analyzed in this study focused on general information about the disease, research and recent advances, and support for health-care professionals and patients. General awareness of the disease accounted for about 10% of all analyzed applications. Cancer prevention wasn't mentioned as the main theme of any application, despite its importance.

Another issue to consider is the clinical validity of the available applications. A study looked at smartphone applications that claim to detect melanoma and found that they are mostly inaccurate (Wolf et al., 2013). This raises serious questions as reliance on these applications can potentially delay the diagnosis of melanoma and harm users. It is essential that app developers use adequate methods to evaluate and validate health applications to ensure quality and prevent harmful effects derived from the use of these mhealth solutions.

HAPPY: HEALTH AWARENESS AND PREVENTION PERSONALIZED FOR YOU

This section will focus on the rationale, methodological process and preliminary results concerning the development of a cancer prevention mobile application named Happy - Health Awareness and Prevention Personalized for You. The main goal of Happy is to persuade users to change their behavior, making healthier choices, thus reducing their personal risk of developing several types of cancer.

Target Population

The target population of this application is healthy Portuguese young adults, with ages between 18 and 35 years. The choice of a young population is based upon two different reasons: (1) Cancer prevention should start at an early stage of life (reducing exposure time to risk factors) (Colditz et al., 2012); (2) Almost all individuals of this population own at least one mobile device (ANACOM, 2014).

As a preliminary study designed to characterize the target population, an online survey concerning sociodemographic characteristics, health and lifestyle, and smartphone user experience was applied to a sample of the target population (n = 862) (Table 1).

Analyzing the results, it is possible to conclude that the great majority of respondents disregarded cancer prevention guidelines. This is particularly true for physical exercise (only 29.1% workout more than 2 hours per week), and fruit and vegetable consumption (only 4.2% eat 5 or more portions per day). Also, tobacco and alcohol consumption were reported by 18.7% and 21.4% of the respondents, respectively. Healthy Portuguese young adults have to improve their behavior if they want to stay healthy in the future. These results emphasize the need to design mhealth interventions that could improve this scenario and provides the best justification for the development of a cancer prevention application.

Interestingly, the majority of respondents (56.0%) use their smartphone more than one hour per day, and 52.2% used their smartphone to monitor health-related behaviors. This shows that this population is already using health-related applications and strengthens the belief that a cancer prevention application might have a widespread use. However, using smartphones to monitor diet, tobacco and alcohol consumption – three behaviors that raise the personal risk of cancer – is less common, which highlights the need of applications that effectively engage users on long-term monitoring of cancer-risk associated behaviors.

Project Development

The development of a successful application designed to prevent cancer is a hard and complex task: several questions regarding the persuasive power of the application, usability and long-term usage emerge and must be answered to ensure that it succeeds. This iterative process involves several steps and different methods (Figure 2).

Table 1. Results of the online survey

Sociodemographic Characteristics	
Gender, n (%)	
Female	**557** (64.6)
Male	**289** (33.5)
No answer	**16** (1.9)
Age, mean ± SD	**23.8** ± 4.6
Education Level, n (%)	
College degree	**657** (76.2)
No college degree	**198** (23.0)
No answer	**7** (0.8)
Health and Lifestyle	
Physical exercise (weekly average), n (%)	
*>2 hours**	**251** (29.1)
1 to 2 hours	**167** (19.4)
<1 hour	**296** (34.4)
None	**146** (16.9)
No answer	**2** (0.2)
Fruit and Vegetable Consumption (Daily Average), n (%)	
*≥5 portions**	**36** (4.2)
3 to 4 portions	**227** (26.4)
1 to 2 portions	**549** (63.7)
None	**46** (5.3)
No answer	**4** (0.4)
Smoking Status, n (%)	
Smoker	**161** (18.7)
Former smoker	**95** (11.0)
*Non smoker**	**600** (69.6)
No answer	**6** (0.7)
Alcohol Consumption (Daily Average), n (%)	
>2 drinks	**3** (0.3)
1 to 2 drinks	**182** (21.1)
*None**	**673** (78.1)

continued in next column

Table 1. Continued

No answer	**4** (0.5)
Body Mass Index (BMI)	
High	**203** (23.5)
*Normal**	**596** (69.2)
Low	**51** (5.9)
No answer	**12** (1.4)
Smartphone User Experience	
Smartphone operating system, n (%)	
Android	**620** (71.9)
iOS	**127** (14.7)
Other	**67** (7.8)
Don't know/ No answer	**48** (5.6)
Smartphone Ownership, n (%)	
>1 year	**547** (63.5)
6 months to 1 year	**143** (16.6)
< 6months	**172** (19.9)
Smartphone Use (Daily Average), n (%)	
>2 hours	**280** (32.5)
1 to 2 hours	**203** (23.5)
<1 hour	**348** (40.3)
No answer	**31** (3.7)
Smartphone Used to Monitor Health-Related Behaviors, n (%)	
Yes	**450** (52.2)
No	**412** (47.8)
Monitored Health-Related Behaviors, n (%)	
Tobacco consumption	**17** (7.7)
Alcohol consumption	**6** (1.3)
Body weight	**135** (30.0)
Diet	**102** (22.6)
Physical exercise	**277** (61.5)
Other health issues (headaches, moods, …)	**199** (44.2)

* Values compliant with cancer prevention guidelines.

Requirement analysis: three focus groups (n=16) were conducted to explore: 1) prior experiences with health-related applications, 2) points of view concerning currently available health-related applications, 3) desired features in a cancer prevention application, and 4) opinions on what influences long term usage of health promotion applications. Based on the focus groups analysis, a questionnaire was designed and applied online to a larger sample (n=798) of healthy Portuguese young adults. The results were analyzed and produced a set of specific guidelines that informed the design and development of the cancer prevention application.

Figure 2. Summary of project development steps involved in the conception of Happy

Project steps	Purpose	Methods used
Requirement analysis	Inform the development of the app	Focus groups Online survey
Prototype development	Develop a functional version of the app (prototype)	Technical development
Pilot study	Test recruitment, registration and data collection processes Test the app (usability and functionality)	Small nonrandomized study
Beta version development	Improve and refine app features based on the feedback provided by the pilot study participants	Focus groups
Implementation	Field-test the app in a large scale intervention Test the effect of the app in comparison with a control group	Quasi-experimental study
Evaluation of implementation impact	Determine the effect of the app on behavior change Refine app development	Focus groups Online survey Semi-structured interviews

- **Prototype Development:** Based on the resulting guidelines of the requirement analysis step, as well as on the scientific literature, a functional prototype of Happy was developed and is ready to be field-tested in a pilot study.
- **Pilot Study:** Happy will be tested in a pilot study. About 50 volunteers will use the application for four weeks. This step will be very important to test essential processes regarding volunteer recruitment, registration and analytical data collection. It will also be used to assess the application in terms of usability and functionality.
- **Beta Version Development:** Randomly selected pilot study participants will discuss their ideas and thoughts in four focus groups (each with 6 to 8 participants) and the results, along with the analytical data, will be used to further develop the cancer prevention application. This version of the application will have to be fully functional and robust enough so that it can be used for a whole year by a large group of volunteers (n>100).
- **Implementation:** A quasi-experimental study with one control group and two experimental groups (each with a minimum of 30 participants) will be implemented to field-test the cancer prevention application. The use of two experimental groups is justified by the need to study the role of social support in behavior change. Therefore, the first experimental group will use a restricted version of the application while the second experimental group will have access to the full version of the application. The control group won't have access to the application but will have access to another application designed specifically to report their health-related behavior. All participants

will be asked to periodically report their health-related behavior (alcohol consumption, physical activity level, skin and breast self-examination, etc.). This periodical input will be essential to pinpoint the exact moments and causes of behavior change. This large-scale intervention will last a full year in order to see long-term usage (and dropout) rates of the application and to allow participants enough time to change behavior. It will also allow the analysis of participant's behavior in summer months, critical for skin cancer prevention.

- **Evaluation:** The final step will allow the in-depth analysis of the implementation results. Four focus groups will be conducted, each with 6 to 8 participants. Randomly selected participants from the quasi-experimental study will form the focus groups, essential to provide the feedback needed to complete the development of the cancer prevention application. Semi-structured interviews to selected participants of the study (high and low achievers) will be conducted to further analyze the advantages and weaknesses of the application in terms of behavior change capabilities.

This project is under development and currently entering the third step (pilot study). The two completed steps will now be described in detail:

Requirement Analysis

Three focus groups with 16 healthy young adults (potential end users of the application) were conducted between December 2013 and January 2014. Participants were encouraged to share prior experiences, points of view and opinions about currently available health-related applications. Desired features in a cancer prevention application, personal health data storing and sharing and important factors for long-term app usage emerged as the recurrent themes on the focus groups discussions (Table 2).

Based on the focus groups results, a questionnaire was designed and applied online to a larger sample of healthy young adults (potential end users of the application). The online survey was available during March 2014. A total of 798 valid questionnaires (out of 1693) were collected. The data was analyzed and confronted with the focus groups results.

Concerning the desired features in a cancer prevention application, the respondents of the online survey tended to agree with the focus group participants (Figure 3).

Regarding personal health data storing and sharing, online respondents also tended to agree with the focus groups participants (Figure 4). They agreed that sharing health information with other users that have similar issues could help them cope with the situation and thus they would share information, although they stated that they would not share any personal info with others. However, contrary to what was stated on the focus groups, sharing information for comparison purposes was ill viewed by respondents. This is more noticeable in the female gender as they tend to disagree more with these statements. Also, female respondents didn't see competition with friends as a very motivating feature.

Concerning data storage, most respondents didn't oppose to having their data stored in a server.

The online respondents identified several other factors (adding to the ones identified by the focus groups participants) that are deemed as important for long-term application usage (Figure 5). According to the online respondents, the quality of health information (validation, updated info, tailoring and detail), behavior tracking, healthy challenges promotion and reminders use are all important factors to be considered.

Again, online respondents didn't see the ability to connect with friends or other users as a very important factor for long-term application use. This was particularly true for female respondents.

Table 2. Overview of the results from the focus groups

Theme	Key Points Identified	FG Sample Transcription
Desired features in a cancer prevention application	*Health behavior tracking* • Potentially motivating feature • Allows the identification of behavior mistakes • Tracking negative behaviors might trigger negative emotions	"A person is able to track and see how we are every day and I think that's an advantage because we can see if we exceeded something or not and that's going to influence our habits." (Participant B, FG#1)
	Health goal setting • Important motivation factor • If associated with a reward system might boost motivation • If goals aren't met, might have a negative effect on user's behavior	"People like to have things to accomplish, goals to achieve. And if the app doesn't have a goal people will… and it has to be interactive and simple." (Participant B, FG#2)
	Tailored information • Information tailoring is essential due to the nature of health information • Excess of information might lead to confusion and hurt user's understanding, particularly concerning cancer	"Not a generic thing. Like, a person has bad eating habits, downloads some app that's going to suggest thousands of healthy things. Even if that person doesn't need them. Instead of just giving the same suggestions to all users, try to figure out how the person is, it's profile, and then use this information to create tailored suggestions." (Participant F, FG#1)
	Use of reminders • Use of reminders to go to medical appointments or to trigger healthy behaviors is very useful for behavior change • This feature should be used with caution and only in relevant contexts to avoid becoming annoying and being deactivated by users.	"When I think about prevention and health the first thing that comes to mind is our eating habits. An app that, I don't know… for instance, uses reminders, that's also very important. Remind us to drink water or eat fruit." (Participant A, FG#1)
Personal health data storing and sharing	• The importance of keeping personal health data private and secure was consensual among participants • Users may feel uncomfortable using an application that stores personal data online • Participants revealed some willingness to share personal data with others, as long as they controlled what is shared • Sharing personal information in specific contexts (to compete with friends or with users with the same health issue, for instance) could be potentially motivating	"One thing is to follow ourselves. Other thing is to have 'our friends from NSA' following us 24/7. And that links to the question of where the data is saved. One thing is keeping it on the phone and being able to delete it. A different thing is keeping it on the other side, in the cloud. Because there you can delete it, what you see, but you won't really delete it. It's like Facebook chat, you delete it but it isn't deleted." (Participant B, FG#1)
Important factors for long-term application usage	*Easiness of use*, quality of the *user interface*, *peer influence* (applications used by friends) and *device optimization* of the application (battery management, for instance) were identified as the most important factors for long-term usage	"I think that, the more information you have to input, less likely it will be to use the app for a long period of time. The first time we will like it and do it, the second also, the third one… right?" (Participant C, FG#2) "The graphic output, the interface. It's… the app might be very good, if it has a horrible interface it can't be, I won't use it, it has to be attractive." (Participant A, FG#3)

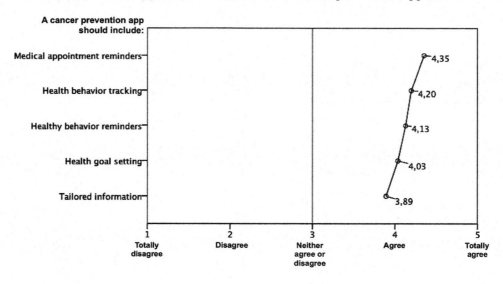

Figure 3. Online survey results of features to include on a cancer prevention application

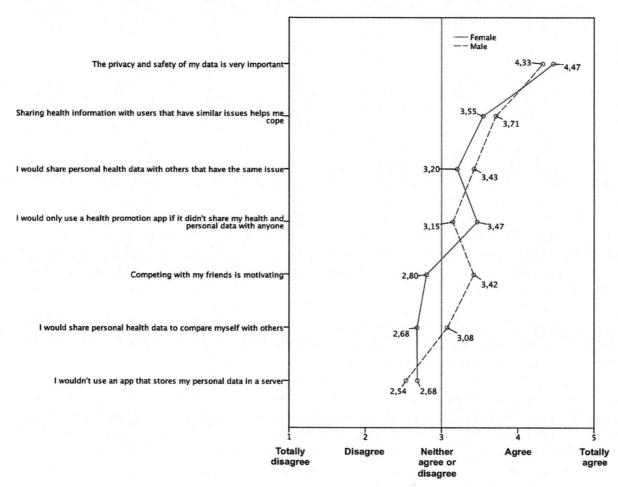

Figure 4. Online survey results of personal health data storing and sharing by gender

Figure 5. Online survey results of the relative importance of factors for long-term application usage by gender (8 or more = very important)

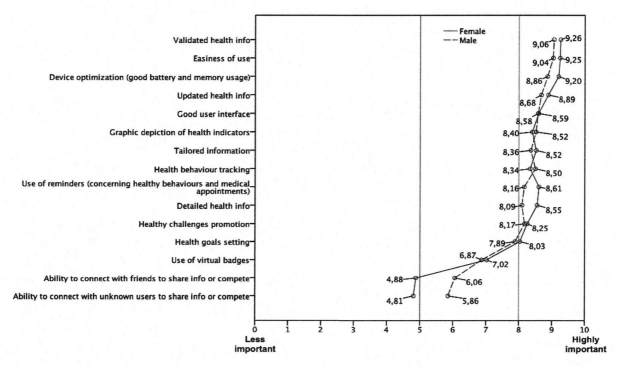

The study participants identified four main features that should be included in a cancer prevention application: health behavior tracking, health goal setting, reminders and tailored information. The first two were seen as more engaging and motivating and could be the core features to support behavior change. It was implied by several participants that seeing how we behave could be a call to action for most people and lead to the desired behavior change. Likewise, most participants considered that having goals to achieve was an important motivational factor and a feature that should be included. This has also been reported in previous studies (Ahtinen et al., 2009; Consolvo, Klasnja, McDonald, & Landay, 2012; Dennison, Morrison, Conway, & Yardley, 2013). The ability to set reminders was viewed as a very important feature, mainly to remind scheduled medical appointments but also to remind to comply with healthy guidelines (eat more fruit, for example). This feature was also highlighted in another study (Ramanathan, Swendeman, Comulada, Estrin, & Rotheram-Borus, 2013). Finally, study participants noted the importance of tailoring health information provided to the user. Several participants highlighted this feature as a way to help users understand what they have to do without being overwhelmed by too much information. This feature was stressed as essential when it concerns cancer, as there are many misconceptions and myths surrounding this disease (Burak & Boone, 2008).

Regarding information sharing, focus group participants showed some openness as long as this was user controlled and only in specific contexts, like between users with similar problems or with friends for competition purposes. However, online respondents seemed less keen on sharing information, despite recognizing its value - the majority agreed that sharing information with similar users would help them cope with a healthy lifestyle. This tendency was particularly apparent in female respondents and regarding information sharing for competition or comparison purposes. As for long-term use of health applications, the study participants identified several dimensions that could influence it. Easiness of use, good user interface, good smartphone resource management, quality of health information (validation, updated information, tailoring and detail), behavior tracking, healthy challenges promotion and use of reminders were highlighted as the most important dimensions. Study results seem to show that, if a user perceives the application as useful, with a good user experience and having an increased value to them (mainly due to the type of information it contains), they will be more likely to use it for a long period of time. This is an important finding because, if we want them to change behavior in a consistent and sustained way, we have to find ways to engage users for a long period of time.

Features associated with gamification (use of virtual badges, competition with others), designed to increase motivation and to further engage users with applications, don't seem to be important dimensions for long-term use of health-related applications. This was more apparent in female respondents even though male respondents also didn't perceive it as so important as other dimensions.

The requirement analysis step allowed the definition of a guideline set for the development of a cancer prevention application (Table 3). The guidelines highlight the focus groups and online survey results and are linked to design and development dimensions. Each dimension provides a possible solution to address the corresponding guideline.

Prototype Development

Happy aims to be a simple and easy-to-use cancer prevention application that attempts to persuade users to change their behavior, making healthier choices, and thus reducing their personal risk of developing several types of cancer. The application was designed bearing in mind the resulting guidelines of the requirement analysis step and uses Fogg Behavior Model (Fogg, 2009, 2011; Stanford Persuasive Tech Lab, 2010) as a theoretical framework.

Happy is based on the principle of tailoring, i.e., using information on a given individual/profile to determine what specific content he or she will receive (Hawkins, Kreuter, Resnicow, Fishbein, & Dijkstra, 2008). Thus, when users access Happy for the first time they need to answer a behavior assessment

Table 3. Guidelines for the development of a cancer prevention application

	Guidelines	**Dimensions**
User experience	Application has to be light, simple to use, and behaviour tracking should be passive or based upon low burden inputs.	Easiness of use User interface Smartphone resource management Data input
Motivation	Application has to be engaging and provide tools to enhance users' motivation. Gamification features aren't considered important.	Behaviour tracking Healthy challenges promotion Health goal setting
Usefulness	Application has to have useful tools that help users make healthier choices and gain insight on their behaviour.	Use of reminders Behaviour tracking Healthy challenges promotion
Application content	Application content must be validated and up to date. Health information provided should be tailored to the users current health status.	Quality and pertinence of content
Social sharing	Application can have social features but they should be optional and user controlled.	Information sharing
Privacy and Safety	Application has to be safe to use and preserve users privacy using secure connections.	Safety Security Data storage

questionnaire (Figure 6A). This assessment allows the definition of the users profile and determines the current level of cancer prevention, called HappyScore (Figure 6B). The HappyScore depicted on the landing page will allow the users to self-monitor their behavior changes. The highest the displayed number, the better the behavior in terms of cancer prevention. This strategy as proven effective in influencing health behaviors in other contexts (Helfer & Shultz, 2014). The score ranges from 0 to 150, having the commonly used 0 to 100 been deliberately avoided to prevent misunderstandings: if the score ranged from 0 to 100 it could be mistaken as a percentage of protection against cancer; thus 100 would mean 100% protection, a vision that is misleading as we can lower our personal risk of cancer but we can't eliminate it completely by having a healthier life.

The user profile is also used to tailor health messages to each individual. Tailored messages (Figure 6C) are the triggers of behavior change. The messages are tailored accordingly to the users profile, influenced by users previous behavior and take into account users context (location, time of day, week and month, weather conditions). There are messages designed to change specific behaviors and reminders to do self-examinations or to enroll in screenings. The goal is to deliver the right message to the right user in the right moment. The effort of tailoring messages to the users profile and context has been proven successful in other behavior change interventions (Campbell et al., 2009; Gerend, Shepherd, & Lustria, 2013) and is, therefore, a core feature of Happy. Messages target specific behaviors and follow the guidelines of the European Code Against Cancer (Boyle et al., 2003).

Happy also allows behavior tracking. Users can track their behavior by answering behavior questions that are sent to them periodically by the application or by deliberately entering behavior data. These behavior assessments are used to recalculate the users HappyScore and change the user profile over time, allowing the tailoring to occur concurrently to the changes in behavior. At any given time, users can explore the Statistics section (Figure 6D) of the application and assess their own behavior evolution. Statistics are the graphic feedback of behavior tracking. It is mainly a self-assessment and motivation tool. Graphic feedback can help people reflect on patterns of their activities and may help them change their behavior (Consolvo et al., 2012). Happy's behavior tracking relies upon low burden inputs. For

Figure 6. Happy main features: behavior assessment questionnaire (A), HappyScore (application's landing page) (B), tailored message (C) and statistics (D)

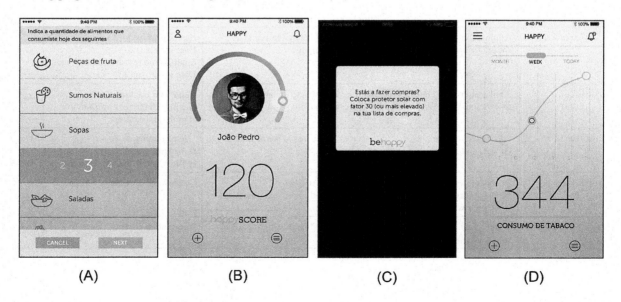

instance, from time to time, users will be prompted to input amounts of fruits and vegetables consumed that day. As users input this data, the correspondent graphic will start to take form, allowing users to track this behavior through time.

In order to further engage users with Happy there are two other sections: Challenges and Social.

Challenges are healthy challenges meant to further engage users with the application. The challenges are optional and users can enroll them at their own will. They are designed to give small achievable goals to boost users motivation and help them reach desired behaviors. Each completed challenge has a score and can be used for comparison purposes with other users in the social section.

Social section displays all users that are added to the user's social network. It allows users to communicate with other users in an individual, group or application community level. This feature is designed to boost online support and competition between users. In order to leverage existing online social interactions, Happy was integrated with the most widely used social networking system: Facebook ("Facebook statistics," 2015). This was done using Facebook's open application-programing interface (API) that allows access to functions for online interaction to third party applications.

Happy's general architecture (Figure 7) consists of the sensors (date and time, GPS and accelerometer) embedded in the smartphone; the smartphone; a server (that acts simultaneously as a web server and a data repository); a message & challenges database; and World Weather Online, Google Maps and Facebook services. The smartphone's embedded sensors detect and feed data (GPS coordinates, device movement, date and time) to Happy. The application then processes this data using the World Weather Online and Google Maps API to generate significant contextual data (weather conditions and location). The smartphone transmits the data to the remote server where it is bundled with the user profile (previously stored in the server). This data set is then used to search the message database and select the message that is best suited to the user profile and current context. The selected message (tailored message) is then sent to the smartphone and presented to the user in the application.

Behavior data entered by users is sent to the server where it is registered and used to recalculate the HappyScore and statistics. These values are then sent to the smartphone and presented graphically to the

Figure 7. Happy's general architecture

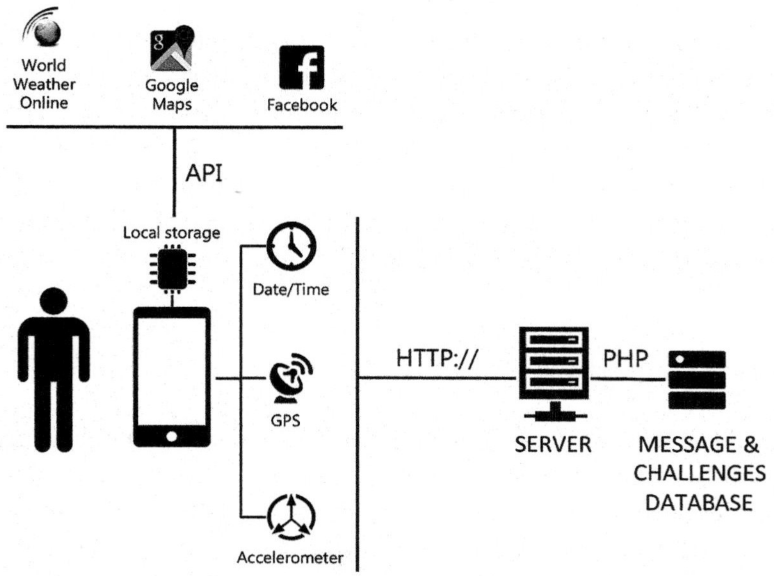

user. All entered data is stored in the server and mapped into the user profile, influencing the subsequent messages sent to the user and the challenges that are suggested to the user by the application. The Facebook API is used to manage all social interactions between the user and his peers. Hypertext Transfer Protocol (HTTP) is used in all data transmission between the smartphone and the server, which means that the smartphone must have an Internet connection service such as General Packet Radio Service (GPRS), 3rd generation (3G), 4th generation (4G) or a wireless local area network. If the smartphone is temporarily disconnected from the Internet, all entered data will be stored locally and sent to the server when the connection is restored, updating all data values. Happy runs on Android OS and iOS, the two most commonly used smartphone platforms.

FUTURE RESEARCH DIRECTIONS

Behavior change interventions using mobile technologies are a new research field. As technology evolves, new and more complex tools can be developed to help users change their behavior towards a healthier lifestyle. Recent developments have led to the commercialization of several electronic activity monitors, known as wearables, that can monitor health indicators (e.g. physical activity or sleep patterns) continuously throughout the day (Ledger & McCaffrey, 2014; Steinhubl, Muse, & Topol, 2015). These devices offer a great opportunity to enhance behavior change interventions. They can track all activity seamlessly, significantly lowering user input burden. Tracked data can be used to further tailor interventions to the users needs. Despite acknowledge potential, wearable devices also have disadvantages. They can't track all types of activities and often misinterpret performed activities (Consolvo et al., 2012). This inaccuracy can lead to user disappointment and might help explain why most users stop using wearables six months after purchase (Ledger & McCaffrey, 2014). There is still a long way to go until most people adopt some type of wearable that can help them improve their lifestyle.

The development of Happy, the cancer prevention application designed to change behavior, will continue as described. The prototype will be tested in a pilot study and refinements to the application will be included. Then, the application will be used in a large-scale intervention and its impact evaluation will allow an in-depth analysis of the real capabilities of Happy to induce behavior change in users and, thus, contribute to cancer prevention.

One major issue to be tackled in this project will be long-term use of the application. Studies have shown that continued active use of health related applications is very low (Consumer Health Information Corporation, n.d.). The value of healthy eating or physical activity arises from performing it in a sustainable way over time. Cancer prevention through behavior change relies upon performing healthy behaviors for the rest of people's lives. Health interventions usually do not approach behavior change from this long-term perspective (Consolvo et al., 2012). This is one of the most important challenges that future behavior change research will have to face.

CONCLUSION

Cancer incidence could be reduced to half if populations adopted healthier behaviors. Behavior change, despite being a very difficult task, can be achieved with proper strategies. Smartphones provide a great opportunity for behavior change. They are personal, connected and always close-at-hand. They follow people around and can sense what they are doing, allowing interventions to occur at the most opportune time. Smartphones have been used successfully in interventions ranging from smoking cessation, to weight loss and disease management. They can be very useful tools to empower people and help them make healthier choices.

Happy is an exploratory approach to cancer prevention using smartphones. The application's main goal is to persuade users to change their behavior, making healthier choices, thus reducing their personal risk of developing several types of cancer. The development process of Happy requires multiple steps and relies upon successive refinements of a prototype involving the target population. The work described shows that users are open to this type of intervention and identifies an opportunity to help people change behavior towards cancer prevention.

REFERENCES

Ahtinen, A., Mattila, E., Vaatanen, A., Hynninen, L., Salminen, J., Koskinen, E., & Laine, K. (2009). User experiences of mobile wellness applications in health promotion: User study of Wellness Diary, Mobile Coach and SelfRelax. In *Proceedings of the 3d International ICST Conference on Pervasive Computing Technologies for Healthcare* (pp. 1–8). ICST. doi:10.4108/ICST.PERVASIVEHEALTH2009.6007

ANACOM. (2014). *Serviços móveis: informação estatística - 1º trimestre de 2014*. ANACOM.

Bert, F., Giacometti, M., Gualano, M. R., & Siliquini, R. (2014). Smartphones and health promotion: A review of the evidence. *Journal of Medical Systems, 38*(1), 9995. doi:10.1007/s10916-013-9995-7 PMID:24346929

Boyle, P., Autier, P., Bartelink, H., Baselga, J., Boffetta, P., Burn, J., & zur Hausen, H. et al. (2003). European Code Against Cancer and scientific justification: Third version (2003). *Annals of Oncology, 14*(7), 973–1005. doi:10.1093/annonc/mdg305 PMID:12853336

Burak, L., & Boone, B. (2008). College Women and Breast Cancer: Knowledge, Behaviour, and Beliefs Regarding Risk Reduction. *American Journal of Health Education, 39*(4), 206–212. doi:10.1080/1932 5037.2008.10599040

Campbell, M. K., Carr, C., Devellis, B., Switzer, B., Biddle, A., Amamoo, M. A., … Sandler, R. (2009). A randomized trial of tailoring and motivational interviewing to promote fruit and vegetable consumption for cancer prevention and control. *Annals of Behavioral Medicine: A Publication of the Society of Behavioral Medicine, 38*(2), 71–85. doi:10.1007/s12160-009-9140-5

Colditz, G. A., & Wei, E. K. (2012). Preventability of cancer: The relative contributions of biologic and social and physical environmental determinants of cancer mortality. *Annual Review of Public Health, 33*(1), 137–156. doi:10.1146/annurev-publhealth-031811-124627 PMID:22224878

Colditz, G. A., Wolin, K. Y., & Gehlert, S. (2012). Applying what we know to accelerate cancer prevention. *Science Translational Medicine, 4*(127), 127. doi:10.1126/scitranslmed.3003218 PMID:22461645

Consolvo, S., Klasnja, P., McDonald, D. W., & Landay, J. A. (2012). Designing for Healthy Lifestyles: Design Considerations for Mobile Technologies to Encourage Consumer Health and Wellness. *Foundations and Trends® in Human–Computer Interaction, 6*(3–4), 167–315. doi:10.1561/1100000040

Consumer Health Information Corporation. (n.d.). *Motivating Patients to Use Smartphone Health Apps*. Retrieved August 26, 2014, from http://www.prweb.com/releases/2011/04/prweb5268884.htm

Davis, S. W., & Oakley-girvan, I. (2014). mHealth Education Applications Along the Cancer Continuum. *Journal of Cancer Education*, 10–15. doi:10.1007/s13187-014-0761-4 PMID:25482319

Dennison, L., Morrison, L., Conway, G., & Yardley, L. (2013). Opportunities and Challenges for Smartphone Applications in Supporting Health Behavior change: Qualitative Study. *Journal of Medical Internet Research*, *15*(4), e86. doi:10.2196/jmir.2583 PMID:23598614

eMarketer. (2014). *2 Billion Consumers Worldwide to Get Smart(phones) by 2016*. Retrieved July 6, 2015, from http://www.emarketer.com/Article/2-Billion-Consumers-Worldwide-Smartphones-by-2016/1011694

European Commission. (2014). *Green Paper on mobile Health ("mHealth")*. Retrieved from http://ec.europa.eu/digital-agenda/en/news/green-paper-mobile-health-mhealth

Facebook Statistics. (2015). Retrieved May 30, 2015, from http://www.statisticbrain.com/facebook-statistics/

Fiordelli, M., Diviani, N., & Schulz, P. J. (2013). Mapping mHealth research: A decade of evolution. *Journal of Medical Internet Research*, *15*(5), e95. doi:10.2196/jmir.2430 PMID:23697600

Fogg, B. J. (2009). A behavior model for persuasive design. *Proceedings of the 4th International Conference on Persuasive Technology - Persuasive '09*. doi:10.1145/1541948.1541999

Fogg, B. J. (2011). *BJ Fogg's Behavior Model*. Retrieved May 29, 2013, from http://www.behaviormodel.org/index.html

Gerend, M. A., Shepherd, M. A., & Lustria, M. L. A. (2013). Increasing human papillomavirus vaccine acceptability by tailoring messages to young adult women's perceived barriers. *Sexually Transmitted Diseases*, *40*(5), 401–405. doi:10.1097/OLQ.0b013e318283c8a8 PMID:23588130

Hawkins, N. A., Berkowitz, Z., & Peipins, L. A. (2010). What does the public know about preventing cancer? Results from the Health Information National Trends Survey (HINTS). *Health Education & Behavior*, *37*(4), 490–503. doi:10.1177/1090198106296770 PMID:17478600

Hawkins, R. P., Kreuter, M., Resnicow, K., Fishbein, M., & Dijkstra, A. (2008). Understanding tailoring in communicating about health. *Health Education Research*, *23*(3), 454–466. doi:10.1093/her/cyn004 PMID:18349033

Helfer, P., & Shultz, T. R. (2014). The effects of nutrition labeling on consumer food choice: A psychological experiment and computational model. *Annals of the New York Academy of Sciences*, *1331*(1), 174–185. doi:10.1111/nyas.12461 PMID:24913496

IARC. (2008). *World Cancer report 2008*. IARC.

International Union Against Cancer. (2004). *Evidence-based Cancer Prevention: Strategies for NGOs*. UICC.

ITU. (2014). *Be He@lthy Be Mobile*. Geneva. Retrieved from http://www.itu.int/en/ITU-D/ICT-Applications/eHEALTH/Be_healthy/Documents/Be_Healthy_Be_Mobile_Annual_Report 2013-2014_Final.pdf

Jemal, A., Bray, F., Ferlay, J., Ward, E., & Forman, D. (2011). Global Cancer Statistics. *CA: a Cancer Journal for Clinicians*, *61*(2), 69–90. doi:10.3322/caac.20107 PMID:21296855

Kaptein, M., De Ruyter, B., Markopoulos, P., & Aarts, E. (2012). Adaptive Persuasive Systems. *ACM Transactions on Interactive Intelligent Systems*, 2(2), 1–25. doi:10.1145/2209310.2209313

Keeney, S., McKenna, H., Fleming, P., & McIlfatrick, S. (2010). Attitudes to cancer and cancer prevention: What do people aged 35-54 years think? *European Journal of Cancer Care*, 19(6), 769–777. doi:10.1111/j.1365-2354.2009.01137.x PMID:19708946

Klasnja, P., & Pratt, W. (2012). Healthcare in the pocket: Mapping the space of mobile-phone health interventions. *Journal of Biomedical Informatics*, 45(1), 184–198. doi:10.1016/j.jbi.2011.08.017 PMID:21925288

Kremers, S. P. J., De Bruijn, G.-J., Schaalma, H., & Brug, J. (2004). Clustering of energy balance-related behaviours and their intrapersonal determinants. *Psychology & Health*, 19(5), 595–606. doi:10.1080/0 8870440412331279630

Ledger, D., & McCaffrey, D. (2014). *Inside Wearables: How the Science of Human Behavior Change offers the Secret to Long-Term Engagement*. Retrieved from http://endeavourpartners.net/assets/Endeavour-Partners-Wearables-White-Paper-20141.pdf

Mata, J., Silva, M. N., Vieira, P. N., Carraça, E. V., Andrade, A. M., Coutinho, S. R., & Teixeira, P. J. et al. (2009). Motivational "spill-over" during weight control: Increased self-determination and exercise intrinsic motivation predict eating self-regulation. *Health Psychology*, 28(6), 709–716. doi:10.1037/a0016764 PMID:19916639

Mosa, A. S. M., Yoo, I., & Sheets, L. (2012). A systematic review of healthcare applications for smartphones. *BMC Medical Informatics and Decision Making*, 12(1), 67. doi:10.1186/1472-6947-12-67 PMID:22781312

Pandey, A., Hasan, S., Dubey, D., & Sarangi, S. (2013). Smartphone apps as a source of cancer information: Changing trends in health information-seeking behavior. *Journal of Cancer Education*, 28(1), 138–142. doi:10.1007/s13187-012-0446-9 PMID:23275239

Ramanathan, N., Swendeman, D., Comulada, W. S., Estrin, D., & Rotheram-Borus, M. J. (2013). Identifying preferences for mobile health applications for self-monitoring and self-management: Focus group findings from HIV-positive persons and young mothers. *International Journal of Medical Informatics*, 82(4), e38–e46. doi:10.1016/j.ijmedinf.2012.05.009 PMID:22704234

Silva, B. M. C., Rodrigues, J. J. P. C., de la Torre Díez, I., López-Coronado, M., & Saleem, K. (2015). Mobile-health: A review of current state in 2015. *Journal of Biomedical Informatics*, 56, 265–272. doi:10.1016/j.jbi.2015.06.003 PMID:26071682

Spring, B., Schneider, K., Mcfadden, H. G., Vaughn, J., Kozak, A. T., Smith, M., & Lloyd-jones, D. M. et al. (2012). Multiple Behavior Changes in Diet and Activity. *Archives of Internal Medicine*, 172(10), 789–796. doi:10.1001/archinternmed.2012.1044 PMID:22636824

Stanford Persuasive Tech Lab. (2010). *Purple Path Behavior Guide*. Stanford Persuasive Tech Lab.

Stein, C. J., & Colditz, G. A. (2004). Modifiable risk factors for cancer. *British Journal of Cancer*, 90(2), 299–303. doi:10.1038/sj.bjc.6601509 PMID:14735167

Steinhubl, S. R., Muse, E. D., & Topol, E. J. (2015). The Emerging Field of Mobile Health. *Science Translational Medicine, 7*(283), 1–6. doi:10.1126/scitranslmed.aaa3487 PMID:25877894

Whittaker, R., Merry, S., Dorey, E., & Maddison, R. (2012). A development and evaluation process for mHealth interventions: examples from New Zealand. *Journal of Health Communication, 17.* doi:10.1080/10810730.2011.649103

WHO. (2011). *mHealth: new horizons for health through mobile technologies: second global survey on eHealth* (Vol. 3). Retrieved from http://www.who.int/goe/publications/goe_mhealth_web.pdf

Wolf, J. A., Moreau, J. F., Akilov, O., Patton, T., English, J. C., Ho, J., & Ferris, L. K. (2013). Diagnostic Inaccuracy of Smartphone Applications for Melanoma Detection. *JAMA Dermatology, 149*(4), 422. doi:10.1001/jamadermatol.2013.2382 PMID:23325302

KEY TERMS AND DEFINITIONS

Behavior Change: Any transformation or modification of human behavior.

Behavior Change Intervention: Broad range of activities and approaches, focused on individual, community and environmental influences on behavior, designed to change behavior.

Cancer Prevention: All the active measures that can be taken to decrease the risk of cancer. Includes actions to lower exposure to known cancer risk factors (*primary prevention*) and diagnose pre-malignant forms of cancer (*secondary prevention*).

Cancer: Term used to describe more than 100 different diseases in which abnormal cells divide without control and are able to invade surrounding tissues.

Healthy Behavior: All behaviors that promote a healthy life. Includes being physically active, having a good diet, not smoking, among other behaviors.

Mobile Phone: Wireless handheld device that can make and receive calls among other features.

Smartphone: A mobile phone that has more advanced computing capability than basic feature phones. Smartphones typically have a relatively large screen and an operating system capable of running general-purpose applications.

Smartphone Application: Computer program designed to run on smartphones. Usually refers to simple programs that perform specific functions on the smartphone.

SmarTV Care:
Benefits and Implications of Smart TVs in Health Care

Eliseo Sciarretta
Link Campus University, Italy

Filippo Benedetti
Link Campus University, Italy

Andrea Ingrosso
Link Campus University, Italy

Roberta Grimaldi
Link Campus University, Italy

INTRODUCTION

The Smart TV is a digital TV set connected to the Internet that offers web-based functions and services. This consumer device offers more advanced computing ability and connectivity than a basic television set and is considered the technological convergence between computers and television with advanced multimedia and interactive features. It provides online services typically intended for normal personal computer (e.g. internet browsing, video on demand, Internet TV, home networking access, streaming services, social networks, etc.), maintains the basic function of broadcasting media and enhances the interactivity of the user with the television set and other connected devices. Smart TVs run complete Operating System and also provide public Software Development Kit (SDK) and/or Native Development Kit (NDK) so that applications can be developed from third-party companies. Apps can be implemented on the browser and ran on the TV screen. Smart TVs technology can also be integrated in set-top boxes (i.e. external devices that enhance basic television features), digital media players, game consoles and other network connected interactive devices. Thanks to the creation of this new convergence area, Smart TV demand is likely to significantly grow and is expected to play a central role in the future smart homes (MoonKoo Kim, 2011). In 2013, global sales of smart TVs have increased 55% over the previous year, with a 33% share of the total number of flat screen TVs purchased during the year. Soon overtaking will come and in 2017 old generation TVs still circulating on the market will be less than a third (Compagnucci, Croce, Da Empoli, & Zambardino, 2014).

The interest in Smart TVs is very high, especially because unlike other devices that may ensure the provision of similar services, such as set-top-boxes, the market growth advances much more quickly (Pant & Greeson, 2013)

The core concept of the device is progressively turning from a convenient use of broadcasting and Internet to a hub of smart life via TV.

In this chapter, the potential of this device to deliver health care services is discussed, by highlighting its strengths and weaknesses and with a focus on usability issues.

DOI: 10.4018/978-1-4666-9978-6.ch082

BACKGROUND

The potential of this technology makes possible to be directly connected to users and patients at home with a wide range of information and services. In this way, a significant impact on the quality, timeliness and availability of health services can be reached. Since it is a rather new topic, researches on it are few and quite lacking at the moment.

When it comes to a target audience with special needs such as elderly and disabled patients, it is also important to plan eHealth services with solutions that allow overcoming the technological barriers (Cashen, Dykes, & Gerber 2004). The employment of an easy-to-use consumer device as Smart TVs can be crucial to address the usability needs of this kind of users who are not familiar with PC or the more recent smart devices. Currently, for this category the TV remains the most well-known technological medium, widely adopted and most familiar as entertainment system and equipped in almost every house. By using this kind of device in the e-Health and Telemedicine area, easily accessible systems can be designed to assist users directly at home. In this way, a Smart TV based telemedicine system can provide a cost effective and user friendly device in terms of interface and acceptance, since the TV is a familiar and the most common household appliance. By taking advantage from this technology, users can easily access medical services from their own environment with comfort, privacy and a significantly positive impact on health condition.

Considering these factors, several services have been proposed by adopting Smart TV sets.

Some applications focus on a telematic rehabilitation exercisers in form of a game for physically limited people (Epelde, et al., 2013; Hinderer, Friedrich, Hobel, & Wolf, 2013; Hinderer, Friederich, & Wolf, 2012). This kind of therapy at home usually aims to preserve or restore mobility. In these cases, gaming is conceived as a tool to objectivise the performance improvements and increase the motivation for a self-directed rehabilitation. Since interaction is also a crucial part of the system, the therapeutic recommendations for further exercises are delivered while monitoring and collecting data during the rehabilitation.

Telemonitoring services have also been deeply embedded in healthcare industry through Smart TV sets. The purpose of this kind of service is on one side to reduce the hospitalisation of patients by taking care and supervise them directly in their own domestic environment, on the other to provide a more independent life while being able to rely on help in case of emergency. Due to chronic illnesses, a continuous monitoring is required with aged patients. Systems can be designed to detect abnormalities, provide temporary advice or send alerts to the medical staff in case of emergency (Sorwar & Hasan, 2012). In order to help care-dependent people to be more independent, television services have been designed so that patients can access their own medical reports (Raffaeli, Gambi, & Spinsante, 2014), receive reminders or check their status displayed on screen (Lorenz & Oppermann, 2009). In all of the different telemonitoring frameworks composed by smart devices, Smart TV technology can be used as the mean of interaction between the user and the health care providers.

Monitoring is a solution that let the aged patients to live in their environment as long as possible. In addition, the social isolation problem has been deeply considered in the design of systems for this population. Regarding this issue, Smart TV applications have been proposed to support socially oriented activities for older people to improve psychological well-being (Alaoui & Lewkowicz, 2013). Providing individuals with the opportunity to use Internet allow them to access information and communicate with others. On one side this contributes to reduce their isolation and on the other makes possible to reconnect to the world in a new way. Projects (e.g. FoSIBLE), Virtual communities (e.g. Australian GreyPath) and Social TV systems (e.g. i.TV, Boxee, Telebuddies, NDS Social TV, iNeighbour TV) (Abreu & Almeida,

2012; Alliez, 2008; Luyten, Thys, Huypens, & Coninx, 2006) have been developed. These systems offer access to services such as forums, blogs, text chat, voice communication, TV recommendations, group video games and support groups. The principal challenge of these kinds of innovative social applications is to promote participation and increase involvement in collective practices and health care (Alaoui, Lewkowicz, & Seffah, 2012).

IMPLICATIONS AND OPEN ISSUES

The analysis of the services that e-Health applications can offer via smart devices has to focus on the implications on the daily lives of people.

Telemedicine systems create a unique relationship with the patient, requiring the attention and adherence to the principles of professional ethics. One of the main risks of the doctor-patient relationship is in the increase of authoritarian and paternalistic attitude of the expert and a corresponding submission of the patient (Papi, 1997). This relationship should not be regulated by strict laws, but modulated onto a true "therapeutic alliance." With regard to this one of the main features of telemedicine is in the continuation of the relationship from the clinical context directly to home. At the same time attention has to be paid at the decrease of the "personal" relationship that can lead to complaints about medical practice. For this reason, a care-at-distance system primarily focuses on clinical-diagnostic aspects, while recognises as fundamental the contextualisation and the accessibility of therapy.

In order to make the connection as direct as possible and achieve a good compliance with patients, especially with the older population, the employment of Smart TV platform based services can be considered an efficient/effective solution. Such a device can better address the needs of people lacking in technological skills. It is important to note that Smart TV is not necessarily easier to use than other devices (neither more difficult), nonetheless it can represent a better solution for elderly people and users who are unfamiliar with new technologies.

Television is well known and frequently used by elderly people, modern TVs have large screens that simplify the reading of the content and therefore the use of services. Moreover, while computers are commonly considered as a working tool, the TVs are more likely to be accepted as a communication media from this population (Lehtinen, Näsänen, & Sarvas, 2009). In this way, the interaction with the medical staff for the monitoring or rehabilitation services and also the social media functions can be easily accessed and accepted in the daily life of patient. Nevertheless, when dealing with the recent smart devices in telemedicine services, it must be remembered that technologies can often be considered as intrusive from older population. With the increase of disability and the loss of independence, increases the need of private information by the new systems to be more effective (Alaoui & Lewkowicz, 2012). Even more so, the acceptability of the device becomes an important issue. Privacy of the user and the security of data transmitted over the device have also to be taken into consideration. The telemedicine systems should adopt protocols and network security software for the protection of patient data, as well as the confidentiality and identification. Privacy should be ensured by adopting a minimum encryption and digital signatures as https protocol, and SSL (Secure Socket Layer) certificates.

The adoption of Smart TV sets has great potential as a medium for telemedicine and e-Health services, especially in terms of acceptability. However, problems of interaction and interface can rise when employing this kind of technology for new purposes in the daily life of older people. The conjunction of physical and cognitive problems, and the lack of motivation, may cause several difficulties in the relation between users and technology. Therefore, this kind of limitations should be kept in mind when the services are designed for aged or disabled population. Enhancing the accessibility to this kind of technology has to be considered a primary aim in order to avoid specific problems of usage.

INTERACTION

Portable devices (e.g. tablets and smart phones) and personal computers are usually adopted for tele-medicine and e-Health systems. However, these can be less efficient for older people, who are not accustomed to the use of such devices in the daily life. The possibility to converge the recent IT devices into the most accepted one has the potential to reduce the intrusiveness of technology in the domestic environment and thus influences positively the acceptance by users. In addition to this, TV screens are generally bigger than PC monitors, this can simplify the access to the e-Health services for older people. These Smart TVs features can make the enjoyment easier not only of health care services, but of all the services that can be offered to the user.

However, a wide range of TV sets is on the market in terms of size and performance, from CRT (i.e. Cathode Ray Tube) to LCD monitors, from 20 up to 60 inches, with a resolution that may vary from HD ready, to Full HD or even Ultra HD. These variables have implications in the design process, for example the proportion between characters and screen size have to be taken into account, as well as the organisation of contents for an efficient utilisation of the available space. The best trade-off between readability, available space on the TV screen, and easy consulting has to be achieved (Raffaeli, et al. 2014).

The main input device used to interact with the Smart TV is the TV remote control. On one hand this entails advantages in terms of familiarity for all the users categories. On the other, with the advance of features available on the Smart TVs, the remote control can result not practical and problematic in the interactive environment. For example, typing text on a virtual QWERTY keyboard, searching or sharing content become complex operations. When the design of devices is addressed to an elderly or disabled population, age-related difficulties must also be taken into account. For many people, the remote control may become a significant barrier due to issues of cognitive processing ability, limited vision and/or manual dexterity. In fact, the remote control requires a combination of sequences of buttons to access the services and significant difficulties are raised about the number, keys layout and size in relation to the navigation process within the applications. These usually involve the excessive number of buttons, their proximity and their inadequate grouping and labeling (Carmichael, Rice, & Sloan, 2005).

With the advancements in the telemedicine area, new types of remote controls and ways to interact with the Smart TV are needed. The user-centered design of these devices should be managed, in order to provide easily accessible services (Lim, 2012). Currently, integrating new interface modes appears to provide a solution for the limitations of the remote control. Motion detection and voice control[1] use can lead to efficient interaction results, as long as the developers of the apps are able to smooth out the complexity of services through an interface that is friendly for users with little or no experience with technology.

Voice interfaces can be very useful for people with motor disabilities to avoid problems with digital interfaces by using the natural language. The use of voice and hearing is a familiar practice that requires minimal physical effort and has no need of eyes and hands. In this way, a direct communication is implemented with devices, which circumvents the problems of coordination of disabled population. This type of interface also makes easier to include users who are not familiar with technology in general.

Users movements can also be detected; in this way gestures become a good interaction system. A possible critical point of this type of interaction is related to the commands that are not voluntary. A further improvement is in the development of interfaces that require no explicit commands from the user, but act instead according to not explicit user messages such as eye movements, gesture recognition and posture.

It is better to avoid indirect input devices (e.g. keyboard and mouse), which are not easy-to-use by this type of users (Wood, Willoughby, Rushing, Bechtel, & Gilbert, 2005). The mouse handling may be not easy to master as it requires high hand-eye coordination and a consequent cognitive effort (Vigouroux, Rumeau, Vella, & Vellas, 2009). The age-related changes in motor skills, the effect of chronic diseases or disabilities caused by strokes or arthritis, interfere with the level of precision in the movement of the hands. The standard keyboards may also cause the same problem with respect to motor skills, although to a lesser extent. More difficulties can be related to sight if there is no familiarity with the symbols placed on the keys. (Czaja & Lee, 2003)

Good results in interaction have been reached by providing adapted input devices in addition to the traditional remote control to make the interaction more attractive and easy-to-use (Alaoui & Lewkowicz, 2013; Alaoui et al., 2012). In these cases gesture recognition and tablets were used to control the TV-based media platform: the motion detection to interact with the menus, and the tablet as an additional control device, input terminal (e.g. enter text during chats or when writing a short article) or a display for messages when the TV is switched off.

Even if the Smart TV doesn't necessarily requires additional devices, for some types of services in the telemedicine area this integration can be an efficient solution to simplify the interaction with the device.

DESIGN GUIDELINES FOR THE INTERFACE

Older adults and disabled patients often have difficulties to cope with the increasingly urgent demand of integration with new technologies. The abandonment in the approach to new devices can be caused by complex menus, small font-size, the fear in handling a new type of object or unwanted feedback. Therefore, the interface should be developed as transparent as possible, taking advantages from its familiarity for the users.

For example, the adoption of an inappropriate color can make a text unreadable or invisible for someone, or the presence of profound hierarchical menus in a Smart TV service can become a significant obstacle for older people with memory problems. A clear design and a simple interface that does not require special efforts to be learned are certainly preferred from this type of users. In the design process of an interface, the user needs have to be put in the first place and the limits of cognitive, sensory and/or physical potential users of the system must be taken into account (Alaoui et al., 2012).

The layout should be stable, with few orderly options, outlining clearly the hierarchy of information and the structure of the system; the presence of moving icons should be avoided; color contrasts have to be high; the typographical choices larger than average, possibly sans-serif in a not justified text, in order to increase the ease of reading; considering the different cultural contexts from which the user can come or any cognitive impairment, the words in the text must be simple and easy to understand.

In the literature there are ergonomic guidelines for the development of easy-to-use applications on Smart TVs (Dickinson, Arnott, & Prior, 2007; Carmichael, 1999). The existing knowledge and methods from user-centered design and usability engineering studies can also be applied. By following these guidelines, references or best practice applications, evaluation results by end users and platform-specific design guidance (Kunert, 2005), the development of e-Health services for the older population can be better addressed to specified user needs.

However, in comparison with other applications in the field of Telemedicine, there are few services concretely implemented through Smart TV, and there is a lack of experience and user feedback. Moreover, the existing knowledge is not focused on sharing and collaboration among different stakeholders (Alaoui et al., 2012). Beside the employment of existing user-centered design methods and guidelines, the participation of the future users - specifically of older adults - in the development of a service can be a solution to this problem. The selection of potential end-users in the design process leads to the identification, classification and modeling of elderly people needs for the TV-based user interface and help stakeholders to be more user-focused.

CONCLUSION

Within the Telemedicine field, the aim of the development of new technologies is in the attempt to access into the domestic context of elderly or disabled people. The Smart TV technology has the potential to become a significant resource among older people. Thanks to its wide adoption in almost every house, the inclusion of vulnerable groups can be promoted by enhancing their possibility to access content and other services available via this expanding medium.

Nevertheless, few steps have been taken in the research to design Smart TV equipment and services on large-scale for older users and disabled patients. A deeper analysis of the wide diversity of their abilities is needed to develop easy-to-use interaction and interface systems. Rethinking this kind of technology from this point of view can give to the medicine system a privileged access directly at home of different patients and help them to concretely pursue a more independent life.

REFERENCES

Abreu, J., & Almeida, P. (2012). A social TV application for senior citizens–iNeighbour TV. *10th European Interactive TV Conference (EuroITV 2012)*. Berlin: ACM New York.

Alaoui, M., & Lewkowicz, M. (2012). Struggling against social isolation of the elderly—the design of smarttv applications. In *From Research to Practice in the Design of Cooperative Systems: Results and Open Challenges* (pp. 261–275). Springer London. doi:10.1007/978-1-4471-4093-1_18

Alaoui, M., & Lewkowicz, M. (2013). A livingLab approach to involve elderly in the design of smart TV applications offering communication services. In *Online Communities and Social Computing* (pp. 325–334). Springer Berlin Heidelberg. doi:10.1007/978-3-642-39371-6_37

Alaoui, M., Lewkowicz, M., & Seffah, A. (2012, January). Increasing elderly social relationships through TV-based services. In *Proceedings of the 2nd ACM SIGHIT International Health Informatics Symposium* (pp. 13-20). ACM. doi:10.1145/2110363.2110369

Alliez, D., & France, N. (2008). Adapt TV paradigms to UGC by importing social networks. In *Adjunct Proceedings of the EuroITV2008 Conference*.

Carmichael, A. (1999). *Style guide for the design of interactive television services for elderly viewers*. Winchester, UK: Independent Television Commission.

Carmichael, A., Rice, M., & Sloan, D. (2005, August). Digital Interactive Television in the UK: is the opportunity for 'inclusivity' being missed. In *Proceedings of the 2005 international conference on Accessible Design in the Digital World* (pp. 8-8). British Computer Society.

Cashen, M. S., Dykes, P., & Gerber, B. (2004). e-Health technology and Internet resources: Barriers for vulnerable populations. *The Journal of Cardiovascular Nursing, 19*(3), 209–214. doi:10.1097/00005082-200405000-00010 PMID:15191264

Compagnucci, S., Croce, L., Da Empoli, S., & Zambardino, B. (2014). *Rapporto I-Com 2014 su reti & servizi di nuova generazione*. I-COM.

Czaja, S. J., & Lee, C. C. (2002, January). Designing computer systems for older adults. In *The human-computer interaction handbook* (pp. 413–427). L. Erlbaum Associates Inc.

Dickinson, A., Arnott, J., & Prior, S. (2007). Methods for human–computer interaction research with older people. *Behaviour & Information Technology, 26*(4), 343–352. doi:10.1080/01449290601176948

Epelde, G., Abascal, J., Jimenez, J. M., Vivanco, K., & Gomez-Fraga, I. (2012). Smart Medical System for the Universal Remote Delivery of Rehabilitation. *InImpact: The Journal of Innovation Impact, 6*(1), 98.

Hinderer, K. U., Friedrich, P., Hobel, O., & Wolf, B. (2013, September). Telematic rehabilitation 2.0. In *Consumer Electronics?? Berlin (ICCE-Berlin), 2013. ICCE Berlin 2013. IEEE Third International Conference on* (pp. 8-12). IEEE.

Hinderer, K. U., Friedrich, P., & Wolf, B. (2012, September). Home care: A Telematic rehabilitation exerciser. In *Consumer Electronics-Berlin (ICCE-Berlin), 2012 IEEE International Conference on* (pp. 15-18). IEEE. doi:10.1109/ICCE-Berlin.2012.6336525

Kim, M., & Park, J. (2011, February). Demand forecasting and strategies for the successfully deployment of the smart TV in Korea. In *Advanced Communication Technology (ICACT)*, 2011 *13th International Conference on* (pp. 1475-1478). IEEE.

Kunert, T. (2009). *User-centered interaction design patterns for interactive digital television applications*. Springer Science & Business Media. doi:10.1007/978-1-84882-275-7

Lehtinen, V., Näsänen, J., & Sarvas, R. (2009, September). A little silly and empty-headed: older adults' understandings of social networking sites. In *Proceedings of the 23rd British HCI Group Annual Conference on People and Computers: Celebrating People and Technology* (pp. 45-54). British Computer Society.

Lim, Y., Park, J., Jung, E. S., Chung, D. H., Kim, T., Choi, K., & Lee, S. (2012, September). Comparative Study on Advanced TV Interface Types in the Smart Media World. In *Ubiquitous Intelligence & Computing and 9th International Conference on Autonomic & Trusted Computing (UIC/ATC), 2012 9th International Conference on* (pp. 342-348). IEEE. doi:10.1109/UIC-ATC.2012.61

Lorenz, A., & Oppermann, R. (2009). Mobile health monitoring for the elderly: Designing for diversity. *Pervasive and Mobile Computing, 5*(5), 478–495. doi:10.1016/j.pmcj.2008.09.010

Luyten, K., Thys, K., Huypens, S., & Coninx, K. (2006, April). Telebuddies: social stitching with interactive television. In CHI'06 extended abstracts on Human factors in computing systems (pp. 1049-1054). ACM.

Pant, V., & Greeson, M. (2013). *In-Home CE and Home Network Ecosystem 2013*. TDG The Diffusion Group.

Papi, G. (1997). La telemedicina per la Sanità del 2000. *TELEMED - Innovazione e tecnologia per la qualità della vita, 5,* 26 - 29.

Raffaeli, L., Gambi, E., & Spinsante, S. (2014, April). Smart TV based ecosystem for personal e-health services. In *Medical Information and Communication Technology (ISMICT), 2014 8th International Symposium on* (pp. 1-5). IEEE. doi:10.1109/ISMICT.2014.6825208

Sorwar, G., & Hasan, R. (2012, March). Smart-TV based integrated e-health monitoring system with agent technology. In *Advanced Information Networking and Applications Workshops (WAINA), 2012 26th International Conference on* (pp. 406-411). IEEE. doi:10.1109/WAINA.2012.155

Vigouroux, N., Rumeau, P., Vella, F., & Vellas, B. (2009). Studying point-select-drag interaction techniques for older people with cognitive impairment. In Universal Access in Human-Computer Interaction. Addressing Diversity (pp. 422-428). Springer Berlin Heidelberg. doi:10.1007/978-3-642-02707-9_48

Wood, E., Willoughby, T., Rushing, A., Bechtel, L., & Gilbert, J. (2005). Use of computer input devices by older adults. *Journal of Applied Gerontology, 24*(5), 419–438. doi:10.1177/0733464805278378

ENDNOTE

[1]   http://www.samsung.com/ph/smarttv/smart_interaction.html

Tele–Care Mobile Sensing Systems:
Technical and Social Barriers

Alvaro Suarez
University de Las Palmas de Gran Canaria, Spain

Elsa Mª Macias
University de Las Palmas de Gran Canaria, Spain

INTRODUCTION

The e-Health is the practice of healthcare supported by *Information and Communications Technologies (ICT)* (Oh, Rizo, Enkin, Jadad, Powell & Pagliari, 2005). One face of e-Health is Tele-care that helps the physicians to tele-monitor the patients using Web technologies for designing and implementing new and exciting services for citizens with improved 4G wireless access (Kyriacoul, Pattichis, Pattichis, Panayides, Pitsillides, 2007) and smart mobile telephones to use services any time and any place. Modern enriched mobile Web interfaces help to use mobile tele-care (m-tele-care) that was envisioned by Istepaninan and Lacal (Istepanian & Lacal, 2003) and refined by Klasnja and Pratt (Klasnja, Pratt, 2012). Web interfaces have led to many subsequent implementations. An example of rich Web interfaces for m-tele-care demonstrated the applicability of m-tele-care to smoking disease (Macías, Suarez, & Calvo, 2013), which is the first cause of avoidable morbidity and mortality in the developed world diseases (WHO, 2001). The Body Area Network and its key component Wearable Light Device of Complete Ambient Assisted Living Experiment system are in charge to control the mobility of elderly people and their biological variables (Rocha, et. al., 2013).

Mobile sensing is a relatively new technique used to solve cooperatively a sensing problem using Mobile Internet (Lane, Miluzzo, Lu, Peebles, Choudhury, Campbell, 2010). The main element in a mobile sensing system is a smart mobile telephone that behaves as an access point for sensors to Web. Moreover, a smart mobile telephone could be a complex multiple-sensor element. Mobile sensing applies for several domains: weather prediction, environmental degradation, energy saving... However, up to our knowledge it has not applied for m-tele-care in the area of infectious disease early control. Modern m-tele-care systems includes mobile smartphones for sensing (Postolache, Girão, Ribeiro, Guerra, Pincho, Santiago & Pena, 2011). Infectious disease in the developed World outbreaks periodically every 4 to 6 years threaten public Health. The control of this kind of disease is very complicated and jeopardizes not only the public Health system but also the entire social and politic system of countries. It is very important to provide solutions to this complex problem. For this reason, we have applied the mobile sensing theory to m-tele-care to provide novel and initial ideas to achieve the early control of outbreaks.

In this chapter, we first present an overview of mobile sensing systems and its application to the control of infectious diseases domain. We argument the possibility that lay people to implement rapidly open hardware for sensors and applications for mobile smart telephones for a particular (traditional or new) infectious disease. We show that the state of the art in technology allows implementing rapidly a Web server or cloud service to process rapidly the data sensed by people. The main social benefit is that

DOI: 10.4018/978-1-4666-9978-6.ch083

rapid detection of outbreaks can be detected and informed to responsible of Health. This allows early controlling the outbreaks and achieving a control official plan. We present our model to develop the mobile sensing system and present technical and social barriers.

The organization of the rest of this chapter is as follows: In Section 2 we present a review of mobile sensing applied to m-tele-care of infectious diseases. In Section 3, we propose a framework for rapid developing of mobile sensing systems applied to infectious diseases and we identify different technical and social barriers. We present further research directions in section 4. Finally, we summarize some conclusions.

MOBILE SENSING SYSTEMS AND INFECTIOUS DISEASES

A mobile sensing system is composed of a mobile smart telephone which is responsible of controlling the sensors (Macias, Suarez & Lloret, 2013); a Web Server that stores the sensed data and makes the fusion and learning processes; and the protocols and services based in modern cloud and social networks.

The objective of personal health mobile sensing (people-centric mobile sensing) is to measure biological variables of runners, fitness, control the daily calories, weight, sleep, nutrition habits (Handel, 2011) (Liu, Zhu, Kenneth, Seng, 2011)... It often consists in a mobile application that optionally publishes information in a social network. Traditionally elderly (Maaser & Ortmann, 2010) and home care (Sashima, Inoue, Ikeda, Yamashita & Kurumatani, 2008) also used sensors to monitor patients using *Java Specification Report* 256 (*JSR 256*) (JSR, 2014) software to control sensors and *Bluetooth* or *Wireless Fidelity* (*WiFi*) technologies to communicate with sensors (Ghose, Bhaumik, Das, & Agrawal, 2012).

The objective of participatory or social mobile sensing is to organize a campaign of sensing to cover the sensing of a geographic area. Collaboration among sensing people is mandatory to accomplish the objective of sensing. For example, Yang et. al. (Yang, Yang, Luo, Gonga, 2009) described the control infectious diseases after an earthquake done by the China Government distributing more than 600 mobile telephones among Health professional. However, the mobile telephones only reported information to a Central of control. We consider participatory mobile sensing system in which people in a determinate geographical area do personal sensing while do their normal live (MIT, 2014). The kind of sensing is discontinuous (for example, every certain amount of time). The Web server will receive health-sensed data, which fuses and learns how to early control the infectious disease. The server would warn Health authorities about an outbreak in a determinate geographic area. The fuse and learning processes demand the formalization of epidemics. Hethcote (Hethcote, 2000) presented a wide study of different models for different diseases. Khöler and Trifa (Köhler, &Trifa, 2007) presented initial ideas for applying mobile smart telephones for sensing infectious diseases data. They reviewed issues such reliability of sensed data, privacy and the minimum size of participating group. We in this chapter present initial ideas about a novel model for m-tele-care presenting a schema for rapid developing of the mobile sensing system. Madan et al. (Madan, Cebrian, Lazer, & Pentland, 2010) developed a study of identification of the behavior changes reflected in mobile phone sensors, when individuals suffer from common colds, influenza, fever, stress and mild depression. Our model is general and it is applied for any infectious disease rapidly implementing sensors and software in the mobile smart telephone and the server.

NOVEL MODEL OF MOBILE SENSING FOR INFECTIOUS DISEASES

Participatory or Social Mobile sensing is appropriate to early detect and manage infectious diseases. However, each infection disease has its own characteristics. These characteristics are normally different from one disease to another. The first question is how to detect an infection in a particular disease. For example for Ebola Virus infection, the procedure to detect a possible infection is to measure the fever of the people. This is very simple to detect with a thermometer sensor. For similar diseases like this, we part from the following assumptions:

1. **Open Sensor Hardware Can Be Rapidly and Easily Built by Normal People**: Sensors like thermometer or similar can be built nowadays rapidly and easily. Each infectious disease has its own documentation in a Web server. This documentation includes the open hardware schemas of the sensors. In this way, any people can consult this information, download the corresponding schema, and build the sensor. The schema of the sensors includes the hardware block (Bluetooth or WiFi) to communicate with the mobile smart telephone. The corresponding software controllers of these communication blocks are standard. Example of sites for open hardware are *berduino*, *phoneblocks, openpicus*... SPARTAN is a framework for rapid implementation of sensors (Wang, Shi, Arnetz & Wiholm, 2010).

2. **Mobile Software Can Be Rapidly and Easily Implemented by Normal People:** Today there are many free platforms for developing mobile software like the one needed for making a sensing application. Well-known examples are *AppInventor* for Android and *Kino for iOS*.

3. **Mobile Sensing Can Apply Easily:** Because the people only must download a mobile application from a Web server and a schema of an open hardware sensor and use them, or introduce in the mobile smart telephone data manually or use a free platform to develop a simple mobile application.

Next, we will discover the stakeholders, the general software and hardware principles for the m- participatory mobile sensing system.

Stakeholders

The different stakeholders of the model are:

1. **ICT Specialists**: They manage the computation and communication processes.
2. **Scientific Specialists**: They formalize model of treatment of infection processes and verify the results of the computing models (fusion and learning in the Web server).
3. **Health Specialists:** They receive notification of the validated results of the participatory mobile sensing system, publish information, and deliver actions for controlling the infection.
4. **Volunteer People**: They build the open hardware sensors (or introduce data in the mobile application), install the mobile application and grant appropriated permission to the mobile application to deliver the sensed data to a central server.

Moreover, the Government members and other important instances of a country have access to the sensed data. This is due to in an emergency all these high instances of a country must collaborate. The administration of specific roles in the access to the sense information and actuation patterns corresponds to the Government.

Principles of the Mobile Sensing System

The central element of our system is the mobile smart telephone. The responsibilities of the mobile smart telephone are:

1. **Execution of the Mobile Application:** It is stored in a mobile memory or any particular Web server owned by an official Health stakeholder. The user can immediately download it at any time and any place. Alternatively, people could program a new application easily.
2. **Managing of the Open Hardware Sensors:** The mobile application has the ability to communicate with the sensors using the Internet protocol stack over Bluetooth or WiFi communication controllers. We in contrast to JSR 256 propose the use of simple Web protocols like *Constrained Application Protocol* (*CoAP*) (Shelby, Hartke & Bormann, 2014) according to the reasons given by (Cecilio & Furtado, 2011).
3. **Communication with Geographically near Mobile Smart Telephones:** Not only physicians but other kind of users could receive the state of other users. This is interesting just in case an emergency takes place. This communication can be implemented with Bluetooth or WiFi technologies.
4. **Communication to the Web Server:** Just in case the accumulated values of sensor values indicate a state of possible infection, the mobile telephone automatically (under the permission of the user), will upload the historic values of the sensor to the Web Server. This Web server can work as a Mobile Cloud system like the one proposed by Hoang and Chen (Hoang & Chen, 2010) or it can offer *Sensing-as-a-Service* (*S²aaS*) (Kantarci & Mouftah, 2014).
5. **Receive Instructions from the Web Server:** Such as periodic information about the diseases under control, download of software and open hardware implementations. It will deliver other emergency instructions. For example, how to control panic in a particular area with infected people, how to clean things and how to dress.

The Web server or a particular official Health stakeholder has the following responsibilities:

1. **Distribution of Sensing Campaigns:** The mobile smart telephones subscribed to that server will receive instructions how to develop a particular campaign. The middleware registers mobile smart telephones only if they will increase the sensing coverage of a geographical area (Hachem, Pathak & Issarny, 2014).
2. **Fusion and Learning:** The Web server processes (fusion) different values received from the mobile smart telephones. From these fused values, the server must learn patterns of infection in a certain geographical zone. Formal models of infection help to do these high computing demand processes. Learning helps to inform the people about the early and estimated propagation of the infection.
3. **Collaborate with Other Cloud Servers:** Fusion and learning will implement processes in a Cloud (*S²aaS*) when the number of possible infectious is large using big data processing techniques.
4. **Presentation of Public Real Time Information:** The server delivers the results of fusion and learning in real time to people. This information is under supervision of a special Commission named by the Government. Health, ICT and scientific specialist compose this Commission.
5. **Deliver Concrete Instructions When a Possible Epidemic Could Probably Occur:** When an individual infection is detected, the individual and appropriated stakeholders will be informed. When the fusion and learning software detect a possible epidemic, the software will immediately inform the official stakeholders.

An example of use case of the mobile telephone and Web server is explained in the following steps:

Step 1: An individual suspects that it has an infection (for example Ebola) because it fever pattern match the one published in existing Ebola information Web Servers.

Step 2: The user downloads the schema of an open hardware thermometer and the mobile application.

Step 3: The user measures his fever three times a day during 4 days. The software of the mobile smart telephone detects high values of fever during these days and communicates all the values to the Web server.

Step 4: The Web server fuses the received values with other stored previously. It learns that there are several similar cases in a particular geographical zone or simply the new values received actually indicate the user is infected.

Step 5: Just in case an infection happens (or detects an outbreak), the Web server will warn the Commission in real time. Each Commission's member will do their work. For example, in less than 30 minutes:

Step 5.1: The ICT specialist will verify all the computing and communication processes and notify this to the Scientists.

Step 5.2: The Scientist will revise the original values and fuse and learn values and will validate the truth of the results and notify the Health specialist.

Step 5.3: The Health specialist will allow automatic publication of information in the Server and notify the corresponding process to evacuate the infected people.

Step 5.4: Other instances of the Government will act appropriately when be informed.

Step 6: In parallel with the above steps, the server and mobile smart telephones continue working in seek of new infection cases.

Technical and Social Barriers

In our previous model, we did not take into account different technical requirements of the mobile application. For example, the reduced capacity of computation and memory capacity of smart mobile telephones conduced us to assign the fusion and learning processes to the Web server. The advantage of that is the people can use any kind of mobile telephone. However, there are other complex barriers, like the energy saving problem: the more measures the mobile smart telephone does, the more battery it will drain. This is an important technical barrier because no people will want to consume their battery measuring and communicating values to the Web server. Mitra et. al. (Mitra, Emken, Lee, Li, Rozgic, Thatte, Vathsangam, Zois, Annavaram, Narayanan, Levorato & Spruijt-Metz, 2012) presented the lessons learnt after they had probed their system with several people during long time implementing continuous measuring. In our mobile sensing system, this is not the case, because we only propose sensing discontinuously. Another technical problem is the observations that sensed values can coincide or contradict among them (Wang, Kaplan & Abdelzaher, 2014). However, this is not a problem in our participatory mobile sensing system because of people read their own personal values.

Social barriers severely reduce the application of mobile sensing applied to m-tele-care. For example, Lim et al. (Lim, 2011) presented an interesting study showing that Singaporean women have difficulties in using their mobiles to seek health information in the Web. More important problem is that we have supposed that all the people measuring their biological variables with the appropriated sensor always send trust values to the server (Giannetsos, Gisdakis & Papadimitratos, 2014). However, unfortunately this is not always the case. For this reason, the server must implement security mechanism to assure the reliability of received data. We propose to implement works like the ones explained in (Gilbert, Cox, Jung, Wetherall, 2010) (Gilbert, Jung, Lee, Qin, Sharkey, Sheth & Cox, 2011) and (Sorber, Shin, Peterson & Kotz, 2012). Amulet (Sorber, Shin, Peterson, Cornelius, Mare, Prasad, Marois, Smithayer & Kotz, 2012) collected users' health information and forwarded it to a health record system in a secure way. Amintoosi and Kanhere (Amintoosi, Kanhere, 2014) have presented a reputation method for assuring trustworthiness that is based on the participation of people in a social network. However, we think our m-tele-care mobile sensing system must assure the anonymous collaboration of people in order to grant their privacy. Other social barriers as difficulty, embarrassment, overload, usefulness, personalization and dangerous can be overcame with the appropriate good programming practices of the mobile application (Cherubini, de Oliveira, Hiltunen & Oliver, 2011). However, another important social barrier is that not always people tend to collaborate with their mobile smart telephones. They find that they incur in a cost (battery drain, network charge, time and effort commitment) but the benefits they will obtain are not clear. Luo et. al. (Luo, Tan & Xia, 2014) presented a strategy to incentive the participators that will be difficult to adapt to our participatory mobile sensing system due to no auction could be provided. Sun and Ma (Sun & Ma, 2014) presented interesting pricing incentive schemes and designed a restless multi-armed bandit process based solution for long-term sensing problems (for example video sensing). This solution is not applicable to our model because of we do not use continuous sensing. We state that the organizations, physicians, politics and other social agents must be involved as recognized by Mori et. al. (Mori, Mazzeo, Mercurio, & Verbicaro, 2013).

FUTURE RESEARCH DIRECTIONS

Theoretical and practical works in the area of mobile sensing endorse the main initial ideas we have presented in this chapter. However, several hotspots must be strengthen in the future:

- We must assure the people will send their data anonymously. An electronic notary must have the possibility to find out when negligent people try to hack the participatory mobile sensing system.
- Gamification mechanisms particular to this kind of mobile sensing system can improve their participation. We will study how to adapt standard gamification mechanism to our model.
- Governments must solve social barriers as culture in the participation of people in our mobile sensing system seeking the appropriate connection between tele-care and teaching at early age.
- Other kind of symptoms (different from the one identified in step one of use case example) must be studied.
- Calibration and accuracy of samples must be assured by the open hardware sensors. This is a topic in our days and must be researched.

CONCLUSION

In this chapter, we have proposed initial ideas for a new way to implement the early control of infectious diseases using participatory mobile sensing. The main idea is to facilitate the collaboration among people with their smart telephones and other Health stakeholders. The rapid development of open hardware and software to develop the sensors and mobile applications that communicate with open Web server software, allow to early control the outbreaks. These benefits contrast with the technical barriers and social barriers we have identified. We plan to develop a prototype for Ebola infectious disease.

REFERENCES

Amintoosi, H., & Kanhere, S. S. (2014). A Reputation Framework for Social Participatory Sensing Systems. *Mobile Networks and Applications, 19*(1), 88–100. doi:10.1007/s11036-013-0455-x

Cecilio, J., & Furtado, P. (2011). Distributed Configuration and Processing for Industrial Sensor Networks. In *Proceedings of the 6th International Workshop on Middleware Tools, Services and Run-time Support for Networked Embedded Systems* (vol. 4). Doi:10.1145/2090296.2090300

Cherubini, M., de Oliveira, R., Hiltunen, A., & Oliver, N. (2011). Barriers and Bridges in the Adoption of Today's Mobile Phone Contextual Services. In *Proceedings of the 13th International Conference on Human Computer Interaction with Mobile Devices and Services (MobileHCI'11)* (pp. 167-176). Doi:10.1145/2037373.2037400

Ghose, A., Bhaumik, C., Das, D., & Agrawal, A. K. (2012). Mobile Healthcare Infrastructure for Home and Small Clinic. In *Proceedings of the 2nd ACM International Workshop on Pervasive Wireless Healthcare (MobileHealth '12)* (pp. 15-20). Doi:10.1145/2248341.2248347

Giannetsos, T., Gisdakis, S., & Papadimitratos, P. (2014). Trustworthy People-Centric Sensing: Privacy, Security and User Incentives Road-Map. In *Proceedings of 13th Annual Mediterranean Ad Hoc Networking Workshop (MED-HOC-NET)*. IEEE Communication Society. doi:10.1109/MedHocNet.2014.6849103

Gilbert, P., Cox, L. P., Jung, J., & Wetherall, D. (2010). Toward Trustworthy Mobile Sensing. In *Proceedings of the 11th Workshop on Mobile Computing Systems & Applications (HotMobile '10)* (pp. 31-36). Doi:10.1145/1734583.1734592

Gilbert, P., Jung, J., Lee, K., Qin, H., Sharkey, D., Sheth, A., & Cox, L. P. (2011). YouProve: Authenticity and Fidelity in Mobile Sensing. In *Proceedings of the 9th ACM Conference on Embedded Networked Sensor Systems (SenSys '11)* (pp. 176-189). Doi:10.1145/2070942.2070961

Hachem, S., Pathak, A., & Issarny, V. (2014). Service-oriented middleware for large-scale mobile participatory sensing. *Pervasive and Mobile Computing, 10*, 66–82. doi:10.1016/j.pmcj.2013.10.010

Handel, M. J. (2011). Mhealth (Mobile Health)—Using Apps for Health and Wellness. *Explore (New York, N.Y.), 7*(4), 256–261. doi:10.1016/j.explore.2011.04.011 PMID:21724160

Hethcote, H. W. (2000). The Mathematics of Infectious Diseases. Society for Industrial and Applied Mathematics (SIAM). *RE:view, 42*(4), 599–563.

Hoang, D. B., & Chen, L. (2010). Mobile Cloud for Assistive Healthcare (MoCAsH). In *Proceedings of IEEE Asia-Pacific Services Computing Conference* (pp. 325-332). Hangzhou, China. IEEE Computer Society.

Istepanian, R. S. H.; Lacal, Jose C. (2003). Emerging Mobile Communication Technologies for Health: Some Imperative notes on m-health. In *Proceedings of Annual International Conference of the IEEE Engineering in Medicine and Biology Society (EMBS)* (pp. 1414-1416). Cancun, México. IEEE Press. doi:10.1109/IEMBS.2003.1279581

JSR 256: Mobile Sensor API. (2014). Retrieved November 04, 2014, from http://jcp.org/en/jsr/detail?id=256

Kantarci, B., & Mouftah, H. T. (2014). Reputation-based Sensing-as-a-Service for Crowd Management over the Cloud. In *Proceedings of the IEEE ICC 2014 - Selected Areas in Communications Symposium*, (pp. 3614-3619). Sydney, Australia: IEEE.

Klasnja, P., & Pratt, W. (2012). Healthcare in the pocket: Mapping the space of mobile-phone health interventions. *Journal of Biomedical Informatics*, *45*(1), 184–198. doi:10.1016/j.jbi.2011.08.017 PMID:21925288

Kuhler, M., & Trifa, V. M. (2007). Epidemic modeling using mobile phones. In *Proceedings of ACM SenSys, 5th ACM Conference on Embedded Networked Sensor Systems*. ACM.

Kyriacoul, E., Pattichis, M. S., Pattichis, I. C. S., Panayides, A., & Pitsillides, A. (2007). m-Health le-Emergency Systems: Current Status and Future Directions. *IEEE Antennas and Propagation Magazine*, *49*(1), 216–231. doi:10.1109/MAP.2007.371030

Lane, N. D., Miluzzo, E., Lu, H., Peebles, D., Choudhury, T., & Campbell, A. T. (2010). A Survey of Mobile Phone Sensing. *IEEE Communications Magazine*, *48*(9), 140–150. doi:10.1109/MCOM.2010.5560598

Lim, S., Xueb, L., Yen, C. C., Changa, L., Chanc, H. C., Tai, B. C., & Choolani, M. et al. (2011). A study on Singaporean women's acceptance of using mobile phones to seek health information. *International Journal of Medical Informatics*, *8*(0), e189–e202. doi:10.1016/j.ijmedinf.2011.08.007 PMID:21956003

Liu, C., Zhu, Q., Kenneth, H. A., & Seng, E. K. (2011). Status and trends of mobile-health applications for iOS devices: A developer's perspective. *Journal of Systems and Software*, *84*(11), 2022–2033. doi:10.1016/j.jss.2011.06.049

Luo, T., Tan, H.-P., & Xia, L. (2014). Profit-Maximizing Incentive for Participatory Sensing. In *Proceedings of INFOCOM 2014*.

Maaser, M., & Ortmann, S. (2010). Remote Medical Treatment at Home Using the Java Mobile Sensor API. In *Proceedings of the IEEE GLOBECOM Workshops* (pp. 2039-2043). Doi:10.1109/GLOCOMW.2010.5700303

Macias, E., Suarez, A., & Lloret, J. (2013). Mobile Sensing Systems. *Sensors (Basel, Switzerland)*, *13*(12), 17292–17321. doi:10.3390/s131217292 PMID:24351637

Macías, E. M., Suarez, A., & Calvo, F. (2013). Improving Health using Therapies 2.0 with Ubiquitous Wireless Access. In M. Cruz-Cunha, I. Miranda, & P. Gonçalves (Eds.), *Handbook of Research on ICTs and Management Systems for Improving Efficiency in Healthcare and Social Care* (pp. 953–970). Hershey, PA: Medical Information Science Reference; doi:10.4018/978-1-4666-3990-4.ch050

Madan, A., Cebrian, M., Lazer, D., & Pentland, A. (2010). Social sensing for epidemiological behavior change. In *Proceedings of the 12th ACM International conference on Ubiquitous computing, Ubicomp*. ACM. doi:10.1145/1864349.1864394

MIT Mobile Experience Laboratory. (2014). *Mobile UV Monitor*. Retrieved November 04, 2014, from http://jbr.org/articles.html http://mobile.mit.edu/portfolio/mobile-uv-monitor/

Mitra, U., Emken, B. A., Lee, S., Li, M., Rozgic, V., Thatte, G., & Levorato, M. et al. (2012). D. KNOWME: A Case Study in Wireless Body Area Sensor Network Design. *IEEE Communications Magazine*, *50*(5), 116–125. doi:10.1109/MCOM.2012.6194391

Mori, A. R., Mazzeo, M., Mercurio, G., & Verbicaro, R. (2013). Holistic health: Predicting our data future (from inter-operability among systems to co-operability among people). *International Journal of Medical Informatics, 8*(2), e14–e28. doi:10.1016/j.ijmedinf.2012.09.003 PMID:23122923

Oh, Rizo, Enkin, Jadad, Powell, & Pagliari. (2005). What is eHealth (3): A Systematic Review of Published Definitions. *Journal of Medical Internet Research, 7*(1).

Postolache, O., Girão, P. S., Ribeiro, M., Guerra, M., Pincho, J., Santiago, F., & Pena, A. (2011). Enabling telecare assessment with pervasive sensing and Android OS Smartphone. In *Proceedings of IEEE International Workshop on Medical Measurements and Applications Proceedings (MeMeA)* (pp. 288-293). Bari, Italia: IEEE. doi:10.1109/MeMeA.2011.5966761

Rocha, A., Martins, A., Juniora, F., Celso, J., & Boulos, K. (2013). Innovations in health care services: The CAALYX system. *International Journal of Medical Informatics, 8*(2), e307–e320. doi:10.1016/j.ijmedinf.2011.03.003 PMID:21481633

Sashima, A., Inoue, Y., Ikeda, T., & Yamashita, T. (2008). K. CONSORTS-S: A Mobile Sensing Platform for Context-Aware Services. In *Proceedings of the International Conference on Intelligent Sensors, Sensor Networks and Information Processing* (pp. 417-422). doi:10.1109/ISSNIP.2008.4762024

Shelby, Z., Hartke, K., & Bormann, C. (2014). *The Constrained Application Protocol (CoAP). Request For Comments (RFC). Internet Engineering Task Force.* IETF.

Sorber, J., Shin, M., Peterson, R., Cornelius, C., Mare, S., Prasad, A., & Kotz, D. et al. (2012). An Amulet for Trustworthy Wearable mHealth. In *Proceedings of the 12th Workshop on Mobile Computing Systems & Applications (HotMobile'12)* (7:1-7:6). Doi:10.1145/2162081.2162092

Sorber, J. M., Shin, M., Peterson, R., & Kotz, D. (2012). Plug-n-Trust: Practical Trusted Sensing for mHealth. In *Proceedings of the 10ᵗʰ International Conference on Mobile Systems, Applications, and Services (MobiSys '12)* (309-322). Doi:10.1145/2307636.2307665

Sun, J., & Ma, H. (2014). Heterogeneous-belief based incentive schemes for crowd sensing in mobile social networks. *Journal of Network and Computer Applications, 42*, 189–196. doi:10.1016/j.jnca.2014.03.004

Wang, D., Kaplan, L., & Abdelzaher, T. F. (2014). Maximum Likelihood Analysis of Conflicting Observations in Social Sensing. *ACM Transactions on Sensor Networks, 10*(2), 30. doi:10.1145/2530289

Wang, S., Shi, W., Arnetz, B. B., & Wiholm, C. (2010). *Proceedings of 6th International Conference on Collaborative Computing: Networking, Applications and Worksharing (CollaborateCom).* Chicago, IL. IEEE Press.

WHO, World Health Organization. (2001). First European Recommendations on the Treatment of Tobacco Dependence. Copenhagen: WHO.

Yang, C., Yang, J., Luo, X., & Gonga, P. (2009). Use of mobile phones in an emergency reporting system for infectious disease surveillance after the Sichuan earthquake in China. *Bulletin of the World Health Organization, 87*(8), 619–623. doi:10.2471/BLT.08.060905 PMID:19705013

Toward a Critically Conscious and Culturally Competent Telepractice in Psychology

Brittany A. Canfield
Fielding Graduate University, USA

INTRODUCTION

As the field of psychology moves closer to implementing improved telehealth practices, it is also challenged by how it continues to make the same mistakes once made in traditional modes of care. An important question is how to remain critically conscious in the practice of psychology while using telehealth as a primary or secondary mode of mental health care delivery. Cultural competency continues to be an issue in traditional mental health practices, from the globalization of psychiatric standards to misdiagnosis within cultural frameworks. In the course of making such cultural considerations, understanding how the field can assess, treat, and implement the vast knowledge of Western psychology practices has been an area of increased development. Achieving a practice that features cultural competency extends far beyond considerations made in treatment, or assessments of language, sexual orientation, gender, tradition, religious/spiritual practices and beliefs, socioeconomic status, or geographical location. In the area of mental health care, there continue to be shortcomings in the global relationship dialogue of cultural competency.

This chapter provides an overview of the challenges inherent in traditional psychology practices, even as practitioners develop a foundation for critical consciousness. References are made to the literature outlining the many challenges and shortcomings made on cultural considerations within the practice of psychiatry, which are not to be mistaken with psychology. Additionally, this chapter explores established global mental health practices related to the use of telehealth, as well as guidelines for making cultural considerations when reaching out to remote or rural populations worldwide. A new standard for cultural competency will be explored within the context of telehealth practices; this will include an emphasis on how we currently understand cultural competency, and the impact it can have when used or not used. Suggestions for future research are made with an eye to furthering our understanding of psychological telepractice in rural communities and global mental health arenas.

BACKGROUND

Franz Fanon posed the notion of "a systemized negation of the other—to deny the other any attribute of humanity" in the social environment of the "colonial type" (Fanon, 1963, p. 182). Thus, describing the experience of the "other" in a tireless search for the meaning of their reality. Kitzinger and Wilkinson (1996) boldly describe Western social constructionism thus: "'We' use the other to define ourselves: 'we' understand ourselves in relation to what 'we' are not" (pp. 1-32). From the social constructionist

DOI: 10.4018/978-1-4666-9978-6.ch084

perspective, there is skepticism of the "categories of knowledge," and there are assertions that the use of those categories leads to "viewing them as accounts shaped in accordance with cultural dictates" (Hare-Mustin & Marecek, 1994, pp. 531-537).

"The attribution of meaning is bound up with power" (Parker et al., 1995, p. 16), which means that "power relations" that are formed around groups subjected to inequality (e.g., gender, racial/ethnic) are influenced by the very definitions of "normal" that ultimately guide various psychological diagnoses. Landrine (1988) asserts that "what is constructed as 'normal' is limited to the experience of dominant cultural groups, and therefore precludes, and excludes, the experiences of women and people of color," for example (pp. 37-44); this assertion can also be applied to individuals from rural and/or indigenous communities. It is important to note, additionally, that this applies to those of "lesser" socioeconomic status more so than to the "creators of the norm" (pp. 37-44).

Social constructionists argue that the mental illness monologue that guides psychological theory and practice is molded by (a) definitions of "normal" that stem from a partial and elite perspective, and (b) stereotypical notions of gender, race/ethnicity, and sexuality (Hare-Mustin & Marecek, 1994). As such, there is an underlying theme in the DSM-IV Casebook of defining "normal" through constructions of race and gender. The Casebook contributes to a "gendered and raced" way of conceptualizing mental illness, and "explicit definitions of pathology" reflect in the use of "implicit definitions of normalcy" (Carmele, Daniels, & Anderson, 2001, pp. 229-247). Further, it is debated "whether the diagnostic categories in the DSM-IV reflect the existence of actual entities of mental disorders" or if they reflect a construct of mental illness based on theory and bias (Caplan, 1995, pp. 1-32). Although the field of Western culture sets a standard for accurate diagnoses that inform care, the very tool developed to be an efficacious resource has failed to make appropriate cultural considerations.

For example, in reviewing national databases from the United States and Britain, it becomes clear that whites are more likely to receive a diagnosis of an affective disorder than blacks, and the latter are more likely to be diagnosed with schizophrenia (Fernando, 1991). Additionally, blacks are more likely to be described as violent, dangerous, or angry, despite an identical symptom presentation between blacks and whites. Fernando (1991) argues that this differentiation allows for opportunities for racism to occur within the assessment and diagnostic process, as well as in treatment—and even that "racism in psychiatry is not an aberration" but the "normal condition" (p. 115). Fernando goes on to describe the very ways in which Western culture has perpetuated differences among individuals, given that the DSM-IV Casebook defines individuals as "white Americans," "non-white," and "non-American." As such, the Casebook once again draws a line of segregation between white Americans and the "other."

Furthermore, a review of the Casebook shows a discrepancy between the cases provided and racial/ethnic marking: of the 90 (55) adult male (female) case studies examined, 80% (87%) went unmarked for racial or ethnic references (Carmele, Daniels, & Anderson, 2001). The issue being presented relates to the need for differentiating between what the Casebook refers to as "non-white" or "non-American"—a need that has vast implications, aside from the most obvious of contributing to cultural construction while using the concept of "whiteness" as the normative point of reference (Carmele, Daniels, & Anderson, 2001).

Social and psychological knowledge that forms from historical and cultural frameworks should contribute to the context and process of scientific psychology, as they reflect societal norms (Moradio & Yoder, 2001). Carmele, Daniels, and Anderson (2001) demonstrate the lack of reference to a social constructionist framework within attempts to make cultural considerations, without being descriptive as to what various cultures are being considered. These readings shed light on the neglect of the field in addressing culture with respect to mental illness. Resources that aim to provide an educational atmosphere for students of psychology and psychiatry continue to fall short of developing and maintaining cultural competency in assessing and diagnosing mental illness across diverse populations.

"Limited knowledge of mental disorders", their lack of "mental health literacy", or the need to "teach" health workers and the people they serve about mental health. Here Western psychobiological discourse is setting out to instruct, regulate, and modernize, presenting as definitive the contemporary Western way of being a person. It is unclear why this should be good for mental health in Africa or Asia. This is medical imperialism, similar to the marginalisation of indigenous knowledge systems in the colonial era, and is generally to the disadvantage of local populations. (Summerfield, 2008, p. 992-994)

There are multiple translations involved in psychiatry; they involve the very "translation of experiences and local idioms of distress into psychiatric categories, into English" and thus into various languages (Mills, 2014, p. 2). Psychiatry has long been viewed as colonial, a discipline that perpetuates the "alienating" or marginalizing process of individuals understanding themselves through foreign terms, hence "a colonization of the mind" (Thiong'o, 1981). If it is indeed true that psychiatry is "already racialized and colonial" (Diamond, 2013, pp. 64-78), then these experiences must be acknowledged as having been felt differently by various groups. Thus, claiming that all who are "psychiatrized" are "simultaneously colonized" would marginalize the realities of those populations who have experienced both (Tam, 2013, pp. 281-297). The literature challenges our preoccupation with the individual and summons a more "collective" view of the individual—in conjunction with the cultural environment from which the "individual" originated—and pushes us to do so within a broader framework of cultural competency.

CULTURAL COMPETENCY IN TELEPRACTICE

For as psychiatry travels, so do the networks, initiatives and movements that fight against psychiatric hegemony, from alternative frames of reference where distress may not be an "illness." (Mills, 2014, p. 11)

Cultural competency extends our collective understanding of how culture is incorporated into psychological practices. Our initial notions are based on what it means to share a therapeutic space with one of another gender, someone of a race or ethnicity different from our own or one of another sexual orientation. The "culture" that needs to be spoken of in this context consists of one's beliefs and perceptions of one's world, which is held individually or shared collectively within a community. From an "etic approach," mental illness originates from pathological or biological processes and is thus universal; the "emic approach" to mental illness, on the other hand, is one that comprises subjective experiences that are influenced by culture and should therefore be studied within their particular cultural context (Mills, 2014).

While the definition of "cultural competence" in psychological treatment has been a topic of interest for decades within the psychological community, multicultural specialists have described the various ways in which mental health professionals have failed to incorporate cultural competency into their mental health practices. For example, "discriminatory practices in mental health delivery systems are deeply embedded in the ways in which the services are organized and in how they are delivered to minority populations"; they also reflect the type of personnel who occupy decision-making roles (Cross et al., 1989, pp. 1-7). Though the term "cultural competency" holds varying definitions in multiple practices, it can be described as a "respect for and understanding of diverse ethnic and cultural groups, their histories, traditions, beliefs, and value system in the provision and delivery of services—in practice—cultural competency converts the knowledge gained from groups and individuals into policies and procedures that result in practices that increase the quality of the services to produce better outcomes" (Benavides & Hernandez, 2007, p. 15). Further, the term "cultural humility" coined to provide an alternative view of the idea of cultural competence and the dangerous waters in which it wades, incorporates a "life-long commitment—to redressing the power imbalances in the patient-physician dynamic, and to developing mutually beneficial and nonpaternalistic advocacy partnerships" (Tervalon & Murray-Garcia, 1998, p. 117).

Thus far, mental health professionals in the United States have been thought to operate from a "monoculturally competent" framework, within a limited segment of the white Euro-American population (Sue & Sue, 2003, p. 9). On a more global mental health scale, concerns vis-à-vis a lack of cultural competence stem from greater forces: psychiatric colonization, in which Western care forms replace alternative methods of healing that are local, religious, or indigenous (Watters, 2010). Those Western forms also tend to overlook the complexity of lived experiences by focusing on a "global norm for mental health" (Shukla et al., 2012, p. 292), and they couch people's experiences in alienating technical terms that deny or otherwise restrict personal or social meaningfulness (Johnstone, 2000; Mills, 2012). In current telemedicine practices in the United States, psychiatric services are provided to rural areas and communities wherever the state is licensed to offer psychiatric telemedicine services. Appointments can last anywhere from 10 to 20 minutes, depending on the psychiatrist and the individual receiving care. How is it possible within this short time to relay cultural competence in the interaction and dialogue to the individual, and thus experience a culture informed interaction?

"Telemedicine," "telehealth," and "telepractice" are terms largely unknown worldwide. They may relay a sense of curiosity, confusion, and often skepticism toward individuals and professionals in fields that are just beginning to incorporate these terms into modern practices. As the telepractice of psychology is an innovative and controversial mode of mental health care, which has recently become a topic of discussion, research in this area is still nascent. In the Practice Guidelines of the New York State Education Department in the United States (NYSED, 2013, Education Law, Section 6509), a number of considerations on the "impact of telepractice on dimensions of mental health practice" are listed; they include (a) awareness and assessment of nonverbal behavior exhibited by the patient, (b) ensuring the privacy of patients and the protection of confidential information through all information transmissions, (c) relational and transferential issues, (d) access issues, such as the distribution of computers and familiarity with technology, (e) temporal factors such as simultaneous communication, time between responses, and formalized "sessions," (f) provisions for emergencies, and (g) the development of technological proficiencies and an online culture/language.

In relating to the subsection on "access issues such as distribution of computers and familiarity," the impact of telepractice in rural communities and global settings needs be evaluated. The telepractitioner is responsible for being aware not only of this "issue," but also of possibly reactionary implications. It is not the individual's or the group's responsibility to understand technology or access the technology needed to receive care, let alone be proficient in its use. However, the telepractitioner must remain critically conscious of the fact that a far greater number of communities within our own countries and around the world have had little to no exposure to technological advances. Thus, telepractitioners bear the responsibility of understanding and mediating possible technical challenges, and of using and/or developing resources to assist in the transmission of telepractice services (e.g., interpreter, on-ground social workers, or on-ground team that works closely with the individual or group to provide assistance).

If telepractices are going to be used in remote settings, we must not assume that our sole responsibility is to "show up"; rather, we must also facilitate the ease of "showing up" for the individual or group that will be receiving care and addressing the challenges inherent in using technology, keeping the responsibility separate from that of the individual. By informing care with an understanding of world events, histories of cultures or peoples within a particular geographical location, and immersing ourselves as telepractitioners in the population to which we intend to provide care, we will, by default, become aware of the so-called "disadvantages" that other societies face. At this point, we may change our viewpoint from one of the perceived disadvantages vis-à-vis items such as technology—not including food, water, clothing, shelter, and medical assistance when needed—and reconsider the superficial privileges that many industrialized societies take for granted.

On a greater global scale—one that can be applied to rural communities within our own countries—cultural competency begins with awareness and understanding of the histories and narratives that people carry. As experiences with various symptomologies (i.e., what have come to be known as symptoms, but rather are symptoms of life, such as trauma, death, disease, oppression) are so unique to every individual, and (ir)relevance to culture is a factor, the rawness of experience remains. Within the cultural competency literature, a fundamental model can be conceptualized to apply critical consciousness to the practice of cultural competency in telepractice settings. The first concept is to "obtain a specific and complete understanding of the individual's chief complaint" (Guindon & Sobhany, 2002, pp. 269-282). In doing so, the clinician can begin to form a dialogue with the individual and contain the intimacy of the individual's struggle, which is unique to him or her.

While keeping in mind cultural context, the clinician can begin to formulate a conceptualization of the individual, with the individual. Second, the clinician should "be aware of discrepancies" in clinician/ individual "perceptions of clinical reality" (Guindon & Sobhany, 2002, pp. 269-282). As mentioned, the critically conscious telepractitioner is responsible for being aware of the individual's collective history, narrative, and social surroundings. While bearing this framework in mind, the clinician works to prevent additional unconscious or conscious oppression or even colonization from being brought to bear on the individual.

A previous deficit in the cultural competency practices in rural communities and/or global settings has been seen in the lack of (or neglectful interpretations of) individual-level "clinical" realities. The literature of the history of psychiatric colonization illustrates how the "profession" has oppressed individuals within the global mental health and rural communities by writing of their own realities of individual's experiences. Within the cultural competency model, third, we can "elicit" clients' clinical realities and explain counselor or clinician "models" (Guindon & Sobhany, 2002). During this process, the clinician can formulate a dialogue with the individual about the beliefs he or she "holds" about his or her suffering, as well as the various "attachments" he or she infuses with personal and/or social meaning.

Developing a cultural competency model specific to telepractice in rural communities and/or global settings should include that which other cultural competency models include—namely, knowledge of the language. One of the most common barriers to individuals seeking help, treatment outcomes, and perceived clinician effectiveness stems from the inability to communicate with a common language, wherein the clinician and the individual can understand the same meanings, contexts, culturally specific idioms, and language-specific terminology. Moreover, in the telepractice setting, cultural competency techniques such as nonverbal behavior (including but not limited to emotional displays, gestures, or eye contact) carry vast implications in themselves. As the "interpretation of affect and its antecedents" plays an integral role in many psychotherapy modalities, the clinician "must consider what personal and cultural group meanings" are associated with such nonverbal expressions (Bassey & Melluish, 2013, pp. 151-173).

FUTURE RESEARCH

As we move forward in the use of telepractice treatment models, the need for an even greater understanding of the rural communities and global mental health settings in which these models are being developed is becoming increasingly evident. If the profession is capable of having a devastatingly deleterious impact on non-Western communities and those within our own countries—which history has shown to be the case—what might the impact be on the implementation of telepractice modes of care on a larger scale? If we are indeed responsible for our use of social generalizations, the development of norms, psychiatric colonization, and the use of oppression while practicing within traditional modes of care, what makes us think we will not do even greater damage when utilizing telepractice treatment models? How are we displacing centuries of cultural practices, beliefs, and social positions? How can we learn about culture to understand the implications of telepractice without being reactionary to the notion of the general "we" in need of understanding the "other?"

An answer to this question is as essential as the need for social awareness, understanding, and critical consciousness, and the need to transform the ignorance and repression we have seen in the histories of psychology and psychiatry. While transitions into telepractice treatment models could potentially deliver a variety of benefits specific to the communities they will be or currently are implemented, the continuation of our current cultural framework must be rewritten. New research should adopt both the social constructionist approach and a systems approach, not only so that we might understand mental illness and possible treatments within a particular cultural setting, but so that we might also understand the intricate social and personal connections woven throughout history. Expansions of telepractice guidelines in remote settings need be addressed and made culture-specific to the area for which telepractice services are intended. Social activism, social justice, and human rights are imperative when incorporating a potential telepractice treatment model into rural communities and global mental health settings, if we are to prevent the perpetuation of conscious or unconscious social marginalization and oppression—especially given that human rights violations are so easily made in remote locations (Mills, 2014).

How does the implementation of telepractice treatment models impact the community at large? How will traditional modes of care be transformed into telepractice treatment models that do not hold the same definition of "normal" as that within the Western world, where telepractice was created? How can we prevent the same oppression, marginalization, and colonization of peoples unexposed to Western ideologies while implementing and providing psychological telepractices? These are questions that must be answered, if we are to ensure the future of viable telepractice in rural communities and global mental health settings.

CONCLUSION

The veritable telepractice in psychology faces challenges far greater than providing accessibility to remote locations around the world. Rather, a critically conscious and culturally competent telepractice in psychology must question the ramifications, potential exploitations, and justification for engaging in telepractices in rural communities or remote locations. History tells us that maintaining cultural awareness or cultural competence extends far beyond than holding awareness or understanding of a general population, awareness of our reactions to those populations, and how we may form a dialogue. Albeit those aspects can serve a purpose and be important within a monocultural framework of cultural competency in Western psychology, the critical practitioner need not be reactionary, but conscious of the people and cultures wherein these ideas and practices are being implemented.

Whom does it serve to generalize human experience? Whom does it serve to delete the other? By broadening a term such as "the human experience," we have given ourselves a clear and present road by which to instruct and modernize all peoples, by incorporating them into the same experiences as "us" or "them." It is incredibly reactionary and dangerous to drown out the cries of centuries of marginalization by further marginalizing those of a lower socioeconomic status, those of a different race, those of different belief systems, and thus those of different cultures, by utilizing a term such as "the human experience." The question must be posed: Is telepractice within the context of psychology dangerous?

REFERENCES

Bassey, S., & Melluish, S. (2013). Cultural competency for mental health practitioners: A selective narrative review. *Counselling Psychology Quarterly*, *26*(2), 151–173. doi:10.1080/09515070.2013.792995

Benavides, A. D., & Hernandez, J. C. T. (2007). Serving diverse communities—cultural competency. *Public Management*, *89*(6), 14–18.

Caplan, P. (1995). *They say you're crazy: How the world's most powerful psychiatrists decide who's normal*. Reading, MA: Addison-Wesley.

Carmele, J. A., Daniels, S., & Anderson, K. L. (2001). Defining normal: Constructions of race and gender in the DSM-IV casebook. *Feminism & Psychology*, *11*(2), 229–247. doi:10.1177/0959353501011002011

Cross, T. L., Bazron, B. J., Dennis, K. W., & Isaacs, M. R. (1989). *Towards a culturally competent system of care*. Washington, DC: Child and Adolescent Service System Program Technical Assistance Center.

Diamond, S. (2013). What makes us a community? Reflections in building solidarity in anti-sanist praxis. In B. A. LeFrancois, R. Menzies, & G. Reaume (Eds.), *Mad matters: A critical reader in Canadian mad studies* (pp. 64–78). Toronto: Canadian Scholars Press.

Fanon, F. (1963). *The wretched of the earth* (C. Farrington, Trans.). London: Penguin Books.

Fernando, S. (1991). *Mental health, race, and culture*. New York, NY: St. Martin's Press. doi:10.1007/978-1-349-21644-4

Guindon, M. H., & Sobhany, M. S. (2002). Toward cultural competency in diagnosis. *International Journal for the Advancement of Counseling*, *23*(4), 269–282. doi:10.1023/A:1014443901294

Hare-Mustin, R. T., & Marecek, J. (1994). Asking the right questions: Feminist psychology and sex differences. *Feminism & Psychology*, *4*(4), 531–537. doi:10.1177/0959353594044007

Johnstone, L. (2000). Users and abusers of psychiatry. London: Routledge Publishing.

Kitzinger, C., & Wilkinson, S. (1996). Theorizing representing the other. In S. Wilkinson & C. Kitzinger (Eds.), *Representing the other: A feminism and psychology reader* (pp. 1–32). London: Sage.

Landrine, H. (1988). Revising the framework of abnormal psychology. In P. Bronstein & K. Quina (Eds.), *Teaching a psychology of people: Resources for gender and sociocultural awareness* (pp. 37–44). Washington, DC: American Psychological Association Press. doi:10.1037/10066-004

Mills, C. (2012). Special "treatment," special rights: Dis/abled children as doubly diminished identities. In M. Freeman (Ed.), *Law and Childhood: Current Legal Issues* (Vol. 14, pp. 862–898). Oxford, UK: Oxford University Press.

Mills, C. (2014). *Decolonizing global mental health: The psychiatrization of the majority world.* London: Routledge Publishing.

Moradio, B., & Yoder, J. D. (2001). Demonstrating social constructionism in psychology courses: The "Who am I?" exercise. *Teaching of Psychology, 28*(3), 201–203. doi:10.1207/S15328023TOP2803_07

New York State Education Department. (2013). *Mental health practitioners: Practice guidelines.* (Education Law, Section 6509). Retrieved from http://www.op.nysed.gov/prof/mhp/mhppg9.htm

Parker, I., Georgaca, E., Harper, D., McLaughlin, T., & Stowell-Smith, M. (1995). *Deconstructing psychopathology.* Thousand Oaks, CA: Sage Publishing.

Shukla, A., Philip, A., Zachariah, A., Phadke, A., Suneetha, A., & Davar, B., CEHAT, et al. (2012). Letter—to global mental health. *Indian Journal of Medical Ethics, 4*(4), 292. PMID:23099610

Sue, D. W., & Sue, D. (2003). *Counseling the culturally diverse: Theory and practice* (4th ed.). New York, NY: John Wiley & Sons Inc.

Summerfield, D. (2008). How scientifically valid is the knowledge base of global mental health? *British Medical Journal, 336*(7651), 992–994. doi:10.1136/bmj.39513.441030.AD PMID:18456630

Tam, L. (2013). Whither indigenizing the mad movement: Theorizing the social relations of race and madness through conviviality. In B. A. LeFrancois, R. Menzies, & G. Reaume (Eds.), *Mad matters: A critical reader in Canadian mad studies* (pp. 281–297). Toronto: Canadian Scholars Press.

Tervalon, M., & Murray-Garcia, J. (1998). Cultural humility versus cultural competence: A critical distinction in defining physician training outcomes in multicultural education. *Journal of Health Care for the Poor and Underserved, 9*(2), 117–125. doi:10.1353/hpu.2010.0233 PMID:10073197

Thiong'o, N. (1981). *Decolonizing the mind: the politics of language in African culture.* Nairobi: East African Educational Publishers.

Watters, E. (2010). *Crazy like us: The globalization of the American psyche.* London: Free Press.

KEY TERMS AND DEFINITIONS

Colonization: The establishment of a Western ideology in remote locations where its understanding, awareness, or cultural beliefs are unknown, or differ; it also references settling within another cultural community through thought, action, beliefs, and practices.

Emic: A personal account of a behavior or belief within a culture.

Etic: An account made by an observer of behavior or belief that can be applied across cultures and is intended to be culturally neutral so as to not place cultural bias or limitations by the observer.

Global Mental Health: The movement to provide or improve mental health services in areas of the world where services do not exist, are sparse, or are not aligned with the evidenced-based practices established in the country of origin.

Marginalization: The act of holding societal beliefs that keep a person and/or group in a powerless, vulnerable, unimportant, or misunderstood position.

Oppression: The occurrence of an action or societal belief that perpetuates the subjection of, cruel, inhumane, or unjust treatment toward, or control of a person and/or group.

Psychiatric Colonization: The establishment of Western psychiatric ideology and practices in mental illness treatments within non-Western cultures where spiritual, religious beliefs, and cultural practices can be overruled if the need for psychiatric treatment is deemed necessary.

Rural Communities: A community within a country of origin that does not have services, resources, or amenities similar to those in the neighboring city or town.

Social Constructionism: Understanding the social perception of a reality unique to a social group or culture, by examining the development of interconnected meanings with the world around it.

Systems Theory Approach: The examination of multiple systems within a larger group that considers interactions among multiple interrelated parts.

Telepractice: The implementation of technological advances in the practice of medicine, psychology, or other services using web-based video interaction, web-based communication, or the use of other multimedia platforms in rendering said service.

Trends of Factors and Theories in Health Information Systems Acceptance:
2002 – 2014 Review

Emre Sezgin
Middle East Technical University, Turkey

Sevgi Özkan Yıldırım
Middle East Technical University, Turkey

INTRODUCTION

Today, Health information systems (HIS) constitute a crucial part of medical and health studies in the literature, and HIS studies have been expanded by the development of health technologies. Providing healthcare services on the mobile platform is also boosted the technological developments by increasing reachability, accessibility and ability to perform tasks on decision making/ diagnostic processes (Nah & Siau, 2005; Sarker, 2003). The term HIS has been interchangeably used with the terms of "e-health" and "health informatics" in the literature, however, they had slight differences by the means of definition. HIS defined as an interdisciplinary field which involve information systems, computer science and health services (Eysenbach & Diepgen, 2001). On the other side, Mitchell (1999) defined health informatics as a supporting healthcare practice which is the combination of electronic and digital processes.

At the time of early developments in health technologies in health and medicine, it was started with improvement in utilities and tools being used in health services. In this context, Reichertz (2006) explained technological developments in hospitals emphasizing the social side of technology. However, it was noticed that technology is required to be learned as Haux (2006) outlined. Haux (2006) elaborated Reichertz's study by increasing use and evaluation of health technologies and emphasized on the need of education and research on HIS. Furthermore, Berg (2001) argued the success in health information systems not limited to specific criteria but depended on implementation itself with inclusion of all parameters as systems and users. On the other side, altruism, individual commitment and motivation were identified as contributing attributes for technology acceptance of health technologies (L. Schaper & Pervan, 2007). Here, it is a fact that Information and Communication Technologies (ICT) provides important assistance to health providers in terms of providing health services. For instance, non-communicable health diseases constituted an important part of health services due to their high degree of fatal results (WHO, 2008). In this context, cardiovascular diseases were estimated to cause death of 17.3 million people in 2008 (WHO, 2011). However, it was estimated that HIS stands as one of the key elements to reduce the risk of fatal results.

The literature presents plenty of studies in the field of HIS. One study reported that HIS have been assisted to healthcare providers for diagnostic processes which increased effectiveness (Piette, Blaya, Sanchis, Box, & Arbor, 2011). Another study about patient safety stated that information technologies in cardiac health services have been assisted physicians in diagnoses and vitally reduced risks in patient security (Daudelin, Kwong, & Beshansky, 2005). Here, it can be deducted that the success in HIS is vitally significant, but here, implementing HIS successfully emerges as another important question.

DOI: 10.4018/978-1-4666-9978-6.ch085

HIS stands as a part of Information Systems (IS) and Information Communication Technology (ICT) domain. Thus, it suffers from several drawbacks of IS applications. Studies demonstrated that around 40% of information technology developments in various industries have been concluded as failures or labeled as inconclusive (Kaplan & Shaw, 2004; Kijsanayotin, Pannarunothai, & Speedie, 2009). Since the implementation of information systems and technologies mostly remained confidential at corporations, there is no specific number of information system implementations that succeeded or failed, however, independent studies demonstrated the big picture. It was outlined that around 20-25% of IS projects in industrialized (developing and developed) countries failed, and an additional %40 of projects remained as partially failed (Heeks, 2002, Peppart et al, 2014). Littlejohns et al (2003) stated the reasons of failure as the result of lack in understandings in a new system and its underestimation due to the complexity of the system. In another study, Lorenzi and Riley (2003) explained the reasons for IS failures as a result of human behavior in underestimation of complexity, ineffective communication, organizational, technological and leadership problems. Considering the health domain, it was outlined that, within the context of healthcare system, EPR system included complex interaction of technical and organizational factors (Jones, 2003, Galliers & Leidner, 2014). On the other side, Taylor and Todd (1995) emphasized on prior use in information technology may resulted with different attitudes towards the system, such as HIS users. As is seen here, the IS applications presented that technology use may show variance among different type of users. Thus, here the moral of the story is not to underestimate human factor in the equation. Studies in ICT and HIS domains demonstrated that understanding human factors is a must as well as developing a system itself. Hence, the socio-technical side of information technology is essential part of success in information technologies (M Berg, Aarts, & Van Der Lei, 2003). In this context, the studies presented the need of involvement human side into the equation of technology use. Regarding to that, there were number of studies conducted to assess health information system use by end users, who were mostly patients, physicians and health professionals. Prominent behavioral theories, such as Technology Acceptance Model (TAM), Innovation Diffusion Theory (IDT), Theory of Planned Behavior (TPB) and Unified Theory of Acceptance and Use of Technology (UTAUT) constitute the majority of the employed theories for acceptance studies.

In the literature, the studies regarding to health professionals' acceptance of particular technologies expands consistently. In this context, this research revealed that HIS acceptance researches have been increasing rapidly for the last 18 years (Figure 1). Since the human factor is important aspect of technology use, here, the question is what are the trends of factors affecting the acceptance of Health Information Systems by health professionals? The answer of this question will reveal the changes in user needs over the time.

In this study, the changes in influencing factors in acceptance of HIS by health professionals are being investigated by following a research procedure, and the implications are demonstrated. The results of this study would assist decision makers and researchers to learn about timely changes in health professionals attitudes towards HIS, and it would contribute to literature.

LITERATURE OF TECHNOLOGY ACCEPTANCE

For a long time, human attitude towards technologies have been assessed and studied in psychology domain (Bandura, 1977; M Fishbein & Ajzen, 1975). But technology acceptance of users and its assessment has gained popularity in the beginning of 1990. By the development of TAM after TRA and TPB, the studies in acceptance field increased dramatically (Ajzen, 1991; Davis, 1989; Venkatesh &

Figure 1. Changes in publications on HIS acceptance studies

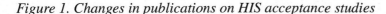

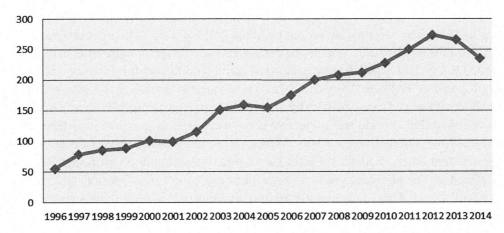

Davis, 2000; Venkatesh, Morris, Davis, & Davis, 2003; Wood & Bandura, 1989). The following theories constitute the majority of technology acceptance theories and they were commonly used in many HIS acceptance studies.

Technology Acceptance Model

The model was developed by Davis (1989) and based on sciences of psychology and human behaviors (Figure 2). In the literature, the studies demonstrated that theories developed which investigated human behavior and those theories were adapted to other disciplines as technology acceptance. The roots of TAM were grounded to Theory of reasoned actions (TRA) of Fishbein ve Ajzen (1972) and TPB of Ajzen (1991). The theory assess user intentions based on two main constructs which are perceived usefulness ("the degree to which a person believes that using a particular system would be free from effort") and perceived ease of use ("the degree to which a person believes that using a particular system would enhance his or her job performance").

At the bottom line, the aim of TAM is to determine behaviors of users towards particular technologies. The model argues that actual system use is affected by two main elements, perceived ease of use (PEOU) and perceived usefulness (PU). However, in e-health domain, it was observed that TAM theory has been successfully applied in variety of studies (Holden & Karsh, 2010)

Figure 2. Technology Acceptance Model (Davis, 1989)

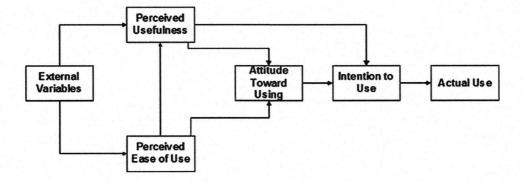

Theory of Planned Behavior

TPB, similar to TAM, was based on Ajzen and Fishbein's (1972) TRA. The most influential factor common in TRA and TPB is "intention" which was defined as main factor for human behavior (Ajzen, 1991). It demonstrated the variables which were defined as influential factors for intention and their relations.

TPB proposed perceived behavioral control as a new variable regarding to TRA, which was defined as "an individual's perceived ease or difficulty of performing the particular behavior" (Ajzen & Fishbein, 1972). In addition to that attitude and subjective norm were also proposed as interdependent variables which affect intention. Subjective norm was defined as "an individual's perception of social normative pressures, or relevant others' beliefs that he or she should or should not perform such behavior" and attitude was defined as "an individual's positive or negative evaluation of self-performance of the particular behavior" (Ajzen, 1991). Thus, TPB investigates the relations of those 3 variables with intention to use.

Innovation Diffusion Theory

The effect of innovation may show varieties in terms of success. It may resulted as failure, high success or need of incubation process (Rogers & Shoemaker, 1971). In this context, Rogers (1995) proposed Diffusion of innovation theory (IDT) in order to explain concept of innovation within the society. This theory aimed to identify acceptance constructs, to ground a mechanism and define the path of success for innovations. Mainly, the theory is all about transformation process of a new innovation or existing technology. It explained that phases of innovation as followings: (1) Knowledge (to be exposed to technology), (2) Persuasion (planting positive attitude), (3) Decision (affirmation of acceptance), (4) Confirmation (support by positive consequences). The most important features of innovation were defined as relative advantage, compatibility, complexity, trialibility and observability (Rogers, 1995). In IDT, different groups were defined considering acceptance process of innovation. These groups were early adapters, early majority, late majority and laggards. The theory outlines 3 main concepts which are features of success in innovations, the importance of communication and networking in society and determining needs of different users (Rogers & Shoemaker, 1971).

Unified Theory of Acceptance and Use of Technology

UTAUT was developed by Venkatesh et al. (2003) as an alternative theory for assessing the factors influencing users' technology acceptance. In the study of UTAUT, eight distinguished model of acceptance were reviewed, compared and utilized to establish a unified model. Those models were TRA, TAM, TPB, motivational model, a model combining TAM and TPB, model of PC utilization, IDT and social cognitive theory. The models were tested on four organizations, which explained up to 53% of variance in user intention to use IT. 8 models were tested within 4 different organizations about 4 different technologies (two of which were subject to mandatory use, the other were voluntary use) by employing a longitudinal survey study (questionnaire). Sample size was between 38 and 65 for each organization. PLS was employed to analyze reliability and validity. Results showed that eight models explained acceptance with 17% to 42% variance in intention. Considering the results and variables of the studies, UTAUT was formed, empirically tested by data from 4 organizations and cross validated by additional data from two other organizations. Preliminary test (215 sample size) presented acceptable internal consistency reliabilities and 70% of variance in usage intention.

The relation between the theories are obvious. Over the time they were evolved considering user needs and changes in technologies. In Figure 3, these changes were briefly demonstrated. Here, Sun et al. (2013) presented the relation of major theories (TAM, TRA, TPB and UTAUT) with changes in influencing factors (PU, PEOU, SN, PBC and Facilitating conditions). TAM was improved by social norms to TAM2, and eventually to UTAUT by including facilitating conditions. Similarly, TRA was utilized to develop TAM and TPB theories.

RESEARCH PROCEDURE

Since the purpose of the study is to reveal trends in influencing factors of HIS for health professionals, a comprehensive literature review is the first step to acquire relevant knowledge from HIS literature. In this study, HIS acceptance studies of last 12 years were investigated. The time interval of 12 years was selected by the time of popularity and increasing significance of the HIS studies. A systematic literature review procedure (Brereton et al, 2007; Creswell, 2003; Kitchenham, 2004) was employed in order to conduct a comprehensive review of the literature. In the study, all major scholar databases were reviewed (IEEE, Scopus, Sciencedirect, ISI Web of Knowledge, Proquest). In addition to that, for latent researches, Google Scholar was reviewed. A set of keywords were selected for database research. The keyword search was maintained progressively considering the result accuracy. The combinations of the following keywords were used: "e-health", "health information system", "m-health", "mobile health", "health informatics" combined with "information system acceptance", "adoption", "acceptance", "technology adoption", "technology acceptance" and "health professional", "employee", "doctor", "practitioner", "physician", "professional", "personnel", "worker", "nurse". Inclusion criteria were determined

Figure 3. Technology acceptance theories and their relations (Sun, Wang, Guo, & Peng, 2013)

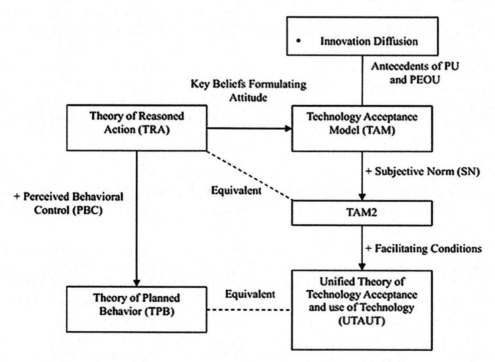

to eliminate redundant and unjustifiable studies. The criteria were as the following: (1) Studies should be in English language, (2) Objective of the papers should be about acceptance or adoption of HIS (3) Studies should be published in peer reviewed journals (4) The target sample of the researches should be health professionals (5) Study results should include quantitative data (6) Publication time interval is 12 years (2002-2014). The results were read, analyzed and categorized by the common parameters.

RESULTS AND DISCUSSION

In the preliminary stage of scholar database search, the databases were searched for HIS acceptance studies following the research procedure, and the quantitative results were recorded. The quantitative search results were cumulated and consolidated. Here, it was found that there is a rising trend of acceptance studies in HIS. Search of HIS acceptance in all major databases demonstrated the fact that since 1996 there were number of studies in HIS acceptance by users (patients, consumers and health professionals), yet it has been on a fast-track in increasing researches after 2000s. As given in Figure 1, in 2013, the studies have peaked in the field. According to Wolters Kluwer and Deloitte reports, health domain adopts new technologies exponentially and health professionals have been using new technologies (Deloitte, 2013; *Wolters Kluwer Health 2013 Physician Outlook Survey*, 2013). Thus, it was concluded that the use of HIS by professionals raised scholar interests in last 10 years.

In the following stages of the research, the implementation of the research procedure resulted with 36 studies from the literature. Keyword research returned +600 studies, and they were eliminated considering the inclusion criteria. The final 36 studies were investigated to seek for trending factors in HIS acceptance. Studies were reported in the Appendix (Table 5) including employed technology acceptance theories, variance explained (R^2), target sample, sample size and significantly related factors. This knowledge was used to analyze and report the changes in studies and user needs over the years, as given in the following paragraphs.

After the implementation of research procedure, the results presented a number of significant influencing factors in HIS acceptance (Appendix). The factors were categorized by their relevance under the common factors from the major theories in Table 1 and, they are grouped considering their significant relations in Table 2. Table 2 summarizes the fundamental factors of technology acceptance theories and their relations with behavioral intention in order to explain user behaviors. Here, it was found that the original factors in technology acceptance relations are still matter of HIS acceptance relations. In this context, PU-BI, PEOU-BI, Attitude-BI and PEOU-PU demonstrate major relations in explaining the health professionals' attitudes in acceptance studies. However, the changes of significant factors over the time proposed that there is a trend in employing factors of Self-efficacy, Trust, Social norms, PU and PEOU in explaining user attitudes towards HIS. Due to increasing need in security and trust in technologies and highly socialized communities, trust and social norms have importance from a global standpoint. In addition to that, PU and PEOU maintain their explanatory power in defining user attitudes towards the new technologies.

On the other hand, variance explained for intention to use (R^2) has similar trend in the studies over the years. The changes in variance explained in intention to use remain in a steady pace over the time, which presents that the studies were not able to explain user attitudes beyond a specific level of relations. It is quite unexpected that variance explained has not showed noticeable increase even though theories and influencing factors have been modified to increase the explanatory power of them. Yet, it can be argued that the explanatory power of researches on acceptance studies may not be able to cover changes in user needs in new technologies due to subtle emerging influences beyond the scene.

Table 1. Categorization and definition of factors (Ajzen, 1991; Davis, 1989; Rogers, 1995; Venkatesh et al., 2003)

Major Factors	Theory	Number of Use (categorized)	Definitions
Perceived Usefulness (PU)	TAM	33	"The degree to which a person believes that using a particular system would enhance his or her job performance"
Behavioral Intention (BI)	TAM	25	"An individual's performing a conscious act, such as deciding to accept (or use) a technology"
Perceived ease of use (PEOU)	TAM	22	"The degree to which a person believes that using a particular system would be free of effort"
Compatibility	IDT	12	"The degree to which the use of the system is perceived to be consistent with health- care professionals' existing values, prior experiences and needs"
Self-Efficacy	TAM3	11	"The healthcare professional's perceptions of his or her ability to use the system in the accomplishment of healthcare task"
Facilitating Conditions	UTAUT	8	"The technical support and the amount of training provided by individuals or groups with the system knowledge"
Attitude	TAM	17	"Individual's positive or negative feeling about performing the target behavior "
Trust	Extended	9	"believe in the reliability, truth and ability of particular technology"
Personal Innovativeness in IT	IDT	5	"Personal innovativeness represents the degree to which an individual is willing to take a risk by trying out an innovation"
Social Norms (SN)	TPB	11	"The degree to which the social environment perceives particular technology as desirable"
Perceived Behavioral Control (PBC)	TPB	15	"Reflects perceptions of internal and external constraints on behavior and encompasses self-efficacy, resource facilitating conditions, and technology facilitating condition"

Table 2. List of significant relations in HIS

Significant Relations*	Number of Relations in HIS Studies (36)
PU- BI	10
PEOU- BI	11
PEOU- PU	12
Attitude –BI	9
PU- Attitude	6
PEOU- Attitude	7
Compatibility -BI	8
Self-Efficacy -BI	6
Facilitating Conditions -BI	9
Trust -PEOU	8
Personal Innovativeness in IT- PU	4
Social Norms (SN)	11
Perceived Behavioral Control (PBC)	5
Others –BI **	14
* The main constructs of technology acceptance theories and their statistically significant relations with each other were presented; ** Others involve constructs of hospital type, self-identity, accessibility of medical records, accessibility of patients, normative factors, perceived readiness, computer level, logical access, image, perceived financial cost and perceived system performance.	

Table 3 presented the theories which were employed by the HIS acceptance studies. It was found that TAM leads as the major theory being employed by the studies for the last 12 years. It was followed by UTAUT, IDT and TPB. Other theories were used to create integrated model with current theories. Here, TAM remained as the flagship of the HIS acceptance studies in sole and integrated model developments. Even though the studies after 2000s modified and integrated these theories to form distinctive models in explaining user attitudes towards technologies, in the very core of them TAM and others constitute the basis of the framework. Figure 4 presented the chart of theories being employed over the years.

Table 4 presented the target samples of studies in HIS. The types were grouped in four as physicians, nurses, others and mixed. Their definitions were given below the table. According to the studies, physicians were found as the popular target samples in the HIS acceptance studies, and it was followed by nurses. The popularity of physicians and nurses are found to be related to two major reasons. The main reason is that they constitute the majority of end users of HIS applications. They constitute a crucial part in diagnostic and decision making processes in healthcare services, thus, this condition increases their importance in use of HIS. Another reason can be argued as the reachability of target samples (convenience sampling). Because they, as the target sample, are employed by hospitals, which are the common reachable institutions, it leads the researchers to easily communicate with physicians and nurses, and to use substantial amount of data in the studies.

In the bottom line, the findings of this study presented that major technology acceptance theories are still employed by the studies of HIS acceptance of healthcare professionals in the literature. Even though

Figure 4. Changes in acceptance theories in 12 years

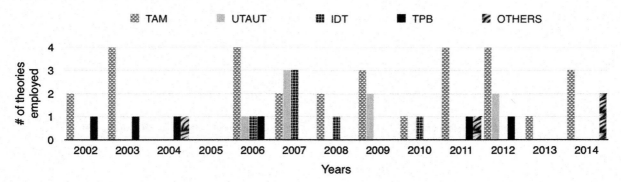

Table 3. List of theories employed in HIS

Theory Employed	Number of Studies in HIS (Out of 36)
TAM*	30
UTAUT	8
IDT	6
TPB	6
Others**	4

* TAM includes TAM and TAM2; ** Others include theories of TRA, IS success model and Task-technology fit and psychosocial model.

Table 4. Professions of target samples participated to HIS

Samples	Number of Studies in HIS (Out of 36)
Physicians*	18
Nurses	9
Healthcare workers**	4
Mixed***	5

* Physicians include physicians, clinicians and pediatricians; ** Healthcare workers involve physiotherapists, caregivers, technicians, ER teams and therapists; *** Mixed samples include a mixed set of participants consist of physicians, nurses and others.

these theories were modified in terms of their frameworks, factors and the relations, they still constitute the core of the methodology. TAM remains as the leading theory, and factors of PU and BI relations remain the most commonly investigated relationship in HIS. Most of the factors were influenced by PU, PEOU and BI. In addition to that, physicians were found as the most commonly used target samples in the studies.

CONCLUSION

Technology acceptance studies are being conducted in continuous manner in HIS domain, and new approaches and models are presented almost in each study. However the trajectory of these studies in terms of model development and determining influencing factors were unclear. In this study, the literature was systematically investigated for the last 12 years, and influencing factors for acceptance of Health Information Systems by health professionals were presented. The trends in employing theories, target samples and relations among the factors were analyzed and discussed. To summarize the study, influencing factors were categorized and results were reported in charts and tables. The findings revealed significant knowledge about use of theories and assessment of user intentions. The findings of this study is believed to assist researchers in model development about HIS acceptance studies, and to provide guidance in investigating trends in acceptance studies conducted on health professionals. It is suggested to conduct further studies on HIS acceptance of patients to broad the perspective in determining trends in HIS use by end users.

REFERENCES

Aggelidis, V. P., & Chatzoglou, P. D. (2009). Using a modified technology acceptance model in hospitals. *International Journal of Medical Informatics*, *78*(2), 115–126. doi:10.1016/j.ijmedinf.2008.06.006 PMID:18675583

Ajzen, I. (1991). The Theory of Planned Behavior. *Organizational Behavior and Human Decision Processes*, *50*(2), 179–211. doi:10.1016/0749-5978(91)90020-T

Bandura, A. (1977). Self-efficacy toward a unifying theory. *Psychological Review*, *84*(2), 191–215. doi:10.1037/0033-295X.84.2.191 PMID:847061

Barker, D. J., Van Schaik, P., Simpson, D. S., & Corbett, W. A. (2003). Evaluating a Spoken Dialogue System for recording clinical observations during an endoscopic examination. *Informatics for Health & Social Care*, *28*(2), 85–97. doi:10.1080/14639230310001600452 PMID:14692586

Berg, M. (2001). Implementing information systems in health care organizations: Myths and challenges. *International Journal of Medical Informatics*, *64*(2-3), 143–156. doi:10.1016/S1386-5056(01)00200-3 PMID:11734382

Berg, M., Aarts, J., & Van Der Lei, J. (2003). ICT in health care: sociotechnical approaches. *Methods of Information in Medicine*. Schattauer GmbH. Retrieved from http://www.ncbi.nlm.nih.gov/pubmed/17466251

Brereton, P., Kitchenham, B., Budgen, D., Turner, M., & Khalil, M. (2007). Lessons from applying the systematic literature review process within the software engineering domain. *Journal of Systems and Software*, *80*(4), 571–583. doi:10.1016/j.jss.2006.07.009

Chang, I.-C., Hwang, H.-G., Hung, W.-F., & Li, Y.-C. (2007). Physicians' acceptance of pharmaco-kinetics-based clinical decision support systems. *Expert Systems with Applications*, *33*(2), 296–303. doi:10.1016/j.eswa.2006.05.001

Chen, C., Wu, J., & Crandall, R. (2007). Obstacles to the adoption of radio frequency identification technology in the emergency rooms of hospitals. *International Journal of Electronic Healthcare*, *3*(2), 193–207. doi:10.1504/IJEH.2007.013100 PMID:18048269

Chen, J., Park, Y., & Putzer, G. J. (2010). An Examination of the Components that Increase Acceptance of Smartphones among Healthcare Professionals. *Electronic Journal of Health Informatics*, *5*(2), 1–12.

Chismar, W. G., & Wiley-patton, S. (2003). Does the Extended Technology Acceptance Model Apply to Physicians? In *Proceedings of the 36th Hawaii International Conference on System Sciences* (pp. 1–8). doi:10.1109/HICSS.2003.1174354

Creswell, J. W. (2003). *Research design: qualitative, quantitative, and mixed method approaches*. Sage Publications. Retrieved from http://books.google.es/books?id=nSVxmN2KWeYC

Daudelin, D., Kwong, M., & Beshansky, J. (2005). Using Specialized Information Technology to Reduce Errors in Emergency Cardiac Care. *Advances in Patient Safety*, *3*, 7–22. Retrieved from http://oai.dtic.mil/oai/oai?verb=getRecord&metadataPrefix=html&identifier=ADA434231

Davis, F. D. (1989). Perceived Usefulness, Perceived Ease of Use, and User Acceptance of Information Technology. *Management Information Systems*, *13*(3), 319–340. doi:10.2307/249008

Deloitte. (2013). *Physician adoption of health information technology: Implications for medical practice leaders and business partners*. Retrieved from http://www.deloitte.com/view/en_US/us/Industries/health-care-providers/index.htm

Dünnebeil, S., Sunyaev, A., Blohm, I., Leimeister, J. M., & Krcmar, H. (2012). Determinants of physicians' technology acceptance for e-health in ambulatory care. *International Journal of Medical Informatics*, 1–15. doi:10.1016/j.ijmedinf.2012.02.002 PMID:22397989

Eysenbach, G., & Diepgen, T. L. (2001). The role of e-health and consumer health informatics for evidence-based patient choice in the 21st century. *Clinics in Dermatology*, *19*(1), 11–17. doi:10.1016/S0738-081X(00)00202-9 PMID:11369478

Fishbein, M., & Ajzen, I. (1972). Attitudes and opinions. In Annual Review of Psychology. Lawrence Erlbaum. Retrieved from http://books.google.com/books?hl=en&lr=&id=wmph8grxWpAC&oi=fnd&pg=PR11&dq=Attitudes+and+opinions&ots=jNtahqVcOz&sig=v0B8lOXn9tRXN8WCjUU7gHqNxgo

Fishbein, M., & Ajzen, I. (1975). *Belief, attitude, intention and behaviour: An introduction to theory and research*. Addison-Wesley. Retrieved from http://www.people.umass.edu/aizen/f&a1975.html

Gagnon, M.-P., Ghandour, E. K., Talla, P. K., Simonyan, D., Godin, G., Labrecque, M., & Rousseau, M. et al. (2014). Electronic health record acceptance by physicians: Testing an integrated theoretical model. *Journal of Biomedical Informatics*, *48*, 17–27. doi:10.1016/j.jbi.2013.10.010 PMID:24184678

Gagnon, M.-P., Godin, G., Gagné, C., Fortin, J.-P., Lamothe, L., Reinharz, D., & Cloutier, A. (2003). An adaptation of the theory of interpersonal behaviour to the study of telemedicine adoption by physicians. *International Journal of Medical Informatics*, *71*(2-3), 103–115. doi:10.1016/S1386-5056(03)00094-7 PMID:14519403

Galliers, R. D., & Leidner, D. E. (Eds.). (2014). *Strategic information management: challenges and strategies in managing information systems*. Chicago: Routledge.

Han, S., Mustonen, P., & Seppanen, M. M. K. (2006). Physicians' acceptance of mobile communication technology an exploratory study. *International Journal of Mobile Communications*, *4*(2), 210–230. Retrieved from http://www.inderscience.com/browse/index.php?journalCODE=ijmc

Haux, R. (2006). Health information systems - past, present, future. *International Journal of Medical Informatics*, *75*(3-4), 268–281. doi:10.1016/j.ijmedinf.2005.08.002 PMID:16169771

Heeks, R. B. (2002). Information Systems and Developing Countries: Failure, Success and Local Improvisations. *The Information Society*, *18*(2), 101–112. doi:10.1080/01972240290075039

Holden, R. J., Brown, R. L., Scanlon, M. C., & Karsh, B.-T. (2012). Pharmacy workers' perceptions and acceptance of bar-coded medication technology in a pediatric hospital. *Research in Social & Administrative Pharmacy*. http://doi.org/<ALIGNMENT.qj></ALIGNMENT>10.1016/j.sapharm.2012.01.004

Horan, T. A., Tulu, B., Hilton, B., & Burton, J. (2004). Use of online systems in clinical medical assessments: an analysis of physician acceptance of online disability evaluation systems. In *Proceedings of the 37th Annual Hawaii International Conference on System Sciences* (p. 10). IEEE. http://doi.org/doi:10.1109/HICSS.2004.1265364

Hung, S.-Y., Ku, Y.-C., & Chien, J.-C. (2012). Understanding physicians' acceptance of the Medline system for practicing evidence-based medicine: A decomposed TPB model. *International Journal of Medical Informatics*, *81*(2), 130–142. doi:10.1016/j.ijmedinf.2011.09.009 PMID:22047627

Hung, S.-Y., Tsai, J. C.-A., & Chuang, C.-C. (2014). Investigating primary health care nurses' intention to use information technology: An empirical study in Taiwan. *Decision Support Systems*, *57*, 331–342. doi:10.1016/j.dss.2013.09.016

Ilie, V., Van Slyke, C., Parikh, M. A., & Courtney, J. F. (2009). Paper Versus Electronic Medical Records: The Effects of Access on Physicians' Decisions to Use Complex Information Technologies*. *Decision Sciences*, *40*(2), 213–241. doi:10.1111/j.1540-5915.2009.00227.x

Jones, M. R. (2003). "Computers can land people on Mars, why can't they get them to work in a hospital?" Implementation of an Electronic Patient Record System in a UK Hospital. *Methods of Information in Medicine*, *42*(4), 410–415. Retrieved from http://www.ncbi.nlm.nih.gov/pubmed/14534642 PMID:14534642

Kaplan, B., & Shaw, N. T. (2004). Future directions in evaluation research: People, organizational, and social issues. *Methods of Information in Medicine*, *43*(3), 215–231. Retrieved from http://www.ncbi.nlm.nih.gov/pubmed/15227551 PMID:15227551

Kijsanayotin, B., Pannarunothai, S., & Speedie, S. M. (2009). Factors influencing health information technology adoption in Thailand's community health centers: Applying the UTAUT model. *International Journal of Medical Informatics*, *78*(6), 404–416. doi:10.1016/j.ijmedinf.2008.12.005 PMID:19196548

Kitchenham, B. (2004). *Procedures for Performing Systematic Reviews*. Joint Technical Report, Keele University TR/SE-0401 and NICTA 0400011T.1, 1–33.

Kummer, T.-F., Schäfer, K., & Todorova, N. (2013). Acceptance of hospital nurses toward sensor-based medication systems: A questionnaire survey. *International Journal of Nursing Studies*, *50*(4), 508–517. doi:10.1016/j.ijnurstu.2012.11.010 PMID:23352607

Liang, H., Xue, Y., & Byrd, T. A. (2003). PDA usage in healthcare professionals: Testing an extended technology acceptance model. *International Journal of Mobile Communications*, *1*(4), 372. doi:10.1504/IJMC.2003.003992

Lin, H.-C. (2014). An investigation of the effects of cultural differences on physicians' perceptions of information technology acceptance as they relate to knowledge management systems. *Computers in Human Behavior*, *38*, 368–380. doi:10.1016/j.chb.2014.05.001

Littlejohns, P., Wyatt, J. C., & Garvican, L. (2003). Evaluating computerised health information systems: Hard lessons still to be learnt. *BMJ (Clinical Research Ed.)*, *326*(7394), 860–863. doi:10.1136/bmj.326.7394.860 PMID:12702622

Liu, L., & Ma, Q. (2006). Perceived system performance: A test of an extended technology acceptance model. *ACM SIGMIS Database*, *37*(2-3), 51. doi:10.1145/1161345.1161354

Lorenzi, N. M., & Riley, R. T. (2003). Organizational issues equals change. *International Journal of Medical Informatics*, *69*(2-3), 197–203. doi:10.1016/S1386-5056(02)00105-3 PMID:12810124

Melas, C. D., Zampetakis, L., Dimopoulou, A., & Moustakis, V. (2011). Modeling the acceptance of clinical information systems among hospital medical staff: An extended TAM model. *Journal of Biomedical Informatics*, *44*(4), 553–564. doi:10.1016/j.jbi.2011.01.009 PMID:21292029

Mitchell, J. (1999). From telehealth to e-health: the unstoppable rise of e-health. Canberra Australia National Office for the Information Technology. Sydney: Commonwealth Department of Communications, Information Technology and the Arts. Retrieved from http://archive.dcita.gov.au/1999/09/rise

Moores, T. T. (2012). Towards an integrated model of IT acceptance in healthcare. *Decision Support Systems*, *53*(3), 507–516. doi:10.1016/j.dss.2012.04.014

Ortega Egea, J. M., & Román González, M. V. (2011). Explaining physicians' acceptance of EHCR systems: An extension of TAM with trust and risk factors. *Computers in Human Behavior*, *27*(1), 319–332. doi:10.1016/j.chb.2010.08.010

Pai, F.-Y., & Huang, K.-I. (2011). Applying the Technology Acceptance Model to the introduction of healthcare information systems. *Technological Forecasting and Social Change*, *78*(4), 650–660. doi:10.1016/j.techfore.2010.11.007

Paré, G., Sicotte, C., & Jacques, H. (2006). The effects of creating psychological ownership on physicians' acceptance of clinical information systems. *Journal of the American Medical Informatics Association : JAMIA*, *13*(2), 197–205. doi:10.1197/jamia.M1930 PMID:16357351

Peppard, J., Galliers, R. D., & Thorogood, A. (2014). Information systems strategy as practice: Micro strategy and strategizing for IS. *The Journal of Strategic Information Systems, 23*(1), 1–10. doi:10.1016/j.jsis.2014.01.002

Piette, J. D., Blaya, J. A., Sanchis, J. B. B., Box, P. O., & Arbor, A. (2011). Experiences in mHealth for Chronic Disease Management in 4 Countries. *Proceedings of the 4th International Symposium on Applied Sciences in Biomedical and Communication Technologies.* doi:10.1145/2093698.2093868

Pynoo, B., Devolder, P., Duyck, W., van Braak, J., Sijnave, B., & Duyck, P. (2012). Do hospital physicians' attitudes change during PACS implementation? A cross-sectional acceptance study. *International Journal of Medical Informatics, 81*(2), 88–97. doi:10.1016/j.ijmedinf.2011.10.007 PMID:22071012

Reichertz, P. L. (2006). Hospital information systems--past, present, future. *International Journal of Medical Informatics, 75*(3-4), 282–299. doi:10.1016/j.ijmedinf.2005.10.001 PMID:16330253

Rho, M. J., Choi, I. Y., & Lee, J. (2014). Predictive factors of telemedicine service acceptance and behavioral intention of physicians. *International Journal of Medical Informatics, 83*(8), 559–571. doi:10.1016/j.ijmedinf.2014.05.005 PMID:24961820

Rogers, E. M. (1995). Diffusion of Innovations. In An integrated approach to communication theory and research (Vol. 65). Free Press. http://doi.org/ doi:<ALIGNMENT.qj></ALIGNMENT>10.1525/aa.1963.65.5.02a00230

Rogers, E. M., & Shoemaker, F. F. (1971). *Communication of Innovations: A Cross-Cultural Approach.* Free Press. Retrieved from http://www.eric.ed.gov/ERICWebPortal/detail?accno=ED065999

Schaper, L., & Pervan, G. (2007). An investigation of factors affecting technology acceptance and use decisions by Australian allied health therapists. In *Proceedings of the 40th Hawaii International Conference on System Sciences* (pp. 141–141). IEEE. http://doi.org/ doi:10.1109/HICSS.2007.69

Schaper, L. K., & Pervan, G. P. (2007). ICT and OTs: A model of information and communication technology acceptance and utilisation by occupational therapists. *International Journal of Medical Informatics, 76*(1), 212–221. doi:10.1016/j.ijmedinf.2006.05.028 PMID:16828335

Sun, Y., Wang, N., Guo, X., & Peng, Z. (2013). Understanding The Acceptance Of Mobile Health Services: A Comparison And Integration Of Alternative Models. *Journal of Electronic Commerce Research, 14*(2), 183–200. Retrieved from http://csulb.edu/journals/jecr/issues/20132/paper4.pdf

Taylor, S., & Todd, P. A. (1995). Assessing IT Usage:The Role of Prior Experience. *Management Information Systems Quarterly, 19*(2), 561–570. doi:10.2307/249633

Tung, F.-C., Chang, S.-C., & Chou, C.-M. (2008). An extension of trust and TAM model with IDT in the adoption of the electronic logistics information system in HIS in the medical industry. *International Journal of Medical Informatics, 77*(5), 324–335. doi:10.1016/j.ijmedinf.2007.06.006 PMID:17644029

Van Schaik, P., Bettany-Saltikov, J. A., & Warren, J. G. (2002). Clinical acceptance of a low-cost portable system for postural assessment. *Behaviour & Information Technology, 21*(1), 47–57. doi:10.1080/01449290110107236

Venkatesh, V., & Davis, F. D. (2000). A Theoretical Acceptance Extension Model : Four Longitudinal Field Studies. *Management Science, 46*(2), 186–204. doi:10.1287/mnsc.46.2.186.11926

Venkatesh, V., Morris, M. G., Davis, G. B., & Davis, F. D. (2003). User Acceptance of Information Technology: Toward a Unified View. *Management Information Systems*, *27*(3), 425–478.

Walter, Z., & Lopez, M. S. (2008). Physician acceptance of information technologies: Role of perceived threat to professional autonomy. *Decision Support Systems*, *46*(1), 206–215. doi:10.1016/j.dss.2008.06.004

WHO. (2008). *World Health Organization: Deaths from NCDs*. Retrieved from http://www.who.int/gho/ncd/mortality_morbidity/ncd_total_text/en/index.html

WHO. (2011). *World Health Organization: Global atlas on cardiovascular disease prevention and control*. World Health Organization. Retrieved from http://www.who.int/cardiovascular_diseases/en/

Wolters Kluwer Health 2013 Physician Outlook Survey. (2013). Retrieved from http://www.wolterskluwerhealth.com/News/Pages/latestnews.aspx

Wood, R., & Bandura, A. (1989). Social Cognitive Theory of Organizational Management. *Academy of Management Review*, *14*(3), 361–384. doi:10.2307/258173

Wu, I.-L., Li, J.-Y., & Fu, C.-Y. (2011). The adoption of mobile healthcare by hospital's professionals: An integrative perspective. *Decision Support Systems*, *51*(3), 587–596. doi:10.1016/j.dss.2011.03.003

Wu, J.-H., Wang, S.-C., & Lin, L.-M. (2007). Mobile computing acceptance factors in the healthcare industry: A structural equation model. *International Journal of Medical Informatics*, *76*(1), 66–77. doi:10.1016/j.ijmedinf.2006.06.006 PMID:16901749

Yi, M. Y., Jackson, J. D., Park, J. S., & Probst, J. C. (2006). Understanding information technology acceptance by individual professionals: Toward an integrative view. *Information & Management*, *43*(3), 350–363. doi:10.1016/j.im.2005.08.006

Yu, P., Li, H., & Gagnon, M.-P. (2009). Health IT acceptance factors in long-term care facilities: A cross-sectional survey. *International Journal of Medical Informatics*, *78*(4), 219–229. doi:10.1016/j.ijmedinf.2008.07.006 PMID:18768345

KEY TERMS AND DEFINITIONS

Behavioral Intention: It is the common factor being employed by all technology acceptance theories. It aims to define individuals' act in use a particular technology.

Health Information Systems (HIS): HIS is a common definition of information systems being used to serve health services. It covers telemedicine, electronic health (e-health), mobile health (m-health) and other healthcare related technologies.

Innovation Diffusion Theory (IDT): IDT proposes a model to investigate the transformation process of emerging innovations or existing technologies.

Technology Acceptance Model (TAM): TAM is one of the pioneering theories which aims to determine behaviors of users towards particular technologies by employing two factors: perceived usefulness and perceived ease of use.

Technology Acceptance: Technology acceptance is an interdisciplinary domain, which employs psychology and information systems fields of study to investigate users' attitudes towards new technologies.

Theory of Planned Behavior (TPB): TPB constitutes the basis of TAM, and it proposes a theory which explains user attitudes towards technologies by investigating their perception of ease or difficulty of performing the particular behavior and social influence.

Unified Theory of Acceptance and Use of Technology (UTAUT): UTAUT is one of the most popular technology acceptance theory which was developed by unifying eight different theories. It aims to explain user intentions by proposing a unified model for information system use.

APPENDIX

Table 5. List of HIS acceptance studies on health professionals (2002-2014)

Study / Reference	Significantly Related Variables	Model /Theory	Target Sample	Sample Size	R²
(Chau, 2002)	PU -BI Attitude-BI PBC-BI	Integrated model TAM-TPB	Physicians of telemedicine	408	0.43
(Van Schaik, Bettany-Saltikov, & Warren, 2002)	PEOU-PU PU-BI	TAM	Physiotherapists	49	0.39
(Gagnon et al., 2003)	Self-Identity- BI Normative Factors- BI Habit- Affect	Theory of Interpersonal Behavior (TPB and TAM)	Physicians of telemedicine	519	0.81
(Barker, Schaik, Simpson, & Corbett, 2003)	Perceived System Response –PEOU	TAM	Clinicians	10	-
(Chismar & Wiley-patton, 2003)	PU-BI Job relevance-PU Output Quality- PU	TAM2	Physicians (pediatricians)	89	0.54
(Liang, Xue, & Byrd, 2003)	Personal Innovativeness- Actual Use PEOU- Actual Use Support-PEOU PEOU-PU Job Relevance- PU Compatibility-PU	TAM	Healthcare professionals	173	0.62
(Horan, Tulu, Hilton, & Burton, 2004)	Perceived Readiness-BI Attitude-BI Work Practice Compatibility- BI PEOU-PU PU-Attitude PEOU-Attitude	Integrated model by TAM, TPB and Task-Technology Fit	Physicians	141	0.44
(Yi, Jackson, Park, & Probst, 2006)	Personal Innovativeness (PIIT)-PBC PIIT-Result Demonstrability (RD) PIIT- SN PIIT- PEOU PBC- BI PEOU- PU PU-BI SN- Image RD- PEOU RD- PU Image- PU	Integrated model by TAM and TPB	Physicians	222	0.57
(Shengnan Han, Pekka Mustonen, Matti Seppanen, 2006)	PU-BI Age on ease of use-BI Age on compatibility-BI	TAM and UTAUT	Professional physicians	151	0.65
(Paré, Sicotte, & Jacques, 2006)	Attitude-Use PU-Use PU-Attitude PEOU-Attitude PEOU-PU Psychological ownership-PU Psychological ownership-PEOU	TAM	Physicians	91	0.55
(Liu & Ma, 2006)	Perceived System Performance- BI Perceived System Performance-PU Perceived System Performance -PEOU PEOU-PU PEOU-BI PU-BI	TAM	healthcare workers (managing patient records)	77	0.52

continued on following page

Table 5. Continued

Study / Reference	Significantly Related Variables	Model /Theory	Target Sample	Sample Size	R²
(C. Chen, Wu, & Crandall, 2007)	-	UTAUT	Emergency room medical teams	81	0.62
(J.-H. Wu, Wang, & Lin, 2007)	Compatibility –Self Efficacy Compatibility- BI Compatibility- PU Compatibility- PEOU Self-Efficacy- PU Self-Efficacy- PEOU Technical support and training- Self efficacy PEOU-PU PEOU-BI PU-BI	TAM and IDT	Physicians, nurses, and medical technicians in Taiwan	123	0.70
(Chang, Hwang, Hung, & Li, 2007)	Performance Expectancy-BI Effort Expectancy-BI	UTAUT	Physicians	140	0.43
(L. K. Schaper & Pervan, 2007)	Effort Expectancy –BI Organizational facilitating conditions- Effort Expectancy Organizational facilitating conditions- Performance Expectancy Compatibility- Performance Expectancy Compatibility- BI Computer Anxiety –Effort Expectancy Performance Expectancy- Attitude Computer Self Efficacy- Effort Expectancy	UTAUT and TAM	Australian therapists	1605	0.63
(Walter & Lopez, 2008)	Perceived threat to autonomy -PU PU- BI PEOU- PU	TAM	Physicians	203,129	0.22, 0.18
(Tung, Chang, & Chou, 2008)	Perceived Financial Cost- BI Compatibility- BI Compatibility- PU PU-BI PEOU-PU PEOU-BI PEOU-Trust Trust- BI	TAM and IDT	Nurses	252	0.70
(Ilie & Slyke, 2009)	Physical and Logical access -PEOU Physical and Logical access –PU Logical access- BI PEOU-PU PU- Attitude PEOU-Attitude PU-BI Attitude-BI	TAM	Physicians	199	0.64
(Kijsanayotin et al., 2009)	Performance Expectancy-BI Effort Expectancy-BI	UTAUT	Health workers, nurses and public health specialists	1607	0.54

continued on following page

Table 5. Continued

Study / Reference	Significantly Related Variables	Model /Theory	Target Sample	Sample Size	R^2
(Yu, Li, & Gagnon, 2009)	Image- BI Image- PEOU Subjective Norm- PU Subjective Norm- PEOU Job Role –PU Computer Level- BI Computer Level-PEOU PU-BI PEOU-BI PEOU-PU	TAM2	Caregivers	134	0.34
(Aggelidis & Chatzoglou, 2009)	PU- Anxiety PU-BI PEOU-PU SN- BI Training- PEOU Training- Facilitating Conditions Facilitating conditions- PU/PEOU/ Anxiety/ Self-Efficacy Anxiety-Self Efficacy Anxiety- Attitudes towards Use PU- Attitudes towards Use PEOU- Attitudes towards Use	TAM and UTAUT	Members of medical, nursing and administrative personnel	283	0.87
(J. Chen, Park, & Putzer, 2010)	Attitude –BI PU- BI PU- Attitude Self-efficacy- PEOU Self-efficacy - BI Compatibility - PU Task- Attitude Compatibility- PEOU	TAM- IDT	Physician and nurses	153	-
(Pai & Huang, 2011)	Information Quality- PU Service Quality- PU Service Quality- PEOU System Quality- PEOU PEOU- PU PU-BI PEOU-BI	TAM2 and IS Success Model	Nurses	366	-
(Melas, Zampetakis, Dimopoulou, & Moustakis, 2011)	ICT feature demands- PU ICT Knowledge- PEOU PEOU- PU PU- Attitude Attitude- BI PEOU- Attitude PU-BI PEOU- BI	TAM	Physicians and medical staff	604	0.83
(Ortega Egea & Román González, 2011)	Information Integrity- Perceived Risk Information Integrity- Trust Perceived Risk- Trust Trust- PU Trust- PEOU Trust- Attitude towards Use PEOU- PU PU- Attitude Attitude- Intention to use	TAM	Physicians	254	0.96

continued on following page

Table 5. Continued

Study / Reference	Significantly Related Variables	Model /Theory	Target Sample	Sample Size	R^2
(I.-L. Wu, Li, & Fu, 2011)	Perceived Service Availability- PU Attitude- BI PEOU-PU PU- BI PU- Attitude Personal Innovativeness in IT- PEOU Personal Innovativeness in IT -PBC SN- BI PBC- BI Hospital type- BI	TAM and TPB	Hospital Professionals	140	0.63
(Dünnebeil, Sunyaev, Blohm, Leimeister, & Krcmar, 2012)	Intensity of IT utilization- PU Importance of Data Security- PU Importance of Documentation- PU e-Health Knowledge- PEOU Importance of Standardization- PEOU Process Orientation- PEOU PU- BI PEOU- BI PEOU-PU	TAM and UTAUT	German Physicians	117	0.55
(Hung, Ku, & Chien, 2012)	PEOU- PU PEOU- Attitude PU- Attitude Attitude- Usage Intention SN- Usage Intention PBC- Usage Intention Interpersonal Influence- SN Personal Innovativeness in IT- PBC Personal Innovativeness in IT- Self efficacy	TAM and TPB	Physicians in Taiwan	224	0.52
(Holden, Brown, Scanlon, & Karsh, 2012)	PU- BI SN- BI	TAM	Pharmacy Technicians	39	0.72
(Moores, 2012)	PEOU -PU Enabling Factors- PEOU Information Quality- PU PU- ATT PEOU-ATT PU – Compatibility PEOU- Compatibility	Integrated TAM	Physicians, nurses, and allied health workers	346	0.23
(Pynoo et al., 2012)	Performance Expectancy-BI Effort Expectancy-BI SN-BI BI- Use Facilitating Conditions- Performance Expectancy Facilitating Conditions- Effort Expectancy Facilitating Conditions- SN	UTAUT	Physicians	46- 61	0.26-0.58
(Kummer, Schäfer, & Todorova, 2013)	Image- PU Demonstrability- PU Personal Innovativeness- PU PU-BI	TAM and TAM2	Nurses	579	0.52

continued on following page

Table 5. Continued

Study / Reference	Significantly Related Variables	Model /Theory	Target Sample	Sample Size	R^2
(Hung, Tsai, & Chuang, 2014)	Compatibility- PU Perceived Trust (PT) - PU Compatibility –PT Social Norms –Attitude PU – Attitude PT- Attitude	TRA	Nurses	768	0.57
(Gagnon et al., 2014)	Professional Norm-BI SN- BI PEOU-BI Demonstrability of the Results (DR)- BI PEOU-PU Self-efficacy- PEOU DR - PU	Integrated model, psychosocial model and extended TAM	Physicians	150	0.44-0.55
(Rho, Choi, & Lee, 2014)	Self-efficacy – PEOU Self-efficacy – PU PEOU-PU Accessibility of medical records- PU Accessibility of patients – PU-BI PEOU-BI	TAM	Physicians	183	-
(Lin, 2014)	PU- BI PEOU- BI Perceived information security- BI SN- BI	Extended TAM	Physicians	106	0.68

Trust and Credibility Perception in E-Health:
Interface Contributions

Andreia Pinto de Sousa
University of Porto, Portugal & Universidade of Aveiro, Portugal

Ana Margarida Pisco Almeida
University of Aveiro, Portugal

INTRODUCTION

Over the past few years there has been a significant increase in e-health information consumption, being the Internet, currently, one of the most important sources to search for health information. In this scenario, it is critical *to understand how people assess the credibility of a site, source, or piece of information, it's a key task in the development of any health education or health promotion undertaking and, thus, an important area of research* (Eysenbach, 2008, p. 125). Aware that Interface is not the only factor that influences trust and credibility perception this study focuses on the Interface influence to fulfill a gap mentioned by authors that are developing research in the e-Health field as Eysenbach (2008): *there is a great deal of high-quality information on the Web that is published by trusted organizations. It is important for these organizations to appear credible enough to initiate a behavior change in consumers* (p.125), Robins et al. (2009) presented results *that showed that health information sites that are rated higher for visual design tend also to be rated higher for perceived credibility* (p. 21). In the same study authors suggested that *it will be valuable for visual designers to know more specifically how to employ tools that promote credibility in websites whose health information is worthy of such a presentation* (p. 28). In 2013 in a study about "User evaluation of Websites" conducted by Thielsch et al. confirmed the importance of aesthetics for the first impression of a website and that importance doesn't disappear even when the information gains importance. The interface is the materialization of all the information, and the behavior of a website.

In this context, nowadays Interface dimensions such as visual design, information architecture, social presence, interaction, and user experience are unavoidable concepts when studying information systems. This study aims to deepen knowledge on online information presentation and on the user and Interface relationships processes, proposing the study of a set of design principles for the credibility and trust, based on a proposed set of Interface dimensions.

The knowledge on the impact of the Interface in a credibility assessment is undoubtedly important in the field of e-health, being fundamental to investigate the processes used by e-health users to select information and make decisions.

This online information credibility analysis has been studied especially in the e-Commerce field, and not so deeply in the e-health area. In Stanford, the Persuasive Lab directed by B. J. Fogg et al., (2003) conducted a study that shows the importance of the design's look in credibility assessment. Later, Robins & Holmes (2008) showed that the average time to respond with a credibility judgment is 2.30 seconds,

DOI: 10.4018/978-1-4666-9978-6.ch086

proving that the Interface plays an important role in this assessment. Acknowledging the impact of the Interface in a credibility assessment is undoubtedly important in the field of e-health, being fundamental to investigate the processes used by e-health users to select information and make decisions.

BACKGROUND

Interface

The Interface is responsible for the mediation between human relationships and human machine interactions. Considering that the Interface is determinant of the type and quality of interactions in which it is involved, it's not limited to an object or space presentation: it's responsible for defining the interactions that happen between people.

In the words of Sá (2010), *Interface is a hybrid space that synthesizes heterogeneities from the entities placed in relation. Their plastic materiality is constituted by the hybridization between the systems being related, limited by them and limiting them, being effective and taking shape by the action* (Sá, 2010, pp. 209–210). From this broad perspective of the Interface that determines how we experience and define the world in which we live, this study focuses mainly on the Interface between the user and the digital platforms, often called a Graphical User Interface, this designation will not be adopted in this study because, in our view, the use of graphic expression seems too limiting to visual or graphical issues. In this context it's important to clarify that when there is reference to the Interface, in the course of this study, it is about a group of dimensions that comprises it, namely: visual, information architecture, social presence, interaction, and the user experience. This suggested group, based in other studies about online credibility and trust that, as can be seen throughout this chapter, reports that one or more of the Interface dimensions have a key role in the perception of online credibility and trust. As Raskin (2000) defines, the Interface is how one accomplishes tasks with a product and how it responds to one's actions. The contact point between information available on the Web and individuals still is the Interface, and it is through the Interface that the starting point is established for the creation of credibility and trust processes.

Related to this issue Fogg (2003) presented a while ago results of a study entitled "How do users evaluate the Credibility of Web sites?" in which, contrary to what was usual at that moment, the analysis of credibility on websites was not only focused on the information. The analysis of comments made by participants reveals the influence of Interface design issues in the perception of credibility. This study has become an essential reference work in the study of online credibility, proving the relevance of design in its process. Also Robins, Holmes, & Stansbury (2009) isolated the analysis of the credibility of the analysis of the information credibility through visual design, demonstrating that the visual design impacts the perception of credibility.

Despite being the focus of attention of different studies, the problem of online trust still needs more research, as evidenced by the survey related to website design and initial trust studies, developed by Karimov, Brussel, Brengman e Hove (2011). From an extensive literature review (from 1996-2010), and focusing on the e-Commerce area, the authors acknowledge that there is no standard for measuring dimensions of websites and propose a conceptual model for the classification of design dimensions that induce the perception of trust which are: visual design, design of social cues and content design. Based on this organization, they gathered all the results found in the literature, demonstrating that the impact of design dimensions on the initial trust of websites is little investigated. Equally important to frame this issue is the study conducted by Wang & Emurian (2005) in which the authors propose a framework of design features that contribute to online trust. They also identified four dimensions of the Interface inducing trust, namely: visual design, design of social cues, design of information architecture and interaction design.

Trust and Credibility

The concept of trust is complex and abstract, being difficult to both define it, and to identify the elements that surround it. It can be described as a belief or dependence in quality or attribute of a person or object (Furman, 2009), it is gradually built through different interactions, allowing people to acquire beliefs about another person or object. Trust is based on interactions and presupposes that there are always two parties involved in the process. It also can be understood as an individual belief that other people are going to behave ethically and socially appropriate and even as an expectation that those who we choose to trust will not take advantage of the situation (Chow & Angie, 2006; Gefen & Karahanna, 2003). In the academic and professional literature, the terms of credibility and trust are used loosely and, although related, they are not synonymous. Credibility is a perceived quality, not residing in an object, a person or a piece of information, compared with trust. Fogg (2003) compares credibility with beauty: in the eye of the spectator, it cannot be touched, seen or even heard, exists only when an assessment of a person, object or a piece of information is made. Is composed of two key dimensions that are trust and expertise these, although both dimensions of credibility, are not directly related to each other and there may be no reliable expertise or vice versa. Computer credibility can be organized in four types: presumed, surface, reputed and earned (Fogg, 2003a).

Trust and Credibility on the Web

Except for a few studies conducted by Fogg, in the Stanford Research Lab, which have used health websites to analyze the impact on superficial credibility, studies on trust and credibility on the Web are mostly focused on the e-Commerce area. For this reason, this section was framed in results obtained from research conducted in this field.

Wang & Emurian (2005) focused on the study of the concept of trust in different disciplines in order to characterize the offline and online trust. The first, referred to as "trust offline", found four characteristics frequently observed and accepted by researchers: the trustor and trustee, vulnerability, produced action and subjective matter. The offline trust shares similar characteristics with the online trust, having, however, an important unique distinction in this environment regarding the trustor and trustee: these two parties remain essential in an online context, being the role of trustee occupied by the user and the role of trustee by a website that represents an entity. In this context it is relevant to remember that the technology (and especially the Web) is itself an object of trust, although the complexity and anonymity

Table 1. Credibility of computing products (Fogg, 2003a)

Type of Credibility	Basis for Credibility
Presumed	General assumptions in the mind of the perceiver
Surface	Simple inspection or initial firsthand experience
Reputed	Third-party endorsements, reports or referrals
Earned	Firsthand experience that extends over time

associated with Web services increases the vulnerability factors (Wang & Emurian, 2005). One element that will always be present in a relationship of trust is subjectivity, as trust offline, and it is directly related to individual differences and contextual factors. The online trust is inherently a subjective matter, since the level of trust required for each individual to make an online transaction is different (Wang & Emurian, 2005). In the case of e-Health, based on the health information available on the websites, this subjectivity applies to the actions produced that may be related with decision-making and health education and prevention.

The online trust and credibility are, therefore, directly related to the structure of the communication medium that, as already mentioned, in the case of digital media, materializes in the Interface through different dimensions. The technological mediation between products and services directly influences the perception of the individual trust.

Models for the Study of Trust in Information Systems

The proliferation of institutional websites and web-enabled sales boosted the emergence of many studies on the processes of perception and evaluation of usability, satisfaction and trust, among others. As mentioned above, many of these studies have been developed in the context of e-commerce, and as Riemenschneider & Leonard (2009) state, focus on one of the most difficult problems to consider: trust and its relationship with other variables that directly influence the perception of the individual. Previous studies (such as DeLone & McLean, 1992; Du & Zhao, 2009; Riemenschneider, Jones, & Leonard, 2009) have tested various different factors that can contribute to the confidence in information systems, namely: usability; ease of use; user satisfaction; quality of information; quality system; the utility; the graphical interface; graphic design; the design of the structure; the design of the content and the design of drawing social cues. In the context of this study, all these factors were considered as members or dependents of the user interface and user experience (User Experience - UX) as key elements and dimensions in the analysis of the quality of that experience. The interface is, from our point of view, a fundamental component of materialization of these processes in the context of the current dynamics of the use of applications and Web services.

E-Health

In the context of the current reconfiguration of health-care models Fortney, Burgess, Bosworth, Booth, & Kaboli (2011) propose four new types of health care delivery, online mediated, which should be considered in addition to the already known encounters face-to-face meeting between the patient and the health care provider: *(i) synchronous digital patient-to-provider encounters, (ii) asynchronous digital patient-to-provider communications, (iii) digital peer-to-peer communications (iv) synchronous digital interactions between patients and computer health applications* (Fortney et al., 2011, p. 640).

The report for communication in social networks, published by the Centers for Disease Control and Prevention, (2011) refers to social networks and other communication technologies *as* aggregators of millions of voices that*: (i) increase the timely dissemination and potential impact of health and safety information; (ii) leverage audience networks to facilitate information sharing; (iii) expand reach to include broader, more diverse audiences; (iv) Personalize and reinforce health messages that can be more easily tailored or targeted to particular audiences; (v) facilitate interactive communication, connection and public engagement.; (vi) Empower people to make safer and healthier decisions* (Centers for Disease Control and Prevention, 2011, p. 1).

The results presented in this report imply a phenomenon called "patient empowerment" a concept that reflects an important change in the patient/ physician relationship: if the patient has not previously questioned the doctor nor his decision, we are doing so today before entering as patients in clinics with a formed idea about our health condition and what treatments to apply (Shneiderman, 2003).

Health information websites, and especially social health networks, allow patients to share information based on their own or others' experiences on topics such as symptoms, diagnoses and treatments, adverse effects of treatments, medical evidence sources, and health care provider experiences and opinions on their quality (Griffiths et al., 2012)

The power of the patient is evident in patient health care provider relationships, which not only actively seeks information, but also the possibility to discuss the matter, sharing or questioning other patients and becoming himself a health content producer.

This new paradigm brings in challenges, including issues of privacy, quality, trust and credibility. Flows and roles relating to communication and information consumption are currently more complex, as the unidirectional flow of health information that departs from health professionals as producers and individuals as consumers is gradually being replaced by a more fluid and evenly distributed where everyone, professional or others may act as consumers and producers of health information (Burton, Tanner, & Giraud-Carrier, 2012)

As stated by Eysenbach (2007), with the ease of access to a huge volume of health information available on the Web, consumers may eventually ignore the intermediation of experts and assume responsibility to assess the credibility of information themselves; this evaluation made by the consumer is based on variables such as autonomy and motivation. The characteristics of the message environment, presentation or attractiveness of the source, as well as its primary decision makers, are perceived as factors in credibility. The same author also refers to new means of information consumption (which are also the new intermediaries) as "apomediaries", a type of mediators that do not necessarily imply the existence of an health professional to stand between consumers or between services and information, as now this could be made by tools and peers.

For this study, the issue of disintermediation or "apomediation" is especially relevant because it is directly related to the perception of credibility and trust online. It has the potential to increase the perception of credibility especially in areas like health, because consumers have a sense of distrust of the system itself (Eysenbach, 2007).

Based on literature review, one can conclude that the interface plays a crucial role in trust and credibility perception on digital platforms. On the other hand, the healthcare field is undergoing profound changes with the amount of information available and shared online. In this new scenario in which the roles of health professionals, health care and patient services are redefined, aiming to understand the contribution of Interface dimensions for trust and credibility perception in e-Health.

Interface Contributes for Trust and Credibility Perception

Based on the literature review described in this chapter and following the question "What are the contributions of the Interface for credibility and trust perception by users in e-Health?", a framework was built (Table 2) to analyze the relationships between different types of credibility, design dimensions, user access and participation with familiarity, reputation and information nature.

The dimensions proposed were defined based on literature review about interface design and some studies presented before. Five dimensions considered relevant in the process of online credibility and trust were defined. The proposed dimensions (Figure 1) are: visual dimension, information architecture dimension, social presence dimension, interaction dimension and the user experience dimension.

Table 2. Analysis model

Dimensions	Concepts	Indicators
Interface	Visual	Acknowledgment of the presence of color, grid, and typography (Prominence)
		Acknowledgement of the importance of color, grid and typography in the building of its credibility (Interpretation)
		Classifying of the relevance of each element.
	Social presence	Acknowledgement of the presence of the social component
		Acknowledgement of the importance of the social component in the building of its credibility (Interpretation)
		Classification of relevance
	Information architecture	Acknowledgement of the presence of the organization (Prominence)
		Acknowledgment of the importance of the organization of the information in the construction of its credibility (Interpretation)
		Classification of relevance.
	Interaction	Acknowledgement of the presence of browsing ease (Prominence)
		Acknowledgement of the presence of browsing ease in the construction of its credibility (Interpretation)
		Classification of relevance
	User experience	Acknowledgement of the presence of a good user experience (Prominence)
		Acknowledgement of the presence of a good user experience in the perception of credibility (Prominence)
		Classification of relevance
Credibility and Trust	Reputation	Classification of relevance
		Recommended by friends or acquaintances
		Presence of partners
	Familiarity	Classification of relevance
		Recommended by friends or acquaintances
	Nature of information	Ease of understanding
		Completeness, link to other sources of information, expertise
e-Health users	Access and Participation	Motivation
		Frequency (Communication, sharing and use)
		Gender
		Age
		Health condition

As mentioned before, the taxonomy for computing products' credibility has four types, which are not mutually exclusive, assuming that the interface plays a crucial role in at least two types of credibility, namely the surface credibility and the credibility gained. Surface credibility is related to the visual dimension and credibility gained is directly related to the other interface dimensions: information architecture, social presence, interaction and user experience dimension.

The survey developed explores this relation between Interface dimensions and types of credibility trying to understand the influence of these dimensions in credibility and trust perception. With this

Figure 1. Interface dimensions framework

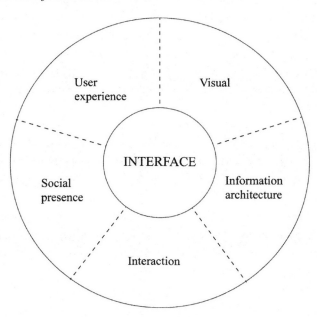

online automated survey, it was possible to get a quick read on user preferences and work with a large sample size.

The first part of the questionnaire presents a set of questions that allow performing a generic characterization of the respondents regarding online health information use, communication, sharing and their habits and perceptions. The formulated questions articulate the access and participation concepts, considering different indicators (such as gender, age, motivation, and health conditions, frequency of use, communication and sharing health information) with the concepts of familiarity, reputation and nature of the information. The respondent is also asked about the ease of understanding of the researched information and its completeness, regarding particularly its connection to other sources of information, and also exploring the concept of expertise.

The second part of the survey is more related with subject focus in this chapter, namely the relation between the Interface dimensions and the perception of credibility and trust. This second part resorts to a set of websites for which selection was based in their number of accesses and in the language, in this case Portuguese. Also, if in the first part the respondent has indicated a preferred website, blog or social network to consume, communicate or share health information this was also shown. The visual dimension explored superficial credibility aspects such as color scheme, typography, contrast and grid referring to the organization of the elements in the page. Then, and only if the respondent indicated familiarity with the websites proposed or a preferred website, social network or blog, the gained credibility was explored by information architecture, interaction, social presence and user experience dimensions. Three indicators, preeminence, interpretation and relevance regarding credibility and trust perception, were used to analyze data. Preeminence and interpretation were used in open questions such as: "Regarding this website, please assess and comment based on your credibility perception justifying whenever possible". In what concerns relevance the questions use an ordinal scale (e.g. 1. Not credible; 2. Not very credible; 3. Credible; 4. Very credible; 5. Completely credible). In these cases, the respondent was asked to indicate the influence of elements related with the Interface dimensions.

Looking for each of the websites presented to respondents to assess the contribute of four elements of the visual dimension, the website Portal do Utente[1]'s visual dimension has more credibility than the other three websites. In 154 responses 133 have evaluated the color scheme, typography, contrast and the organization of elements in the page as credible, very credible or completely credible.

In what concerns the website Medicina NET[2], in the same amount of responses, 96 have considered this website credible, very credible or completely credible. The website Biblioteca Virtual em Saúde[3] has 91 positive responses for the influence of visual elements in credibility and trust perception. In the whole group, the website Manual Merk[4] was considered the less credible with only 86 of the responses considering the elements positive in terms of influence to website's credibility.

Looking with more detail at the relevance of which element, the most relevant element is typography (Figure 2): in 154 responses, 110 considered typography as credible, very credible or completely credible in websites.

The second element that has significant influence in credibility is the color scheme (Figure 3), in 154 responses 101 has considered this element as credible, very credible or completely credible.

Contrast (Figure 4) follows color scheme with 99 in 154 responses considering this element as credible, very credible or completely credible.

Figure 2. Typography contribution to credibility and trust

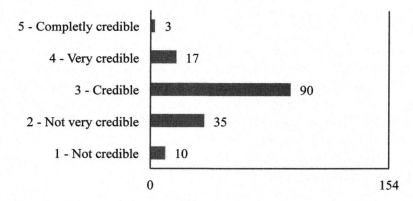

Figure 3. Color scheme contribution to credibility and trust

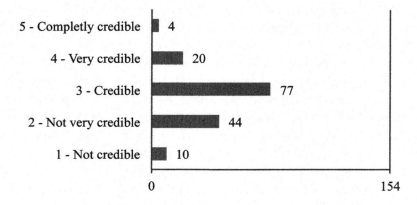

Figure 4. Contrast contribution to credibility and trust

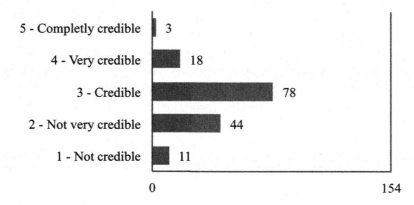

The composition of elements (Figure 5) in the page was the less credible element, with 98 in 154 positive responses. But it's important to refer that this represents more that 50% of the responses, meaning that this also has relevance in credibility and trust.

With these results one can conclude that the visual dimension has a strong influence in credibility and trust perception, obtaining 102 positive responses in 154, and that between the four elements analyzed (color scheme, typography, contrast and the organization of elements in the page) typography is the most influent followed by the color scheme, contrast and the organization of elements.

Regarding the other Interface dimensions, as mentioned before, the second part was only available for the respondents that indicated familiarity with one of the websites analyzed before or if they indicated a preferred website. For that reason, there are different numbers of respondents for each website. In a total of 154 respondents, 99 indicated familiarity with the websites presented, and the most familiar is Portal do Utente with 71 responses, followed by Manual Merk with 17 responses, Medicina NET has 6 responses and Biblioteca Virtual de Saúde 5 responses. In what concerns preferred websites, only 9 in 154 indicated a preferred website that was used in this part of the survey. In total, were obtained 108 responses related to the information architecture, interaction, social presence and user experience Interface dimensions.

The influence of the dimensions in credibility from a global perspective, was analyzed trying to understand which elements have more influence and the results showed that the "information architec-

Figure 5. Composition of elements contribution to credibility and trust

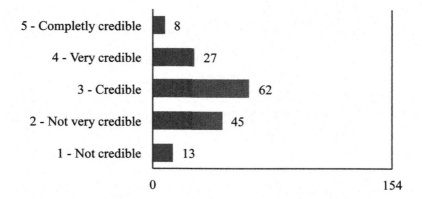

ture" and the "user experience" are the most influent, obtaining 96 positive responses in 108 followed by "interaction" with 91 and "social presence" with 62. Table 3 shows the number of positive responses about credibility influence in different elements of social presence, interaction and user experience dimensions for each website. It is important to refer that the low result of Biblioteca Virtual de Saúde in social presence dimension is due to this website not having the analyzed social elements.

An easy content navigation and a clear and easy to understand language has had 100 positive responses, followed by easy search and navigation through information structure, with 97 responses.

Table 3. Influence of social presence, information architecture and interaction dimensions in credibility per website

Dimension	Website	Elements	Credibility Influence	Average Influence/ Number of Responses
Social presence	Preferred	Other user comments	3	5/9
		Health professionals presence	5	
		Sharing between users (social network)	6	
		User testimony (videos)	5	
		Ability to communicate with other users and/or health professionals via instant message chat	5	
	Biblioteca Virtual de Saúde	Other user comments	1	1/5
		Health professionals presence	2	
		Sharing between users (social network)	1	
		User testimony (videos)	1	
		Ability to communicate with other users and/or health professionals via instant message chat	1	
	Medicina NET	Other user comments	5	5/6
		Health professionals presence	5	
		Sharing between users (social network)	5	
		User testimony (videos)	4	
		Ability to communicate with other users and/or health professionals via instant message chat	4	
	Manual Merk	Other user comments	5	7/17
		Health professionals presence	8	
		Sharing between users (social network)	7	
		User testimony (videos)	6	
		Ability to communicate with other users and/or health professionals via instant message chat	10	
	Portal do utente	Other user comments	38	43/71
		Health professionals presence	44	
		Sharing between users (social network)	40	
		User testimony (videos)	40	
		Ability to communicate with other users and/or health professionals via instant message chat	53	

continued on following page

Table 3. Continued

Dimension	Website	Elements	Credibility Influence	Average Influence/ Number of Responses
Information architecture	Preferred	Information categorization	8	9/9
		Use of clear and easy to understand language	9	
		Information structured to facilitating the search and navigation	9	
	Biblioteca Virtual de Saúde	Information categorization	4	4/5
		Use of clear and easy to understand language	4	
		Information structured to facilitating the search and navigation	3	
	Medicina NET	Information categorization	5	6/6
		Use of clear and easy to understand language	6	
		Information structured to facilitating the search and navigation	6	
	Manual Merk	Information categorization	13	13/17
		Use of clear and easy to understand language	12	
		Information structured to facilitating the search and navigation	14	
	Portal do Utente	Information categorization	61	64/71
		Use of clear and easy to understand language	68	
		Information structured to facilitating the search and navigation	64	
Interaction	Preferred	Ease of navigation between content	9	7/9
		Ease in performing tasks (e.g. content search, to register, subscribe newsletter, etc.)	7	
		Ease in contacting other people via the website (e.g. instant messaging, sending emails to authors, questions, etc.)	6	
	Biblioteca Virtual de Saúde	Ease of navigation between content	3	3/5
		Ease in performing tasks (e.g. content search, to register, subscribe newsletter, etc.)	4	
		Ease in contacting other people via the website (e.g. instant messaging, sending emails to authors, questions, etc.)	3	
	Medicina NET	Ease of navigation between content	6	6/6
		Facility to perform tasks (e.g. content search, to register, subscribe newsletter, etc.)	6	
		Ease in contacting with other people via the website (e.g. instant messaging, sending emails to authors, questions, etc.)	6	
	Manual Merk	Ease of navigation between content	15	12/17
		Ease in performing tasks (e.g. content search, to register, subscribe newsletter, etc.)	12	
		Ease in contacting other people via the website (e.g. instant messaging, sending emails to authors, questions, etc.)	10	
	Portal do Utente	Ease of navigation between content	66	61/71
		Ease in performing tasks (e.g. content search, to register, subscribe newsletter, etc.)	63	
		Ease in contacting other people via the website (e.g. instant messaging, sending emails to authors, questions, etc.)	54	

After verifying the relevance of the Interface dimensions in e-Health credibility websites, is important to know and understand a variety of factors that contribute to these dimensions. In order to reduce the effort necessary to design an Interface based on an extensive literature review, a framework of design principles by dimension has been organized and presented in Table 4. Due to the nature of this chapter, will only be present a selected group of those principles that some how are related with the results here presented.

Table 4. Principles of design by dimension

Dimension		Principle
Visual dimension	Consistency	In the visual or aesthetic layer the consistency refers to a consistency of style and appearance (e.g. the image of a company which uses a consistent typography, color and graphic language). The visual consistency facilitates recognition and defines emotional expectations (Lidwell, Holden, & Butle, 2003, p. 46). One way to guarantee consistency in the visual dimension of the Interface is using a grid, which helps the users foresee where specific information can be found in different pages.
	Scale and Contrast	Must be used to draw attention. These strategies allow the defining of the importance of the elements in a page. According to White there must always be a main element (White, 2011). According to Lidwell et al. (2003), one should not put in evidence more than 10% of the elements because the effect decreases as one increases the percentage
	Typography	Typography has a fundamental role in communicating information. Its form determines character, emotional attributes and directly affects the reader's accessibility and (Ambrose & Harris, 2009; Cullen, 2007). The choice of the typography must be made consciously and according to the communicational goals of the project.
	Hierarchy	It is used to differentiate the relevance of the elements. There should be no more than three levels of hierarchy because otherwise it becomes difficult to understand the hierarchies that are beyond what is more important and less important (White, 2011). The hierarchy can be created on characters by varying the size and weight or created through colors. The location of the elements on the page should follow the Gutenberg Diagram[5] (Lidwell et al., 2003). Our eyes respond to similar elements so it must be used the same shapes, colors and typography to be perceived as related to each other.
Information architecture dimension	Readability	Refers to the level of understanding of information along with readability. Should present the information in the simplest possible form and adjust the level of understanding of the audience (Lidwell et al., 2003).
	Legibility	Text must be organized in a way that is easy and comfortable to read. The factors that affect this principle are, among others: the alignment and justification of the text, the length of its lines, the space between the lines, the size of the text and etc. (Lidwell et al., 2003);
	Recognition instead of recall	Our memory recognizes better than it remembers. One must minimize the need to memorize information as much as possible, offering readable and easy to understand menus, decision helpers and other strategies that make the options clearly available (Lidwell et al., 2003; Wodtke & Govella, 2009);
	Presentation of results	The presentation of results should take into account two main issues: (i) how to present the results, (ii) how to list or group results (Rosenfeld & Morville, 2007).
Social presence dimension	Share of personal experiences	A large part of our conversations its about our personal experiences. One must design ways to make people share memories creating opportunities that help people remember their past experiences (Adams, 2013).
	Meta or generative design	The website should not be drawn as closed system but rather a path giving instructions for users to build their own network. The Interface should involve the user in the community, so that they, through their individual and collective choices, define the shared environment (Crumlish & Malone, 2009).
	Networks	Should be drawn Human-Human Interactions and not Human-Computer Interactions. People live on the network and the networks are transforming our society (Adams, 2013).
	Talk like a person	The website communication for the users should be as if you were chatting informally with a person so that people feel confortable. The adoption of this type of language must cross the entire interface (Crumlish & Malone, 2009).

continued on following page

Table 3. Continued

Dimension	Principle	
Interaction dimension	Perceived affordance	Property through witch the characteristics of an object influence the perception of its function. In digital systems buttons and links should look clickable (Lidwell et al., 2003; Norman, sem data).
	Mapping	Refers to the relationship between the items of interaction (buttons, menus, links) and its movements or effects. A good relationship between these items and their behavior result in a more user-friendly system. These items should be placed so that the behavior and its position correspond to the structure of the device. Each item should be no more than one behavior (Lidwell et al., 2003).
	System consistency	One must create a language and patterns in the structure of the website to facilitate and increase their efficiency. Once the user learns how to achieve a goal or accomplish a task, they should be able to transfer this ability to other parts of the website (Lidwell et al., 2003; Usability.Gov, 2014).
	Predictability	The website should be designed in order to support the user in determining the effect of action based on previous interactions (Dix, Finlay, Abowd, & Beale, 2004).
User experience dimension	Affinity	It is a feeling that we create with the Interface when it is easy to understand, regardless the complexity of the system and the operations that occur behind the Interface. This feeling helps users to focus on their goals and tasks, becoming the Interface invisible. The Interface should be designed in order to create this feeling of affinity: as a mediator of communicating its role is to facilitate and be invisible (Gong, 2009).
	Gratification	The first requirement for an exemplary user experience is to respond to user needs, without noise or annoyance. Later comes the simplicity and elegance that produce an effect of gratification. Products and systems should be designed to go beyond compliance with the requirements, they should produce this gratification effect in its users (Nielsen & Norman, sem data).
	Invite to participation by ensuring trust	Users tend to perform more online transactions and relationships with organizations if they receive strong guarantees that are engaging in a relationship of trust. They seek for reliable reports on past performance and truthful statements about future guarantees. The branding is very important in this process. One should use logos and names of familiar brands whose integrity is respected (Shneiderman, 2000).
	Easy of use	The credibility of a website will increase if it is easy to use (Fogg, 2003a).

FUTURE RESEARCH DIRECTIONS

The proposal of a validated group of design principles for credibility and trust requires the use of more instruments to better characterize user's behaviors and perceptions and to validate a final proposal. Besides the development of deeper broader surveys, it is believed that real-time monitoring data concerning e-health users' web practices are relevant to this analysis. Under this context, and along with the survey, web browsers plugin were developed for rating e-Health websites in terms of trust and credibility TrueH [6] This plugin is different from other reputation and review plugins, like WOT,[7] as it is specially dedicated to healthcare websites. With this plugin, users can evaluate and recommend health websites from a trust and credibility perspective, during real-time use and navigation of the sites as shown in Figure 6.

The rating is based on the same concepts and dimensions presented in the analysis model (Table 2), focusing primarily on the Interface dimension. The data collected with the plugin will also perform the monitoring and management of all information collected in a Web platform. With this tool, a greater volume of data about user behavior will be collected on the use of healthcare websites and their perceptions about credibility and trust and the data collected will be triangulated with results from the survey.

Additionally, to the survey and the web plugin, two other complementary tools will be used to enrich our research: the analysis of interaction with eye tracker and also the discussion of opinions and perceptions with focus groups. These two methodologies will be used at different stages and goals: in the case

Figure 6. TrueH plugin

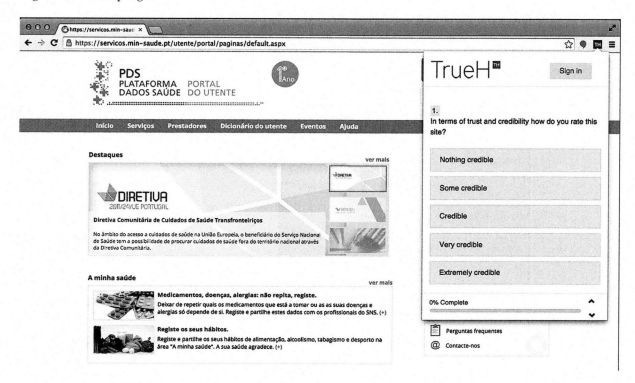

of the eye tracker, further analysis of the use and evaluation of websites with health information and, in the case of the focus group, to obtain qualitative information about the impact of the dimensions of the interface perception of credibility and trust. Based on the collected data analysis and in the group of principles collected from the literature review, a prototype will be developed and submitted to users and experts' reviews. Depending on the evaluation results, this phase will consist of several iterations between the development of the prototype and its evaluation leading us to the prototyping phase until the results are satisfactory and it will able to propose a set of design principles for the credibility and trust.

In what concerns future research related with the Interface dimensions one can explore different types of elements such as in visual dimension the element of typography to specify which is the most influent in credibility and trust perception.

CONCLUSION

Based in an extensive literature review, the work developed to systematize the problem of the influence of Interface in credibility and trust, resulted in its division into three main concepts: "Interface", "credibility and trust" and "e-Health users". This results in an analysis model presented in Table 2 and is drawn from the methodological proposal of Quivy & Campenhoudt, (2005) from which it was possible to associate a set of dimensions and indicators to the main concepts of the study and at this moment were fundamental in helping to structure the analysis instruments as the survey or the web browser plugin.

For the concept of "Interface" five dimensions were considered, believing that they constitute the main dimensions of an interface: visual, information architecture, interaction, social presence and user experience dimensions. The presented results focus in relevance on these dimensions in a health website credibility and trust perception. Previous studies have shown that the visual design has an impact in credibility and trust (Fogg et al., 2003; Karimov et al., 2011; Kelly, 2010; Robins & Holmes, 2008) and this study goes further in the specification of what influences credibility and trust perception. Information architecture and user experience dimensions are the most influent Interface dimensions obtaining 89% positive responses followed by interaction, with 84%, visual design, with 66%, and the social presence, with 58%. Based on the Interface dimensions and on the analyzed elements, a framework of design principles was made based in literature review believing that this information will allow institutions to strengthen their communication skills and users / clients to increase their autonomy in decisions regarding health.

REFERENCES

Adams, P. (2013). *A Set of Principles for Designing Social Experiences*. London: UX London.

Ambrose, G., & Harris, P. (2009). *The Fundamentals of Graphic Design*. AVA Publishing.

Burton, S. H., Tanner, K. W., & Giraud-Carrier, C. G. (2012). *Leveraging social networks for anytime-anyplace health information*. Network Modeling Analysis in Health Informatics and Bioinformatics. doi:10.1007/s13721-012-0016-4

Centers for Disease Control and Prevention. (2011, July). The Health Communicator's Social Media Toolkit. *Electronic Media*.

Chow, W., & Angie, N. (2006). A study of trust in e-shopping before and after first-hand experience is gained. *Journal of Computer Information Systems*.

Crumlish, C., & Malone, E. (2009). *Designing Social Interfaces* (M. Treseler, Ed.). Sebastopol, CA: O'Reilly Media, Inc.

Cullen, K. (2007). *Layout Workbook: A Real-World Guide to Building Pages in Graphic Design (Google eBook)*. Rockport Publishers.

DeLone, W. H., & McLean, E. R. (1992). *Information Systems Success: The Quest for the Dependent Variable*. Academic Press.

Dix, A., Finlay, J., Abowd, G. D., & Beale, R. (2004). Human–Computer Interaction (3rd ed.). Pearson.

Du, Y., & Zhao, J. (2009). An empirical study of end-user trust in a web information system. *2009 International Conference on Information Managment, Innovation Management and Industrial Engineering*, (pp. 561–564). doi:10.1109/ICIII.2009.293

Eysenbach, G. (2007). From Intermediation to Desintermediation and Apomediation: New Models for Consumers to Acess and Assess the Credibility of Health Information in the Age of Web 2.0. *Medinfo*, *2007*, 162–166.

Eysenbach, G. (2008). Credibility of health information and digital media: new perspectives and implications for youth. In M. Metzger & A. Flanagin (Eds.), Digital media, youth, and credibility (pp. 123–154). MIT Press. doi:10.1162/dmal.9780262562324.123

Fogg, B. (2003a). *Persuasive Technology - Using Computers to Change What We Think and Do* (A. Druin & J. Hendler, Eds.). San Francisco: Morgan Kaufman.

Fogg, B. (2003b). Prominence-interpretation theory: explaining how people assess credibility online. *CHI'03 extended abstracts on human factors in ...*, (pp. 722–723). ACM.

Fogg, B., Soohoo, C., Hall, C., Danielson, D. R., Tauber, E. R., Stanford, J., ... Marable, L. (2003). How Do Users Evaluate the Credibility of Web Sites? A Study with Over. *ACM International Conference Proceeding Series*, (pp. 1–15). ACM.

Fortney, J., Burgess, J., Bosworth, H., Booth, B., & Kaboli, P. (2011). A re-conceptualization of access for 21st century healthcare. *Journal of General Internal Medicine*, *26*(S2), 639–647. doi:10.1007/s11606-011-1806-6 PMID:21989616

Furman, S. (2009, Junho 13). Building Trust. *Usability.Gov*. Department of Health and Human Services. Retrieved from http://www.usability.gov/get-involved/blog/2009/09/building-trust.html

Gefen, D., & Karahanna, E. (2003). Trust and TAM in Online Shopping: An Integarted Model. *Management Information Systems Quarterly*, *27*(1), 51–90.

Gong, C. (2009). Human-Machine Interface: Design Principles of Visual Information in Human-Machine Interface Design. *2009 International Conference on Intelligent Human-Machine Systems and Cybernetics*, (pp. 262–265). doi:10.1109/IHMSC.2009.189

Griffiths, F., Cave, J., Boardman, F., Ren, J., Pawlikowska, T., Ball, R., & Cohen, A. et al. (1982). Social networks - The future for health care delivery. *Social Science & Medicine*, *75*(12), 2233–2241. doi:10.1016/j.socscimed.2012.08.023 PMID:22985490

Karimov, F. P., Brussel, V. U., Brengman, M., & Van Hove, L. (2011). The Effect of Website Design Dimensions on Initial Trust: A Synthesis of the empirical Literature. *Journal of Electronic Commerce Research*, *12*(2), 272–301.

Kelly, K. (2010). Consumer Health Information Websites with High Visual Design Ratings Likely to Be also Highly Rated for Perceived Credibility. *Evidence Based Library and Information Practice*, 42–45.

Lidwell, W., Holden, K., & Butle, J. (2003). Universal Principles of Design. Rockport Publishers, Inc.

Nielsen, J., & Norman, D. (n.d.). The Definition of User Experience (UX). *Nielsen Norman Group*. Retrieved from http://www.nngroup.com/articles/definition-user-experience/

Norman, D. (n.d.). Affordances and Design - jnd.org. *jnd.org*. Retrieved from http://www.jnd.org/dn.mss/affordances_and.html

Quivy, R., & van Campenhoudt, L. V. L. (2005). *Manual de investigação em Ciências Sociais (4ᵗʰ ed.)*. Lisboa: Gradiva - Publicações, Lda.

Raskin, J. (2000). *The Humane Interface: New Directions for Designing Interactive Systems*. Addison-Wesley Professional.

Riemenschneider, C., Jones, K., & Leonard, L. N. K. (2009). Web trust—A moderator of the web's perceived individual impact. *Journal of Computer Information Systems*.

Robins, D., & Holmes, J. (2008). Aesthetics and credibility in web site design. *Information Processing & Management, 44*(1), 386–399. doi:10.1016/j.ipm.2007.02.003

Robins, D., Holmes, J., & Stansbury, M. (2009). Consumer health information on the Web: The relationship of visual design and perceptions of credibility. *Conference on Designing for User Experiences, 61*(1), 13–29. doi:10.1002/asi

Rosenfeld, L., & Morville, P. (2007). *Information Architecture for the World Wide Web*. Sebastopol, CA: O'Reilly Media, Inc.

Sá, C. F. A. (2010). *O que é um Interface? Da Entificação à Identificação do Interface equanto complexo Mediador*. Universidade Nova de Lisboa.

Shneiderman, B. (2000). Designing Trust into Online experiences. *Communications of the ACM, 43*(12), 57–59. doi:10.1145/355112.355124

Shneiderman, B. (2003). *Leonardo's Laptop: Human Needs and the New Computing Technologies*. Cambridge, MA: MIT Press.

Thielsch, M. T., Blotenberg, I., & Jaron, R. (2013). User Evaluation of Websites: From First Impression to Recommendation. *Interacting with Computers*. doi:10.1093/iwc/iwt033

Usability.Gov. (2014). User Interface Design Basics. *Usability.Gov*. Department of Health and Human Services. Retrieved from http://www.usability.gov/what-and-why/user-interface-design.html

Wang, Y. D., & Emurian, H. H. (2005). An overview of online trust: Concepts, elements, and implications. *Computers in Human Behavior, 21*(1), 105–125. doi:10.1016/j.chb.2003.11.008

White, A. (2011). *The Elements of Graphic Design (2ⁿᵈ ed.)*. New York: Allworth Press.

Wodtke, C., & Govella, A. (2009). *Information architecture: Blueprints for the Web (2ⁿᵈ ed.)*. New Riders.

ADDITIONAL READING

Csikszentmihalyi, M. (1990). Flow: the psychology of optimal experience. (Harper & Row, Ed.) (First.). New York, NY: HarperCollins.

Dix, A., Finlay, J., Abowd, G. D., & Beale, R. (2004). Human–Computer Interaction (Third Edit.). Pearson.

Jones, P. H. (2013). *Design for Care: Innovating Healthcare Experience* (L. Rosenfeld Media, Ed.). United States of America: Rosenfeld, Louis.

Norman, D. (2005). *Emotional Design: Why We Love (or Hate) Everyday Things*. New York: Basic Books New York.

Röcker, C. (2010). *Human-Centered Design of E-Health Technologies: Concepts, Methods and Applications* (p. 550). IGI Global.

KEY TERMS AND DEFINITIONS

Information Interface Architecture Dimension: Concerns the organization, structuring and names of the contents with the goal of helping users find and understand the content.

Interaction Interface Dimension: Responsible for creating functionality or behavior to provide essentially interactions between people through computers or machines.

Social Presence Interface Dimension: Allows the representation of presence, the connection and communication between individuals and organizations.

User Experience Interface Dimension: Is related to the perception of use of the use or expectation of use of a product or service. Encompasses aspects such as warmth, feeling and significance of this interaction in everyday user.

Visual Interface Dimension: Ensures visual communication between the parties involved in the process communication. It is responsible for the visual materialization of all sizes that make up the interface.

ENDNOTES

[1]   Portal do Utente - https://servicos.min-saude.pt/utente/portal/paginas/default.aspx

[2]   Medicina NET - http://www.medicinanet.com.br

[3]   Biblioteca Virtual em Saúde - http://www.bireme.br/php/index.php

[4]   Manual Merk - http://www.manualmerck.net

[5]   Diagram or Gutenberg rule: This is a diagram with the shape of the letter Z that has a page split into quadrants that define the strongest and weakest in terms of visual attention in reading elements on the page areas. Should consider this diagram in defining the elements to put on the page (Lidwell et al., 2003).

[6]   TrueH - http://trueh.web.ua.pt/

[7]   WOT - www.mywot.com

Verification and Validation of Medical Cyber–Physical Systems

Lenardo Chaves e Silva
UFCG, Brazil

Hyggo Oliveira de Almeida
UFCG, Brazil

Angelo Perkusich
UFCG, Brazil

INTRODUCTION

In recent years, the health care services have followed the evolution of Information and Communication Technologies (ICTs). Telemedicine has been using ICTs, such as computers, internet and smart phones, to overcome geographical barriers and expand access of these services to remote areas and areas that need to improve the quality of care to the population. The idea of Telemedicine is to provide Electronic Health Records (EHR) on an individual and to allow the exchange of such information between health-care professionals for distance clinical support (WHO, 2010).

To make these applications possible it is necessary to integrate computation with physical processes, yielding a class of systems called *Cyber-Physical Systems* (CPS). Helen Gill, from the *National Science Foundation* (NSF) - U.S., was the researcher responsible for coining the term CPS in 2006, claiming the need for understanding the joint dynamics of the components of these systems, such as computers, software, networks, and physical processes. In CPS, feedback loops between physical processes and computing occur. Likewise, computing interferes in physical processes (LEE and SESHIA, 2011).

In this context, some trends and challenges are related to modeling and control of hybrid systems, networks of sensors and actuators, computational abstraction and architectures of these systems (PARK, ZHENG and LIU, 2012). All these factors relate to the mode of dealing with intrinsic aspects of systems focused on physical processes, such as the diversity and amount of information to be captured and processed, the heterogeneity of the elements interacting and the simultaneity of events occurring.

With the increasing elderly population and the high costs associated with quality of life, health has become one of the main application domains of a CPS, these applications are named *Medical Cyber-Physical Systems - MCPS* (LEE et al., 2012). As a distinct class of CPS, MCPS introduces additional computational entities to help the caregivers in the decision support regarding the control of the health of patients. In these systems, the data acquired by monitoring devices are analyzed to determine the condition of the patient and to provide information about the current situation to the experts. Moreover, the most appropriate treatment can be automated by means of actuator devices connected directly to the subject.

The main concern of an MCPS is to ensure patient safety, and therefore its development is considered complex because of insufficient understanding of the dynamics of the human body in response to any treatment. Thus, it is essential to verify if the developed system maintains compliance with its specification as well as to validate that its features meet the needs of professionals who will make use of MCPS.

DOI: 10.4018/978-1-4666-9978-6.ch087

The aim of this chapter is to provide the tools and approaches currently adopted in the MCPS Verification and Validation (V&V), in order to discuss the state-of-the-art related to this research challenge. In this way, we will provide a survey that will identify and compare proposed solutions regarding different aspects such as contribution, formalisms, tool support and testing procedures for these systems. In addition, we will present the systematic review process used in this research.

BACKGROUND

In this section, we introduce the fundamental concepts and main approaches applied to MCPS testing, such as V&V activities and Model-Based Testing (MBT). In addition, we will present some related works.

Verification and Validation Activities

Software verification and validation is an important stage of the system development life cycle. It is intended to show that a system both conforms to its specification and that it meets the expectation of the system customer (SOMMERVILLE, 2011).

Verification and validation are activities that complement each other to achieve a common purpose, which is to ensure that the system must be good enough for its intended use. Verification is concerned to checking if the developer is building the product right. Validation, however, aims to evaluate if the developer is building the right product.

The main activity of V&V process is system testing. In accordance with Utting and Legeard (2007) "Testing is an activity performed for evaluating product quality and for improving it, by identifying defects and problems". Summarizing, *Testing* means to execute a system in order to detect *undesirable behaviors* (failures).

With the advent of model-based development approaches, artifacts and the models themselves, the properties formalized and results of verification and tests may be used as evidence of the MCPS quality (LEE et al., 2012). In MCPS, the patient safety is the main concern. Hence, these systems must be completely tested.

Model-Based Testing

The *Model-Based Testing (MBT)* term have been constantly adopted to describe a variety of techniques used to generate tests (UTTING and LEGEARD, 2007). The four main approaches known in this group are: *1)* generation of test input data from a domain model; *2)* generation of test cases from an environment model; *3)* generation of test cases with information about their outputs (oracles) from a behavior model; and, *4)* generation of test scripts from abstract tests.

Since each clinical scenario of an MCPS encompasses a heterogeneity of medical devices, all controlled by computer systems to support decision making, often with automated interventions, the safety patient must be assured by the system. Thus, it becomes essential that MCPS developers make use of the approaches and tools more adequate to verify and validate such systems. Hence, this is the motivation to perform this research.

MATERIALS AND METHODS

In this section will be described the steps carried out to identify the main approaches and tools, which represent the state of art in testing of MCPS design.

The Systematic Literature Review (SLR) method used in this research is based on five steps described by Khan et al. (2011):

1. Defining the research questions for a review;
2. Identifying relevant work;
3. Assessing the quality of studies;
4. Summarizing the evidence by means of tabulation of study characteristics, quality and effects;
5. Interpreting the findings.

The support tool to conduct the SLR process was the StArt $_{v2.0}$ - *State of the Art through Systematic Review* (Zamboni et al., 2010). Its goal is to help the researcher to apply the SLR method by means of the information management related to research, as well as to evaluate the studies. In addition to make the qualitative analysis easier, the *StArt* tool also provide some features that summary the research data in a quantitative way. This minimizes the researcher's effort in the stage of summarizing of study evidences.

Systematic Literature Review

In order to meet of this research, a systematic review protocol was defined (see supplementary material available at web page containing the supplementary material for this chapter (https://sites.google.com/site/vvmcps/). Its elements are described in this section and grouped in according to each step of the SLR method suggested by Khan et al. (2011). In addition, it was taken into account the information organization in the *StArt* tool, in other words, following the stages of *planning*, *execution* and *summarization* (Hernandes, 2012).

Planning

This stage is characterized by the definition of the research protocol that will support the next steps in the review process. The protocol must contain all information and procedures necessary to conduct the research. Silva, Almeida and Perkusich (2014) detailed the protocol defined for this research. At this moment will be presented only the goal, the research questions by means of the free description method, in addition to the search terms that were grouped according to discipline related to research:

1. Defining the research questions:
    a. **Research Goal:** Identifying the approaches found in the literature to define and generate test cases for MCPS validation. Specifically, we aim at evaluating the approaches and tools to improve the testing practices for these systems, while reducing costs (e.g., effort, financer and time-to-market) associated with the testing process.
    b. Research Questions (RQ):
        i. RQ1: What are the main techniques for testing MCPS design?
        ii. RQ2: What are the main tools used to provide support to the software testing in MCPS?

2. Search Terms:
   a. Medical Systems Terms: "medical cyber-physical systems";
   b. Software Testing Terms: "testing" or "test";
   c. General Terms: "technique" or "approach" or "methodology" or "method".

Execution

Given that the SLR protocol was structured and the research questions were defined in *Step 1* of the review process, the researcher is able to perform the execution stage. This consists of:

1. Identifying the studies related to research questions using Web search engines with search sources list in which the systematic review will be run, and their respective refinements.
2. Selecting or rejecting the studies in according to respective inclusion and exclusion criteria specified in research protocol, and presented here:
   a. Inclusion Criteria (I):
      i. Studies published in Conferences, Journals and/or Magazines;
      ii. Publication year between 2006 and 21 Jan. 2014;
      iii. The full-text of the study must to be accessible;
      iv. Studies with overview of (Medical) Cyber-Physical Systems, discussing its challenges and trends;
      v. Studies that presents formalisms and/or testing strategies for Hybrid Systems.
   b. Exclusion Criteria (E):
      i. Results in that the search terms found are present at: *Demo-abstract, Author index, Table of contents, Technical program, Index Proceedings,* and *References.*
      ii. The study is present in more than one search source (duplicate).
      iii. The study was reorganized and republished.
      iv. The study is not in accordance with the research questions.
      v. The study is not related to the medical domain.
3. Extracting information about the studies selected after full reading of the whole text, and following the form fields into the review protocol.

Summarization

Given the information diversity of the results obtained in the execution stage, the data synthesis carried out in this research aims to not only classify the studies according to approaches of software testing and support tools to the V&V process of an MCPS, but also confront them.

Complementing the summarization stage, these studies were analyzed quantitatively and qualitatively. Lastly, the evidences found in the studies are characterized and tabulated, ending the process with the interpretation of results.

RESULTS AND DISCUSSIONS

The results of the execution of the aforementioned method are presented and discussed in this section.

Identification Results

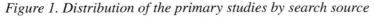

At the preliminary stage of reviewing, we identify 43 studies. This means that these studies met the initial criteria of our SLR protocol. Five search sources of scientific papers were used: *IEEE Xplore DL, ACM DL, Science Direct, Portal de Periódicos CAPES (Scopus, Web of Science, and SpringerLink),* and *Manuallly* (*please*, see the Supplementary Material to know the refinements applied for each search source). Some studies were manually incorporated to the review process. Therefore, this source does not have an explicit search refinement, but its studies meet the SLR protocol adopted in this research. These studies are related work to the research area of MCPS, which were not returned in searches performed by Web search engines listed in the review protocol.

Figure 1 shows the total number of studies found after this step. Most of these studies were indexed by IEEE (63%) and ACM (21%). The remaining search engines together account for only 16% of the total studies identified.

Throughout the various steps of the systematic review process, the studies identified in this research are analyzed and labeled according to their status at each stage of this process. A label may assume the following values: "Accepted"; "Rejected"; "Duplicated"; or, "Unclassified". In the case of duplicated studies, the *Start tool* allows to identify them automatically through a comparative analysis of the references of respective studies.

Selection Results

Taking into account the inclusion and exclusion criteria presented in the SLR protocol, this stage resulted in 25 studies accepted for the *extraction* stage. For the remaining studies, 10 were rejected and 8 considered duplicates. The criteria used to assign the status for each study can be seen on the supplementary material.

Figure 1. Distribution of the primary studies by search source

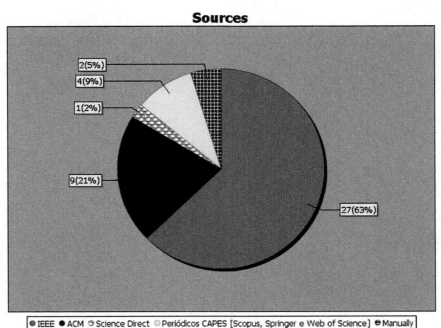

At this stage, it was also possible to determine the priority order of reading the studies based on the evaluation of the metadata: *title, abstract* and *keywords*. The data from this quantitative analysis can be visualized by means of charts related to the *Status* and *Reading Priority*, as shown in the Figure 2.

The priority order of reading can be classified as "Very High", "High", "Low" and "Very Low". It is noteworthy that these data are derived from the execution of *Step 2* of the SLR process, whose goal is to identify and select relevant papers for research.

As can be seen in Figure 2, only 58% of the studies identified in initial search were selected for the next stage of analysis. At the information extraction stage, a full reading of the text is performed to obtain relevant data about each study.

Extraction Results

After the full reading of the 25 studies selected in the previous stage, and extraction of the main information of each study, only 16 studies were considered for qualitative analysis that was performed in the *Step 3* of the SLR process. Others seven studies were rejected and two considered duplicates, as depicted in Figure 3.

The identification of the studies considered duplicates has only been possible after the full reading of the same, which justifies the non-exclusion of such studies in the previous stage. Again, the criteria used to select the studies that will be analyzed in this step can be seen on the supplementary material.

Figure 2. Quantitative analysis in the selecting stage

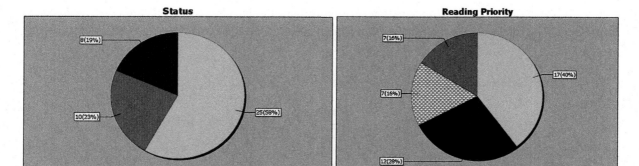

Figure 3. Quantitative analysis in the extraction stage

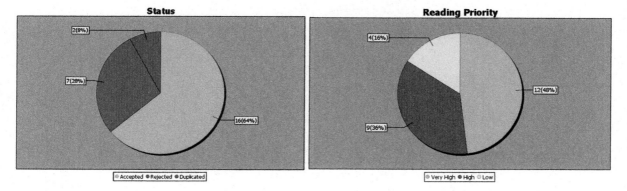

Four categories of information to be extracted from the full reading of the 25 selected studies were created: 1 - *Main Contribution*; 2 - *Formalism*; 3 - *Support Tools*; 4 - *Test Strategies*. This taxonomy was developed to facilitate the distinction among the testing approaches and tools identified in this survey. It is worth remembering that the same study can be contained in more than one subcategory. As for the contributions of the studies, it was decided to choose just the main contribution. The results of quantitative analysis of the information extraction stage also can be seen on the supplementary material.

The *Step 3* of the SLR process aims to evaluate the quality of the 16 accepted in the *extraction* stage. The purpose was to explore the heterogeneity and other details that would allow to analyze the adequacy of the research studies and to verify the evidence of their effectiveness. Table 1 shows the results of the evaluation of these studies. The *Ranking* column is derived information from satisfaction of the quality criteria of the SLR protocol, whose function is to measure the suitability of each study to the research goal (*for more details, see the supplementary material*).

With the ranking of the 16 studies, it becomes possible to identify those that respond better the research questions, as well as performing the *Step 4* of the SLR process (i.e., *Summarizing* stage). At this stage the evidence of the studies are summarized by means of their particularities and their effectiveness.

Summarization Results

Table 2 summarizes the data obtained through the execution of *Step 3* of the SLR process. Furthermore, this stage consists in classifying the studies with regard to testing approaches and support tools for the V&V process of an MCPS. Complementing the summarization stage, studies were analyzed both quantitatively and qualitatively.

Table 1. Ranking of the selected studies in the extraction stage

Study ID	Reference	Ranking
8	Jiang et al. (2011)	1
18	Li et al. (2013)	2
26	Kang et al. (2013)	3
6	Pajic et al. (2014)	4
51	Murugesan et al. (2013)	5
79	Khan et al. (2013)	6
14	Li, Raghunathan and Jha (2013)	7
31	King et al. (2013)	8
27	Simalatsar and De Micheli (2012)	9
9	Miller et al. (2012)	10
13	Lee et al. (2012)	11
19	Sokolsky et al. (2011)	12
16	Alur (2011)	13
12	Canedo et al. (2013)	14
20	Kim et al. (2013)	15
11	Don et al. (2012)	16

Table 2. Synthesis of data from studies at the end of Step 3 of the RSL process

Study ID	Study Characteristics			
	Main Contribution	Formalisms	Support Tools	Testing Techniques
6	Approach	Model-Based; Automata.	UPPAAL; Simulink.	Simulation; Model Checking.
8	System	Model-Based; Automata.	Simulink.	Monitors.
9	Approach	Mockup.	Others.	Others (ad-hoc).
11	Framework	Event-Driven.	None.	Others (ad-hoc).
12	Approach	Model-Based; Others.	Modelica.	Simulation.
13	Literature Review	Model-Based; Automata.	UPPAAL; Simulink; Others.	Simulation; Model Checking.
14	Approach	Others (ad-hoc).	Others.	Model Checking.
16	Literature Review	Model-Based; Automata; Others.	Simulink; Modelica; Others.	Simulation; Model Checking; Others.
18	Approach	Automata; ODE.	PHAVer.	Model Checking.
19	Literature Review	Model-Based; Automata; Others.	UPPAAL; Simulink; Others.	Simulation; Model Checking.
20	Framework	Others.	Others.	Simulation.
26	Approach	Model-Based; Others.	Simulink; Others.	Simulation; Model Checking.
27	Approach	Automata.	Others.	Model Checking; Others.
31	Approach	Model-Based; Others.	Others.	Others.
51	Approach	Model-Based.	Simulink; Others.	Model Checking; Others.
79	System	Model-Based; Automata; ODE.	UPPAAL; Simulink.	Simulation; Model Checking.

According to Table 2, 62.5% of the studies using the model-based approach as main formal method to represent the behavior of MCPS. In general, these models are supported and/or are integrated with other formalisms such as Automata and its variants (e.g., *timed, hybrid* and *task*) that occur in 60% of the studies.

In relation to tool support for V&V of MCPS, the *Simulink[1]* of Mathworks® is a favorite among designers and researchers. It was used by 50% of the analyzed studies. Half of the studies that made use of the *Simulink* also used the *UPPAAL[2]* tool for verification of the proposed models. Another interesting aspects were perceived as, for example, the use of *Stateflow[3]* tool, also from Mathworks®, to represent how these systems react to events, to time-based conditions and to external input signals. In addition, the *TIMES[4]* tool is one of the main tools for code generation from models.

About strategies for testing of MCPS, *model checking* and simulation represent, respectively, the verification and validation process in 62.5% and 50% of the studies. Both techniques were used together in 37.5% of the analyzed studies. Lastly, 56.25% of the studies whose contribution is an approach claim the need to ensure the patient safety in an MCPS.

The classification of the approaches took into account the goals for which they have been proposed within the context of MCPS designs, as also in relation to the use case to demonstrate their application. Table 3 summarizes this classification, identifying such approaches by their respective studies in which they were published.

In the classification process of the tools noted the presence of two major groups: (1) that operate on the level of simulation of the behavior system model; and, (2) those with the capacity to provide mechanism for the verification of such models. The remaining tools identified play other roles in the MCPS design, such as code generation or analysis of requirements and certain properties of the system. These tools were categorized in a third group called "*Support*" tools. We show the classification result in Table 4.

Finally, in *Step 5* of the SLR process, whose aim is to interpret the results obtained from the review, we conclude that the main focus of the studies is to check security properties of the proposed medical device or system. In this sense, the authors present specific usage scenarios to demonstrate proof of concept for each project.

The heterogeneity and low quality of some analyzed studies made it difficult to interpret the results presented in this survey. This is because these approaches were not designed specifically to test for MCPS, but to support the design as a whole.

Table 3. Classification of the design approaches of a Medical CPS

Study ID	Goal in the CPS Design			Use Case
	System	**Devices**	**Others**	
6	Checking the security properties	-	-	PCA (*Patient-Controlled Analgesia*) Infusion Pump Systems integrated to the patient model
9	-	Automating software testing	-	Mechanical ventilation system integrated to the lung model
12[1]	Generating executable functional models for simulation	-	-	Electromechanical popcorn machine
14	-	Checking the security properties	-	Software for cardiac pacemaker
18	Checking the security properties (*online*)	-	-	Laser surgical procedure of the airway with mechanical ventilation system
26	Checking the security properties	-	-	Laser surgical procedure of the airway with mechanical ventilation system
27	-	-	Validating the structural properties of medical protocols formally represented; Checking the properties of their life cycles and real time	Protocol for administration of medications in the treatment of certain kinds of cancers
31	Checking the security properties at the level of requirements	Checking the security properties at the level of requirements	-	PCA Infusion Pump Systems, providing an interface for interaction with the patient
51	Checking the security properties at the level of requirements	-	-	Generic PCA Infusion Pump Systems

[1] Study is related to the industrial systems domain, but its approach may be used in the medical systems domain.

Table 4. Classification of the main tools used in the V&V process of a Medical CPS

Tools	Groups		
	Simulation	Verification	Support
AGREE Framework			●
CBMC			●
MAP			●
Modelica	●		
PHAVer		●	
Simulink	●		
Simulink's Design Verifier		●	
Stateflow	●		
TIMES			●
UPPAAL		●	

Similarly, specific contributions to MCPS design are proposed in these studies, making it difficult to compare these approaches with respect to matters that are inherently related to the testing of this class of systems, such as testing types, testing process and coverage level. Also because of the diversity of approaches identified themselves, and they are not alternative solution for a single problem, it becomes impossible to perform meta-analysis of studies. However, some high-quality studies among the 16 studies in our analysis help to overcome these problems.

FUTURE RESEARCH DIRECTIONS

The results presented in this systematic literature review do not guarantee the presence of all relevant studies to answer the research questions of this survey. However, it is ensured that most of the available studies has been obtained and examined, given the research effort expended and research sources included in this review.

Therefore, although a careful search has been made following the defined review protocol for this research, it is suggested to extend the search terms related to medical systems (e.g., "medical applications" and "e-health systems"), as well as to the technical aspects inherent in testing systems (e.g., "test case", "systems verification" and "systems validation"). Other restrictions that may be removed in future research are the search for terms only in the English language and Web search engines, also including printed materials such as books and reports.

CONCLUSION

This chapter presented a survey of the recent works related to verification and validation of *Medical Cyber Physical Systems* (MCPS). The survey aimed to identify and evaluate the main approaches and support tools used for testing MCPS. To achieve this goal, we define a Systematic Literature Review Protocol.

We initially identified 43 studies, but only 16 were selected for the qualitative analysis of the review process. After the full reading and final analysis of the 16 studies identified in this survey, we highlight the works *6, 8, 18, 31,* and *51,* because they describe in detail the issues related to testing in MCPS.

The results presented here demonstrate the research efforts in the context of MCPS, which in the last three years (2010-2013) has become an important research area. Especially in search of how to provide mechanisms to ensure the patient safety and help caregivers in making correct decision of patient monitoring during treatment, according to each clinical scenario in question. Based on the results it can be state that the goals this research was achieved, since the main approaches and support tools were successfully identified.

REFERENCES

Alur, R. (2011). Formal Verification of Hybrid Systems. In *Proceedings of the Ninth ACM International Conference on Embedded Software* (pp. 273-278). New York, NY: ACM. doi:10.1145/2038642.2038685

Canedo, A., Schwarzenbach, E., & Al Faruque, M. A. (2013). Context-sensitive synthesis of executable functional models of cyber-physical systems. In *Proceedings of the ACM/IEEE International Conference on Cyber-Physical Systems* (pp. 99-108). New York, NY: ACM. doi:10.1145/2502524.2502539

Don, S., Choi, E., & Min, D. (2012). Event driven adaptive awareness system for Medical Cyber Physical Systems. In *Proceedings of the 4th International Conference on Awareness Science and Technology* (pp. 238-242). Seoul, Korea: IEEE. doi:10.1109/iCAwST.2012.6469620

Hernandes, E. M., Zamboni, A., Fabbri, S. and Thommazo, A. D. (2012). Using GQM and TAM to evaluate StArt - a tool that supports Systematic Review. *CLEI Electronic Journal, 15*(1).

Jiang, Z., Pajic, M., & Mangharam, R. (2011). Model-Based Closed-Loop Testing of Implantable Pacemakers. In *Proceedings of the IEEE/ACM International Conference on Cyber-Physical Systems* (pp. 131-140). Chicago, IL: IEEE.

Kang, W., Wu, P., Rahmaniheris, M., Sha, L., Berlin, R. B., & Goldman, J. M. (2013). Towards organ-centric compositional development of safe networked supervisory medical systems. In *Proceedings of the 26th IEEE International Symposium on Computer-Based Medical Systems* (pp. 143-148). Porto: IEEE. doi:10.1109/CBMS.2013.6627779

Khan, K., Kunz, R., Kleijnen, J., & Antes, G. (2011). *Systematic Reviews to Support Evidence-Based Medicine: How to Review and Apply findings of Health Care Research*. London: Hodder Arnold.

Khan, S. H., Khan, A. H., & Khan, Z. H. (2013). Artificial Pancreas Coupled Vital Signs Monitoring for Improved Patient Safety. *Arabian Journal for Science and Engineering, 38(11), 3093-3102*. doi:10.1007/s13369-012-0456-2

Kim, M.-J., Kang, S., Kim, W.-T., & Chun, I.-G. (2013). Human-interactive hardware-in-the-loop simulation framework for cyber-physical systems. In *Proceedings of the Second International Conference on Informatics and Applications* (pp. 198-202). Lodz: IEEE. doi:10.1109/ICoIA.2013.6650255

King, A. L., Feng, L., & Sokolsky, O. and Insup Lee. (2013). Assuring the safety of on-demand medical cyber-physical systems. In *Proceedings of the IEEE 1st International Conference on Cyber-Physical Systems, Networks, and Applications* (pp. 1-6). Taipei, Taiwan: IEEE. doi:10.1109/CPSNA.2013.6614238

Lee, E. A., & Seshia, S. A. (2011). *Introduction to Embedded Systems – A Cyber-Physical Systems Approach*. Retrieved July 06, 2012 from http://LeeSeshia.org

Lee, I., Sokolsky, O., Chen, S., Hatcliff, J., Jee, E., Kim, B., & Venkatasubramanian, K. K. et al. (2012). Challenges and Research Directions in Medical Cyber–Physical Systems. *Proceedings of the IEEE, 100*(1), 75–90. doi:10.1109/JPROC.2011.2165270

Li, C., Raghunathan, A., & Jha, N. K. (2013). Improving the Trustworthiness of Medical Device Software with Formal Verification Methods. IEEE Embedded Systems Letters, 5(3), 50-53. doi:10.1109/LES.2013.2276434

Li, T., Tan, F., Wang, Q., Bu, L., Cao, J., & Liu, X. (2013). From Offline Toward Real-Time: A Hybrid Systems Model Checking and CPS Co-Design Approach for Medical Device Plug-and-Play Collaborations. IEEE Transactions on Parallel and Distributed Systems, (99), 1-1.

Miller, B., Vahid, F., & Givargis, T. (2012). MEDS: Mockup Electronic Data Sheets for Automated Testing of Cyber-physical Systems Using Digital Mockups. In *Proceedings of the Conference on Design, Automation and Test in Europe (DATE '12)*. San Jose, CA: EDA Consortium. doi:10.1109/DATE.2012.6176585

Murugesan, A., Whalen, M. W., Rayadurgam, S., & Heimdahl, M. P. E. (2013). Compositional Verification of a Medical Device System. In *Proceedings of the 2013 ACM SIGAda Annual Conference on High Integrity Language Technology* (pp. 51-64). New York, NY: ACM. doi:10.1145/2527269.2527272

Pajic, M., Mangharam, R., Sokolsky, O., Arney, D., Goldman, J., & Lee, I. (2014). Model-Driven Safety Analysis of Closed-Loop Medical Systems. *IEEE Transactions on Industrial Informatics, 10*(1), 3–16. doi:10.1109/TII.2012.2226594 PMID:24177176

Park, K.-J., Zheng, R., & Liu, X. (2012). Cyber-physical systems: Milestones and research challenges. *Computer Communications, 36*(1), 1–7. doi:10.1016/j.comcom.2012.09.006

Silva, L. C., Almeida, H. O., & Perkusich, A. (2014). *Relatório de Projeto de Tese de Doutorado.* Campina Grande, PB: UFCG. Retrieved Aug. 12, 2014, from http://1drv.ms/1qvnAxX

Simalatsar, A., & De Micheli, G. (2012). Medical guidelines reconciling medical software and electronic devices: Imatinib case-study. In *Proceedings of the IEEE 12th International Conference on Bioinformatics Bioengineering* (pp. 19-24). Larnaca: IEEE. doi:10.1109/BIBE.2012.6399700

Sokolsky, O., Lee, I., & Heimdahl, M. (2011). Challenges in the regulatory approval of medical cyber-physical systems. In *Proceedings of the 2011 International Conference on Embedded Software* (pp. 227-232). Taipei, Taiwan: IEEE. doi:10.1145/2038642.2038677

Sommerville, I. (2011). *Software Engineering* (9th ed.). Boston, MA: Pearson Education, Inc.

Utting, M., & Legeard, B. (2007). *Practical model-based testing: a tools approach.* San Francisco, CA: Morgan Kaufmann Publishers Inc.

WHO. (2010). Telemedicine – Opportunities and developments in Member States: report on the second global survey on eHealth. *Global Observatory for eHealth Series.* Retrieved May 16, 2014, from http://www.who.int/goe/publications/ehealth_series_vol2/en/

Zamboni, A. B., Thommazo, A. D., Hernandes, E. C. M., & Fabbri, S. C. P. F. (2010). StArt - Uma Ferramenta Computacional de Apoio à Revisão Sistemática. In *Congresso Brasileiro de Software: Teoria e Prática - Tools Session,* (pp. 91-96). Salvador, BA: Academic Press.

KEY TERMS AND DEFINITIONS

Medical Cyber-Physical Systems: Safety critical systems that consist of introducing additional computational entities in the traditional clinical scenarios to help the caregivers in the decision support regarding the control of the health of patients.

Metadata: Term used to provide data about others data, whose purpose is to facilitate the understanding of the data themselves.

Model-Based Testing: Set of techniques used to generate test cases from models of the system under test.

Software Testing: Any activity that consists at evaluating the system's behavior in order to detect failures.

Systematic Review: It is a research that identifies relevant studies, evaluates the quality the studies and summarizes their results using a scientific methodology.

Validation: Stage of the software design process that aim to evaluate if the developer is building the right product.

Verification: Stage of the software design process that aim to checking if the developer is building the product right.

ENDNOTES

[1]   http://www.mathworks.com/products/simulink/
[2]   http://www.uppaal.org/
[3]   http://www.mathworks.com/products/stateflow/
[4]   http://www.timestool.com/

The Worker Perspective in Telehealth

Yvette Blount
Macquarie University, Australia

Marianne Gloet
University of Melbourne, Australia

INTRODUCTION

Globally, the adoption of telehealth service delivery has been slow and disappointing. The potential of telehealth, for example to reduce health care costs, increase efficiency and effectiveness, provide better quality and more equitable access to health services, has not yet been realized (Jang-Jaccard, Nepal, Alem, & Li, 2014; van Dyke, 2014). The stated benefits of telehealth adoption include patients not having to travel long distances to access health services, reduced costs for both the patients and the public health system, access to expertise and training by remote health care workers and better connection of services (Beatriz Alkmim et al., 2012; Jang-Jaccard et al., 2014).

There are many stakeholders involved in the successful adoption of telehealth. Jang-Jaccard et al. (2014, p. 496) identified four main stakeholders: 1) governments; 2) telehealth application developers and service providers; 3) health professionals; and 4) patients (including family and community support). There are numerous research studies that attempt to identify both the barriers and facilitators of telehealth adoption. The overarching theme is that adoption of telehealth is more complex and time-consuming than had previously been anticipated (S Mair et al., 2012). Indeed, the adoption, use and diffusion of information and communications technology (ICT) in health care is generally much lower than in other areas of our lives such as work and leisure (Christensen and Remler, 2009; Cho et al., 2007).

There is limited research on the implications of telehealth delivery from the perspective of the health care professionals (workers). Telehealth health care providers work from a variety of locations such as their homes, from call centres, family doctor surgeries and health clinics. Roberts, Mort, and Milligan (2012) note that workers that interact with clients (patients) to provide ICT enabled health care services have specific skills and capabilities to be able to provide the required level of care effectively and efficiently.

This chapter examines the perspectives of telehealth delivery from the perspectives of the health care professionals in this field.

BACKGROUND

Definitions

There are a number of terms in the literature, for example ehealth, mhealth, telehealth, telemedicine and telecare that refer to the flexible delivery of healthcare using various forms of ICT. eHealth encompasses all uses of ICT used in providing health care (van Dyke, 2014; Wade, Eliott, & Hiller, 2014). Telehealth is a subset of ehealth and refers to preventative, promotive and curative health care delivered over a

DOI: 10.4018/978-1-4666-9978-6.ch088

distance (van Dyke, 2014). The technology includes the transmission of data, voice, images and video as well as web and mobile applications and telephony often in real time (Standing, Gururajan, Standing, & Cripps, 2014; Wade et al., 2014). Telemedicine is a subset of telehealth and uses communications networks for delivery of healthcare services and medical education from one geographical location to another (Sood et al., 2007). Mhealth utilizes mobile devices and applications to access eHealth services (van Dyke, 2014). Telecare, a subset of telehealth, uses ICT to monitor emergency or ongoing health conditions to support independent living(van Dyke, 2014). The term 'telehealth' is used in this chapter to refer to the delivery of health services using ICT, which includes the transmission of data, voice, images and video, and can also involve mobile and web technologies.

The objective of telehealth is to improve the accessibility of health care and to reduce costs (Armfield, Edirippulige, Bradford, & Smith, 2014). Telehealth programs usually begin with trials or pilot studies, often funded by governments (Wade et al., 2014). Telemedicine and ehealth applications are predominantly driven from a technology perspective rather than the clinical problem (Armfield et al., 2014). The adoption of ICT in telehealth is also constrained by the lack of integration of new technologies in clinical practice workflow and daily activities (Ackerman, Filart, Burgess, Lee, & Poropatich, 2010). Although the choice of technology is critical for sustainable telehealth adoption, the uptake of telehealth is complex and involves more than just technology. Issues that should be carefully considered include managing stakeholder expectations, integrating telehealth processes with standard work processes, developing effective knowledge sharing and social communication patterns, as well as dealing with the challenges of working in a virtual team environment (Standing et al., 2014; Cho et al.,2007).

Success Factors and Barriers

A number of factors have been found to facilitate the adoption and diffusion of telehealth delivery. These include sufficient levels of technology and infrastructure support, user training, change management, development of protocols, acceptance by health care providers, support for health care provider collaboration, business models and supporting policies and legislation (Wade et al., 2014). A European study that examined diffusion of innovations in telehealth found that telehealth deployment relied on both technological and organizational innovation Another study in the UK found that some health care professionals, often general practitioners (GPs) were reluctant to use ICT enabled health care delivery because they were concerned about losing touch with their patients. In such circumstances, nurses became the main coordinators of ICT enabled health care because they took responsibility for interacting and networking with GPs, other health care providers, call handlers and with the technology itself (Lluch and Abadie, 2013). Another study reports that successful telehealth adoption requires a combination of cultural and behavioral changes in order to be successful (Ackerman et al., 2010).

Barriers to the successful adoption of telehealth delivery include technical problems, insufficient or lack of technical support, usability issues, health care provider concerns about quality, ethical and legal issues, absence of protocols, lack of a business model and regulatory issues (Wade et al., 2014). Many issues with the use of telehealth arise because of the problems relating to virtual work (Standing et al., 2014) including resistance to new work processes (Beatriz Alkmim et al., 2012) and resistance to new technologies (S Mair et al., 2012). A UK study examining telehealth adoption from the perspective of nurses found that the disruption of the technology related to three key areas. The first was the daily work routines, the second was the interaction with their patients and the third was skill set and expertise. The skill set and expertise issue was particularly troubling because nurses felt that they were undermined and not adequately trained (Sharma et al., 2014), thus indicating that sufficient levels of training are a necessary requirement of successful telehealth adoption.

Indeed, the success of information and communication technology (ICT) enabled health care delivery, once the technology infrastructure is in place, depends on the clinical and administration systems supporting it (Smith and Gray, 2009), as well as the applications and the needs of patients and health care professionals (van den Berg, Schumann, Kraft, & Hoffmann, 2012). Moffatt and Eley's (2010) study of rural health professionals in Australia, reported various benefits of telework uptake for health workers, including local access to continuing education and professional development activities, the ability to provide an enhanced local service, and indirect benefits through experiential learning from close contact with specialists in clinical work. Additional benefits reported included the reduced perception of social isolation, improved communication and increased skills and confidence with ICT, all of which may lead to more effective rural health workforce recruitment and retention. However, service workers based in call centres appear to have a different experience. Work is highly controlled by practice protocols and is time-managed through computerized performance monitoring and call recording. These types of jobs can be very demanding and clients can often be verbally abusive and make complaints (Standing et al., 2014).

A Brazilian study (funded by the State Government of Minas Gerais, Brazil) examined the constraints and opportunities of the Telehealth Network, a network that connected teaching hospitals of five public universities with municipal health departments (Beatriz Alkmim et al., 2012). Minas Gerais has some similarities to Australian situation. Minas Gerais and Australia have similar population sizes (approximately 20 million and 23 million respectively). Both populations are unevenly distributed, leading to inequities in health care. One important difference is that the Brazilian public health system does not reimburse for telehealth activities, relying on local health department budgets for funding telehealth. In Australia, some telehealth activities are reimbursed in the public health system. Some financial incentives were previously offered by the Australian government to encourage some health professionals, specifically specialists, to adopt telehealth services; however, these financial incentives were withdrawn as at 30 June 2014. Allied health professionals do not receive any reimbursement for telehealth services. Allied health services must be offered face to face to receive government funding.

Wade et al. (2014), in an Australian study, found that the key factor for successful telehealth adoption was health care provider acceptance, that is, the willingness to engage in telehealth service delivery. One of the lessons learnt from the Brazilian study was that telehealth must meet the needs of all users, health professionals, managers and patients to be successful (Beatriz Alkmim et al., 2012). If the acceptance of the health care provider is the most important influence for adoption of sustainable telehealth services, a more comprehensive understanding of health care providers experience is necessary to develop a conceptual framework that will address the barriers to telehealth adoption both real and perceived.

THE HEALTH PRACTITIONER PERSPECTIVE

Exploratory Study

To better understand the barriers and issues of telehealth adoption from the perspectives of health care professionals, qualitative interview research was undertaken to investigate the broad themes around technology, productivity, barriers/limitations and the quality of service delivery. The purpose of this exploratory study was to explore the perceptions and experiences of teleworkers engaged in ICT enabled health care delivery in Australia. We sought to identify major themes concerned with ICT enabled telehealth delivery from the perspective of telehealth workers. Rather than pre-empting the dialogue, such an investigation allows for the perspective of telehealth workers (as opposed to other stakeholders) to be revealed, including feedback regarding telehealth workers' perceptions of both the benefits and limitations of ICT enabled telehealth delivery for a variety of stakeholders. This includes patients, telehealth workers and other medical professionals, organizations, government and society as a whole.

This research was undertaken in two phases. In the first phase we interviewed telehealth workers from three organizations offering all or part of their services using telehealth, including aged care, patient monitoring and medical advice/referral services. Most telehealth workers in the first phase of this study were registered nurses. Many of them felt there was a lack of uptake on telehealth delivery by other medical professionals, particularly physicians (general practitioners). There was a strong feeling that the potential of ICT enabled health care delivery could be realized to a much higher degree, if physicians were more enthusiastic about adopting telehealth delivery. Issues relating to work, health and safety were also raised by respondents in all the case study organizations.

The second phase involved 23 in-depth interviews with nine general practitioners, ten specialists and three allied health professionals. GPs reported using psychiatry, cardiology, dermatology, neurology, palliative care, pain specialists, orthopaedic surgeons, rheumatologists and urologists. The specialist participants included psychiatry, endocrinology, rheumatology, ophthalmology, sexual health and an environmental specialist. The allied health participants were two speech therapists and a physiotherapist. The final interview was with a manager of a non-government organisation (NGO) cancer support organization. The interviews were conducted between August and December 2014. A set of stem questions guided participant discussion during the interview. These included the following:

- How are ICTs utilized to support telehealth delivery in your organization?
- What is the technology that you use that supports telehealth delivery?
- What are the benefits and limitations of ICT to support telehealth delivery?
- How does telehealth delivery impact on the level of service delivery to patients/clients?
- How does telehealth impact on your productivity?

Themes

All health practitioners in both phases did not find that technology itself was a barrier to telehealth service delivery. In some areas, fast, ubiquitous broadband was available; however, in many rural and remote areas access to fast broadband can be an issue, particularly if video conferencing is required. All health practitioners used Skype because it is free, most people know how to use it and it can be used anywhere on any device. The first barrier is bandwidth as sometimes the voice is sacrificed for image or vice versa. The second barrier is technology support, that is, help for when the technology doesn't function as intended, an issue identified in the first phase of the study.

One of the major themes arising from the study concerned the need for training and support relating to the use of various technologies involved in telehealth service delivery. This included training for telehealth workers, for managers and in some cases for patients who required training to use equipment such as computers, tablets, blood pressure or blood glucose monitors and the like. Without adequate training, the effective use of technology to support telehealth could be compromised. In order to support telehealth workers, strong IT support is necessary, and many of the health professionals stressed the importance of having IT support available on a 24 hour, seven day a week time frame. This was considered essential in order to ensure seamless telehealth service delivery, because most of the organizations represented in this study were involved in around the clock delivery of some or all of their services.

Communication was another significant issue raised by interview participants. Technology to support communication between clients and telehealth workers, between workers and management, and across the organization was considered an essential part of the service delivery model. In terms of interaction between telehealth workers and clients, there was a strong feeling that the quality of the interaction is dependent on effective communication. Technology has the potential to either enhance or detract from communication exchanges, thereby affecting the relationship between workers and clients as well as the overall perception of the quality of the telehealth delivery. For instance, the technology allows workers to keep in touch with colleagues and managers, and allows them to make contact with patients on a more regular basis. However, a phone or skype call cannot replace a face-to-face meeting with a patient, particularly when a diagnosis involving a physical examination is required. Clearly, clients will have expectations regarding the nature of the telehealth delivery, as well as the service quality. These expectations need to be carefully managed.

Several issues related to employee management were raised by both managers and telehealth workers. There was a strong perception that the use of technology increased productivity across the various forms of service delivery, except in instances where the technology failed or where high speed digital broadband was not available. The flexibility associated with telehealth delivery also contributed to better work-life balance for many of the participants, particularly those with families or other responsibilities outside work. Some participants at a later career stage reported that the technology allowed them to remain in the profession and continue working from home, even if they were no longer able to respond to the physical demands of working in a clinical nursing environment. Still, many raised concerns over the real possibility of on-the-job stress, leading to a negative impact on their sense of wellbeing. Various reasons for on-the-job stress were cited, including difficult cases and clients, isolation in the job and lack of support (social and professional isolation). However, the technology was also cited as a cause of stress when there were breakdowns or technical difficulties.

Some 35% of telehealth workers in the first phase of the study reported feeling a sense of social isolation due to working largely on their own, either from home or on the road. For some, there was a big transition required from working in clinical team settings to working alone. However, this did not pose an issue for the majority of the participants who seemed satisfied with the mechanisms in place in their organizations for keeping in touch with managers and co-workers. This included use of social media, phone calls, emails, as well as face-to-face opportunities to meet on a regular basis. Employee support was considered an essential part of telehealth workers' motivation and wellbeing, and strengthened both communication processes and the organizational culture as a whole.

It would appear that the most successful and satisfying telehealth work arrangements are those that allow for regular interaction with managers and co-workers as well as with clients/patients. This included providing opportunities to debrief, particularly after a difficult client interaction. Telehealth workers expected such support to come from management. In one of the case study organizations, workers reported that management did an exceptional job in this regard, but in the other two organizations, management were less highly regarded, particularly in terms of valuing staff and providing support. Several respondents were unhappy with feedback mechanisms in their respective organizations, expressing a desire to obtain more feedback on their own performance, as well as on patient status, on a regular basis.

Respondents generally reported high levels of client satisfaction with telehealth delivery. ICT enabled health care delivery resulted in lower costs of delivery, less travel and disruption for clients, and an overall reduction in hospital and physician visits. Moreover, telehealth services allowed aged clients and those managing chronic health conditions to remain in their homes for longer, thus delaying the need for residential aged care and admissions to hospital. However, health professionals stated that telehealth delivery could not replace face-to-face interaction 100% of the time, and suggested that a balance needs to be struck in this regard. It also became clear in speaking with telehealth workers that adoption of technology to support health care delivery requires new and different ways to monitor and measure service delivery; in many instances, the technology itself could be used for the purposes of monitoring, measurement and evaluation.

The health care professionals in the second phase of this study all expressed their motivation for adopting telehealth consultations as providing a more equitable service, particularly for those patients in rural and regional areas. An important finding in this phase was that telehealth cannot just be a cost saving exercise, the patient or client circumstances need to be taken into account. A number of physicians commented that it often was a choice for patients for some specialties to either go on a long waiting list or have a telehealth consultation. A telehealth consultation was more likely to happen in a timely way. Physicians in rural and remote areas believed that saving the patient from a long trip to a larger center or city, both from a cost (petrol/airfares/accommodation/time off work for both patient and sometimes carer) and stress perspective provided a better quality service. For some patients, travel to see a specialist is not an option for a variety of reasons (cost, inconvenience, can't cope with a city) and telehealth provides access to a specialist in the physician's rooms.

The technology infrastructure in some cases had to be upgraded and some health professionals did not have the expertise to implement the most appropriate technology. In the second phase of the study, each health care professional had to work out how to set up the technology, the workflow and business model. There is no external help available to deal with these issues and provide help to develop a telehealth practice. When asked about privacy and security issues, this was considered as low risk compared to the many advantages of telehealth.

Health practitioners were concerned about the funding model for telehealth services. A number of specialists started telehealth consultations when the financial incentives from the government were in place, around two years ago. This financial incentive had ceased from June 2014. This may be a disincentive for those health professionals that are keen to adopt telehealth but cannot justify the cost. Allied health professionals get no funding from public sources for telehealth consultations. Moreover, private health insurers do not provide rebates for telehealth consultations, so this provides a clear example of how policy decisions can have an important bearing on whether or not telehealth delivery is adopted in the first instance and if telehealth is a sustainable model in the second instance.

The health care professionals in the second phase interviews did not advertise their telehealth services to any great extent and there did not appear to be any great consumer demand for these services; however, this may be because patients are not aware of these services. Most health care professionals are only doing a limited number of telehealth consultations in addition to their regular practice in their rooms. Telehealth consultations are an 'add on' rather than integrated in the practice workflow. The most common theme arising out of the second phase of the research was the collaboration and relationship with local support requirement. The specialists and allied health professionals are mostly located in the cities or in larger towns. A telehealth consultation needs good support from the local health care providers to both manage risk and ensure there is an appropriate management plan in place for the patient.

The business model or process needs to be well considered to ensure that the process is efficient for the physician, the specialist and the patient. In the case of the physicians and the specialist, the consultation takes place in the physician's rooms. This requires efficient scheduling of time from all three because the physician needs to be involved in the consultation, sometimes for part of the time and sometimes for the whole consultation. It also requires organizing any tests (e.g. pathology, imaging) prior to the consultation. This requires discretion on the part of the physician to know to what extent they need to be involved, for example, in some situations the patient may feel more comfortable not having the physician for the entirety of the consultation.

A barrier to engaging in telehealth consultations is the risk of not having enough information to make an accurate diagnosis. In the allied health area, the mitigation of risk can be done by ensuring that diagnosis and management plans are carefully documented, the terms and conditions are clear and that the payment encompasses access to the right level of expertise. For example, a physiotherapist telehealth service offered online services with a payment that included access to physiotherapists (via phone, email and the web) for a three month period.

RECOMMENDATIONS

There needs to be incentives for health practitioners to develop telehealth practices. This should be from both the public and private health sectors (health insurance companies), including appropriate ongoing funding models.

The telehealth practitioners in this study all found ways to develop a business model and work practices that worked successfully for themselves and their patients. At present there is no support available from the government or professional bodies that provides assistance and/or advice regarding technology requirements, how to develop a sustainable telehealth business model or how to develop relationships and collaborate with other practitioners to deliver the right quality of service for the patient.

This is a multi-disciplinary area that involves technology, an understanding of client/patient needs, service quality issues, and most importantly the skills and capabilities of the clinicians and other health care providers in delivering health care using telehealth systems. The conceptual model should include the following components:

1. Technology.

The technology used in telehealth delivery has to be universally available, flexible and affordable. The technology should provide access to everyone who needs to use it. The limitations of insufficient broadband may limit some applications. Privacy and security issues need careful consideration to mitigate any risk to both the health professionals involved in telehealth and the patient.

Telehealth in public hospitals is supported by technologies such as Polycom and Cisco. Training and support for these technologies including the security and privacy issues should be included in the implementation of telehealth applications.

2. Business Model.

Health practitioners have to have some certainty with income. There is an opportunity cost for a physician to be in a telehealth consultation instead of a normal consultation in their rooms.

3. Business Practice.

The skills and capabilities of health care professionals must now include excellent collaboration skills with other health care professionals. All components of the health care service delivery model should be included: assessing if a telehealth consultation is appropriate for the particular patient, booking the consultation, electronic scripting so management of the patient can begin immediately, follow-up consultations and the education of health professionals using telehealth.

Physicians need to be upskilled to be able to refer patients to specialists and allied health professionals engaged in telehealth delivery.

Productivity of telehealth delivery was perceived to be the same as a face to face interaction. The difference was the timeliness of the consultation. Physicians tend to be overworked, particularly in rural and remote areas and have little time to develop business practices around telehealth. Many of the physicians interviewed used the term 'conservative' when talking about their colleagues and their reluctance to utilize telehealth services.

Education and upskilling of physicians is a significant benefit when there is fruitful collaboration between specialists and physicians. The specialist, in diagnosing and providing management plans for the patient, also provides knowledge and training to the physician involved in the case.

Training and support for all telehealth workers (nurses, physicians, specialists and allied health professionals) on the best use of technology, work processes and collaboration for a specific telehealth consultation will be important as telehealth reaches critical mass and becomes a sustainable way to develop health services.

Employee management of telehealth workers is also critical. This includes work, health and safety considerations, communication between management, telehealth practitioners and patients, managing expectations as well as issues relating to productivity and employee wellbeing.

4.   Quality of consultation/interaction.

The perception of the quality of the consultation is important from the perspective of the telehealth practitioner because this will determine whether this mode of interaction between patient and health care provider is sustainable. Health professionals we interviewed for this study cautioned that it would be inappropriate to use telehealth as a replacement for all health care services. On the other hand, telehealth provides access to health services, particularly specialist and allied health services that may otherwise be inaccessible. Telehealth should be a complementary health service that adds value to patient care.

FUTURE RESEARCH DIRECTIONS

While this exploratory study is limited to the Australian context, it provides a much needed perspective, as the telehealth worker perspective is usually not taken into consideration in various analyses of the effectiveness of telehealth services. Broadening the research, particularly in an international context, will provide deeper insights into the implications of telehealth adoption for health care practitioners and other stakeholders. A conceptual model should also be developed using these insights so that health care practitioners, both in primary care and allied health care, can implement telehealth services that are both viable and sustainable.

Our findings show that if a health care practitioner is patient-centered, they will find a way to deliver the service for the patient. Health care practitioners will find ways around any issues or problems with the technology. The technology itself is not perceived as a barrier, although lack of satisfactory bandwidth and technology support may be disincentives. The issue of viable funding models and appropriate telehealth strategies certainly warrants further investigation. Will the future of telehealth provide a more patient-centered approach where the outcomes of equity of access to health care services in a cost effective way? This will very much depend on whether the health care professionals accept and adopt new ways of working, particularly collaborating with other health care professionals to provide the best service for the patient in the most efficient and cost effective way.

CONCLUSION

As we have seen, there are a number of challenges and limitations for telehealth delivery from the point of view of telehealth workers. For as many problems as ICT-enabled technology adoption may be able to address in health care delivery, new challenges related to the use of that technology arise constantly. Many of these issues do not involve the technology itself, but rather the users of the technology. With most developed economies facing a rapidly ageing population and a sharp rise in chronic disease, governments are struggling to respond to the increasing demands on existing health care systems. Given this societal trend of ageing populations and people living longer in general, health care costs are rapidly increasing. Telehealth delivery of certain health services may be a viable means of addressing these challenges; however, a holistic approach is needed in response to this situation, involving consideration of ICT, employee-client interaction, employee management and service quality.

REFERENCES

Armfield, N. R., Edirippulige, S. K., Bradford, N., & Smith, A. C. (2014). Telemedicine — is the cart being put before the horse? *The Medical Journal of Australia, 200*(9), 530–533. doi:10.5694/mja13.11101 PMID:24835716

Beatriz Alkmim, M., Minelli Figueira, R., Soriano Marcolino, M., Silva Cardoso, C., Pena de Abreu, M., Rodrigues Cunha, L., Luiz Pinho Ribeiro, A. (2012). *Improving patient access to specialized health care: the Telehealth Network of Minas Gerais, Brazil*. Academic Press.

Cho, S.C., Mathiassen, L.M. and Robey, D.R. (2007). Dialectics of resilience: a multi-level analysis of a telehealth innovation. *Journal of Information Technology, 22*(1), 24-35.

Christensen, M. C., & Remler, D. (2009). Information and Communications Technology in U.S. Health Care: Why is Adoption So Slow and is Slower Better? *Journal of Health Politics, Policy and Law, 34*(6), 1011–1034. doi:10.1215/03616878-2009-034 PMID:20018989

Jang-Jaccard, J., Nepal, S., Alem, L., & Li, J. (2014). Barriers for Delivering Telehealth in Rural Australia: A Review Based on Australian Trials and Studies. *Telemedicine Journal and e-Health, 20*(5), 496–504. doi:10.1089/tmj.2013.0189 PMID:24801522

Mair, F., May, C., O'Donnell, C., Finch, T., Sullivan, F., & Murray, E. (2012). *Factors that promote or inhibit the implementation of e-health systems: An explanatory systematic review*. Academic Press.

Roberts, C., Mort, M., & Milligan, C. (2012). Calling for Care: 'Disembodied' Work, Teleoperators and Older People Living at Home. *Sociology, 46*(3), 490–506. doi:10.1177/0038038511422551

Sood, S., Mbarika, V., Jugoo, S., Dookhy, R., Doarn, C. R., Prakash, N., & Merrell, R. C. (2007). What Is Telemedicine? A Collection of 104 Peer-Reviewed Perspectives and Theoretical Underpinnings. *Telemedicine Journal and e-Health, 13*(5), 573–590. doi:10.1089/tmj.2006.0073 PMID:17999619

Standing, C., Gururajan, R., Standing, S., & Cripps, H. (2014). Making the Most of Virtual Expertise in Telemedicine and Telehealth Environment. *Journal of Organizational Computing and Electronic Commerce, 24*(2-3), 138–156. doi:10.1080/10919392.2014.896714

van Dyke, L. (2014). A Review of Telehealth Service Implementation Frameworks. *International Journal of Environmental Research and Public Health, 11*(2), 1279–1298. doi:10.3390/ijerph110201279 PMID:24464237

Wade, V. A., Eliott, J. A., & Hiller, J. E. (2014). Clinician Acceptance is the Key Factor for Sustainable Telehealth Services. *Qualitative Health Research, 24*(5), 682–694. doi:10.1177/1049732314528809 PMID:24685708

KEY TERMS AND DEFINITIONS

Business Model: A plan on to successfully operate a business including revenue sources and customer demographics/specialties.

Business Practice: The human experience and skills required for delivering a service repeatedly.

eHealth: All uses of ICT used in providing health care.

ICT: Information and Communications Technology

Telehealth: Is a subset of eHealth and refers to preventative, promotive and curative health care delivered over a distance.

Telemedicine: Telemedicine being a subset of telehealth, uses communications networks for delivery of healthcare services and medical education from one geographical location to another.

About the Contributors

For full contributors' biographies, please visit the book's website at:
http://www.igi-global.com/book/encyclopedia-health-telemedicine/141916

Index

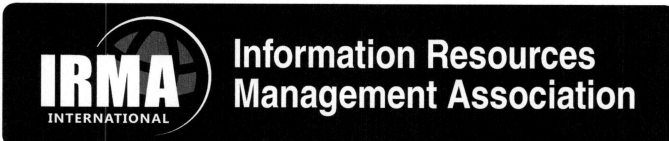
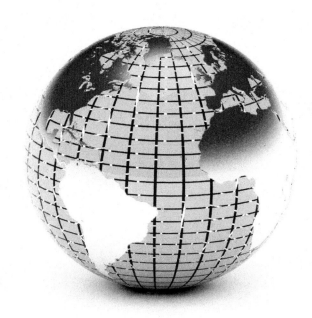

CPSIA information can be obtained
at www.ICGtesting.com
Printed in the USA
BVOW10*0754080616

450279BV00017B/16/P